Systemic Autoinflammatory Diseases—Clinical Rheumatic Challenges

Systemic Autoinflammatory Diseases—Clinical Rheumatic Challenges

Editor

Eugen Feist

MDPI • Basel • Beijing • Wuhan • Barcelona • Belgrade • Manchester • Tokyo • Cluj • Tianjin

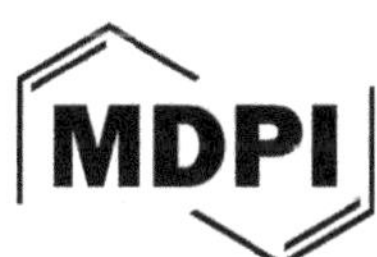

Editor
Eugen Feist
Helios Department for Rheumatology
Cooperation partner of the Otto-von-Guericke University
Germany

Editorial Office
MDPI
St. Alban-Anlage 66
4052 Basel, Switzerland

This is a reprint of articles from the Special Issue published online in the open access journal *Journal of Clinical Medicine* (ISSN 2077-0383) (available at: https://www.mdpi.com/journal/jcm/special_issues/Systemic_Autoinflammatory_Diseases).

For citation purposes, cite each article independently as indicated on the article page online and as indicated below:

LastName, A.A.; LastName, B.B.; LastName, C.C. Article Title. *Journal Name* **Year**, *Volume Number*, Page Range.

ISBN 978-3-0365-2560-0 (Hbk)
ISBN 978-3-0365-2561-7 (PDF)

Contents

About the Editor

Eugen Feist studied medicine at the Institute of Medicine, Kiev, Ukraine, and the Charité, Humboldt-University of Berlin, Germany, from 1989 to 1995. He became a Consultant in Internal Medicine at the Department of Internal Medicine and Rheumatology at the Charité-Universitätsmedizin in 2003. Two years later he became a Rheumatologist and in 2021 an Immunologist. Professor Feist's clinical work and research activities are focused on systemic autoimmune and autoinflammatory diseases, with special interests in rheumatoid arthritis and adult onset Still's disease. He has been awarded the MSD grant for Arthritis and the Wolfgang Schulze prize of the Deutsche Rheuma-Liga. In 2009, he received a postdoctoral lecture qualification for his work on the topic of proteasomes and autoimmunity. Since 2019, Professor Feist is medical director of the Helios Clinic for Rheumatology in Vogelsang-Gommern, a leading center in Saxony-Anhalt. He has acted as Investigator in numerous phase I to IV clinical studies in the field of rheumatology.

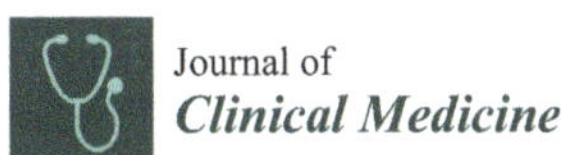
Journal of
Clinical Medicine

MDPI

Editorial

Autoinflammation It Is!

Eugen Feist

Department of Rheumatology, Helios Clinic Vogelsang-Gommern, Cooperation Partner of the Otto-von-Guericke University, Sophie-von-Boetticher-Straße 1, 39245 Vogelsang-Gommern, Germany; Eugen.Feist@helios-gesundheit.de

In recent years, we have entered a new era full of insights into exciting pathways and improved management of a distinct class of inflammatory conditions. Under the umbrella of auto-inflammation, several so far seemingly unconnected diseases have been summarized and separated from autoimmune conditions in particular. Initially, the striking difference became clear for classical monogenetic periodic fever syndromes, where the innate immune system plays a dominant role via the impact of a specific cytokine signature.

In this Special Issue of the *Journal of Clinical Medicine*, we find a diverse spectrum of excellent contributions to this topic. Articles on the current knowledge of cryopyrin-associated periodic syndromes [1] and proteasome-associated autoinflammatory syndromes [2] provide us with valuable advice for diagnosis and treatment of these rare conditions in clinical practice.

The field of auto-inflammation has further extended to more complex polygenetic disorders. In this context, two diseases, namely adult-onset Still's disease [3] and gouty arthritis [4], are focused on in this Special Issue. Both contributions show that in these clinically and mechanistically diverse diseases, the main symptoms are caused by a very similar cytokine signature referring to interleukin 1 as the main driver. This knowledge has also paved the way for new targeted and highly effective therapies.

This Special Issue on auto-inflammation also contains relevant contribution that have been rarely addressed in such detail elsewhere. To highlight just a few points, one can read about the current options of imaging in auto-inflammation [5] with special attention to IgG4 related diseases [6] or about the issue of dysphagia in myositis [7]. Furthermore, this Special Issue also contains valuable original work, such as studies providing basic data on a novel variant of TNF receptor-associated periodic syndrome [8], drug hepatotoxicity in the treatment of gouty arthritis [9], the impact of certain anti-rheumatic drugs on DNA repair [10], genetic background in association with response to anti-rheumatic drugs [11], and the impact of IL1-inhibition on the cytokine milieu in adult-onset Still's disease [12].

Auto-inflammation can also cause life-threatening complications often in association with hyper-inflammation or cytokine storm. Nowadays, everyone is familiar with the issue of severe COVID-19 infections due to an overwhelming and disturbed cytokine signaling. Of note, during this pandemic disaster, special attention has been attributed to the group of patients receiving immunosuppressive therapy, which typically includes those with auto-immune and -inflammatory diseases. In this Special Issue, we are able to publish one of the earliest observations with respect to rare auto-inflammatory diseases. The risk for severe acute COVID-19 disease was mild to moderate in these patients [13]. However, even after resolution of infection, there was an impact on disease activity in these cases. With respect to hyper-inflammation, the critical role of interferons has recently been highlighted. In this context, we can also learn a lot from complications in auto-inflammatory diseases, such as macrophage activation syndrome [14].

Research in the field of auto-inflammation remains in its infancy. Currently, we cannot place each manifestation in a distinct category. To solve this problem, the concept of systemic undefined recurrent fevers has recently been introduced [15]. We should be aware that many of these diseases are still under-recognized, which requires our special

Citation: Feist, E. Autoinflammation It Is! *J. Clin. Med.* **2021**, *10*, 5157. https://doi.org/10.3390/jcm10215157

Received: 26 October 2021
Accepted: 2 November 2021
Published: 3 November 2021

attention. Overall, this Special Issue on auto-inflammation is of valuable interdisciplinary information. I am very thankful to the authors for their contribution to this constantly growing field and wish you a fruitful reading.

Conflicts of Interest: The author declares no conflict of interest.

References

1. Welzel, T.; Kuemmerle-Deschner, J.B. Diagnosis and Management of the Cryopyrin-Associated Periodic Syndromes (CAPS): What Do We Know Today? *J. Clin. Med.* **2021**, *10*, 128. [CrossRef] [PubMed]
2. Goetzke, C.C.; Ebstein, F.; Kallinich, T. Role of Proteasomes in Inflammation. *J. Clin. Med.* **2021**, *10*, 1783. [CrossRef] [PubMed]
3. Mitrovic, S.; Fautrel, B. Clinical Phenotypes of Adult-Onset Still's Disease: New Insights from Pathophysiology and Literature Findings. *J. Clin. Med.* **2021**, *10*, 2633. [CrossRef] [PubMed]
4. Galozzi, P.; Bindoli, S.; Doria, A.; Oliviero, F.; Sfriso, P. Autoinflammatory Features in Gouty Arthritis. *J. Clin. Med.* **2021**, *10*, 1880. [CrossRef] [PubMed]
5. Ziegeler, K.; Eshed, I.; Diekhoff, T.; Hermann, K.G. Imaging of Joints and Bones in Autoinflammation. *J. Clin. Med.* **2020**, *9*, 4074. [CrossRef] [PubMed]
6. Yuan, W.-H.; Li, A.F.-Y.; Yu, S.-Y.; Chen, Y.-Y.; Wu, C.-H.; Hsu, H.-C.; Lirng, J.-F.; Guo, W.-Y. Evaluate the Differences in CT Features and Serum IgG4 Levels between Lymphoma and Immunoglobulin G4-Related Disease of the Orbit. *J. Clin. Med.* **2020**, *9*, 2425. [CrossRef] [PubMed]
7. Labeit, B.; Pawlitzki, M.; Ruck, T.; Muhle, P.; Claus, I.; Suntrup-Krueger, S.; Warnecke, T.; Meuth, S.G.; Wiendl, H.; Dziewas, R. The Impact of Dysphagia in Myositis: A Systematic Review and Meta-Analysis. *J. Clin. Med.* **2020**, *9*, 2150. [CrossRef] [PubMed]
8. Zegarska, J.; Wiesik-Szewczyk, E.; Hryniewiecka, E.; Wolska-Kusnierz, B.; Soldacki, D.; Kacprzak, M.; Sobczynska-Tomaszewska, A.; Czerska, K.; Siedlecki, P.; Jahnz-Rozyk, K.; et al. Tumor Necrosis Factor Receptor-Associated Periodic Syndrome (TRAPS) with a New Pathogenic Variant in *TNFRSF1A* Gene in a Family of the Adult Male with Renal AA Amyloidosis—Diagnostic and Therapeutic Challenge for Clinicians. *J. Clin. Med.* **2021**, *10*, 465. [CrossRef] [PubMed]
9. Oh, Y.-J.; Moon, K.W. Combined Use of Febuxostat and Colchicine Does Not Increase Acute Hepatotoxicity in Patients with Gout: A Retrospective Study. *J. Clin. Med.* **2020**, *9*, 1488. [CrossRef] [PubMed]
10. Reddig, A.; Voss, L.; Guttek, K.; Roggenbuck, D.; Feist, E.; Reinhold, D. Impact of Different JAK Inhibitors and Methotrexate on Lymphocyte Proliferation and DNA Damage. *J. Clin. Med.* **2021**, *10*, 1431. [CrossRef] [PubMed]
11. Favoino, E.; Urso, L.; Serafino, A.; Misceo, F.; Catacchio, G.; Prete, M.; Perosa, F. HLA Allele Prevalence in Disease-Modifying Antirheumatic Drugs-Responsive Enthesitis and/or Arthritis Not Fulfilling ASAS Criteria: Comparison with Psoriatic and Undifferentiated Spondyloarthritis. *J. Clin. Med.* **2021**, *10*, 3006. [CrossRef] [PubMed]
12. Ghannam, K.; Zernicke, J.; Kedor, C.; Listing, J.; Burmester, G.-R.; Foell, D.; Feist, E. Distinct Effects of Interleukin-1β Inhibition upon Cytokine Profile in Patients with Adult-Onset Still's Disease and Active Articular Manifestation Responding to Canakinumab. *J. Clin. Med.* **2021**, *10*, 4400. [CrossRef] [PubMed]
13. Welzel, T.; Samba, S.D.; Klein, R.; van den Anker, J.N.; Kuemmerle-Deschner, J.B. COVID-19 in Autoinflammatory Diseases with Immunosuppressive Treatment. *J. Clin. Med.* **2021**, *10*, 605. [CrossRef] [PubMed]
14. Di Cola, I.; Ruscitti, P.; Giacomelli, R.; Cipriani, P. The Pathogenic Role of Interferons in the Hyperinflammatory Response on Adult-Onset Still's Disease and Macrophage Activation Syndrome: Paving the Way towards New Therapeutic Targets. *J. Clin. Med.* **2021**, *10*, 1164. [CrossRef] [PubMed]
15. Papa, R.; Penco, F.; Volpi, S.; Sutera, D.; Caorsi, R.; Gattorno, M. Syndrome of Undifferentiated Recurrent Fever (SURF): An Emerging Group of Autoinflammatory Recurrent Fevers. *J. Clin. Med.* **2021**, *10*, 1963. [CrossRef] [PubMed]

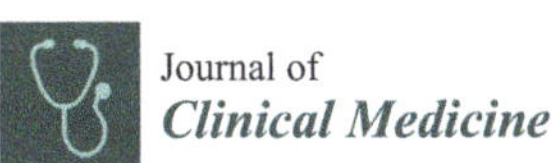

Journal of *Clinical Medicine*

MDPI

Article

Distinct Effects of Interleukin-1β Inhibition upon Cytokine Profile in Patients with Adult-Onset Still's Disease and Active Articular Manifestation Responding to Canakinumab

Khetam Ghannam [1,*], Jan Zernicke [1], Claudia Kedor [1], Joachim Listing [2], Gerd-R. Burmester [1], Dirk Foell [3] and Eugen Feist [1,4]

1 Department of Rheumatology and Clinical Immunology, Charité—Universitätsmedizin Berlin, 10117 Berlin, Germany; jan.zernicke@charite.de (J.Z.); claudia.kedor@charite.de (C.K.); gerd.burmester@charite.de (G.-R.B.); Eugen.Feist@helios-gesundheit.de (E.F.)
2 Epidemiology Unit, German Rheumatism Research Centre, 10117 Berlin, Germany; j.listing@posteo.de
3 Pediatric Rheumatology and Immunology, University Hospital Muenster, 48149 Muenster, Germany; dfoell@uni-muenster.de
4 Helios Department for Rheumatology Vogelsang-Gommern GmbH, 39245 Gommern, Germany
* Correspondence: khetam.ghannam@charite.de; Tel.: +49-(0)30-4505-13356; Fax: +49-(0)30-4505-13957

Abstract: Adult-onset Still's disease (AOSD) is a systemic auto-inflammatory disease characterized by the presence of immunologically mediated inflammation and deficient resolution of inflammation. Canakinumab is an approved IL-1β inhibitor in the treatment of AOSD with a balanced efficacy and safety profile. Since inflammatory cytokines play a major role in the pathogenesis of AOSD, we investigated the effects of canakinumab on the cytokine profile of AOSD patients from a randomized controlled trial. Multiplex analysis and ELISA were used to test the concentrations of several cytokines at three time points—week 0 (baseline), week 1 and week 4—in two patient groups—placebo and canakinumab. Two-way repeated-measures analysis of variance revealed a significant temporal effect on the concentrations of MRP 8/14, S100A12, IL-6 and IL-18 with a significant decrease at week 4 in the canakinumab group exclusively. Comparing responders with non-responders to canakinumab showed a significant decrease in MRP 8/14, IL-1RA, IL-18 and IL-6 in responders at week 4, while S100A12 levels decreased significantly in responders and non-responders. In summary, canakinumab showed a striking effect on the cytokine profile in patients with AOSD, exhibiting a clear association with clinical response.

Keywords: adult-onset Still's disease; canakinumab; cytokines

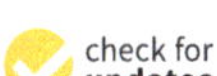

Citation: Ghannam, K.; Zernicke, J.; Kedor, C.; Listing, J.; Burmester, G.-R.; Foell, D.; Feist, E. Distinct Effects of Interleukin-1β Inhibition upon Cytokine Profile in Patients with Adult-Onset Still's Disease and Active Articular Manifestation Responding to Canakinumab. *J. Clin. Med.* **2021**, *10*, 4400. https://doi.org/10.3390/jcm10194400

Academic Editor: Santos Castañeda

Received: 11 August 2021
Accepted: 21 September 2021
Published: 26 September 2021

Publisher's Note: MDPI stays neutral with regard to jurisdictional claims in published maps and institutional affiliations.

1. Introduction

Adult-onset Still's disease (AOSD) is a rare multi-systemic auto-inflammatory disease of unknown etiology, which commonly affects young adults. It is characterized by a high spiking fever, macular and salmon-colored rash, arthritis, sore throat, neutrophilic leukocytosis and hyperferritinemia [1]. AOSD was first defined by Bywaters in 1971 [2] in fourteen patients presenting with clinical manifestations very similar to childhood-onset Still's disease, described a century ago by Sir Still, today called systemic juvenile idiopathic arthritis (sJIA) [3]. Although the etiology of AOSD remains largely elusive, there is evidence that various mechanisms contribute to the pathogenesis of AOSD; genetic susceptibility is considered as a main contributor to AOSD. Associations with distinct HLA alleles including HLA-Bw35, Cw4, DR4, DRw6, B17, B18, B35, and DR2 have been described in different ethnic groups [4–6]. Infections [7–9], as well as other immunological stimuli and a deficient resolution of inflammation, have also been implicated in the pathogenesis of AOSD [10].

Activation and amplification of inflammation are mainly driven by innate immune cells, with macrophage and neutrophil activation representing the hallmark of AOSD pathogenesis. However, adaptive immune cells including natural killer (NK) cells and T cells are also reported to be involved in the inflammatory amplification [11]. Macrophage-colony stimulating factor and interferon-γ (IFN-γ), as biomarkers reflecting macrophage activation, are both increased in patients with AOSD and correlated with disease activity [12,13]. Most circulating leukocytes expressed L-selectin, which is a cell adhesion molecule involved in their rolling on inflamed vascular endothelium prior to transmigration and is, therefore, of interest in this context [14].

The innate immune response in macrophages and neutrophils in AOSD starts with danger or pathogen signals, termed pathogen-associated molecule patterns (PAMPs) and endogenous damage-associated molecular patterns (DAMPs). Several DAMPs including high-mobility group box-1, advanced glycation end products, S100 proteins, soluble CD163, macrophage migration inhibitory factor (MIF), and neutrophil extracellular traps have been well described in the pathogenesis of AOSD [15]. These danger signals are transmitted to macrophages and neutrophils via specific Toll-like receptors and activate NACHT, LRR, and PYD domains-containing protein 3 (NLRP3) inflammasome. The NLRP3 inflammasome is a complex of proteins that activates caspase-1 activity, leading to the proteolytic cleavage of pro-interleukin (IL)-1 and IL-18 to its bioactive and mature forms [16–18]. IL-1β and IL-18 play a central role in AOSD pathophysiology and further promote immune cells to produce a large amount of pro-inflammatory cytokines, including IL-6, IL-8, IL-17, and tumor necrosis factor (TNF)-α, type I interferons (IFN-α and IFN-β), as well as IL-1β and IL-18 themselves, leading to an amplified inflammatory response. Moreover, macrophage activation leads to increased release of ferritin as a common marker of disease activity in Still's disease, including AOSD [19]. The role of adaptive immune cells in the pathogenesis of AOSD was illustrated by different studies, contributing to the activation of macrophages and neutrophils and induction of IFN-γ and IL-17 [11,20]. Moreover, activation of dendritic cells through Toll-like receptor (TLR)-7 induced Th17 response and neutrophil recruitment in AOSD patients [21]. Notably, as a marker of T cell activation, soluble Interleukin-2 Receptor (sIL-2R) was also reported as a potential marker of disease activity in AOSD [22,23].

In addition to inflammatory amplification, a deficiency in the resolution of inflammation has been suggested to play a role in the pathogenesis of AOSD. Besides a deficiency of NK cells, diminished circulating regulatory T cells (Treg) were described in AOSD [24]. However, the levels of the immune-suppressive cytokine IL-10 were elevated in the serum of AOSD and correlated with disease activity [25]. Additionally, several chemokines including C-X-C motif chemokine ligands 9 (CXCL 9) MIG, (CXCL10) IP-10, and CXCL13 have been found to be potential biomarkers in AOSD [10].

Previously, IL-1, IL-6 and TNF-α antagonists have been used as biologic therapies in patients with AOSD refractory to corticosteroids or conventional disease-modifying antirheumatic drugs (c-DMARDs) in clinical practice, but results from controlled clinical trials were missing [26]. Evidence of effectiveness was available for anakinra in particular [27], as an IL-1 receptor antagonist, as well as for canakinumab, as a human antibody against IL-1β, in refractory patients with AOSD [28]. At present, both drugs are approved by the European Medicines Agency (EMA) for sJIA and AOSD with a beneficial efficacy–safety profile [29]. Canakinumab has also been approved by the Food and Drug Administration (FDA) for treatment of sJIA and AOSD. Furthermore, canakinumab is also approved for autoinflammatory periodic fever syndromes including cryopyrin-associated periodic syndrome (CAPS), tumor necrosis factor receptor-associated periodic syndrome (TRAPS), mevalonate kinase deficiency (MKD) and familial Mediterranean fever (FMF) [29]. Since no predictive or associated markers for response to IL1 inhibitors have been established in patients with AOSD so far, this study investigated the cytokine profile in AOSD patients in more detail. To correlate biomarkers to outcome, we used samples from the only randomized controlled trial (RCT) with canakinumab performed so far [30].

2. Patients

Patient materials were taken from the phase II Canakinumab for Treatment of Adult-Onset Still's Disease to Achieve Reduction of Arthritic Manifestation (CONSIDER) study, which was performed as a multicenter, double-blind, randomized, placebo-controlled trial in patients with AOSD and active joint involvement. Randomization, stratified by pre-treatment status with biological disease-modifying antirheumatic drugs (bDMARDs) and study center, was performed in a 1:1 ratio to the canakinumab or the placebo arm according to Atkinsons' DA-optimal biased coin algorithm. In patients treated with nonsteroidal anti-inflammatory drugs (NSAIDs), glucocorticoids or conventional DMARDs, a stable dose prior to randomization and throughout study treatment was required (≥2 weeks (NSAIDs), ≥1 week (glucocorticoids with a dose of ≤10 mg/day prednisolone equivalent) and ≥6 weeks (conventional DMARDs)). Depending on the pharmacokinetic properties of the respective bDMARDs, a washout period between 1 week and 9 months was required [30]. Plasma from 31 adult-onset Still's disease (AOSD) patients was analyzed. Seventeen of the patients (ten female and seven male) had been treated subcutaneously with canakinumab at a dose of 4 mg/kg body weight up to a maximum of 300 mg every 4 weeks. The other 14 patients (10 female and 4 male) had been randomized to placebo and used as a control group. Samples were analyzed at three time points: baseline week 0, at week 1 and at week 4. The CONSIDER study (CACZ885GDE01T) was conducted according to the ethical principles of the Declaration of Helsinki. The study protocol and all amendments were reviewed by the Independent Ethics Commission of the State of Berlin (Ethik-Kommission des Landes Berlin, LAGeSo), and Independent Ethics Committees for each center. An approval from the German regulatory authority was received prior to the start of the study. The reference number at the LAGeSo is: 11/0561-ZS EK 11. All patients provided written informed consent prior to the screening visit.

The additional collection of research samples for this biomarker analysis was a sub-project to the main study. The ethics committee also approved the additional patient consent and a separate signed patient consent form was used for all samples analyzed in this report.

A detailed description of patients analyzed in this study is shown in Table 1.

Table 1. Detailed characteristics of patients investigated in the study.

Patients			**Placebo**			**Canakinumab**		
			Men	**Women**	**Total**	**Men**	**Women**	**Total**
Number			4	10	14	7	10	17
Mean age in years (average)			35 (28–40)	46 (24–70)	40	41 (22–63)	45 (24–61)	43
CRP mg/L baseline mean			48	37	39	33	37	35
CRP mg/L week 12 mean			21	25	24	14	25	21
Ferritin ng/mL baseline mean			883	718	751	514	811	689
Ferritin ng/mL week 12 mean			322	633	576	278	548	437
Medication before study	c-DMARDs		2	5	7	6	7	13
	biological	Anti-IL1 (anakinra)	2	8	10	6	5	11
		Anti-TNF		4	4	1	2	3
		Anti-IL6		2	2	2	2	4
	steroidal	Prednisolone	2	9	11	7	10	17
	NSAIDs	COXIB				2	2	4

Table 1. *Cont.*

Patients		Placebo			Canakinumab		
		Men	**Women**	**Total**	**Men**	**Women**	**Total**
DAS28-ESR baseline	Remission						
	Low		1	1			
	Moderate	1	3	4	5	6	11
	High	1	5	6	2	2	4
DAS28-ESR week 12	Remission		2	2	2	3	5
	Low		3	3	1	2	3
	Moderate	1	3	4	4	2	6
	High	1	1	2		1	1
DAS28-ESR Improvement by at least 1.2	Yes		5	5	4	6	10
	No	2	4	6	3	2	5

CRP: C-reactive protein, NSAIDs: nonsteroidal anti-inflammatory drugs, c-DMARDs: conventional disease-modifying antirheumatic drugs, DAS28-ESR: disease activity score uses 28 joint counts—erythrocyte sedimentation rate.

3. Methods

To investigate the exclusive effect of canakinumab on the expression of inflammatory cytokines, multiplex analysis and ELISA were used to test the concentrations of several cytokines in two patient groups (placebo versus canakinumab) at three time points (baseline week 0, week 1 and week 4) and multiple comparisons were applied between the two groups.

sCD163, IFN-α2 and BAFF/TNFSF13B were tested by Bio-Plex Pro Human Inflam 1 3plx EXP; IFN-γ, interleukin-1 receptor antagonist (IL-1RA), interleukin-2 receptor alpha (IL-2RA), IL-6, IL-10, IL-17, IL-18, MIG (CXCL 9), IP-10 (CXCL 10), and TNF-α were tested using Bio-Plex Pro Hu Screening Panel 10plx EXP, both from BioRad, Hercules, CA, USA. Soluble (s)L-Selectin and CXCL 13 were tested using Human sL-Selectin and Human CXCL 13 (BLC) ELISA Kits, respectively, both from Invitrogen, Waltham, Massachusetts, USA. Legend Max ELISA Kit Human MRP8/14 (Calprotectin) from Biolegend, San Diego, CA, USA was used to test MRP8/14 and levels of S100A12 were measured using Circulex S100A12/EN-RAGE ELISA Kit Ver.2 from MBL International, Woburn, MA, USA.

4. Statistics

As the primary outcome of the study, the 28-joint Disease Activity Score based on erythrocyte sedimentation rate (DAS28-ESR) was used to evaluate disease activity for all patients at week 0, week 1, week 4 and week 12. After discussion with the EMA, DAS28 was used as an established score in rheumatology to measure response with respect to arthritic manifestation. Of note, the Pouchot score was not fully validated at initiation of the CONSIDER study [31]. DAS28 $\leq$ 3.2 was interpreted as low, 3.2 < DAS28 $\leq$ 5.1 as moderate and DAS28 > 5.1 as high disease activity [32], whereas DAS28 < 2.6 corresponds to disease remission [33]. A good EULAR response to treatment was defined as an improvement of DAS28-ESR > 1.2 from baseline to week 12 (responders) [32]. For statistical analysis, logarithmic normally distributed data were used for all values that did not fully fit a normal distribution and extreme outliers were removed. Two-way repeated-measures analysis of variance (ANOVA) with Tukey's multiple comparisons tests (95% confidence interval) and Sidak's multiple comparisons test (95% confidence interval) was used to analyze whether time, treatment (placebo or canakinumab) or the interaction between both factors had a statistically significant effect on the expression of cytokines. The effect of the response rate (responder or non-responder) during treatment in canakinumab patients was analyzed in the same way. For all positive results, one-way repeated-measures ANOVA with Tukey's multiple comparisons test (95% confidence interval) was applied to determine the simple main effect of time on the expression of cytokines in each treatment group. For responder and non-responder groups, repeated measures *t*-test was used. Spearman's correlation coefficient was used to analyze the correlation between all analyzed cytokines and acute phase reactants, C-reactive protein (CRP) and ferritin. GraphPad Prism 7 software (San Diego, CA, USA) was used for all statistical analyses, and statistical significance was set at $p < 0.05$.

5. Results

5.1. Statistically Significant Differences in the Concentrations of MRP8/14 (Calprotectin), S100A12, IL-2RA, IL-6, IL-18 and sL-Selectin between Placebo and Canakinumab Groups

By two-way repeated-measures ANOVA, no significant differences were detected in the biomarkers CXCL13, BAFF, sCD163, IP-10, MIG, TNF-α and IL-1RA between the samples of patients treated with placebo or canakinumab.

Two-way repeated-measures ANOVA revealed a statistically significant effect of interaction between treatment type (placebo or canakinumab) and time (F (2, 30) = 3.744, $p = 0.0353$) on MRP8/14 concentrations. There was no difference between the two treatment groups with respect to MRP8/14 concentrations, but there was a statistically significant difference between time points (F (2, 30) = 8.983, $p = 0.0009$) between the two groups, with a significant reduction in MRP8/14 in the canakinumab group at week 4 (Figure 1a). An additional Tukey's multiple comparisons test showed significant decreases between weeks 0 and 1 (adjusted $p = 0.0065$) and weeks 0 and 4 (adjusted $p \leq 0.0001$) in the canakinumab group, while no significant differences could be detected in the placebo group.

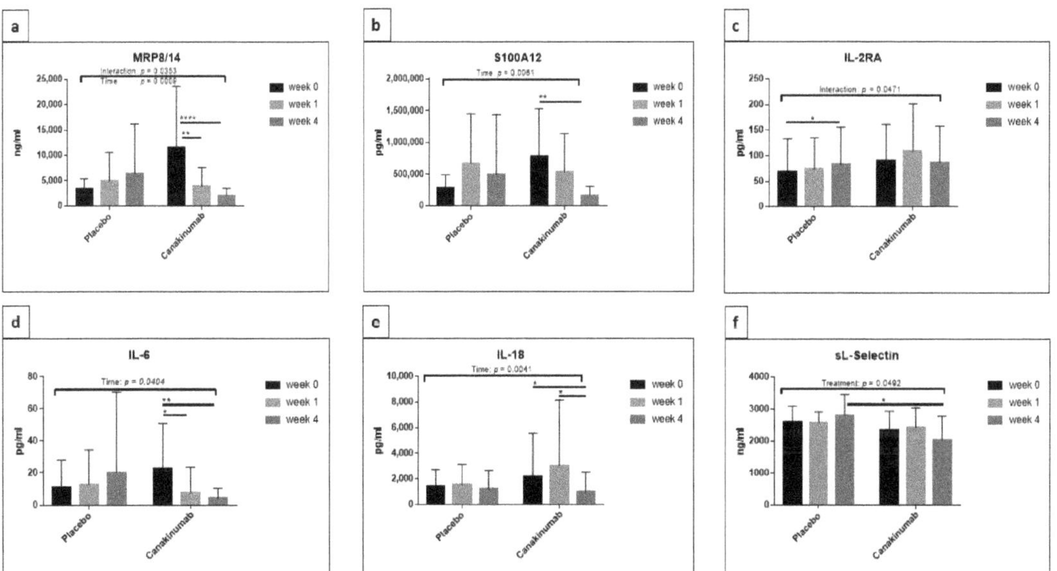

Figure 1. Representative cytokines that showed a significant reduction under the effect of canakinumab. A comparison of the concentrations of MRP8/14 (**a**), S100A12 (**b**), IL-2RA (**c**), IL-6 (**d**), IL-18 (**e**) and sL-Selectin (**f**) between placebo and canakinumab patients at week 0, week 1 and week 4 was applied. The bar plots represent the mean with SD. Two-way repeated-measures ANOVA with Tukey's multiple comparisons test and Sidak's multiple comparisons test was performed using GraphPad Prism 7 and statistical significance was set at $p < 0.05$. * $p < 0.05$, ** $p < 0.01$ and **** $p < 0.0001$.

This result was further confirmed by applying one-way repeated-measures ANOVA for each treatment group separately with three time points. Canakinumab showed a significant decrease in MRP8/14 between weeks ($p = 0.0014$); Tukey's multiple comparisons test showed significant reductions in MRP8/14 between weeks 0 and 1 (adjusted $p = 0.0035$) and weeks 0 and 4 (adjusted $p = 0.0064$) in the canakinumab group in contrast to the placebo (Figure 2a,b).

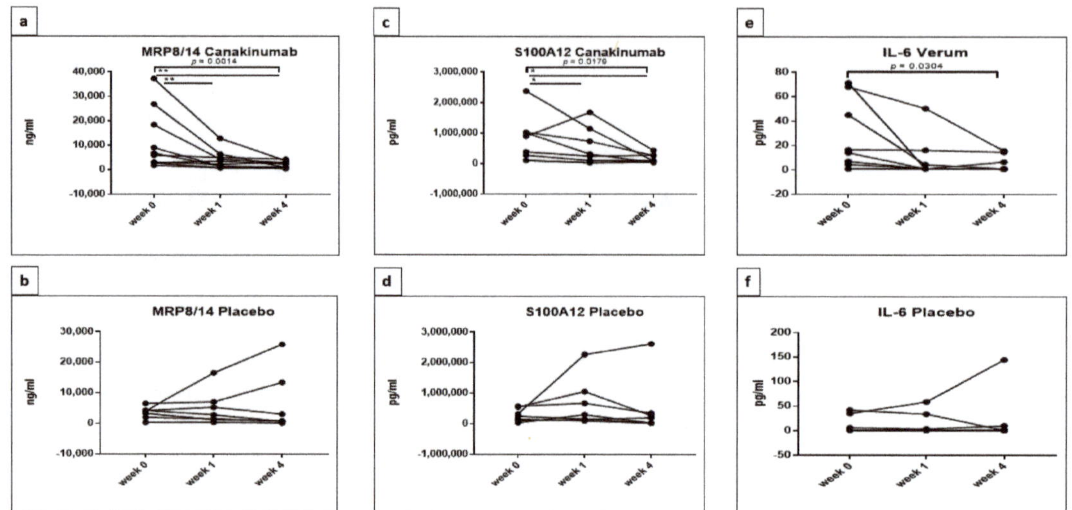

Figure 2. Confirmed significant reduction in MRP8/14 (**a**,**b**), S100A12 (**c**,**d**) and IL-6 (**e**,**f**) in canakinumab patients analyzing each group separately. One-way repeated-measures ANOVA with Tukey's multiple comparisons test was used to investigate the effect of treatment (placebo or canakinumab) on the concentrations of cytokines during three time points (week 0, week 1 and week 4) in each group separately. GraphPad Prism 7 was used and statistical significance was set at $p < 0.05$. * $p < 0.05$, ** $p < 0.01$.

By applying two-way repeated-measures ANOVA on S100A12 concentrations, only a significant effect of time could be detected (F (2, 26) = 6.245, $p = 0.0061$); following this, a Tukey's multiple comparisons test showed a significant decrease in S100A12 levels between weeks 0 and 4 (adjusted $p = 0.0041$) in the canakinumab group exclusively (Figure 1b). One-way repeated-measures ANOVA for each treatment group separately confirmed this result and showed a significant decrease in the concentrations of S100A12 in the canakinumab group only ($p = 0.0179$). The analysis between time points by Tukey's multiple comparisons testing reflected a significant decrease between weeks 0 and 1 and between weeks 0 and 4 ($p = 0.0417$ and 0.0321, respectively) (Figure 2c,d).

The analysis of IL-2RA by two-way repeated-measures ANOVA demonstrated a significant interaction between treatment type and time (F (2, 30) = 3.388, $p = 0.0471$), with decreased expression in canakinumab at week 4. Neither time nor treatment type solely showed a significant effect on the concentrations of IL-2RA. An additional Tukey's multiple comparisons test showed a significant increase between weeks 0 and 4 (adjusted $p = 0.0429$) in the placebo group, while no significant differences could be detected in canakinumab-treated patients (Figure 1c).

The concentrations of IL-6 differed significantly with respect to time (F (2, 32) = 3.555, $p = 0.0404$) in statistical analysis using a two-way repeated-measures ANOVA. As can be seen in Figure 1d, the concentrations of IL-6 decreased in patients treated with canakinumab, while they increased in patients treated with placebo. Additional Tukey's multiple comparisons testing revealed a significant difference in patients treated with canakinumab, in which the concentrations of IL-6 decreased between weeks 0 and 1 (adjusted $p = 0.0133$) and weeks 0 and 4 (adjusted $p = 0.008$).

The significantly decreased concentrations of IL-6 over time in patients treated with canakinumab and not in the placebo group were further demonstrated by one-way repeated-measures ANOVA ($p = 0.0304$) (Figure 2e,f).

The two-way repeated-measures ANOVA of IL-18 concentrations revealed a significant difference with respect to time (F (2, 30) = 6.634, $p = 0.0041$), with a significant decrease in canakinumab at week 4. Further Tukey's multiple comparisons testing revealed a significant decrease in the concentrations of IL-18 between week 0 and 4 (adjusted $p = 0.0436$) and between weeks 1 and 4 (adjusted $p = 0.0118$) only in canakinumab patients (Figure 1e). One-way repeated-measures ANOVA showed no significant differences of IL-18 in both groups.

Two-way repeated-measures ANOVA revealed a significant difference in concentrations of sL-selectin related to type of treatment (placebo or canakinumab) (F (1, 15) = 4.578), $p = 0.0492$), whereas increased concentrations of sL-selectin could be seen in the placebo group at week 4; an obvious decrease was observed only in canakinumab-treated patients. Comparison of the concentrations of sL-selectin between two groups at each time point by Sidak's multiple comparisons test showed that the concentrations at week 4 were significantly decreased in canakinumab patients when compared to placebo (adjusted $p = 0.0361$) (Figure 1f). Further one-way repeated-measures ANOVA for each treatment group separately with three time points showed no significant differences in sL-selectin concentrations between different weeks in both groups.

IFN-γ, IL-10, IL-17A and IFN-α2 were below the lower detection limit of the multiplex assay (1.57, 1.06, 2.44 and 0.95 pg/mL, respectively); therefore, no statistical analyses were applied.

Detailed results of two-way and one-way repeated-measures ANOVA for significantly different cytokines are shown in Tables 2 and 3, respectively.

Table 2. Detailed results of two-way repeated-measures ANOVA with Tukey's and Sidak's multiple comparisons tests for placebo and canakinumab groups. * $p < 0.05$, ** $p < 0.01$, *** $p < 0.001$ and **** $p < 0.0001$.

Cytokine	Source of Variation	*p* Value	Summary	F (DFn, DFd)	Tukey's Multiple Comparisons Test	Adjusted *p* Value	Summary
MRP8/14	Interaction	0.0353	*	F (2, 30) = 3.744	Placebo		ns
	Treatment	0.5932	ns		Canakinumab		
	Time	0.0009	***	F (2, 30) = 8.983	week 0 vs. week 1	0.0065	**
					week 0 vs. week 4	<0.0001	****
					week 1 vs. week 4	0.157	ns
S100A12	Interaction	0.0757	ns		Placebo		ns
	Treatment	0.8699	ns		Canakinumab		
	Time	0.0061	**	F (2, 26) = 6.245	week 0 vs. week 1	0.2236	ns
					week 0 vs. week 4	0.0041	**
					week 1 vs. week 4	0.1746	ns
IL-2RA	Interaction	0.0471	*	F (2, 30) = 3.388	Placebo		
	Treatment	0.6039	ns		week 0 vs. week 1	0.0972	ns
	Time	0.086	ns		week 0 vs. week 4	0.0429	*
					week 1 vs. week 4	0.9209	ns
					Canakinumab		ns

Table 2. *Cont.*

Cytokine	Source of Variation	*p* Value	Summary	F (DFn, DFd)	Tukey's Multiple Comparisons Test	Adjusted *p* Value	Summary
IL-6	Interaction	0.1085	ns		Placebo		ns
	Treatment	0.7974	ns		Canakinumab		
	Time	0.0404	*	F (2, 32) = 3.555	week 0 vs. week 1	0.0133	*
					week 0 vs. week 4	0.008	**
					week 1 vs. week 4	0.9779	ns
IL-18	Interaction	0.6183	ns		Placebo		ns
	Treatment	0.9114	ns		Canakinumab		
	Time	0.0041	**	F (2, 30) = 6.634	week 0 vs. week 1	0.8451	ns
					week 0 vs. week 4	0.0436	*
					week 1 vs. week 4	0.0118	*
					Sidak's multiple comparisons test	Adjusted *p* Value	Summary
sL-Selectin	Interaction	0.2684	ns		Placebo-Canakinumab		
	Treatment	0.0492	*	F (1, 15) = 4.578	week 0	0.8361	ns
	Time	0.6646	ns		week 1	0.9326	ns
					week 4	0.0361	*

Table 3. Detailed results of one-way repeated-measures ANOVA with Tukey's multiple comparisons test for placebo and canakinumab separately for three time points. * $p < 0.05$, ** $p < 0.01$.

Cytokine	Group	*p* Value	Summary	Tukey's Multiple Comparisons Test	Adjusted *p* Value	Summary
MRP8/14	Placebo	0.3967	ns	Placebo		ns
	Canakinumab	0.0014	**	Canakinumab		
				week 0 vs. week 1	0.0035	**
				week 0 vs. week 4	0.0064	**
				week 1 vs. week 4	0.0758	ns
S100A12	Placebo	0.1282	ns	Placebo		ns
	Canakinumab	0.0179	*	Canakinumab		
				week 0 vs. week 1	0.0417	*
				week 0 vs. week 4	0.0321	*
				week 1 vs. week 4	0.2709	ns
IL-6	Placebo	0.6997	ns	Placebo		ns
	Canakinumab	0.0304	*	Canakinumab		ns

5.2. Response Rate Has an Effect on the Concentrations of MRP8/14, S100A12, IL-1RA, IL-18 and IL-6 in Canakinumab Group

To analyze the effect of rate of response on the concentrations of cytokines, canakinumab patients were classified into responders and non-responders based on their DAS28-ESR improvement, and the concentrations of biomarkers were statistically analyzed. Since there were fewer samples at week 1, only concentrations at weeks 0 and 4 were evaluated. Two-way repeated-measures ANOVA showed no significant differences between responders and non-responders for the biomarkers CXCL13, BAFF, sCD163, MIG, IP-10, TNF-α, IL-2RA, sL-selectin and IL-6.

For MRP8/14, two-way repeated-measures ANOVA determined a significant difference with respect to time ($F(1, 13) = 13.61$, $p = 0.0027$). Further Sidak's multiple comparisons testing showed a significant decrease in responders between weeks 0 and 4 (adjusted $p = 0.0023$), as shown in Figure 3a. There was no significant decrease in concentrations of MRP8/14 in non-responders. By applying *t*-test for each group separately, a significant decrease in MRP8/14 between week 0 and week 4 could be detected in the responder group ($p = 0.0023$) exclusively (Figure 4a,b).

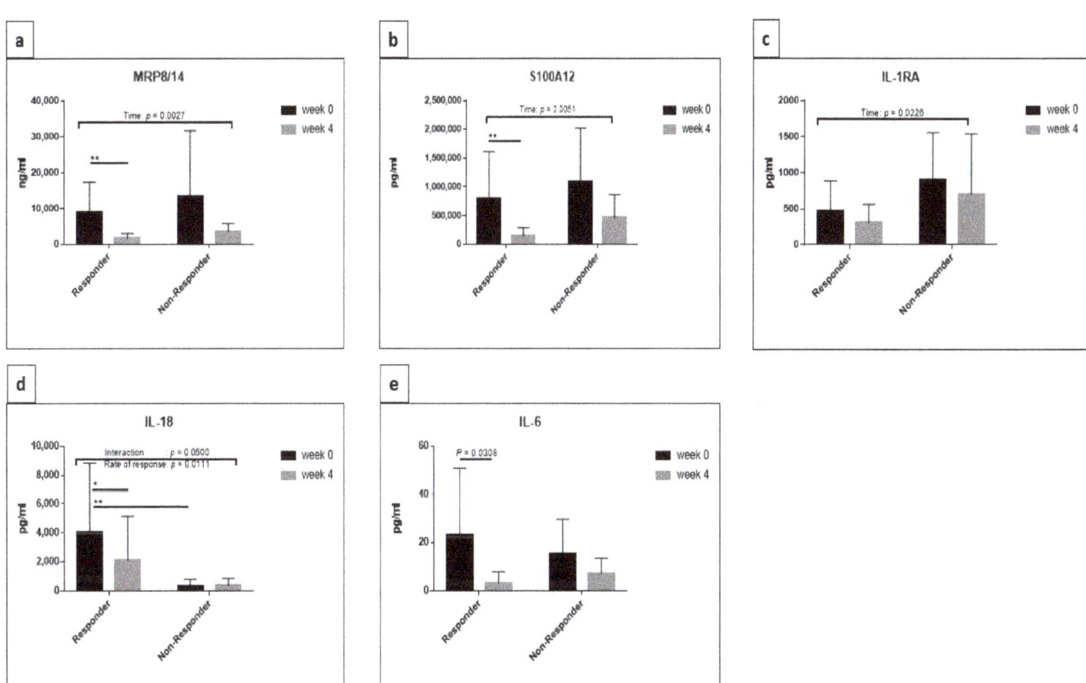

Figure 3. Representative cytokines that showed a significant reduction in response to canakinumab. A comparison of the expression of MRP8/14 (**a**), S100A12 (**b**), IL-1RA (**c**), IL-18 (**d**) and IL-6 (**e**) between responders and non-responders of canakinumab patients at week 0 and week 4 was applied. The bar plots represent the mean with SD. Two-way repeated-measures ANOVA with Tukey's multiple comparisons test and Sidak's multiple comparisons test was performed using GraphPad Prism 7 and statistical significance was set at $p < 0.05$. * $p < 0.05$, ** $p < 0.01$.

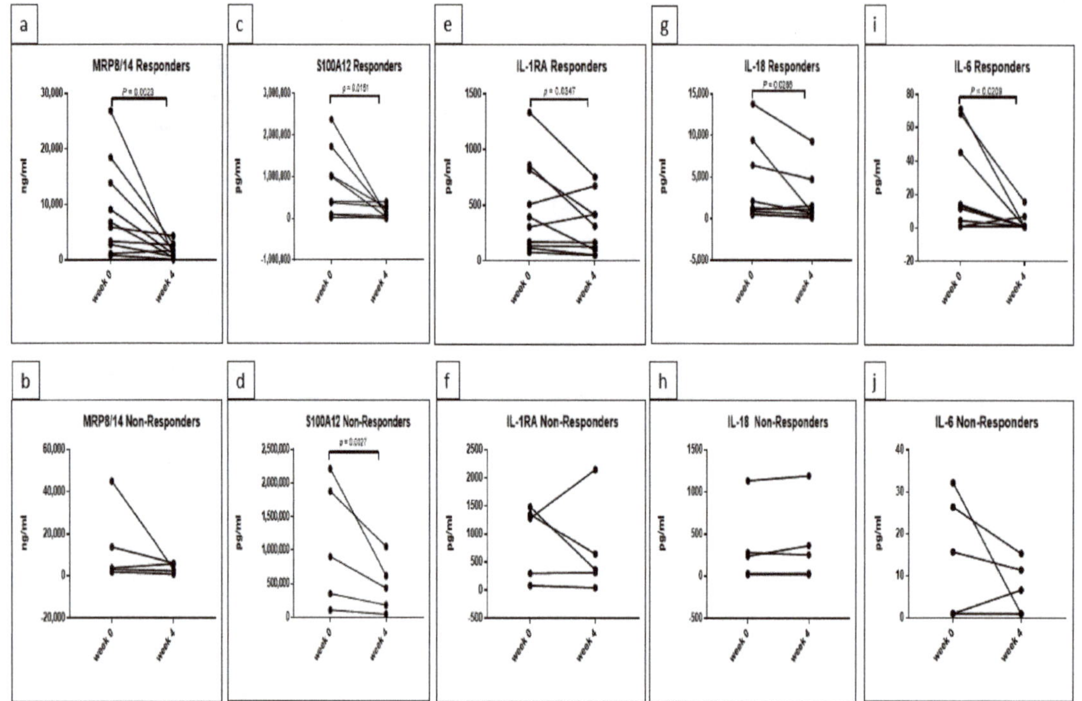

Figure 4. Confirmed significant reduction in MRP8/14 (**a**,**b**), S100A12 (**c**,**d**), IL-1RA (**e**,**f**), IL-18 (**g**,**h**) and IL-6 (**i**,**j**) in responders of canakinumab patients. Investigation of the effect of response rate in each responder and non-responder groups separately. Repeated-measures *t*-test was applied using GraphPad Prism 7 and statistical significance was set at $p < 0.05$.

Two-way repeated-measures ANOVA detected significant differences in the concentrations of S100A12 with respect to time (F (1, 12) = 11.65 $p = 0.0051$); when applying comparison between time points by Sidak's multiple comparisons test, a significant decrease in the concentrations of S100A12 could be detected in the responder group exclusively (adjusted $p = 0.0056$) (Figure 3b). Additional *t*-test in each group separately showed a significant decrease in responders and non-responders at week 4 ($p = 0.0151$ and 0.0027, respectively) (Figure 4c,d).

A significant effect of time was also observed for IL-1RA concentrations by two-way repeated-measures ANOVA (F (1, 13) = 6.688, $p = 0.0226$) (Figure 3c). Although a decrease was observed in both groups, no significant difference was determined by Sidak's multiple comparisons test. *t*-test for each group revealed significant decrease in IL-1RA in responders exclusively ($p = 0.0347$) (Figure 4e,f).

Two-way repeated-measures ANOVA determined a significant effect of the interaction between time and response rate on the concentrations of IL-18 (F (1, 12) = 4.749, $p = 0.05$), with a significant decrease at week 4 detected by Sidak's multiple comparisons test in the responder group exclusively (adjusted $p = 0.0132$). Two-way repeated-measures ANOVA also detected a significant effect regarding the rate of response (responders versus non-responders) (F (1, 12) = 8.989, $p = 0.0111$) with observable reduction in the concentrations of IL-18 in non-responders at both time points when comparing to responders. Sidak's multiple comparisons testing showed a significant decrease in the concentrations of IL-18 in the non-responder group compared to the responder group at week 0 (adjusted $p = 0.0042$) (Figure 3d). Applying *t*-test for each group separately demonstrated a significant decrease in IL-18 at week 4 only in the responder group ($p = 0.0266$) (Figure 4g,h).

Although two-way repeated-measures ANOVA applied on IL-6 concentrations revealed no significant differences between responder and non-responders, further Sidak's multiple comparisons testing showed significant reduced concentrations of IL-6 in responders at week 4 (adjusted $p = 0.0308$) (Figure 3e). The *t*-test confirmed the result and showed a significant decrease in responder group exclusively ($p = 0.0209$) (Figure 4i,j).

Detailed results of two-way repeated-measures ANOVA followed by *t*-test for significantly different cytokines are shown in Tables 4 and 5, respectively.

Table 4. Detailed results of two-way repeated-measures ANOVA with Sidak's multiple comparisons test for responders and non-responders. * $p < 0.05$, ** $p < 0.01$.

Cytokine	Source of Variation	*p* Value	Summary	F (DFn, DFd)	Sidak's Multiple Comparisons Test	Adjusted *p* Value	Summary
MRP8/14	Interaction	0.2892	ns		week 0–week 4		
	DAS28 improvement	0.3022	ns		Responder	0.0023	**
	Time	0.0027	**	F (1, 13) = 13.61	Non-Responder	0.2562	ns
S100A12	Interaction	0.3104	ns		week 0–week 4		
	DAS28 improvement	0.1944	ns		Responder	0.0056	**
	Time	0.0051	**	F (1, 12) = 11.65	Non-Responder	0.3075	ns
IL-1RA	Interaction	0.9816	ns		week 0–week 4		
	DAS28 improvement	0.3475	ns		Responder	0.0877	ns
	Time	0.0226	*	F (1, 13) = 6.688	Non-Responder	0.2501	ns
IL-18	Interaction	0.05	*	F (1, 12) = 4.749	week 0–week 4		
	DAS28 improvement	0.0111	*	F (1, 12) = 8.989	Responder	0.0132	*
	Time	0.108	ns		Non-Responder	0.9548	ns
					Responder-Non-Responder		
					week 0	0.0042	**
					week 4	0.0523	ns
IL-6	Interaction	0.275	ns		week 0–week 4		
	DAS28 improvement	0.5756	ns		Responder	0.0308	*
	Time	0.0585	ns		Non-Responder	0.8209	ns

5.3. Significant Correlations between Certain Cytokine/Chemokine Levels and CRP as well as Ferritin Were Detected at Week 4

To analyze if cytokine/chemokine levels correlated with the activity of disease, Spearman's correlation coefficient was calculated for acute phase reactants such as C-reactive protein (CRP) and ferritin. The analyses were applied in all patients as one group at baseline (week 0) and week 4. At baseline, a correlation with CRP was only observed for CXCL-13 and IL-6 (r values 0.4072 and 0.4368, with *p* values 0.035 and 0.0227, respectively). At week 4, we found significant correlations with CRP for MRP8/14 (r = 0.6667, $p = 0.0003$), S100A12 (r = 0.4497, $p = 0.0275$), BAFF (r = 0.4274, $p = 0.0233$), IL-1RA (r = 0.6229, $p = 0.0004$), IL-2RA (r = 0.6297, $p = 0.0006$), IL-6 (r = 0.7752, $p = <0.0001$), MIG (r = 0.5399, $p = 0.003$), IP-10 (r = 0.541, $p = 0.003$) and TNF-α (r = 0.4189, $p = 0.0297$) (Figure 5a–i), respectively. Likewise, ferritin levels also correlated with several additional cytokines at week 4 compared to baseline. In detail, significant correlations were observed for MRP8/14 (r = 0.6919, $p = 0.0002$), BAFF (r = 0.4537,

$p = 0.0175$), IL-6 ($r = 0.4808$, $p = 0.0129$) and IL-8 ($r = 0.4293$, $p = 0.0322$) at baseline. In contrast, at week 4, a significant correlation was found with MRP8/14 ($r = 0.6275$, $p = 0.0008$), BAFF ($r = 0.5212$, $p = 0.0045$), sCD163 ($r = 0.4402$, $p = 0.0216$), IL-1RA ($r = 0.4469$, $p = 0.0171$), IL-6 ($r = 0.5087$, $p = 0.0067$), IL-18 ($r = 0.4121$, $p = 0.0364$), MIG ($r = 0.5907$, $p = 0.0009$) and IP-10 ($r = 0.5699$, $p = 0.0015$) (Figure 6a–h), respectively.

Table 5. Detailed results of *t*-test between week 0 and week 4 for responder and non-responder groups separately. * $p < 0.05$, ** $p < 0.01$.

Cytokine	Group	*p* Value	Summary
MRP8/14	Responders	0.0023	**
	Non-Responders	0.196	ns
S100A12	Responders	0.0151	*
	Non-Responders	0.0027	**
IL-1RA	Responders	0.0347	*
	Non-Responders	0.2558	ns
IL-18	Responders	0.0266	*
	Non-Responders	0.3871	ns
IL-6	Responders	0.0209	*
	Non-Responders	0.601	ns

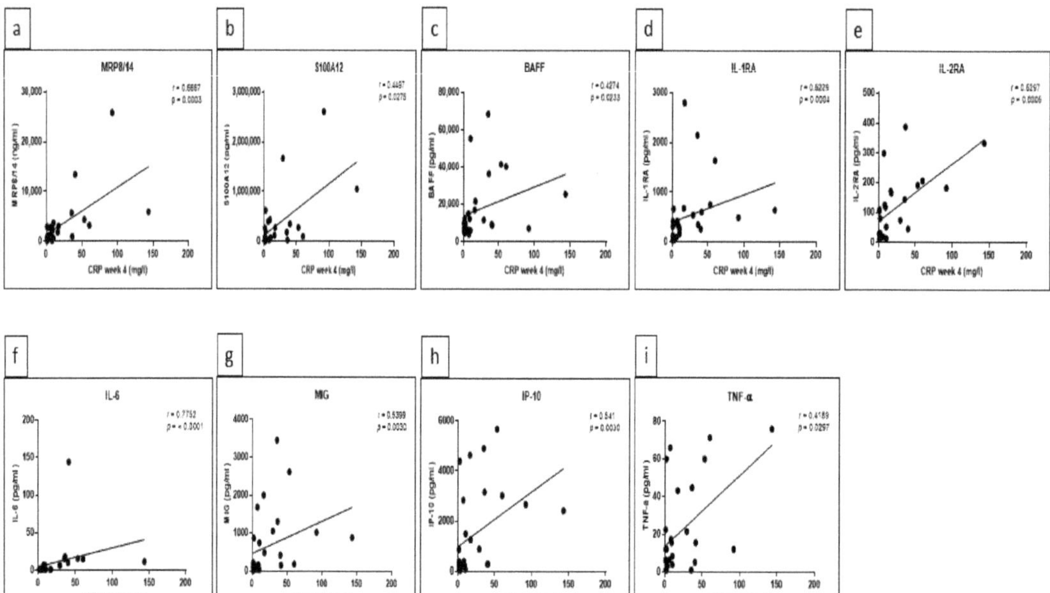

Figure 5. Significant correlations between cytokines/chemokines and C-reactive protein (CRP) at week 4. Spearman's correlation coefficient r and *p* values of correlation analyses between CRP and MRP8/14 (**a**), S100A12 (**b**), BAFF (**c**), IL-1RA (**d**), IL-2RA (**e**), IL-6 (**f**), MIG (**g**), IP-10 (**h**), and TNF-α (**i**) in all patients. GraphPad Prism 7 was used and statistical significance was set at $p < 0.05$.

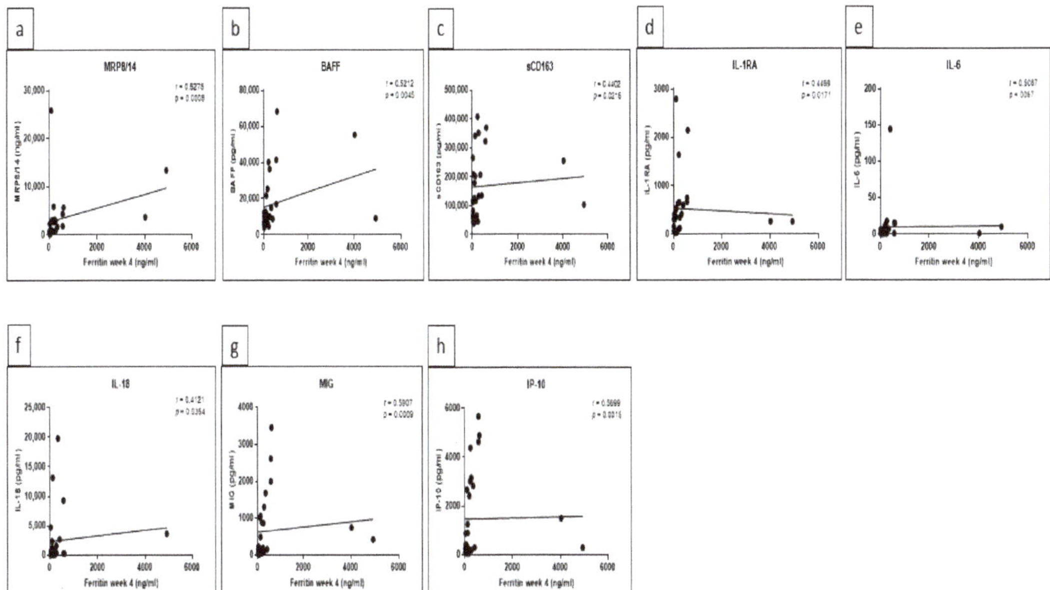

Figure 6. Significant correlations between certain cytokines/chemokines and ferritin at week 4. Spearman's correlation coefficient r and p values of correlation analyses between ferritin and MRP8/14 (**a**), BAFF (**b**), sCD163 (**c**), IL-1RA (**d**), IL-6 (**e**), IL-18 (**f**), MIG (**g**) and IP-10 (**h**) in all patients. GraphPad Prism 7 was used and statistical significance was set at $p < 0.05$.

6. Discussion

In this study, we compared the inflammatory profile of well-characterized patients with AOSD treated with canakinumab to those treated with placebo in a controlled setting. For this purpose, we measured the concentrations of pro-inflammatory cytokines (IFN-α2, IFN-γ, TNF-α, BAFF, IL-6, IL-17 and IL-18), anti-inflammatory cytokine (IL-10), soluble cell adhesion molecule sL-selectin (CD62L), soluble CD163 (a monocyte/macrophage activation biomarker), alarmins (MRP8/14, S100A12) and chemokines (MIG (CXCL 9), IP-10 (CXCL10), and CXCL13). Additionally, we measured IL-1 receptor antagonist (IL-1RA), a natural receptor antagonist for IL-1 and efficient therapeutic molecule in AOSD, and soluble interleukin-2 receptor alpha (sIL-2RA), a marker of T-cell activation. We confirmed the effectiveness of canakinumab on modulating the concentrations of alarmins (MRP 8/14 and S100A12), IL-1RA, IL-18 and IL-6 in patients with AOSD with the strongest association with response rate. As known, alarmins seem to have an important function in AOSD pathogenesis; of those, calcium binding proteins MRP8/14 (S100A8/A9) and S100A12 showed to be useful markers of disease activity and severity in AOSD [34,35]. Our results showed that under treatment with canakinumab, concentrations of both S100 proteins were significantly reduced in AOSD patients when compared to placebo. Moreover, when we classified canakinumab patients by treatment response, MRP 8/14 showed a significant decrease in responders, and S100A12 was significantly decreased in responders and non-responders.

Moreover, a significant increase in the soluble form of IL-2RA at week 4 was also detected in the placebo group, whereas it decreased in canakinumab-treated patients. This is in agreement with previous studies that showed increased soluble IL-2RA in association with disease activity in chronic articular AOSD [23], and serum levels of sIL-2RA were significantly higher in patients with active versus inactive AOSD and decreased significantly with anti inflammatory therapy [22]. IL-1RA is a natural inhibitor of the pro-inflammatory effect of IL-1; it binds IL-1 receptors without inducing a cellular response, thereby modulating a variety of interleukin-1-related immune and inflammatory responses [36]. IL-1RA levels are elevated in different diseases including auto-immune diseases [37,38]. Of note, it was elevated in AOSD patients [39] and significantly higher in patients with AOSD than SLE [40]. Although anakinra, a recombinant version of the interleukin-1 receptor antagonist is used in the treatment of AOSD [39,41], the increase in in vivo circulating IL-1RA levels corresponds to a delayed event in response to IL-1 production and may represent a preventive mechanism in excessive inflammatory response. Moreover, IL-1RA could be considered as an acute phase protein because its expression is regulated by pro-inflammatory cytokines in hepatocytes [42]. In our analysis, canakinumab, an IL-1β inhibitor, could significantly reduce levels of IL-1RA in responders, confirming that AOSD is an IL-1-mediated disease. Significantly higher levels of IL-6 were seen in both sera and skin tissues of patients with active AOSD when compared to healthy donors and quiescent AOSD patients, respectively [43]. Additionally, serum levels of free and total IL-18 were significantly higher in patients with AOSD than healthy donors and control patients with other diseases, including rheumatoid arthritis (RA), systemic lupus erythematosus (SLE) and psoriasis [40]. Furthermore, both cytokines (IL-6 and IL-18) showed an association with clinical activity and declined significantly in the remission phase [43]. This is consistent with the efficiency of canakinumab in significantly reducing the concentrations of both cytokines in our patients and more intensely in the responder group. Notably, the reduction effect of canakinumab on the concentrations of IL-1RA, IL-6, IL-18 and S100A12 in our cohort had been confirmed recently in a systemic juvenile idiopathic arthritis cohort. Moreover, in both cohorts, responders showed higher levels of IL-18 at baseline [44]. L-selectin is a cell adhesion molecule expressed on most leukocytes and is involved in their trafficking to sites of inflammation [14]. The level of soluble L-selectin is used as a surrogate biomarker for leukocyte activity triggered during different autoimmune diseases [45,46]. Our comparison between canakinumab and placebo patients showed a significant effect of canakinumab on lowering the concentrations of sL-selectin at week 4, and significant reduction could be detected in canakinumab when compared to the placebo group at week 4. Although the concentrations of TNF-α were higher in the active untreated AOSD patients when compared to healthy donors [43], canakinumab showed no effect on the concentrations of TNF cytokines used in this study (TNF-α and BAFF).

The concentrations of INF-γ [22], IL-17 [20] and IFN-α2 [21] and a classical anti-inflammatory cytokine IL-10 [25] were higher in AOSD patients than in healthy controls. In our patients, the levels of these cytokines were below the detection limit of the multiplex assay and this consistent with a previous study [40] that also showed undetectable levels of INF-γ, IL-17 and IFN-α. Despite the higher levels of CXCL10 and CXCL13 in AOSD than RA and healthy donors and the confirmed potential role of CXCL9, CXCL10 and CXCL13 as clinical biomarkers for disease activity in AOSD [47,48], our analysis showed no difference between concentrations of these CXC chemokine ligands before and after canakinumab treatment. Moreover, although higher levels of sCD163 in AOSD compared to healthy donors and correlation with disease activity were identified previously [49], no effect of canakinumab could be detected in our analysis. However, despite the robust observations in our study with a well-characterized cohort of patients, there are several limitations to consider. According to the inclusion and exclusion criteria and the outcome measurements as defined by the study protocol, our results are based on a selected cohort of patients with predominant articular disease manifestation. The sample size was small and the biomarker measurements were performed only at two time points over a short time period. Thus, further validations of our results are needed in another larger patient cohort over a longer observation period. Furthermore, it would be of utmost interest to investigate the same biomarker profile in patients with a predominant systemic manifestation of AOSD.

7. Conclusions

In this study, we provide evidence that canakinumab treatment in AOSD has a diverse impact on the cytokine profile of responding patients. Furthermore, we identified a potential biomarker profile for follow-up analyses consisting of S100 proteins, IL-2RA, IL1RA, IL-6 and IL-18 and sL-selectin.

Author Contributions: Conceptualization, E.F.; Methodology, K.G., E.F., D.F., J.Z. and C.K.; Validation, K.G., E.F., J.L., D.F. and G.-R.B.; Formal Analysis, K.G. and J.L.; Investigation, K.G.; Resources, E.F., J.Z., C.K. and G.-R.B.; Data Curation, K.G., E.F., J.Z., C.K. and J.L.; Writing—Original Draft Preparation, K.G.; Writing—Review and Editing, K.G., E.F., D.F., G.-R.B., J.Z., C.K. and J.L. Visualization, K.G., E.F., D.F., J.Z., C.K. and G.-R.B.; Supervision, E.F.; Project Administration, E.F. All authors have read and agreed to the published version of the manuscript.

Funding: This work was sponsored by Novartis Pharma GmbH, contract number: MACZ885A_FVDB003.

Institutional Review Board Statement: The CONSIDER study (CACZ885GDE01T) was conducted according to the ethical principles of the Declaration of Helsinki. The study protocol and all amendments were reviewed by the Independent Ethics Commission of the State of Berlin (Ethik-Kommission des Landes Berlin, LAGeSo), and Independent Ethics Committees for each center. An approval from the German regulatory authority was received prior to the start of the study. The reference number at the LAGeSo is: 11/0561—ZS EK 11. The additional collection of research samples for this biomarker analysis was a sub-project to the main study. The ethics committee also approved the additional patient consent.

Informed Consent Statement: Informed consent was obtained from all subjects involved in the study.

Data Availability Statement: The datasets used and/or analyzed for the current study are available from the corresponding author on reasonable request.

Conflicts of Interest: J.Z. has worked on the study CACZ885GDE01T, which was funded by Novartis Pharma GmbH. C.K. has received personal advisory board and congress fees from Novartis, Pfizer, Roche and Sobi. G.-R.B. Honoraria for lectures from Novartis. D.F. received grant support, honoraria as speaker and adviser from Novartis, Pfizer and Sobi. E.F. received grant support, honoraria as speaker and adviser from Novartis, Roche, Sanofi and Sobi.

References

1. Mahroum, N.; Mahagna, H.; Amital, H. Diagnosis and classification of adult Still's disease. *J. Autoimmun.* **2014**, *48–49*, 34–37. [CrossRef]
2. Bywaters, E.G. Still's disease in the adult. *Ann. Rheum. Dis.* **1971**, *30*, 121–133. [CrossRef] [PubMed]
3. Still, G.F. On a form of chronic joint disease in children. *Med.-Chir. Trans.* **1897**, *80*, 47–60. [CrossRef]
4. Terkeltaub, R.; Esdaile, J.M.; Décary, F.; Harth, M.; Lister, J.; Lapointe, N. HLA—Bw35 and Prognosis in Adult Still's Disease. *Arthritis Rheum.* **1981**, *24*, 1469–1472. [CrossRef] [PubMed]
5. Wouters, J.M.G.W.; Reekers, P.; van de Putte, L.B.A. Adult-onset still's disease. Disease course and HLA associations. *Arthritis Rheum.* **1986**, *29*, 415–418. [CrossRef] [PubMed]
6. Pouchot, J.; Sampalis, J.S.; Beaudet, F.; Carette, S.; Décary, F.; Salusinsky-sternbach, M.; Hill, R.O.; Gutkowski, A.; Harth, M.; Myhal, D.; et al. Adult Still's Disease: Manifestations, Disease Course, and Outcome in 62 Patients. *Medicine* **1991**, *70*, 118–136. [CrossRef]
7. Perez, C.; Artola, V. Adult Still's disease associated with Mycoplasma pneumoniae infection. *Clin. Infect. Dis.* **2001**, *32*, E105–E106. [CrossRef]
8. Escudero, F.J.; Len, O.; Falcó, V.; de Sevilla, T.F.; Sellas, A. Rubella infection in adult onset Still's disease. *Ann. Rheum. Dis.* **2000**, *59*, 490. [CrossRef]
9. Mavragani, C.P.; Spyridakis, E.G.; Koutsilieris, M. Adult-Onset Still's Disease: From Pathophysiology to Targeted Therapies. *Int. J. Inflamm.* **2012**, *2012*, 879020. [CrossRef]
10. Wang, M.Y.; Jia, J.C.; Yang, C.D.; Hu, Q.Y. Pathogenesis, disease course, and prognosis of adult-onset Still's disease: An update and review. *Chin. Med. J.* **2019**, *132*, 2856–2864. [CrossRef]
11. Gerfaud-Valentin, M.; Jamilloux, Y.; Iwaz, J.; Seve, P. Adult-onset Still's disease. *Autoimmun. Rev.* **2014**, *13*, 708–722. [CrossRef] [PubMed]
12. Matsui, K.; Tsuchida, T.; Hiroishi, K.; Tominaga, K.; Hayashi, N.; Hada, T.; Higashino, K. High serum level of macrophage-colony stimulating factor (M-CSF) in adult-onset Still's disease. *Rheumatology* **1999**, *38*, 477–478. [CrossRef] [PubMed]

13. Hoshino, T.; Ohta, A.; Yang, D.; Kawamoto, M.; Kikuchi, M.; Inoue, Y.; Kamizono, S.; Ota, T.; Itoh, K.; Oizumi, K. Elevated serum interleukin 6, interferon-gamma, and tumor necrosis factor-alpha levels in patients with adult Still's disease. *J. Rheumatol.* **1998**, *25*, 396–398. [PubMed]
14. Smalley, D.M.; Ley, K. L-selectin: Mechanisms and physiological significance of ectodomain cleavage. *J. Cell. Mol. Med.* **2005**, *9*, 255–266. [CrossRef]
15. Jung, J.-Y.; Suh, C.-H.; Kim, H.-A. The role of damage-associated molecular pattern for pathogenesis and biomarkers in adult-onset Still's disease. *Expert Rev. Mol. Diagn.* **2019**, *19*, 459–468. [CrossRef] [PubMed]
16. Feist, E.; Mitrovic, S.; Fautrel, B. Mechanisms, biomarkers and targets for adult-onset Still's disease. *Nat. Rev. Rheumatol.* **2018**, *14*, 603–618. [CrossRef]
17. Church, L.D.; Cook, G.P.; McDermott, M.F. Primer: Inflammasomes and interleukin 1beta in inflammatory disorders. *Nat. Clin. Pract. Rheumatol.* **2008**, *4*, 34–42. [CrossRef]
18. Hsieh, C.-W.; Chen, Y.-M.; Lin, C.-C.; Tang, K.-T.; Chen, H.-H.; Hung, W.-T.; Lai, K.-L.; Chen, D.-Y. Elevated Expression of the NLRP3 Inflammasome and Its Correlation with Disease Activity in Adult-onset Still Disease. *J. Rheumatol.* **2017**, *44*, 1142–1150. [CrossRef]
19. Cush, J.J. Autoinflammatory syndromes. *Dermatol. Clin.* **2013**, *31*, 471–480. [CrossRef]
20. Chen, D.Y.; Chen, Y.M.; Lan, J.L.; Lin, C.C.; Chen, H.H.; Hsieh, C.W. Potential role of Th17 cells in the pathogenesis of adult-onset Still's disease. *Rheumatology* **2010**, *49*, 2305–2312. [CrossRef]
21. Chen, D.Y.; Lin, C.C.; Chen, Y.M.; Lan, J.L.; Hung, W.T.; Chen, H.H.; Lai, K.L.; Hsieh, C.W. Involvement of TLR7 MyD88-dependent signaling pathway in the pathogenesis of adult-onset Still's disease. *Arthritis Res. Ther.* **2013**, *15*, R39. [CrossRef]
22. Choi, J.H.; Suh, C.H.; Lee, Y.M.; Suh, Y.J.; Lee, S.K.; Kim, S.S.; Nahm, D.H.; Park, H.S. Serum cytokine profiles in patients with adult onset Still's disease. *J. Rheumatol.* **2003**, *30*, 2422–2427.
23. Fujii, T.; Nojima, T.; Yasuoka, H.; Satoh, S.; Nakamura, K.; Kuwana, M.; Suwa, A.; Hirakata, M.; Mimori, T. Cytokine and immunogenetic profiles in Japanese patients with adult Still's disease. Association with chronic articular disease. *Rheumatology* **2001**, *40*, 1398–1404. [CrossRef]
24. Chen, D.Y.; Chen, Y.M.; Chen, H.H.; Hsieh, C.W.; Lin, C.C.; Lan, J.L. The associations of circulating CD4+CD25 high regulatory T cells and TGF-β with disease activity and clinical course in patients with adult-onset Still's disease. *Connect. Tissue Res.* **2010**, *51*, 370–377. [CrossRef] [PubMed]
25. Sun, Y.; Wang, Z.; Chi, H.; Hu, Q.; Ye, J.; Liu, H.; Cheng, X.; Shi, H.; Zhou, Z.; Teng, J.; et al. Elevated serum levels of interleukin-10 in adult-onset Still's disease are associated with disease activity. *Clin. Rheumatol.* **2019**, *38*, 3205–3210. [CrossRef] [PubMed]
26. Castañeda, S.; Blanco, R.; González-Gay, M.A. Adult-onset Still's disease: Advances in the treatment. *Best Pract. Res. Clin. Rheumatol.* **2016**, *30*, 222–238. [CrossRef] [PubMed]
27. Castañeda, S.; Atienza-Mateo, B.; Martín-Varillas, J.L.; López-Matencio, J.M.S.; González-Gay, M.A. Anakinra for the treatment of adult-onset Still's disease. *Expert Rev. Clin. Immunol.* **2018**, *14*, 979–992. [CrossRef]
28. Junge, G.; Mason, J.; Feist, E. Adult onset Still's disease—The evidence that anti-interleukin-1 treatment is effective and well-tolerated (a comprehensive literature review). *Semin. Arthritis Rheum.* **2017**, *47*, 295–302. [CrossRef]
29. Sfriso, P.; Bindoli, S.; Doria, A.; Feist, E.; Galozzi, P. Canakinumab for the treatment of adult-onset Still's disease. *Expert Rev. Clin. Immunol.* **2020**, *16*, 129–138. [CrossRef]
30. Kedor, C.; Listing, J.; Zernicke, J.; Weiß, A.; Behrens, F.; Blank, N.; Henes, J.C.; Kekow, J.; Rubbert-Roth, A.; Schulze-Koops, H.; et al. Canakinumab for Treatment of Adult-Onset Still's Disease to Achieve Reduction of Arthritic Manifestation (CONSIDER): Phase II, randomised, double-blind, placebo-controlled, multicentre, investigator-initiated trial. *Ann. Rheum. Dis.* **2020**, *79*, 1090–1097. [CrossRef]
31. Kedor, C.; Listing, J.; Zernicke, J.; Feist, E. Response to: 'Changing the outcome measures, changing the results? The urgent need of a specific Disease Activity Score to adult-onset Still's disease' by Ruscitti et al. *Ann. Rheum. Dis.* **2020**, *2020*, 218143.
32. van Gestel, A.M.; Haagsma, C.J.; van Riel, P.L. Validation of rheumatoid arthritis improvement criteria that include simplified joint counts. *Arthritis Rheum.* **1998**, *41*, 1845–1850. [CrossRef]
33. Fransen, J.; Creemers, M.C.W.; Van Riel, P.L.C.M. Remission in rheumatoid arthritis: Agreement of the disease activity score (DAS28) with the ARA preliminary remission criteria. *Rheumatology* **2004**, *43*, 1252–1255. [CrossRef] [PubMed]
34. Jung, S.-Y.; Park, Y.-B.; Ha, Y.-J.; Lee, K.-H.; Lee, S.-K. Serum Calprotectin as a Marker for Disease Activity and Severity in Adult-onset Still's Disease. *J. Rheumatol.* **2010**, *37*, 1029–1034. [CrossRef]
35. Bae, C.-B.; Suh, C.-H.; An, J.-M.; Jung, J.-Y.; Jeon, J.-Y.; Nam, J.-Y.; Kim, H.-A. Serum S100A12 May Be a Useful Biomarker of Disease Activity in Adult-onset Still's Disease. *J. Rheumatol.* **2014**, *41*, 2403–2408. [CrossRef]
36. Perrier, S.; Darakhshan, F.; Hajduch, E. IL-1 receptor antagonist in metabolic diseases: Dr Jekyll or Mr Hyde? *FEBS Lett.* **2006**, *580*, 6289–6294. [CrossRef] [PubMed]
37. Chikanza, I.C.; Roux-Lombard, P.; Dayer, J.-M.; Panayi, G.S. Dysregulation of the in vivo production of interleukin-1 receptor antagonist in patients with rheumatoid arthritis pathogenetic implications. *Arthritis Rheum.* **1995**, *38*, 642–648. [CrossRef]
38. Suzuki, H.; Takemura, H.; Kashiwagi, H. Interleukin-1 receptor antagonist in patients with active systemic lupus erythematosus: Enhanced production by monocytes and correlation with disease activity. *Arthritis Rheum.* **1995**, *38*, 1055–1059. [CrossRef] [PubMed]

39. Fitzgerald, A.A.; LeClercq, S.A.; Yan, A.; Homik, J.E.; Dinarello, C.A. Rapid responses to anakinra in patients with refractory adult-onset Still's disease. *Arthritis Rheum.* **2005**, *52*, 1794–1803. [CrossRef]
40. Girard, C.; Rech, J.; Brown, M.; Allali, D.; Roux-Lombard, P.; Spertini, F.; Schiffrin, E.J.; Schett, G.; Manger, B.; Bas, S.; et al. Elevated serum levels of free interleukin-18 in adult-onset Still's disease. *Rheumatology* **2016**, *55*, 2237–2247. [CrossRef]
41. Ortiz-Sanjuán, F.; Blanco, R.; Riancho-Zarrabeitia, L.; Castañeda, S.; Olivé, A.; Riveros, A.; Velloso-Feijoo, M.L.; Narváez, J.; Jiménez-Moleón, I.; Maiz-Alonso, O.; et al. Efficacy of Anakinra in Refractory Adult-Onset Still's Disease: Multicenter Study of 41 Patients and Literature Review. *Medicine* **2015**, *94*, e1554. [CrossRef] [PubMed]
42. Gabay, C.; Smith, M.F.; Eidlen, D.; Arend, W.P. Interleukin 1 receptor antagonist (IL-1Ra) is an acute-phase protein. *J. Clin. Investig.* **1997**, *99*, 2930–2940. [CrossRef] [PubMed]
43. Chen, D.-Y.; Lan, J.-L.; Lin, F.-J.; Hsieh, T.-Y. Proinflammatory cytokine profiles in sera and pathological tissues of patients with active untreated adult onset Still's disease. *J. Rheumatol.* **2004**, *31*, 2189–2198. [PubMed]
44. Hinze, T.; Kessel, C.; Hinze, C.H.; Seibert, J.; Gram, H.; Foell, D. A dysregulated interleukin-18/interferon-γ/CXCL9 axis impacts treatment response to canakinumab in systemic juvenile idiopathic arthritis. *Rheumatology* **2021**. online ahead of print. [CrossRef]
45. Font, J.; Pizcueta, P.; Ramos-Casals, M.; Cervera, R.; García-Carrasco, M.; Navarro, M.; Ingelmo, M.; Engel, P. Increased serum levels of soluble l-selectin (CD62L) in patients with active systemic lupus erythematosus (SLE). *Clin. Exp. Immunol.* **2000**, *119*, 169–174. [CrossRef]
46. Haznedaroglu, E.; Karaaslan, Y.; Büyükaşik, Y.; Koşar, A.; Ozcebe, O.; Haznedaroglu, I.C.; Kirazli, E.; Dündar, S.V. Selectin adhesion molecules in Behçet's disease. *Ann. Rheum. Dis.* **2000**, *59*, 61–63. [CrossRef] [PubMed]
47. Han, J.H.; Suh, C.-H.; Jung, J.-Y.; Nam, J.-Y.; Kwon, J.E.; Yim, H.; Kim, H.-A. Association of CXCL10 and CXCL13 levels with disease activity and cutaneous manifestation in active adult-onset Still's disease. *Arthritis Res. Ther.* **2015**, *17*, 260. [CrossRef]
48. Bracaglia, C.; De Graaf, K.; Marafon, D.P.; Guilhot, F.; Ferlin, W.; Prencipe, G.; Caiello, I.; Davì, S.; Schulert, G.; Ravelli, A.; et al. Elevated circulating levels of interferon-γ and interferon-γ-induced chemokines characterise patients with macrophage activation syndrome complicating systemic juvenile idiopathic arthritis. *Ann. Rheum. Dis.* **2017**, *76*, 166–172. [CrossRef]
49. Colafrancesco, S.; Priori, R.; Alessandri, C.; Astorri, E.; Perricone, C.; Blank, M.; Agmon-Levin, N.; Shoenfeld, Y.; Valesini, G. sCD163 in AOSD: A biomarker for macrophage activation related to hyperferritinemia. *Immunol. Res.* **2014**, *60*, 177–183. [CrossRef]

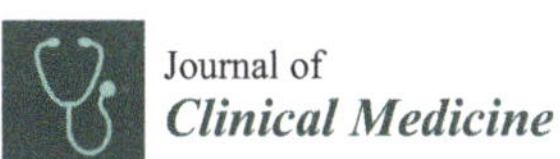
Journal of
Clinical Medicine

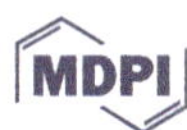

Article

HLA Allele Prevalence in Disease-Modifying Antirheumatic Drugs-Responsive Enthesitis and/or Arthritis Not Fulfilling ASAS Criteria: Comparison with Psoriatic and Undifferentiated Spondyloarthritis

Elvira Favoino, Livio Urso, Alessandra Serafino, Francesca Misceo, Giacomo Catacchio, Marcella Prete and Federico Perosa *

Department of Biomedical Science and Human Oncology (DIMO), Rheumatic and Systemic Autoimmune Diseases Unit, University of Bari Medical School, Piazza G. Cesare 11, I-70124 Bari, Italy; elvira.favoino@uniba.it (E.F.); livio.urso@gmail.com (L.U.); aleserafik@gmail.co (A.S.); franc.misceo@gmail.com (F.M.); giaco.catacchio@gmail.com (G.C.); marcella.prete@uniba.it (M.P.)
* Correspondence: federico.perosa@uniba.it; Tel.: +39-80-547-88-91; Fax: +39-80-547-88-20

Abstract: Spondyloarthritis (SpA) is a group of inflammatory rheumatic diseases characterized by common clinical features, such as inflammatory enthesitis, arthritis and/or back pain. SpA is strongly associated with human leukocyte antigen (HLA) class I allotype B27. Ankylosing spondylitis has historically been the SpA subgroup with one of the strongest, best-proven associations with HLA-B27. The remaining SpA subgroups, namely psoriatic arthritis (PsA), inflammatory bowel diseases-associated arthritis/spondylitis, reactive arthritis, and undifferentiated SpA (uSpA), have also been associated with HLA allotypes other than HLA-B27. In this retrospective study, we analyzed the association between the HLA class I and II haplotypes and the susceptibility to enthesitis and/or arthritis (E/A). Special attention was paid to E/A responding to disease-modifying antirheumatic drugs (DMARDs) not fulfilling ASAS classification criteria (ASAS$^-$), as compared to ASAS$^+$ forms including PsA and uSpA. The whole E/A group showed significant independent associations with HLA-A28(68), B27, Cw3, Cw12, and DQ1; taken singly, PsA was associated with HLA-B27 and DQ1, uSpA with HLA-B16(38,39) and B27, and E/A ASAS$^-$ with HLA-A28(68), Cw8, and Cw12. This study identified novel risk HLA allotypes for different SpA subgroups in an Italian population. HLA typing could aid the diagnosis and treatment of E/A subgroups, including DMARDS-responsive forms not fulfilling ASAS classification criteria.

Keywords: spondyloarthritis; human leukocyte antigen; undifferentiated enthesitis and/or arthritis; ASAS classification criteria; clinical management

Citation: Favoino, E.; Urso, L.; Serafino, A.; Misceo, F.; Catacchio, G.; Prete, M.; Perosa, F. HLA Allele Prevalence in Disease-Modifying Antirheumatic Drugs-Responsive Enthesitis and/or Arthritis Not Fulfilling ASAS Criteria: Comparison with Psoriatic and Undifferentiated Spondyloarthritis. *J. Clin. Med.* **2021**, *10*, 3006. https://doi.org/10.3390/jcm10143006

Academic Editor: Eugen Feist

Received: 28 May 2021
Accepted: 3 July 2021
Published: 6 July 2021

1. Introduction

Spondyloarthritis (SpA) is a heterogeneous group of chronic inflammatory rheumatic diseases encompassing different clinical subgroups, namely ankylosing spondylitis (AS), psoriatic arthritis (PsA), inflammatory bowel diseases-associated arthritis/spondylitis (enteropathic arthritis), reactive arthritis, and undifferentiated SpA (uSpA). The latter includes patients with enthesitis and/or arthritis (E/A) fulfilling ASAS classification criteria [1] (E/A ASAS$^+$) but who cannot be included under the classification criteria of any of the single well-defined ASAS subgroups. SpA can also be clinically classified as axial, peripheral, or combined forms, depending on whether axial or peripheral joints or both [1–3] are the predominant sites affected by clinical manifestations.

SpA and its subgroups share common clinical manifestations, namely enthesitis, inflammatory back pain, sacroiliitis, peripheral arthritis, uveitis, and/or gut inflammation [4,5]. Among these, enthesitis is the most peculiar to SpA [6].

In daily practice, the rheumatologist is very often faced with patients showing signs and symptoms consistent with E/A. Even in the presence of ultrasound-documented E/A, the diagnosis of SpA is not always straightforward when 2011 ASAS criteria are not fulfilled [1] (i.e., patients with only E/A; E/A ASAS$^-$), ASAS$^+$ patients' disease features do not satisfy any of the classification criteria related to SpA subgroups (uSpA), and/or patient-reported symptoms are not clearly inflammatory [7]. In these cases, the possibility of a mechanical/metabolic E/A cannot be ruled out [6]. Even so, a subgroup of E/A ASAS$^-$ patients can still respond efficiently to DMARDs. Due to this uncertainty, it would be helpful to rely on markers to (a) better define E/A ASAS$^-$ patients and/or (b) predict a good response to DMARDs and eventually to more advanced therapies [8].

The etiology of SpA is unknown, although it is believed to be multifactorial, with a major genetic predisposition, mostly consisting of the presence of human leukocyte antigen (HLA) alleles such as HLA-B27 [9]. The HLA-B27 prevalence varies markedly according to the SpA subtype and ethnicity [10,11], ranging from about 15% to 20% in PsA patients to over 95% in AS patients [12]. The same applies to uSpA, although in this case the prevalence of HLA-B27 ranges from 25% to 70% [13]. Besides HLA-B27, other major histocompatibility complex (MHC) alleles have been implicated in SpA susceptibility, including HLA-B8 [14], HLA-B15 [15–17], HLA-B16 with its splits, namely HLA-B38 and -B39 [14,18], HLA-DR1 [15,17] and DR4 [17].

The aim of this study was to investigate the HLA profile in a Caucasian cohort of patients affected by E/A, paying particular attention to the ASAS$^-$ as compared to the ASAS$^+$ subgroups, namely PsA and uSpA.

2. Patients and Methods

From 2013 to 2018, 113 consecutive patients with symptomatic peripheral E/A confirmed through ultrasound were recruited at the Rheumatology Research program Unit of the University of Bari. Patients with rheumatoid arthritis (fulfilling the 2010 ACR/EULAR classification criteria), as well as patients with AS, enteropathic, or reactive arthritis, were excluded. Patients with PsA were defined according to CASPAR criteria [19], while uSpA were defined according to the ASAS criteria for peripheral SpA in the absence of a more definite diagnosis (E/A ASAS$^+$). Patients with E/A, responding to DMARDs, but not fulfilling ASAS criteria, were defined as E/A ASAS$^-$. For each patient, data related to gender, age, and age at the onset of first symptoms, and medical history, including the presence of cardiovascular risk, metabolic syndrome, other autoimmune diseases (systemic or organ specific), fibromyalgia and malignancies, were recorded. Response to DMARDs was assessed according to DAPSA criteria, considering a minimum improvement of 50% from baseline [20,21]. Controls included a total of 318 HLA-I and -II serotyped healthy donors (HD) (female to male ratio 1:1). The study was approved by the Ethics Committees of the University of Bari. All participants gave written informed consent to enrollment as part of a project to study HLA disease markers.

3. Statistical Analysis

Statistical analyses were performed using Statistical Package for Social Sciences (SPSS) software (v21 for Windows). The Mann–Whitney *U* test was used to compare the differences between groups for continuous variables. Comparisons between groups for nominal variables were performed using Fisher's exact test. Variables with statistically significant associations were analyzed by multivariate logistic regression, adjusting for gender as confounding variable. Multivariable logistic regression was performed to define the independent association between variables and SpA. For all tests, a p-value < 0.05 was taken to indicate statistical significance.

4. Results

In this retrospective study, 113 patients with E/A were enrolled, of which 73 ASAS$^+$ (54 patients with PsA, 19 patients with uSpA), and 40 ASAS$^-$, responsive to conventional DMARDS. The clinical characteristics of the study population are described in Table 1. The female to male ratio in the whole E/A cohort (wE/A) was 4:1, mean age ± SD was 53.8 ± 11.4, and mean age at the onset of the first symptoms was 44.5 ± 12.7. The mean body mass index (BMI) was 26.7 ± 4.4. No individuals in the uSpA or E/A ASAS$^-$ groups had cutaneous psoriasis (Table 1). In addition, the HD group female to male ratio was 1:1 with a mean age ± SD of 34.82 ± 12.21.

Table 1. Clinical characteristics of the 113 patients with peripheral seronegative enthesitis/arthritis (E/A), in the whole cohort, and the ASAS$^+$ and ASAS$^-$ subgroups.

Variable	Whole Cohort $n = 113$	ASAS$^+$		ASAS$^-$ $n = 40$
		PsA $n = 54$	uSpA $n = 19$	
Female (n; %)	92; 81.4	42; 79.2	19; 84.2	34; 85.0
Age (mean ± SD; median)	53.8 ± 11.4; 54	53.2 ± 9.5; 54.5	50.8 ± 15.2; 55	56.2 ± 11.8; 54
Age at the onset of first symptoms (mean ± SD; median)	44.5 ± 12.7; 44.6	43.4 ± 12.0; 42.15	40.8 ± 14.1; 43.2	47.6 ± 12.6; 46.9
Weight (mean ± SD; median)	72.4 ± 14.4; 70	72.9 ± 15.1; 70	70.7 ± 15.0; 75	71.7 ± 12.5; 70
High (mean ± SD; median)	164.1 ± 8.4; 164	165.1 ± 7.6; 165	163.7 ± 7.5; 165	162.8 ± 9.5; 165
BMI (mean ± SD; median)	26.7 ± 4.4; 26	26.7 ± 4.8; 26	26.2 ± 4.7; 26	26.9 ± 3.7; 27
BMI > 29.9 (n; %)	29; 25.6	12.0; 22. 6	5; 26.3	11.0; 27.5
Familiarity for psoriasis (n; %)	45; 39.8	39; 73.6	3; 18.79	3.0; 7.5
Cutaneous psoriasis (n; %)	26; 23.0	26; 49.1	0	0
Peripheral arthritis only (n, %)	103; 91.2	47; 88.7	16; 84.2	39; 97.5
Peripheral and axial arthritis (n; %)	10; 8.8	6; 11.3	3; 15.78	1; 2.5
Smoking (n; %)	26; 23.0	8; 15.1	7; 26.8	10; 25
Hypertension (n; %)	46; 40.7	26; 49.1	4; 21	15; 37.5
Cardiovascular risk (n; %) [a]	37; 32.7	20; 37.7	5; 26.3	11; 27.5
Metabolic syndrome [b] (n; %)	5; 4.4	2; 3.8	2; 10.5	1; 2.5
Autoimmune thyroiditis (n; %)	16; 14.1	10; 18.9	2; 10.5	4;10
Fibromyalgia (n; %)	24; 21.2	12; 22.6	4; 21.0	8; 20
Malignancy (n; %)	10; 8.8	6; 11.3	1; 11.1	3; 7.5

BMI, body mass index; ASAS$^-$, E/A patients responding to DMARDs, but not fulfilling ASAS criteria; PsA, psoriatic arthritis; uSpA, patients fulfilling ASAS classification criteria but not satisfying any of the classification criteria related to SpA subgroups. [a] Categorized as positive in the presence of any of the followings: diabetes, obesity, hypercholesterolemia, and metabolic syndrome. [b] Defined by the National Cholesterol Education Program (NCEP) Adult Treatment Panel III (ATP III) criteria.

As expected, the item "family history of psoriasis" was statistically higher in the PsA than in the uSpA ($p < 0.001$) or ASAS$^-$ ($p < 0.001$) subgroups (Table 2). Variables such as "peripheral and axial arthritis," "smoking," "hypertension," "cardiovascular risk," "metabolic syndrome," "autoimmune thyroiditis," "fibromyalgia," and "malignancy" were similarly distributed between subgroups (Table 2). Interestingly, significant differences in age at the onset of symptoms were found between PsA and ASAS$^-$ ($p = 0.03$), being higher in ASAS$^-$. As expected, the HLA-B27 distribution percentage in the wE/A group ($p = 0.001$) and its subgroups, PsA ($p = 0.001$) and uSpA ($p < 0.001$), was significantly higher than in the HD group (Table 3).

Fisher's exact test was performed to define the association between HLA allotypes and wE/A or its subgroups (Table 4). wE/A was directly associated with HLA-A28(68) ($p = 0.001$), B27 ($p = 0.001$), Cw3 ($p = 0.022$), Cw8 ($p = 0.023$), Cw12 ($p = 0.004$), DQ1 ($p = 0.005$), and DQ3 ($p = 0.038$), and inversely with Cw7 ($p = 0.004$) and DR3 ($p = 0.008$).

Table 2. Fisher's exact test to define clinical characteristics showing a statistically higher (odds ratio; OR > 1) or lower (OR < 1) prevalence in peripheral seronegative enthesitis/arthritis (E/A) ASAS$^+$ (PsA and uSpA) vs. ASAS$^-$ clinical subgroups.

Variable	PsA vs. uSpA	PsA vs. ASAS$^-$	uSpA vs. ASAS$^-$
		p; OR [a]	
Female	0.745; 0.6	0.607; 0.7	1; 1.06
Age	0.355	0.329	0.221
Age at the onset of first symptoms	0.580	**0.03**	0.09
Weight	0.554	0.880	0.662
Height	0.465	0.058	0.425
BMI	0.811	0.671	0.685
BMI > 29.9	1; 0.88	0.817; 0.89	1; 1.06
Familiarity for psoriasis	<0.001; 13.86	<0.001; 33.8	0.072; 0.83
Cutaneous psoriasis	<0.001; NA	<0.001; NA	NA
Peripheral and axial arthritis	0.69; 0.66	0.132; 5.12	0.094; 0.13
Smoking	0.098; 0.31	0.216; 0.52	0.366; 0.56
Hypertension	0.033; 3.75	0.214; 1.80	0.247; 2.25
Cardiovascular risk	0.41; 1.78	0.275; 1.79	1; 1.06
Metabolic syndrome	0.276; 0.32	1; 1.57	0.240; 0.21
Autoimmune thyroiditis	0.72; 1.93	0.256; 2.15	1; 0.94
Fibromyalgia	1; 1.07	0.80; 1.21	1; 0.93
Malignancy	0.67; 2.25	0.727; 1.62	1; 1.45

ASAS$^-$, patients responding to DMARDs, but not fulfilling ASAS criteria; BMI, Body Mass Index; NA, not applicable; OR, odds ratio; PsA, psoriatic arthritis; uSpA, patients fulfilling ASAS classification criteria but not satisfying any of the classification criteria related to SpA subgroups; [a] significance was assessed by Mann–Whitney *U* test for continuous variables (p), and Fisher's exact test for nominal variables (p; OR). A $p < 0.05$ was considered statistically significant.

Table 3. HLA-B27 percentage in patients with peripheral seronegative enthesitis/arthritis (E/A) in the whole cohort (wE/A), in ASAS$^+$ psoriatic arthritis (PsA) and uSpA, and in ASAS$^-$ patients.

Group (*n* of Patients)	B27$^+$ (*n*; %)	*p* [a]
wE/A (113)	12; 10.61	0.001
PsA (54)	7; 13	0.001
uSpA (19)	5; 26.3	<0.001
ASAS$^-$ (40)	0; 0	1
Healthy donors (318)	7; 2.2	NA

ASAS$^-$, patients responding to DMARDs, but not fulfilling ASAS criteria; NA, not applicable; uSpA, patients fulfilling ASAS classification criteria but not satisfying any of the classification criteria related to SpA subgroups. [a] Fisher's exact test for each group vs. healthy donors; $p < 0.05$ was considered statistically significant.

PsA was directly associated with HLA-B17(57.58) ($p = 0.035$), B27 ($p = 0.001$), DQ1 ($p = 0.036$), and DQ3 ($p = 0.030$), whereas Cw7 ($p = 0.016$) and DQ7 ($p = 0.015$) were found to be protective alleles (Table 4). In addition, HLA-Cw6 was found to be positively associated with cutaneous psoriasis (OR = 2.50, $p = 0.036$) in the PsA subgroup (data not shown).

Alleles directly associated with uSpA were HLA-B16(38,39) ($p = 0.02$) and B27 ($p < 0.001$), whereas the protective alleles were Cw7 ($p = 0.034$) and DQ5 ($p = 0.04$), the latter not being recorded in any uSpA. In the ASAS$^-$ subgroup, a direct association was found with HLA-A28(68) ($p = 0.002$), B15(62) ($p = 0.049$), Cw8 ($p = 0.006$), and Cw12 ($p = 0.001$) (Table 4).

With the only exception of HLA-DQ5 (not recorded in any uSpA), all statistically significant alleles in Fisher's exact test were then subjected to multivariate (logistic regression) and multivariable analyses (Table 5).

Table 4. Fisher's exact test to define HLA allotypes showing a statistically higher (odds ratio; OR > 1) or lower (OR < 1) prevalence in peripheral seronegative enthesitis/arthritis (E/A) patients than in healthy donors (HD).

E/A Patients Grouping	Allotype	p [a]	OR (95% CI)
Whole	A28(68)	0.001	11.12 (2.32–53.22)
	B27	0.001	5.27 (2.02–13.77)
	Cw3	0.022	2.29 (1.17–4.47)
	Cw7	0.004	0.50 (0.31–0.79)
	Cw8	0.023	4.44 (1.23–16.04)
	Cw12 [b]	0.004	N/A
	DR3	0.008	0.16(0.03–0.71)
	DQ1	0.005	2.39 (1.32–4.31)
	DQ3	0.038	2.67 (1.09–6.26)
PsA	B17(57,58)	0.035	2.19 (1.05–4.33)
	B27	0.001	6.76 (2.22–19.71)
	Cw7	0.016	0.45 (0.25–0.90)
	DQ1	0.036	2.23 (1.08–4.61)
	DQ3	0.030	3.14 (1.15–8.54)
	DQ7	0.015	0.40 (0.20–0.82)
uSpA	B16(38,39)	0.02	3.61 (1.29–10.10)
	B27	<0.001	15.86 (4.47–56.29)
	Cw7	0.034	0.30 (0.09–0.94)
	DQ5 [c]	0.04	NA
ASAS$^-$	A28(68)	0.002	16.22 (2.86–91.71)
	B15(62)	0.049	5.07(1.16–22.10)
	Cw8	0.006	8.97 (2.14–37.46)
	Cw12	0.001	NA

ASAS$^-$, patients responding to DMARDs, but not fulfilling ASAS criteria, CI, confidence interval; NA, not applicable; NI, not included; OR, odds ratio; PsA, psoriatic arthritis; uSpA, patients fulfilling ASAS classification criteria but not satisfying any of the classification criteria related to SpA subgroups; [a] Fisher's exact test; a $p < 0.05$ was considered statistically significant. [b] Not recorded in any HD. [c] Not recorded in any uSpA.

In the former analysis, in which each single allele was analyzed using "gender" as confounding variable (Table 5), besides HLA-B27 (p = 0.003), the wE/A group showed a significant direct association with HLA-A28(68) (p = 0.005), Cw3 (p = 0.022), Cw8 (p = 0.018), and DQ1 (p = 0.003), while Cw7 (p = 0.014) and DR3 (p = 0.044) were confirmed to be protective.

In the PsA subgroup, alleles other than HLA-B27 (p = 0.002) showing a significant direct association were HLA-B17(57,58) (p = 0.017), DQ1 (p = 0.024), and DQ3 (p = 0.036), while Cw7 (p = 0.037) and DQ7 (p = 0.011) were protective, as found with the previous Fisher's exact test.

The uSpA subgroup showed a significant association with HLA-B16(38,39) (p = 0.025) and B27 (p < 0.001) and the ASAS$^-$ subgroup with HLA-A28(68) (p = 0.005) and Cw8 (p = 0.004).

At multivariable logistic regression analyses, the wE/A group showed significant independent associations with HLA-A28(68) (p = 0.047), B27 (p = 0.026), Cw3 (p = 0.004) and DQ1 (p = 0.008) (Table 5). When the same type of analysis was applied to E/A subgroups, the results showed that PsA was associated with HLA-B27 (p = 0.035) and DQ1 (p = 0.042), uSpA with HLA-B16(38,39) (p = 0.003) and B27 (p < 0.001), and E/A ASAS$^-$ with HLA-28(68) (p = 0.006), and Cw8 (p = 0.006).

Table 5. Logistic regression analyses to assess the interdependency of variables found to be statistically associated with peripheral seronegative enthesitis/arthritis (E/A) in the whole cohort or clinical subgroups (odds ratio; OR > 1), as compared to healthy donors (HD).

Disease and Subgroup	Allotype	Multivariate [a]		Multivariable [b]	
		OR (95% CI)	p	OR (95% CI)	p
Whole E/A	A28(68)	10.26 (2.02–51.94)	0.005	10.17 (1.03–100.02)	0.047
	B27	4.58 (1.69–12.44)	0.003	12.20 (1.34–111.00)	0.026
	Cw3	2.26 (1.25–4.56)	0.022	11.21 (2.18–57.6)	0.004
	Cw7	0.55 (0.34–0.88)	0.014	0.95 (0.44–1.84)	0.784
	Cw8	5.18 (1.32–20.32)	0.018	4.48 (0.33–59.81)	0.256
	Cw12 [c]	NA	0.999	NA	0.999
	DR3	0.20 (0.04–0.95)	0.044	0	0.999
	DQ1	2.66 (0.94–5.92)	0.003	2.68 (1.29–5.55)	0.008
	DQ3	2.33 (0.94–5.92)	0.066	3.27 (1.01–10.61)	0.048
PsA	B17(57,58)	2.43 (1.17–5.07)	0.017	2.59 (0.87–7.67)	0.085
	B27	6.09 (1.96–18.92)	0.002	14.99 (1.29–186.25)	0.035
	Cw7	0.51 (0.27–0.96)	0.037	0.83 (0.36–1.91)	0.669
	DQ1	2.41 (1.12–5.17)	0.024	2.37 (1.03–5.46)	0.042
	DQ3	3.05 (1.07–8.68)	0.036	2.12 (0.60–7.52)	0.244
	DQ7	0.38 (0.18–0.80)	0.011	0.50 (0.21–1.16)	0.110
uSpA	B16(38,39)	3.81 (1.16–9.44)	0.025	5.63 (1.78–17.81)	0.003
	B27	13.56 (3.65–50.31)	<0.001	20.96 (5.08–86.36)	<0.001
	Cw7	0.34(0.10–1.05)	0.062	0.31 (0.09–1.04)	0.059
ASAS⁻	A28(68)	13.48 (2.19–82.68)	0.005	14.72 (2.18–99.28)	0.006
	B15(62)	4.27 (0.92–19.77)	0.063	7.54 (1.46–38.78)	0.016
	Cw8	9.96 (2.12–46.80)	0.004	9.97 (1.90–52.24)	0.006
	Cw12	NA	0.999	NA	0.999

ASAS$^-$, E/A patients responding to DMARDs, but not fulfilling ASAS criteria; CI, confidence interval; NA, not applicable; NI, not included; OR, odds ratio; PsA, psoriatic arthritis; uSpA, patients fulfilling ASAS classification criteria but not satisfying any of the classification criteria related to SpA subgroups; [a] Alleles found statistically associated with E/A in Fisher's exact test were analyzed by multivariate logistic regression, in which each single variable, tested for E/A vs. HD, was adjusted for gender. [b] Variables found statistically associated with E/A in Fisher's exact test were analyzed by multivariable logistic regression. [c] Not recorded in any HD.

5. Discussion

To the best of our knowledge, this is the first study to investigate the association between HLA class I and class II alleles and E/A ASAS$^-$(vs. ASAS$^+$ PsA and uSpA) in a cohort of Caucasian patients (n = 113) as compared to an HLA-typed HD cohort (n = 318).

While previous studies investigated the association between PsA [22] and HLA-B27 only, our analysis was focused on alleles other than HLA-B27 in E/A patients and its subgroups, PsA, uSpA, and ASAS$^-$.

In addition to HLA-B27, in the wE/A cohort, our data revealed a significant association with HLA-A28(68), Cw3, Cw12, and DQ1. All these associations, except the one with HLA-Cw12, were independent of HLA-B27, as demonstrated by multivariable regression analysis. Regarding HLA-Cw12, it was not possible to establish the interdependence with HLA-B27, because this allele was not present in any HD.

Interestingly, we found that both HLA-A28(68) and Cw12 were also associated with ASAS$^-$ but not with PsA or uSpA, suggesting that these alleles can confer susceptibility to ASAS$^-$. While HLA-A28, with its splits 68 and 69, has been demonstrated to be significantly associated with B27 risk-related diseases, including AS [23], reactive arthritis [23], juvenile chronic polyarthropathy [23], and intermediate uveitis [24], only a minimal predisposition to cutaneous psoriasis has been reported for HLA-Cw12 [25,26].

ASAS$^-$, which was the only E/A subgroup not associated with HLA-B27, presented an additional association with HLA-Cw8, never previously found to be associated with E/A or its subgroups.

Regarding HLA-Cw3 and HLA-DQ1, both of which favor wE/A, the former was reported to have a statistically high prevalence in other immune-mediated diseases such as rheumatoid arthritis-associated vasculitis [27,28], while HLA-DQ1 was shown to be a predisposing factor for autoimmune uveitis, the most common extra-articular manifestation of SpA, in a cohort of Caucasian Italian patients [29]. Furthermore, HLA-DQ1 and HLA-DQ2 have been associated with the presence of anti-Ro/SSA antibodies in both Sjögren's syndrome [30] and systemic lupus erythematosus patients [31].

In our study population, HLA-DQ1, along with HLA-B27, was also associated with PsA.

The prevalence of PsA patients positive for HLA-B27 in our investigation was 13%, comparable to the 12% reported by Paladini et al. [22] in an Italian Caucasian cohort.

Several studies have shown that HLA-Cw6 is strongly associated with cutaneous psoriasis, but not with PsA [32,33]. The lack of an established diagnosis of cutaneous psoriasis in 51% of our PsA group can explain the absence of this subgroup association with HLA-Cw6.

Another finding of this study is the association of HLA-B16 (38,39) with uSpA, although earlier reports suggested an HLA-B39 association with PsA [34,35], HLA-B27-negative AS [36,37], and pauci-articular juvenile chronic arthritis [37,38].

A major study limitation is the lack of longitudinal observations that could establish whether ASAS$^-$ forms could eventually evolve into any other E/A subgroup, although the peculiar association of ASAS$^-$ with HLA-Cw8 makes this possibility unlikely.

The role of gender in influencing some HLA associations deserves some comment in that certain HLA allotypes, found to be significantly associated with wE/A (HLA-DQ3), uSpA (HLA-Cw7) or ASAS$^-$ (HLA-B15(62)) by Fisher's exact test, lost their significant association when "gender" was included as covariate in the multivariate analyses. These findings suggest that gender had an impact on the expression of certain HLA alleles in the E/A groups in our study, in agreement with previous studies showing gender-related HLA differences in different autoimmune diseases [39–42].

Finally, our work paves the way for further investigation aimed at genotyping the HLA alleles found in this study to be associated with uSpA or ASAS$^-$.

6. Conclusions

Our study revealed that HLA-B27 and HLA-B16(38,39) are significantly more frequent in uSpA patients, while HLA-A28(68), HLA-Cw8, and HLA-Cw12 were found to be associated with ASAS$^-$ in the general population in Italy. These alleles can thus be associated with a diagnosis of ASAS$^-$, and HLA typing may contribute to correct clinical management, as well as to identifying family members at risk, in particular those patients with enthesitis and/or arthritis who do not meet the criteria for a uSpA diagnosis. These findings warrant confirmation in further large, multicenter cohort studies.

Author Contributions: Conceptualization, E.F., L.U. and F.P.; methodology, E.F., L.U., A.S., F.M., G.C. and F.P.; validation, E.F., L.U., M.P. and F.P.; formal analysis, E.F., A.S., F.M., G.C., M.P. and F.P.; investigation, E.F., L.U., A.S., F.M., G.C., M.P. and F.P.; data curation, E.F., L.U., M.P. and F.P.; writing—original draft preparation, E.F., F.P.; writing—review and editing, E.F., L.U., A.S., F.M., G.C., M.P. and F.P. All authors have read and agreed to the published version of the manuscript.

Funding: This work was supported by a grant from the University of Bari Medical School 2020. The funder had no role in study design, data collection and analysis, decision to publish, or preparation of the manuscript.

Institutional Review Board Statement: All procedures performed in studies involving human participants were conducted in accordance with the ethical standards of the institutional and/or national research committee (Ethical Committee of the University of Bari Medical School, no. A31580/DS) and with the 1964 Helsinki declaration and its later amendments or comparable ethical standards.

Informed Consent Statement: Informed consent was obtained from all subjects involved in the study.

Data Availability Statement: The data presented in this study are available on request from the corresponding author. The data are not publicly available due to privacy restrictions.

Acknowledgments: The authors thank Maria Daniele and Giuseppina Dammacco for their excellent secretarial assistance.

Conflicts of Interest: The authors declare no conflict of interest.

References

1. Rudwaleit, M.; van der Heijde, D.; Landewe, R.; Akkoc, N.; Brandt, J.; Chou, C.T.; Dougados, M.; Huang, F.; Gu, J.; Kirazli, Y.; et al. The Assessment of SpondyloArthritis International Society classification criteria for peripheral spondyloarthritis and for spondyloarthritis in general. *Ann. Rheum. Dis.* **2011**, *70*, 25–31. [CrossRef] [PubMed]
2. Rudwaleit, M.; Landewe, R.; van der Heijde, D.; Listing, J.; Brandt, J.; Braun, J.; Burgos-Vargas, R.; Collantes-Estevez, E.; Davis, J.; Dijkmans, B.; et al. The development of Assessment of SpondyloArthritis international Society classification criteria for axial spondyloarthritis (part I): Classification of paper patients by expert opinion including uncertainty appraisal. *Ann. Rheum. Dis.* **2009**, *68*, 770–776. [CrossRef] [PubMed]
3. Rudwaleit, M.; van der Heijde, D.; Landewe, R.; Listing, J.; Akkoc, N.; Brandt, J.; Braun, J.; Chou, C.T.; Collantes-Estevez, E.; Dougados, M.; et al. The development of Assessment of SpondyloArthritis international Society classification criteria for axial spondyloarthritis (part II): Validation and final selection. *Ann. Rheum. Dis.* **2009**, *68*, 777–783. [CrossRef]
4. Bakker, P.; Molto, A.; Etcheto, A.; Van den, B.F.; Landewe, R.; van, G.F.; Dougados, M.; van der, H.D. The performance of different classification criteria sets for spondyloarthritis in the worldwide ASAS-COMOSPA study. *Arthritis Res. Ther.* **2017**, *19*, 96. [CrossRef]
5. Kiltz, U.; van der, H.D.; Boonen, A.; Akkoc, N.; Bautista-Molano, W.; Burgos-Vargas, R.; Wei, J.C.; Chiowchanwisawakit, P.; Dougados, M.; Duruoz, M.T.; et al. Measurement properties of the ASAS Health Index: Results of a global study in patients with axial and peripheral spondyloarthritis. *Ann. Rheum. Dis.* **2018**, *77*, 1311–1317. [CrossRef] [PubMed]
6. Schett, G.; Lories, R.J.; D'Agostino, M.A.; Elewaut, D.; Kirkham, B.; Soriano, E.R.; McGonagle, D. Enthesitis: From pathophysiology to treatment. *Nat. Rev. Rheumatol.* **2017**, *13*, 731–741. [CrossRef]
7. Balint, P.V.; Terslev, L.; Aegerter, P.; Bruyn, G.A.W.; Chary-Valckenaere, I.; Gandjbakhch, F.; Iagnocco, A.; Jousse-Joulin, S.; Moller, I.; Naredo, E.; et al. Reliability of a consensus-based ultrasound definition and scoring for enthesitis in spondyloarthritis and psoriatic arthritis: An OMERACT US initiative. *Ann. Rheum. Dis.* **2018**, *77*, 1730–1735. [CrossRef]
8. Favoino, E.; Prete, M.; Catacchio, G.; Ruscitti, P.; Navarini, L.; Giacomelli, R.; Perosa, F. Working and safety profiles of JAK/STAT signaling inhibitors. Are these small molecules also smart? *Autoimmun. Rev.* **2021**, *20*, 102750. [CrossRef]
9. Busch, R.; Kollnberger, S.; Mellins, E.D. HLA associations in inflammatory arthritis: Emerging mechanisms and clinical implications. *Nat. Rev. Rheumatol.* **2019**, *15*, 364–381. [CrossRef]
10. Khan, M.A. HLA-B27 and its subtypes in world populations. *Curr. Opin. Rheumatol.* **1995**, *7*, 263–269. [CrossRef]
11. Lopez de Castro, J.A. HLA-B27 and the pathogenesis of spondyloarthropathies. *Immunol. Lett.* **2007**, *108*, 27–33. [CrossRef] [PubMed]
12. Gonzalez, S.; Garcia-Fernandez, S.; Martinez-Borra, J.; Blanco-Gelaz, M.A.; Rodrigo, L.; Sanchez del, R.J.; Lopez-Vazquez, A.; Torre-Alonso, J.C.; Lopez-Larrea, C. High variability of HLA-B27 alleles in ankylosing spondylitis and related spondyloarthropathies in the population of northern Spain. *Hum. Immunol.* **2002**, *63*, 673–676. [CrossRef]
13. Kavadichanda, C.G.; Geng, J.; Bulusu, S.N.; Negi, V.S.; Raghavan, M. Spondyloarthritis and the Human Leukocyte Antigen (HLA)-B(*)27 Connection. *Front Immunol.* **2021**, *12*, 601518. [CrossRef] [PubMed]
14. Winchester, R.; Minevich, G.; Steshenko, V.; Kirby, B.; Kane, D.; Greenberg, D.A.; FitzGerald, O. HLA associations reveal genetic heterogeneity in psoriatic arthritis and in the psoriasis phenotype. *Arthritis Rheum.* **2012**, *64*, 1134–1144. [CrossRef]
15. Vargas-Alarcon, G.; Londono, J.D.; Hernandez-Pacheco, G.; Pacheco-Tena, C.; Castillo, E.; Cardiel, M.H.; Granados, J.; Burgos-Vargas, R. Effect of HLA-B and HLA-DR genes on susceptibility to and severity of spondyloarthropathies in Mexican patients. *Ann. Rheum. Dis.* **2002**, *61*, 714–717. [CrossRef]
16. Londono, J.; Santos, A.M.; Pena, P.; Calvo, E.; Espinosa, L.R.; Reveille, J.D.; Vargas-Alarcon, G.; Jaramillo, C.A.; Valle-Onate, R.; Avila, M.; et al. Analysis of HLA-B15 and HLA-B27 in spondyloarthritis with peripheral and axial clinical patterns. *BMJ Open.* **2015**, *5*, e009092. [CrossRef] [PubMed]
17. Santos, A.M.; Pena, P.; Avila, M.; Briceno, I.; Jaramillo, C.; Vargas-Alarcon, G.; Rueda, J.C.; Saldarriaga, E.L.; Angarita, J.I.; Martinez-Rodriguez, N.; et al. Association of human leukocyte A, B, and DR antigens in Colombian patients with diagnosis of spondyloarthritis. *Clin. Rheumatol.* **2017**, *36*, 953–958. [CrossRef]
18. Eder, L.; Chandran, V.; Pellet, F.; Shanmugarajah, S.; Rosen, C.F.; Bull, S.B.; Gladman, D.D. Human leucocyte antigen risk alleles for psoriatic arthritis among patients with psoriasis. *Ann. Rheum. Dis.* **2012**, *71*, 50–55. [CrossRef]
19. Taylor, W.; Gladman, D.; Helliwell, P.; Marchesoni, A.; Mease, P.; Mielants, H. Classification criteria for psoriatic arthritis: Development of new criteria from a large international study. *Arthritis Rheum.* **2006**, *54*, 2665–2673. [CrossRef]
20. Schoels, M.M.; Aletaha, D.; Alasti, F.; Smolen, J.S. Disease activity in psoriatic arthritis (PsA): Defining remission and treatment success using the DAPSA score. *Ann. Rheum. Dis.* **2016**, *75*, 811–818. [CrossRef]
21. Smolen, J.S.; Schols, M.; Braun, J.; Dougados, M.; FitzGerald, O.; Gladman, D.D.; Kavanaugh, A.; Landewe, R.; Mease, P.; Sieper, J.; et al. Treating axial spondyloarthritis and peripheral spondyloarthritis, especially psoriatic arthritis, to target: 2017 update of recommendations by an international task force. *Ann. Rheum. Dis.* **2018**, *77*, 3–17. [CrossRef] [PubMed]

22. Paladini, F.; Taccari, E.; Fiorillo, M.T.; Cauli, A.; Passiu, G.; Mathieu, A.; Punzi, L.; Lapadula, G.; Scarpa, R.; Sorrentino, R. Distribution of HLA-B27 subtypes in Sardinia and continental Italy and their association with spondylarthropathies. *Arthritis Rheum.* **2005**, *52*, 3319–3321. [CrossRef] [PubMed]
23. Arnett, F.C.; Hochberg, M.C.; Bias, W.B. HLA-C locus antigens in HLA-B27 associated arthritis. *Arthritis Rheum.* **1978**, *21*, 885–888. [CrossRef]
24. Martin, T.; Weber, M.; Schmitt, C.; Weber, J.C.; Tongio, M.M.; Flament, J.; Sahel, J.; Pasquali, J.L. Association of intermediate uveitis with HLA-A28: Definition of a new systemic syndrome? *Graefes Arch. Clin. Exp. Ophthalmol.* **1995**, *233*, 269–274. [CrossRef]
25. Liao, H.T.; Lin, K.C.; Chang, Y.T.; Chen, C.H.; Liang, T.H.; Chen, W.S.; Su, K.Y.; Tsai, C.Y.; Chou, C.T. Human leukocyte antigen and clinical and demographic characteristics in psoriatic arthritis and psoriasis in Chinese patients. *J. Rheumatol.* **2008**, *35*, 891–895. [PubMed]
26. Onsun, N.; Pirmit, S.; Ozkaya, D.; Celik, S.; Rezvani, A.; Cengiz, F.P.; Kekik, C. The HLA-Cw12 Allele Is an Important Susceptibility Allele for Psoriasis and Is Associated with Resistant Psoriasis in the Turkish Population. *Sci. World J.* **2019**, *2019*, 7848314. [CrossRef]
27. Yen, J.H.; Moore, B.E.; Nakajima, T.; Scholl, D.; Schaid, D.J.; Weyand, C.M.; Goronzy, J.J. Major histocompatibility complex class I-recognizing receptors are disease risk genes in rheumatoid arthritis. *J. Exp. Med.* **2001**, *193*, 1159–1167. [CrossRef] [PubMed]
28. Turesson, C.; Schaid, D.J.; Weyand, C.M.; Jacobsson, L.T.; Goronzy, J.J.; Petersson, I.F.; Dechant, S.A.; Nyahll-Wahlin, B.M.; Truedsson, L.; Sturfelt, G.; et al. Association of HLA-C3 and smoking with vasculitis in patients with rheumatoid arthritis. *Arthritis Rheum.* **2006**, *54*, 2776–2783. [CrossRef] [PubMed]
29. Prete, M.; Guerriero, S.; Dammacco, R.; Fatone, M.C.; Vacca, A.; Dammacco, F.; Racanelli, V. Autoimmune uveitis: A retrospective analysis of 104 patients from a tertiary reference center. *J. Ophthalmic Inflamm. Infect.* **2014**, *4*, 17. [CrossRef]
30. Harley, J.B.; Reichlin, M.; Arnett, F.C.; Alexander, E.L.; Bias, W.B.; Provost, T.T. Gene interaction at HLA-DQ enhances autoantibody production in primary Sjogren's syndrome. *Science* **1986**, *232*, 1145–1147. [CrossRef]
31. Fujisaku, A.; Frank, M.B.; Neas, B.; Reichlin, M.; Harley, J.B. HLA-DQ gene complementation and other histocompatibility relationships in man with the anti-Ro/SSA autoantibody response of systemic lupus erythematosus. *J. Clin. Investig.* **1990**, *86*, 606–611. [CrossRef] [PubMed]
32. Gudjonsson, J.E.; Karason, A.; Antonsdottir, A.A.; Runarsdottir, E.H.; Gulcher, J.R.; Stefansson, K.; Valdimarsson, H. HLA-Cw6-positive and HLA-Cw6-negative patients with Psoriasis vulgaris have distinct clinical features. *J. Invest Dermatol.* **2002**, *118*, 362–365. [CrossRef] [PubMed]
33. Chen, L.; Tsai, T.F. HLA-Cw6 and psoriasis. *Br. J. Dermatol.* **2018**, *178*, 854–862. [CrossRef] [PubMed]
34. Salvarani, C.; Macchioni, P.; Cremonesi, T.; Mantovani, W.; Battistel, B.; Rossi, F.; Capozzoli, N.; Baricchi, R.; Portioli, I. The cervical spine in patients with psoriatic arthritis: A clinical, radiological and immunogenetic study. *Ann. Rheum. Dis.* **1992**, *51*, 73–77. [CrossRef] [PubMed]
35. Trabace, S.; Cappellacci, S.; Ciccarone, P.; Liaskos, S.; Polito, R.; Zorzin, L. Psoriatic arthritis: A clinical, radiological and genetic study of 58 Italian patients. *Acta Derm. Venereol. Suppl.* **1994**, *186*, 69–70.
36. Khan, M.A.; Kushner, I.; Braun, W.E. B27-negative HLA-BW16 in ankylosing spondylitis. *Lancet* **1978**, *1*, 1370–1371. [CrossRef]
37. Yamaguchi, A.; Tsuchiya, N.; Mitsui, H.; Shiota, M.; Ogawa, A.; Tokunaga, K.; Yoshinoya, S.; Juji, T.; Ito, K. Association of HLA-B39 with HLA-B27-negative ankylosing spondylitis and pauciarticular juvenile rheumatoid arthritis in Japanese patients. Evidence for a role of the peptide-anchoring B pocket. *Arthritis Rheum.* **1995**, *38*, 1672–1677. [CrossRef]
38. Hall, P.J.; Burman, S.J.; Laurent, M.R.; Briggs, D.C.; Venning, H.E.; Leak, A.M.; Bedford, P.A.; Ansell, B.M. Genetic susceptibility to early onset pauciarticular juvenile chronic arthritis: A study of HLA and complement markers in 158 British patients. *Ann. Rheum. Dis.* **1986**, *45*, 464–474. [CrossRef]
39. Queiro, R.; Sarasqueta, C.; Torre, J.C.; Tinture, T.; Lopez-Lagunas, I. Comparative analysis of psoriatic spondyloarthropathy between men and women. *Rheumatol. Int.* **2001**, *21*, 66–68.
40. Megiorni, F.; Mora, B.; Bonamico, M.; Barbato, M.; Montuori, M.; Viola, F.; Trabace, S.; Mazzilli, M.C. HLA-DQ and susceptibility to celiac disease: Evidence for gender differences and parent-of-origin effects. *Am. J. Gastroenterol.* **2008**, *103*, 997–1003. [CrossRef] [PubMed]
41. Eder, L.; Thavaneswaran, A.; Chandran, V.; Gladman, D.D. Gender difference in disease expression, radiographic damage and disability among patients with psoriatic arthritis. *Ann. Rheum. Dis.* **2013**, *72*, 578–582. [CrossRef] [PubMed]
42. Flesch, B.K.; Konig, J.; Frommer, L.; Hansen, M.P.; Kahaly, G.J. Sex Alters the MHC Class I HLA-A Association With Polyglandular Autoimmunity. *J. Clin. Endocrinol. Metab.* **2019**, *104*, 1680–1686. [CrossRef] [PubMed]

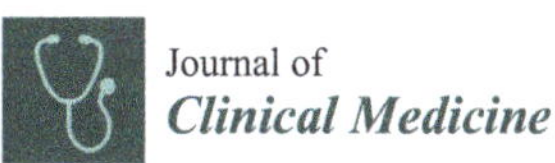

Journal of
Clinical Medicine

MDPI

Article

Impact of Different JAK Inhibitors and Methotrexate on Lymphocyte Proliferation and DNA Damage

Annika Reddig [1,*], Linda Voss [1], Karina Guttek [1], Dirk Roggenbuck [2,3], Eugen Feist [4] and Dirk Reinhold [1]

1 Institute of Molecular and Clinical Immunology, Otto-Von-Guericke-University Magdeburg, 39120 Magdeburg, Germany; linda.voss@med.ovgu.de (L.V.); karina.guttek@med.ovgu.de (K.G.); dirk.reinhold@med.ovgu.de (D.R.)
2 Institute of Biotechnology, Faculty Environment and Natural Sciences, Brandenburg University of Technology Cottbus-Senftenberg, 01968 Senftenberg, Germany; dirk.roggenbuck@b-tu.de
3 Faculty of Health Sciences, Joint Faculty of the Brandenburg University of Technology Cottbus-Senftenberg, the Brandenburg Medical School Theodor Fontane and the University of Potsdam, 01968 Senftenberg, Germany
4 Helios-Department of Rheumatology, Cooperation Partner of the Otto-Von-Guericke-University, 39245 Vogelsang-Gommern, Germany; eugen.feist@helios-gesundheit.de
* Correspondence: annika.reddig@med.ovgu.de; Tel.: +49-391-67-17842

Abstract: Janus kinase inhibitors (JAKis) represent a new strategy in rheumatoid arthritis (RA) therapy. Still, data directly comparing different JAKis are rare. In the present in vitro study, we investigated the immunomodulatory potential of four JAKis (tofacitinib, baricitinib, upadacitinib, and filgotinib) currently approved for RA treatment by the European Medicines Agency. Increasing concentrations of JAKi or methotrexate, conventionally used in RA therapy, were either added to freshly mitogen-stimulated or preactivated peripheral blood mononuclear cells (PBMC), isolated from healthy volunteers. A comparable, dose-dependent inhibition of lymphocyte proliferation was observed in samples treated with tofacitinib, baricitinib, and upadacitinib, while dosage of filgotinib had to be two orders of magnitude higher. In contrast, antiproliferative effects were strongly attenuated when JAKi were added to preactivated PBMCs. High dosage of upadacitinib and filgotinib also affected cell viability. Further, analyses of DNA double-strand break markers γH2AX and 53BP1 indicated an enhanced level of DNA damage in cells incubated with high concentrations of filgotinib and a dose-dependent reduction in clearance of radiation-induced γH2AX foci in the presence of tofacitinib or baricitinib. Thereby, our study demonstrated a broad comparability of immunomodulatory effects induced by different JAKi and provided first indications, that (pan)JAKi may impair DNA damage repair in irradiated PBMCs.

Keywords: JAK inhibitor; proliferation; DNA damage repair; γH2AX; PBMCs; T lymphocytes

Citation: Reddig, A.; Voss, L.; Guttek, K.; Roggenbuck, D.; Feist, E.; Reinhold, D. Impact of Different JAK Inhibitors and Methotrexate on Lymphocyte Proliferation and DNA Damage. *J. Clin. Med.* **2021**, *10*, 1431. https://doi.org/10.3390/jcm10071431

Academic Editor: Mitsuhiro Takeno

Received: 2 February 2021
Accepted: 29 March 2021
Published: 1 April 2021

1. Introduction

Rheumatoid arthritis (RA) is a chronic, autoimmune disease, characterized by inflammation and progressive damage of synovial joints, when treated insufficiently [1]. With increasing knowledge about disease pathophysiology, new pharmaceutical strategies and compounds are available. After the application of conventional synthetic disease-modifying antirheumatic drugs (csDMARDs), such as methotrexate (MTX) in late 1980s, and biological DMARDs since late 1990s, small-molecule Janus kinase inhibitors (JAKis), classified as targeted synthetic DMARDs, represent a new milestone in RA treatment [1–3]. Clinical studies with JAKi demonstrated similar efficacy and safety compared to biological DMARDs [4,5]. However, long-term data for JAKi covering several years are still missing.

Janus kinases (JAKs) are cytoplasmic tyrosine kinases comprising four different types of JAK enzymes in humans: JAK1, JAK2, JAK3, and tyrosine kinase 2 (TYK2) [6]. While JAK1, JAK2, and TYK2 are expressed ubiquitously, JAK3 is predominantly detectable in hematopoietic tissue [7,8]. Upon extracellular ligand binding, JAKs associate as homo- or heterodimers with type I and type II cytokine receptors. Subsequently, JAK dimers become activated by auto- and transphosphorylation and phosphorylate the cytoplasmic tail of the cytokine receptor [6,8]. This induces the recruitment and binding of signaling molecules, such as the members of the signal transducer and activator of transcription (STAT) family (seven members: STAT1/2/3/4/5A/5B/6). After JAK-mediated STAT phosphorylation, dimerization, and activation, STAT dimers translocate to the nucleus where they act as transcription factors for multiple target genes, modulating, i. a., survival, proliferation, or differentiation of T lymphocytes [9,10]. More than 50 different cytokines and growth factors are known ligands of type I/II cytokine receptors. Depending on the cytoplasmic chains of the receptor, they are able to associate either with only one type of JAK enzyme or with different JAK isoforms. Hence, this creates a high degree of specificity regarding different JAK and STAT combinations [9–11].

Sufficient JAK-STAT signaling is essential in the regulation of immunological processes. Polymorphisms and loss- or gain-of-function mutations within this pathway are associated with immunodeficiency, autoimmune disease, and hematological malignancy [9,12]. Therefore, JAK-targeting agents represent a new class of immunomodulatory drugs [11]. After first approval of JAK inhibiting drugs for the treatment of neoplastic diseases, several JAKi are also authorized for the treatment of RA by the U.S. Food and Drug Administration (FDA) and European Medicines Agency (EMA) [13,14]. The two approved first-generation JAK inhibitors tofacitinib (JAK3 > JAK1 > JAK2) and baricitinib (JAK1 > JAK2 > JAK3) are classified as pan-JAK inhibitors, targeting multiple JAK isoforms, but with different affinities. In contrast, the two second-generation JAKi upadacitinib and filgotinib (not yet approved by the FDA) show high selectivity for JAK1 and primarily inhibit its associated cytokine-receptors [10,15]. However, selectivity of JAKi towards specific JAK isoforms is not absolute and depends on dosage and cell type [16]. An overview of reported mean half-maximal inhibitory concentrations (IC_{50}) obtained by enzymatic assays is provided in Table S1.

Although already approved for RA treatment, in vivo and in vitro head-to-head studies of all four JAKi are rare. Therefore, we evaluated the immunomodulatory and cytotoxic potential of tofacitinib, baricitinib, upadacitinib, and filgotinib on human PBMCs freshly isolated from healthy donors. For comparison with conventional synthetic DMARDs, samples treated with MTX were investigated in parallel. JAKi or MTX were either added directly to freshly PHA-stimulated PBMCs or 48 h after PBMC activation, to investigate their impact on preactivated T lymphocytes, as this might be more relevant regarding inflammatory conditions in vivo [17]. Compared to healthy controls, peripheral blood isolated from patients with active RA revealed an enhanced level of activated PBMCs, which may play a direct role in disease pathogenesis [18]. Furthermore, Kitanaga et al. stated constitutive activation of JAK/STAT signaling in PBMCs from patients with systemic sclerosis or RA [19].

JAK/STAT signaling is involved in regulation of multiple fundamental cellular processes. Additionally, there is increasing evidence suggesting that JAK/STAT signaling also modulates molecules involved in DNA damage response pathways [20–24]. To investigate the impact of JAKi on DNA double-strand break (DSB) formation and on repair of radiation-induced DNA damage we quantified nuclear foci stained by γH2AX or 53BP1 (p53-binding protein 1) antibodies. These markers have been described as sensitive molecular indicators for DNA DSBs [25–27].

The objective of the present in vitro study was to compare the immunomodulatory potential of all four JAKi currently approved for RA treatment in Europe. Therefore, we treated freshly and preactivated PBMCs with rising concentrations of either tofacitinib, baricitinib, upadacitinib, filgotinib, and MTX and determined the effect on cell proliferation, activation (CD25) and apoptosis. Furthermore, we investigated the impact of different JAKi and MTX on DNA damage induction and repair by fluorescence microscopic analysis of DNA DSB markers γH2AX and 53BP1. Our study indicates a broad comparability of the immunomodulatory effects induced by different JAKi and offers a first indication, that (pan)JAKi may impair DNA damage repair in radiated lymphocytes.

2. Experimental Section

2.1. Ethics Statement

The study was performed in accordance with the Declaration of Helsinki and was approved by the local ethics committee (No. 183/20). All 14 healthy blood donors (10 female and 4 male; mean age: 35 ± 12 years) who agreed to participate in this study provided written informed consent.

2.2. Cell Culture

Human peripheral blood mononuclear cells (PBMCs) were isolated from heparinized blood by density gradient centrifugation using Pancoll separating solution (PAN-Biotech, Aidenbach, Germany). Afterwards, PBMCs were washed twice and suspended to a final density of 1×10^6 PBMCs per mL in serum-free AIM-V culture medium (Invitrogen, Eggenstein, Germany). Activation of T lymphocytes among PBMCs was achieved by mitogen stimulation with 2 µg/mL phytohemagglutinin (PHA, life technologies/Gibco, London, UK).

JAK inhibitors tofacitinib, baricitinib, upadacitinib, and filgotinib and methotrexate (MTX) were all purchased from Selleckchem (Houston, TX, USA). These agents (stock solution: 10 mM in dimethyl sulfoxide (DMSO)) were either added simultaneously with PHA into cell culture plates or 48 h after PHA-stimulation, to investigate their impact on preactivated PBMCs. Cells treated with DMSO, diluted 1:1000, served as corresponding vehicle controls.

2.3. Proliferation Analysis by ^{3}H-Thymidine Incorporation

Cell proliferation was analyzed by ^{3}H-thymidine incorporation assay. For T cell activation, PHA was added to PBMC suspension and 1×10^5 PBMCs/well were seeded into flat bottom 96-well plates. Different concentration (1 nM–10 µM, 1:10 serial dilution) of the four investigated JAKi were added as triplicates either directly to the cell culture or 48 h after PHA-stimulation (preactivated lymphocytes). After 72 h of PHA activation, PBMCs were pulsed with [^{3}H]-thymidine at a dose of 0.2 µCi/well for additional 6 h. At the end of the incubation period cells were harvested and ^{3}H-thymidine incorporation was quantified using the microplate liquid scintillation counter Wallac MicroBeta TriLux from Perkin Elmer (Waltham, MA, USA).

2.4. Proliferation Analysis by the CFSE Dilution Assay

Additionally, cell proliferation was assessed by the cell trace carboxyfluorescein succinimidyl ester (CFSE) cell proliferation kit (Invitrogen, Carlsbad, CA, USA). Therefore, freshly isolated PBMCs were washed in phosphate buffers saline (PBS; PAN-Biotech) and resuspended in 1 mL PBS containing 5% inactivated fetal calf serum (FCS). Subsequently, 5 µM CFSE solution was added and incubated for 5 min at room temperature in the dark. Afterwards, cells were washed twice in PBS-FCS and were resuspended to a final concentration of 1×10^6 PBMC/mL in AIM-V medium. CFSE loaded unstimulated cells served as control sample, representing CFSE^{high}, non-divided cell population. For activation PHA was added to remaining CFSE-stained PBMC suspension, which was subsequently plated into 24-well cell culture plates. Increasing concentrations of JAKi or MTX were either added directly or 48 h after PHA-stimulation. After an incubation period of 96 h PBMCs were transferred into 5 mL round bottom polystyrene tubes and washed once in cold PBS containing 0.5% BSA. Subsequently, CFSE intensity of living cells (gating based on forward/side scatter signal) was determined in FITC channel by flow cytometry (LSRFortessa cell analyzer, BD Biosciences, Mountain View, CA, USA) and FlowJo software (version 7.6.4, Tree Star Inc., Ashland, OR, USA).

2.5. Analysis of CD25 Expression

Activation status was assessed by CD25 expression. Therefore, 1×10^6 PBMCs/sample were simultaneously treated for 48 h with PHA and different JAKi at various concentrations as indicated. Afterwards, cells were transferred into 5 mL round bottom polystyrene tubes, washed twice with PBS containing 0.5% bovine serum albumin (BSA; AppliChem, Darmstadt, Germany) and incubated for 30 min at 4 °C with 1:200 diluted phycoerythrin(PE)-coupled anti-human CD25 antibody (BioLegend, San Diego, CA, USA). Subsequently, samples were washed with PBS containing 2 mM ethylenediaminetetraacetic acid (EDTA) and resuspended in PBS-BSA. Samples were kept cold until flow cytometry analysis using a BD LSRFortessa cell analyzer. Data were acquired by FACSDiva 6.0 software (BD Biosciences) and analyzed by FlowJo software.

2.6. Viability Assessment

JAKi- and MTX- induced cell death was determined after 72 h in unstimulated, freshly PHA-stimulated and preactivated PBMCs using a FITC Annexin V/propidium iodide (PI) apoptosis detection kit (BioLegend, San Diego, CA, USA). In brief, 1×10^6 PBMC were transferred into 5 mL round bottom polystyrene tubes, washed once in cold PBS-BSA and resuspended in 50 μL staining solution, comprising Annexin V and PI diluted 1:20 in Annexin V binding buffer. After 15 min incubation at room temperature in the dark cellular staining was terminated by addition of 200 μL binding buffer. Ratio of viable (Annexin V^-/PI^-), early apoptotic (Annexin V^+/PI^-), late apoptotic (Annexin V^+/PI^+), and necrotic (Annexin V^-/PI^+) cells was determined of 20,000 cells/sample by BD LSRFortessa cell analyzer and subsequent analysis utilizing FlowJo software. Unstained, single- and double-stained cells treated with camptothecin were included as control samples.

2.7. Detection of γH2AX and 53BP1 Foci

Automated quantification of intranuclear γH2AX and 53BP1 foci, described as sensitive indicators for DNA double-strand breaks (DSB), was performed to study JAKi-induced DNA DSB and their impact on DNA repair of radiation-induced DSBs [25–27]. Therefore, unstimulated PBMCs were treated with indicated concentrations of JAKi or MTX. Additionally, one fraction was exposed to γ-rays at a dose of 2 Gy (Biobeam 8000, Cs 137, Gamma-Service Medical, Leipzig, Germany) to induce DNA damage. After an incubation period of 24 h non-irradiated and radiated samples were harvested, washed in PBS and fixed for 15 min with 1% formaldehyde on silanized glass slides, as described in detail elsewhere [28,29]. Subsequently, cells were permeabilized in 0.2% Triton X-100, washed in blocking buffer (PBS containing 1% BSA) and incubated for 60 min at room temperature simultaneously with 1:1000 diluted γH2AX (anti-phosphohistone H2AX mouse monoclonal IgG primary antibody, clone JBW301, Millipore, Schwalbach, Germany) and 53BP1 primary antibodies (anti-53BP1 rabbit polyclonal IgG (NB 100–305), Novus Biologicals, Centennial, CO, USA). Afterwards, slides were washed and incubated for 1 h at room temperature with 1:500 diluted polyclonal goat anti-mouse IgG antibody conjugated to Alexa Fluor 488 and polyclonal goat anti-rabbit IgG antibody conjugated to Alexa Fluor 647 (Lifetechnologies, Darmstadt, Germany). After a final washing cycle in PBS, slides were covered with DAPI (4′,6-diamidino-2-phenylindole)-containing mounting medium (Medipan, Berlin/Dahlewitz, Germany). Directly after staining procedure slides were analyzed by an automated digital microscopy system (AKLIDES, Medipan, Berlin/Dahlewitz, Germany) quantifying the number of γH2AX and 53BP1 foci in 300 nuclei per sample [28,29].

2.8. Statistical Analysis

Quantitative data analysis was performed by GraphPad Prism software version 5.01 (Graph Pad Software, La Jolla, CA, USA). Half-maximal inhibitory dose (IC_{50}) was calculated by non-linear regression from logarithm-transformed data. Significance levels among samples treated with the same JAKi or MTX were calculated by repeated measures ANOVA (analysis of variance) with 95% confidence interval ($\alpha = 0.05$) followed by the Dunnett's post-hoc test, to compare the results with DMSO-treated control group. Data in text and figures are displayed as the mean ± standard error of the mean (SEM), and p values are indicated by asterisks (*** $p \leq 0.001$; ** $p \leq 0.01$; * $p \leq 0.05$).

3. Results

3.1. Impact of JAKi and MTX on Lymphocyte Activation and Proliferation

3.1.1. ^{3}H-Thymidine Incorporation

To assess the impact of different JAKi on lymphocyte proliferation DNA synthesis was analyzed by ^{3}H-thymidine incorporation 72 h after PHA-stimulation (Figure 1). As expected, lymphocyte proliferation was significantly inhibited in freshly stimulated PBMCs by all four investigated JAKi in a dose-dependent manner (Figure 1a). However, whereas tofacitinib, baricitinib, and upadacitinib showed significantly inhibitory effects already at the nanomolar dose range, higher concentrations of filgotinib were required to reduce lymphocyte proliferation to a similar extent. Though, treatment of PBMCs with 10 µM filgotinib showed the strongest decrease in ^{3}H-thymidine incorporation (5.5% ± 1.0%) when compared to cell cultures treated with 10 µM tofacitinib (38.6% ± 7.6%), baricitinib (19.8% ± 3.3%), or upadacitinib (19.4% ± 4.6%).

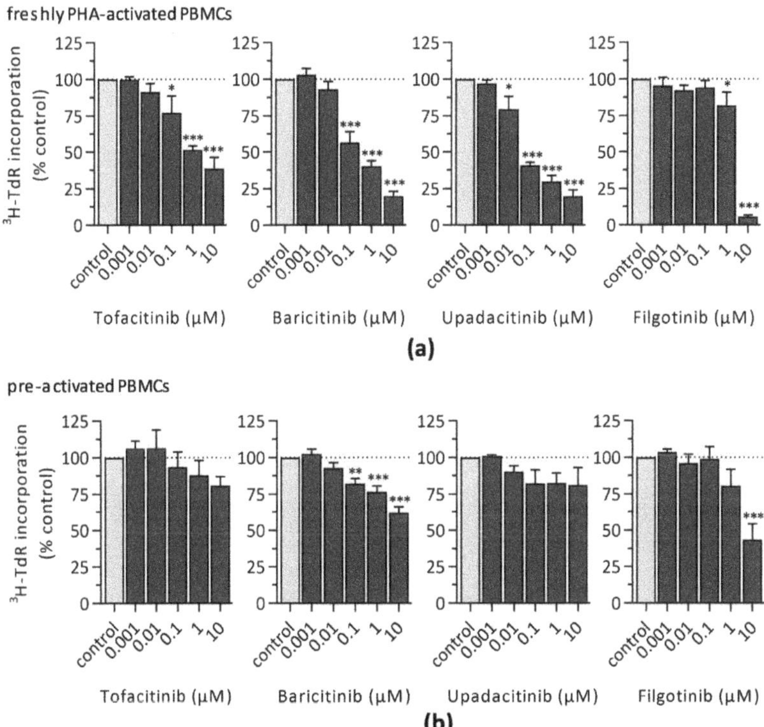

Figure 1. Proliferation analysis by ^{3}H-thymidine incorporation assay 72 h after PHA-stimulation of PBMCs treated with indicated concentrations of JAKi either (**a**) immediately after activation or (**b**) 48 h after PHA-stimulation. Diagrams display the mean ± SEM of five independent experiments normalized to the DMSO control (*** $p \leq 0.001$; ** $p \leq 0.01$; * $p \leq 0.05$).

Additionally, we investigated the immunomodulatory potential of these four JAKi on preactivated PBMCs. Therefore, increasing concentrations of JAKi were added to the cell culture 48 h after PHA-stimulation (Figure 1b). Assessment of ^{3}H-thymidine incorporation revealed no significant inhibitory effects in preactivated lymphocytes treated with tofacitinib or upadacitinib, whereas baricitinib decreased cell proliferation in a dose-dependent manner. Filgotinib significantly reduced the level of incorporated ^{3}H-thymidine only when the highest dose (10 μM) was applied. Of note, inhibitory potential of JAKi was strongly attenuated in preactivated cell cultures compared to freshly stimulated PBMCs.

However, due to assay limitations, data obtained from PBMCs treated with MTX had to be excluded from this proliferation analysis. MTX led to a concentration dependent increase of ^{3}H-thymidine incorporation (Figure S1), as also observed by others [30]. This effect is caused by MTX-induced blockage of internal thymidine biosynthesis. The lack of available endogenous thymidine was overcome by enhanced incorporation of external radiolabeled thymidine provided in the cell culture medium, as reflected by an increase in counted radioactivity.

To confirm results obtained by ^{3}H-thymidine incorporation and to include samples treated with MTX, proliferation was additionally analyzed by the CFSE dilution assay.

3.1.2. CFSE Dilution Assay

In line with our data obtained by ^{3}H-thymidine incorporation, CFSE dilution analysis demonstrated a dose-dependent decrease in lymphocyte proliferation, when JAKi were added to freshly stimulated lymphocytes (Figure 2a). Filgotinib significantly reduced the percentage of dividing cells only when PBMCs were treated with 10 μM filgotinib (36.8% $\pm$ 15.7%), yet representing the strongest effect compared to samples cultured with 10 μM tofacitinib (42.4% $\pm$ 3.4%), baricitinib (38.3% $\pm$ 3.7%), or upadacitinib (55.5% $\pm$ 2.9%), respectively. Treatment with MTX $\geq$ 0.1 μM also significantly reduced cell proliferation by more than 50%.

In preactivated cell cultures, the antiproliferative impact of JAKi was reduced. Still, JAKi significantly diminished the fraction of dividing cells after treatment with either 1 μM (93.3% $\pm$ 0.3%) or 10 μM (92.4% $\pm$ 0.4%) tofacitinib, 1 μM (92.5% $\pm$ 1.0%) or 10 μM (92.9% $\pm$ 0.4%) baricitinib, and 10 μM filgotinib (94.0% $\pm$ 1.0%) (Figure 2b). In contrast, MTX strongly reduced ratio of dividing cells (<50%) at a dose range $\geq$ 0.1 μM when added to freshly and to preactivated PBMCs.

3.1.3. CD25 Expression

Lymphocyte activation was assessed 48 h after simultaneous incubation of PBMCs with PHA and JAKi by the flow cytometric measurement of CD25 expression (Figure 3). Similar to proliferation analyses, JAKi and MTX induced a dose-dependent reduction of CD25 expression. Since data from CFSE analysis were insufficient to calculate half maximal inhibitory concentration (IC_{50}) for all JAKi investigated, we compared IC_{50} based on the CD25 expression level. Upadacitinib (IC_{50}: 0.0149 μM) showed the strongest inhibitory effect, followed by baricitinib (IC_{50}: 0.0284 μM), tofacitinib (IC_{50}: 0.0522 μM), and filgotinib (IC_{50}: 2.4378 μM). Due to an attenuated effect of MTX on CD25 expression respective IC_{50} value could not be calculated. Nevertheless, a significant reduction of CD25 was observed for PBMCs treated with 0.1 μM (77.3% $\pm$ 8.6%), 1 μM (73.9% $\pm$ 6.4%), or 10 μM (75.3% $\pm$ 7.8%) MTX.

3.2. Impact of JAKi and MTX on Lymphocyte Viability

Further, we investigated JAKi-induced cytotoxicity in unstimulated (Figure 4a), freshly stimulated (Figure 4b), and preactivated (Figure 4c) PBMCs using Annexin V/PI staining. Statistical analysis revealed a small but significant rise of apoptotic cell fraction already in unstimulated PBMCs (control: 17.9% $\pm$ 0.9%) treated either with 1 μM baricitinib (22.7% $\pm$ 2.7%), 1 μM (21.5% $\pm$ 2.3%), or 10 μM upadacitinib (21.8% $\pm$ 2.1%) or after incubation with 10 μM filgotinib (21.7% $\pm$ 2.3%) (Figure 4a). Tofacitinib and MTX did not affect viability in unstimulated PBMCs.

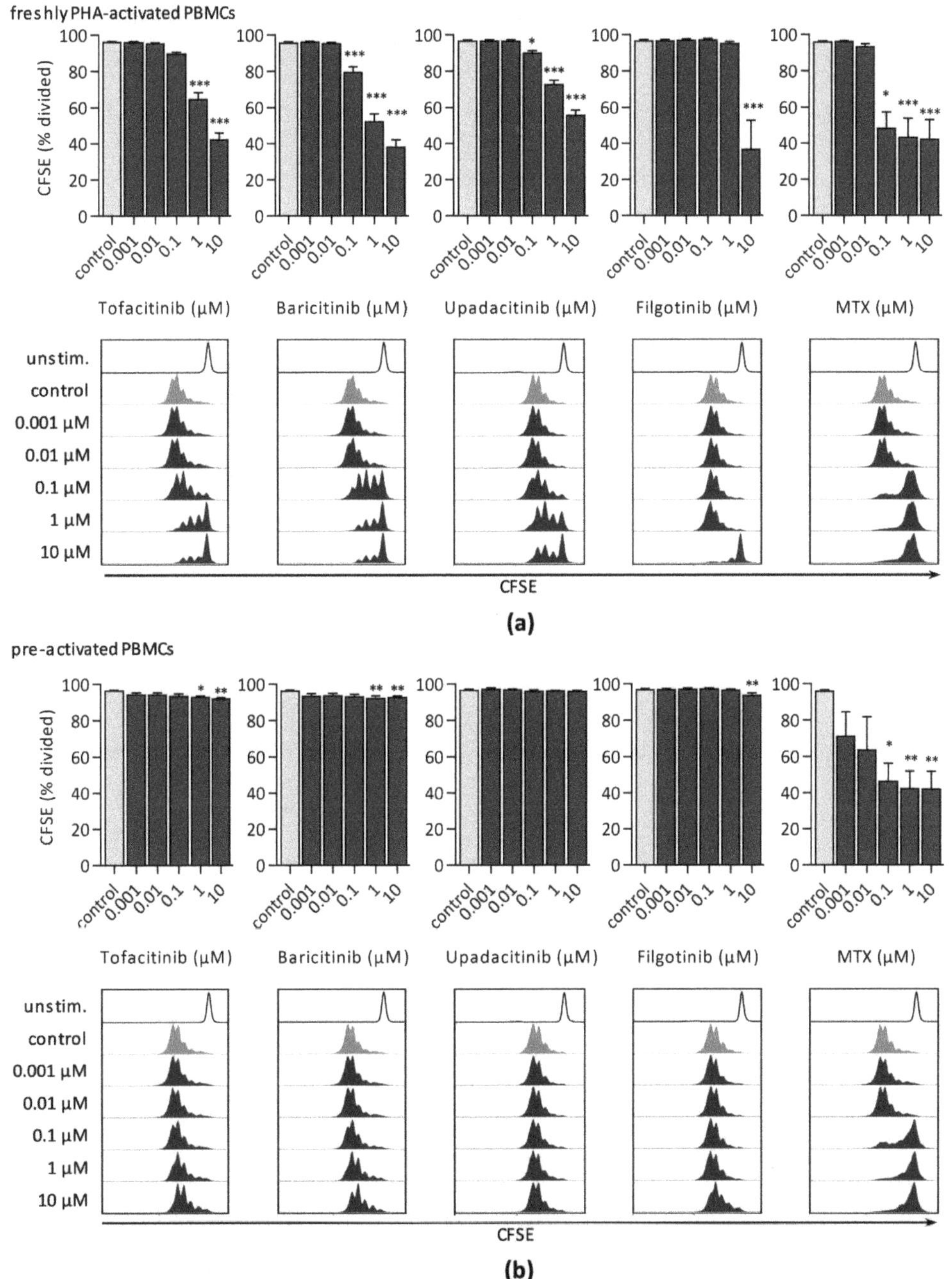

Figure 2. Proliferation analysis by CFSE dilution assay 96 h after PHA-stimulation of PBMCs treated with indicated concentrations of JAKi or MTX either (**a**) immediately after activation or (**b**) 48 h after PHA-stimulation. Percentage of divided cell population was quantified. Diagrams display the mean ± SEM of three independent experiments (*** $p \leq 0.001$; ** $p \leq 0.01$; * $p \leq 0.05$). Representative histograms of CFSE intensity are shown below.

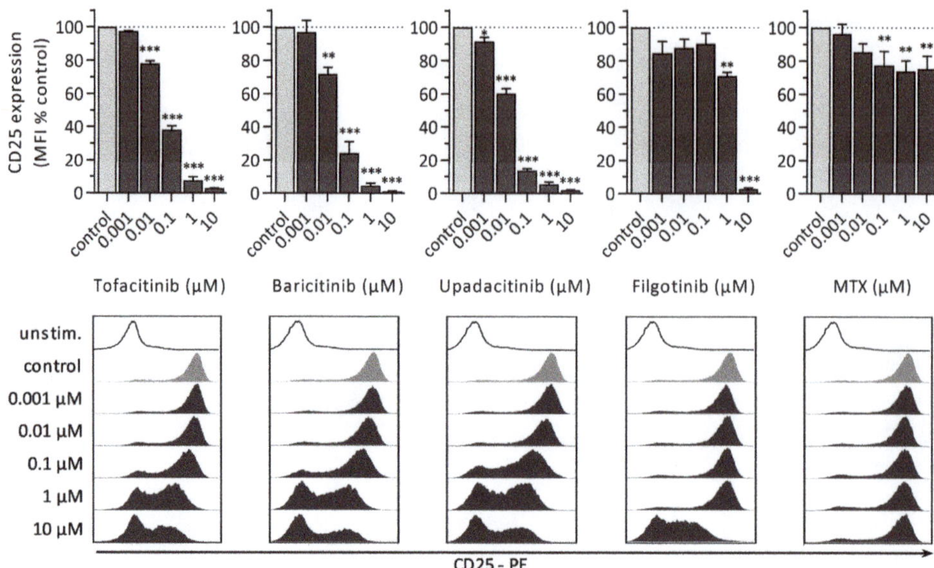

Figure 3. Assessment of lymphocyte activation by CD25 expression 48 h after PHA-stimulation and combined treatment of indicated JAKi or MTX concentrations. Median fluorescence intensity of CD25 expression was quantified. Diagrams display the mean ± SEM of three independent experiments (*** $p \leq 0.001$; ** $p \leq 0.01$; * $p \leq 0.05$). Representative histograms of CD25 intensity are shown below.

PHA-activation itself significantly increased the apoptotic cell population (control: 35.5% ± 2.2%) (Figure 4b). Apoptotic fraction further rose 72 h after treatment with 10 μM tofacitinib (52.8% ± 4.9%), 10 μM upadacitinib (53.2% ± 4.1%), or 10 μM filgotinib (53.2% ± 3.3%). In contrast to JAKi, simultaneous incubation of PBMCs with PHA and 0.1 μM MTX already induced a high proportion of apoptotic cells (89.7% ± 2.1%), which did not further grow with increasing MTX concentrations.

Addition of tofacitinib or baricitinib to preactivated PBMCs did not affect cell viability. However, high doses of JAK1-selective JAKi upadacitinib (1 μM: 37.2% ± 2.5%; 10 μM: 37.32% ± 2.3%) or filgotinib (10 μM: 42.5% ± 2.7%) induced a significant rise in apoptotic cell fraction. Treatment of preactivated PBMCs with MTX also strongly induced cell death (0.1 μM: 62.5% ± 5.4%).

3.3. Impact of JAKi and MTX on DNA Double-Strand Break Formation and DNA Repair

To analyze the impact of JAKi on DNA DSB formation we investigated the induction of γH2AX and 53BP1 foci 24 h after drug treatment (Figure 5). In general, incubation of unstimulated PBMCs with JAKi or MTX did not induce γH2AX foci, only samples treated with 10 μM filgotinib revealed a significant increase in γH2AX foci formation (control: 0.41 ± 0.04 foci/cell; 10 μM filgotinib: 0.63 ± 0.06 foci/cell). This enhanced level of DNA DSB marker after 10 μM filgotinib treatment was further confirmed by a significant rise of 53BP1 foci (control: 0.59 ± 0.05 foci/cell; 10 μM filgotinib: 0.72 ± 0.04 foci/cell). Additionally, an increase of 53BP1 foci was also observed in cells treated with 10 μM baricitinib (0.82 ± 0.09 foci/cell).

Assessment of residual γH2AX and 53BP1 foci 24 h after radiation was applied to analyze DNA repair efficacy by means of foci clearance. Therefore, JAKi or MTX were added to cell cultures, which were subsequently irradiated with 2 Gy γ-radiation. Remaining foci were determined 24 h after irradiation (Figure 6). A significant, dose-dependent enrichment of residual γH2AX was determined in samples treated with pan-JAKi tofacitinib (control: 3.50 ± 0.37 foci/cell; 1 μM tofacitinib: 3.96 ± 0.41 foci/cell; 10 μM tofacitinib: 3.93 ± 0.51 foci/cell) or baricitinib (control: 3.33 ± 0.32 foci/cell; 1 μM baricitinib: 3.84 ± 0.39 foci/cell; 10 μM baricitinib: 4.12 ± 0.29 foci/cell). Radiated PBMCs incubated in the presence of 10 μM baricitinib also revealed a significant increase in the 53BP1 foci level (control: 3.25 ± 0.23 foci/cell; 10 μM baricitinib: 3.60 ± 0.29 foci/cell). Furthermore, treatment of irradiated PBMCs with 10 μM filgotinib correlated with enhanced level of residual γH2AX foci (control: 2.71 ± 0.27 foci/cell; 10 μM filgotinib: 3.85 ± 0.32 foci/cell) and 53BP1 foci (control: 2.48 ± 0.10 foci/cell; 10 μM filgotinib: 2.79 ± 0.09 foci/cell). Of note, differences in foci levels of DMSO controls among groups were caused by individual variance among blood donors, since some additional experiments investigating the impact of upadacitinib and filgotinib had to be performed separately.

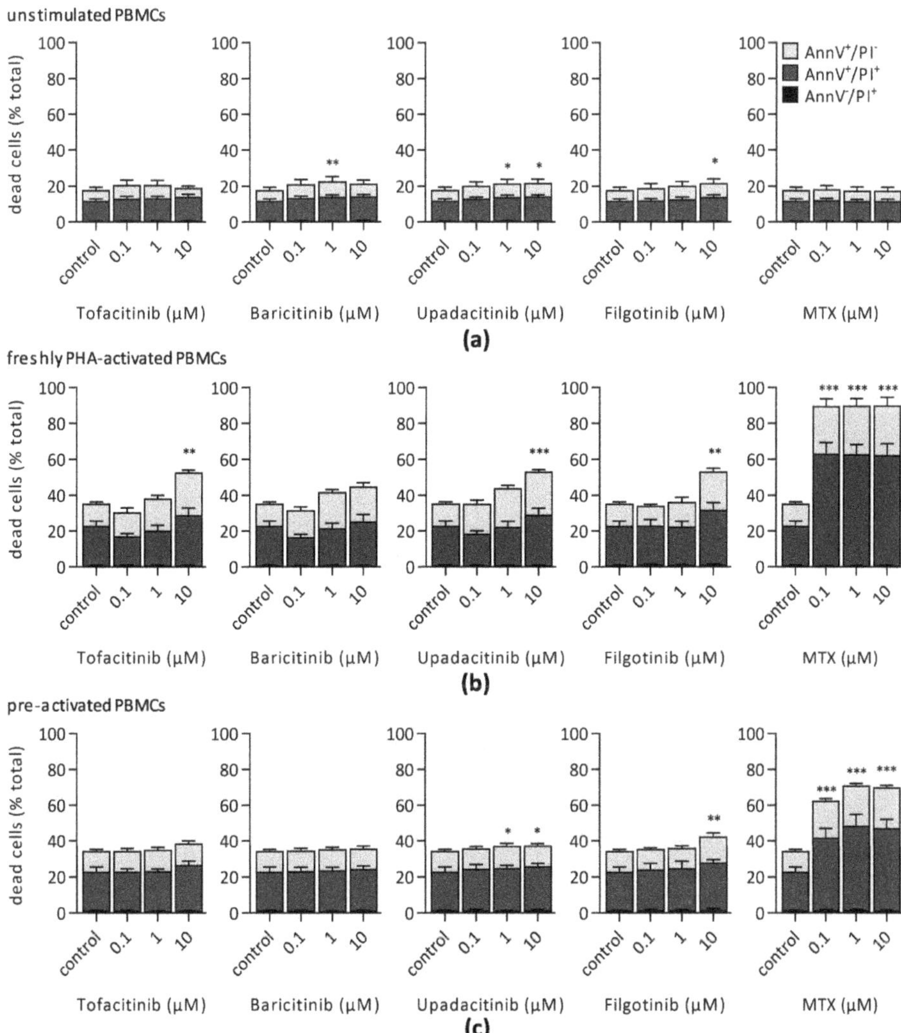

Figure 4. Cell viability was assessed after 72 h by Annexin V/PI staining of (**a**) unstimulated, (**b**) freshly PHA-stimulated, or (**c**) preactivated PBMCs treatment with indicated concentrations of JAKi or MTX. Percentage of Annexin V$^+$/PI$^-$ (light grey), Annexin V$^+$/PI$^+$ (dark grey), and Annexin V$^-$/PI$^+$ (black; <2%) population were quantified. Diagrams display the mean ± SEM of five independent experiments (*** $p \leq 0.001$; ** $p \leq 0.01$; * $p \leq 0.05$).

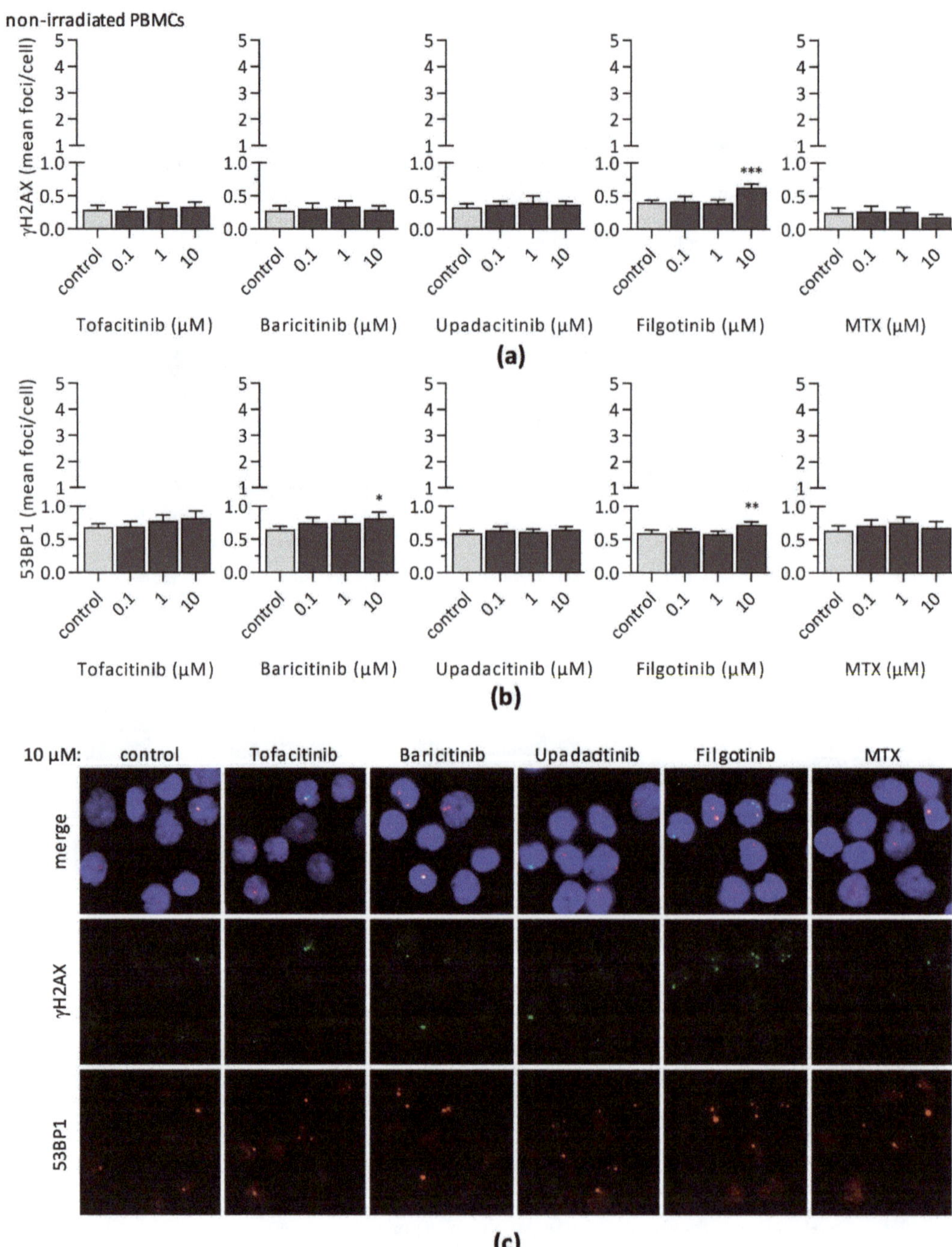

Figure 5. The mean number of (**a**) γH2AX and (**b**) 53BP1 foci per cell were assessed, as markers for induced DNA double-strand breaks, 24 h after treatment of unstimulated PBMCs with indicated JAKi or MTX concentration. Diagrams display the mean ± SEM of seven independent experiments (*** $p \leq 0.001$; ** $p \leq 0.01$; * $p \leq 0.05$). (**c**) Representative immunofluorescence microscopy images of PBMCs from one donor treated with either 10 μM JAKi or MTX. Colors indicate DNA/DAPI (blue), γH2AX (green), and 53BP1 (red).

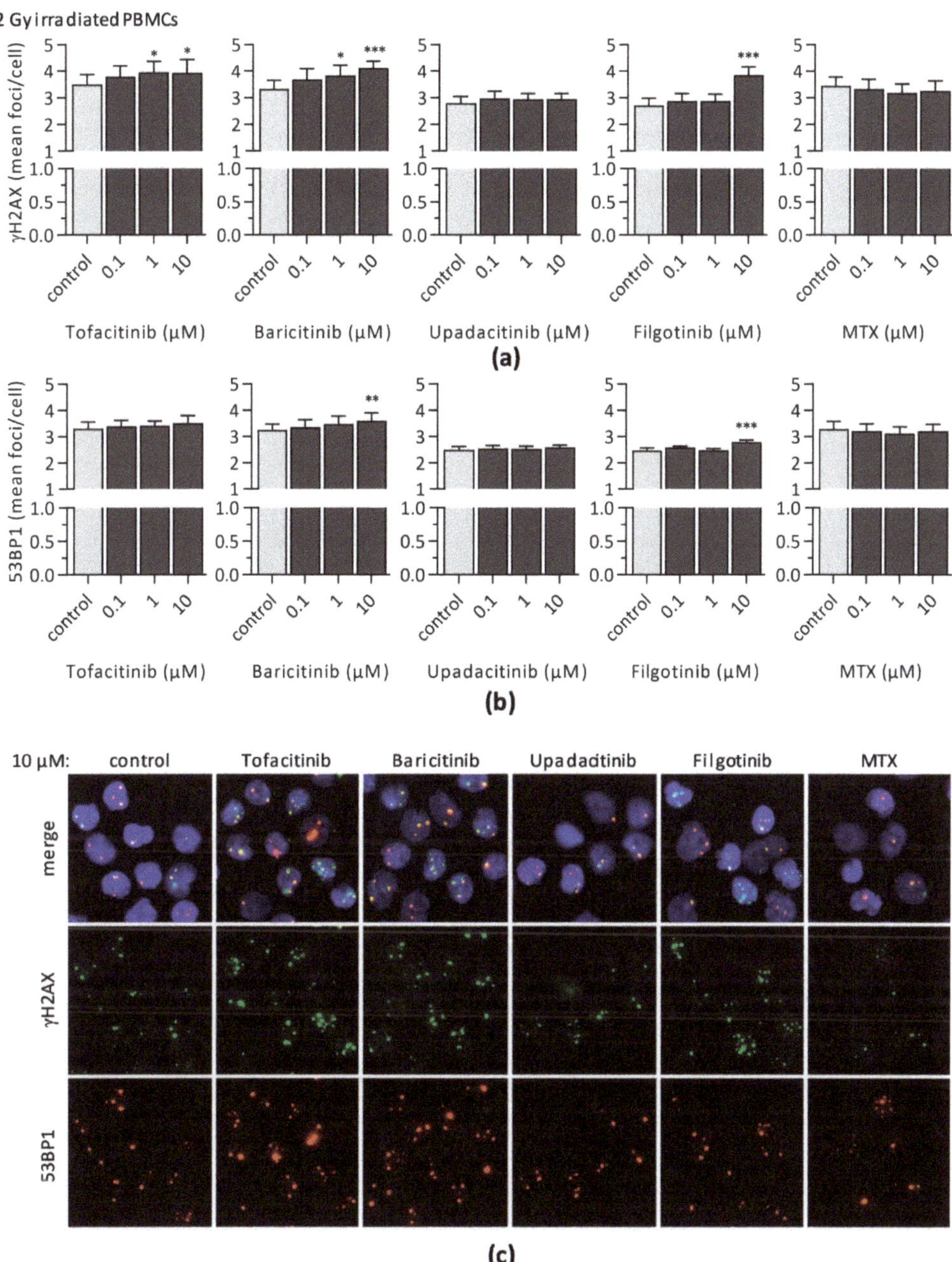

Figure 6. The mean number of residual (**a**) γH2AX and (**b**) 53BP1 foci per cell were assessed 24 h after 2 Gy irradiation of unstimulated PBMCs in the presence of indicated JAKi or MTX to analyze DNA repair by means for foci clearance. Diagrams display the mean ± SEM of seven independent experiments (*** $p \leq 0.001$; ** $p \leq 0.01$; * $p \leq 0.05$). (**c**) Representative immunofluorescence microscopy images of PBMCs from one donor treated with either 10 µM JAKi or MTX. Colors indicate DNA/DAPI (blue), γH2AX (green), and 53BP1 (red).

4. Discussion

JAK inhibitors represent a new class of immunomodulatory drugs, currently being approved for therapy of cancer and inflammatory diseases [10,11]. In comparison to biological DMARDs, which are expensive to manufacture, require cold storage, and have to be administered parenterally, small molecular JAKi circumvent these limitations. Furthermore, JAKi are compounds that can be taken orally and typically exhibit a dose-proportional pharmacokinetic profile and a short half-life in the range of hours [4,31]. This allows rapid reversal of immunosuppressive or potential drug-induced adverse effects [4]. Although not just targeting one specific cytokine, but rather signaling pathways of multiple cytokine receptors, JAKi show similar efficacy and safety profiles compared to biological DMARDs, like TNF inhibitors [4,5,13]. However, analysis of currently available data revealed, e.g., an increased frequency of herpes zoster infection and thromboembolic adverse events in RA patients receiving JAKi, while the incidence of respiratory or urinary tract infections and recorded malignancies were similar compared to other DMARDs [4,9,13]. Completion of ongoing long-term extension studies and increasing prescription rates of JAKi will provide more pharmacovigilance data also concerning potential long-term effects [32].

Currently, leading pharmaceutical authorities, such as the FDA (United States), the EMA (Europe), and the Pharmaceuticals and Medical Devices Agency (PMDA) in Japan licensed the three JAKi tofacitinib (Xeljanz®), baricitinib (Olumiant®), and upadacitinib (Rinvoq®) for the treatment of patients with active RA, who responded inadequately to conventional therapies [13,14]. In September 2020 a fourth JAKi, filgotinib (Jyseleca®), received approval by the EMA and PMDA. In contrast, the FDA has rejected filgotinib for RA treatment, raising concerns, e.g., regarding its impact on sperm parameters and the risk–benefit profile of 200 mg dose [14,33]. In Asian countries, such as Japan and Korea, an additional pan-JAKi, peficitinib (Smyraf®), has also been approved for the treatment of patients with moderate RA [34,35].

Due to the absence of head-to-head trials, direct comparison of JAKi with respect to their efficacy in RA treatment is limited [36,37]. In the present in vitro study, we investigated all four JAKi currently approved by the EMA for RA treatment to gain more information about their immunomodulatory potential. In contrast to previous studies, which analyzed different JAKi and their inhibitory profile concerning specific cytokine receptor signaling pathways, we determined their inhibitory potential with regard to overall lymphocyte proliferation and activation [17,38].

Therefore, PBMCs were isolated from healthy volunteers and T cells contained therein were activated by addition of PHA. Increasing concentrations of tofacitinib, baricitinib, upadacitinib, filgotinib, or MTX were added to cell cultures either directly or 48 h post PHA-stimulation, to analyze the impact on preactivated lymphocytes. Proliferation and activation were assessed by ^{3}H-thymidine incorporation analysis, CFSE dilution assay, and CD25 expression. Although small numerical differences have been observed, freshly activated lymphocytes incubated with tofacitinib, baricitinib, or upadacitinib exhibited a comparable, dose-dependent inhibition of T lymphocyte proliferation and CD25 expression. In contrast, concentrations of filgotinib had to be approximately two orders of magnitude higher to induce significant inhibitory effects. This deviation also reflects the higher dosage of filgotinib regarding IC_{50} values of JAK1-enzymatic inhibition and administered concentrations in clinical studies [16,38].

As JAKi are also administered under inflammatory conditions, it is of interest to investigate their immunomodulatory potential on previously activated lymphocytes [17]. Therefore, different JAKi were added to cell cultures 48 h after PHA-stimulation. Compared to direct JAKi exposure, inhibitory effects of JAKi on lymphocyte proliferation of preactivated cells were strongly attenuated. While the CFSE assay revealed a small but significant dose-dependent decrease in cultures treated with high doses of tofacitinib, baricitinib, or filgotinib, no alterations were observed in preactivated samples incubated with upadacitinib. Data obtained from ^{3}H-thymidine incorporation only revealed a significant, dose-dependent reduction of DNA synthesis in preactivated cells subsequently incubated with baricitinib or treated with 10 µM filgotinib. However, in the highest concentration of 10 µM, filgotinib among all four JAKi induced the strongest proliferation inhibition in freshly stimulated and in preactivated PBMCs.

Furthermore, behavior of JAKi on lymphocyte proliferation is also reflected by data obtained from CD25 analysis, supporting an antiproliferative rather than a cytotoxic impact of JAKi. Of note, CD25 represents the interleukin-2 receptor α-chain (IL-2Rα) being part of the high-affinity IL-2 receptor [39]. Its surface expression is regulated by initial T cell receptor (TCR) activation and delayed IL-2 receptor stimulation [40]. Since IL-2R signal transduction depends on JAK/STAT pathways, impairment of JAK/STAT signaling inhibited CD25 expression and T cell proliferation [40,41]. Further, it was reported that application of JAK1/2 inhibitor ruxolitinib suppressed IL-2-induced STAT5 phosphorylation and CD25 expression, whereas phosphorylation of molecules associated with early T cell receptor signaling was not affected [42].

Our data obtained from MTX-treated samples (≥0.1 µM) demonstrated reduced CD25 expression, but to a lesser extent compared to JAKi-application, while MTX caused a strong proliferation inhibition of freshly stimulated and preactivated PBMCs. These results are in line with values obtained from 3-(4,5-dimethylthiazol-2-yl)-2,5-diphenyl-2H-tetrazolium bromide (MTT) assay by Nesher et al., stating a significant proliferation inhibition of mitogen-stimulated PBMCs when treated with MTX concentrations > 10 nM for 72 h [43].

To further distinguish proliferation inhibition from cytotoxicity, we additionally performed cell death analysis by Annexin V/PI staining. Treatment of freshly activated PBMCs with a high dose (10 µM) of tofacitinib, upadacitinib, or filgotinib induced a significant increase of apoptotic cells from 36% to 53%. Cell death was also enhanced in preactivated PBMCs treated with high concentrations of JAK1-selective JAKi upadacitinib or filgotinib. Therefore, the decreased proliferation rate after high dose JAKi exposure might at least partly be due to induced cell death. Whereas viability of unstimulated PBMCs treated with MTX was not significantly affected in the applied setting, a strong increase of apoptosis was determined for MTX treatment of freshly and preactivated lymphocytes, leading to the conclusion that this reduced lymphocyte proliferation was mainly due to cytotoxicity. As already shown in publications from the 1990s, MTX primarily targets highly proliferating lymphocytes, mainly in the S phase of the cell cycle, while resting T cells were only little affected [44,45]. Therefore, only low-dose MTX therapy is applied in patients suffering from RA. Nevertheless, also this approach can induce drug toxicity, forcing patients to change the treatment method [46–48].

Cell death can be induced by enhanced cytotoxic but also by genotoxic stress, when DNA lesions cannot be repaired efficiently. DNA DSBs are among the most lethal types of DNA damage. A widely used marker to analyze DNA DSBs and DNA repair is γH2AX, a core histone protein rapidly phosphorylated on serin-139 by ataxia telangiectasia mutated protein (ATM), ATM- and Rad3-related (ATR), or DNA-dependent protein kinase (DNA-PK) in chromatin surrounding the break site [25,27]. Immunofluorescence staining followed by quantification of individual γH2AX foci represents the most sensitive method to detect DSBs [25,27,28]. DNA DSBs are repaired by two major pathways—non-homologous end joining (NHEJ) and homologous recombination (HR). Due to its simplicity NHEJ is the preferred pathway throughout the cell cycle, directly ligating two adjacent DNA DSB ends. In contrast, HR provides higher fidelity but requires a homologues DNA template. Thus, HR is primarily activated in the S/G2 phase of the cell cycle [49,50].

There is increasing evidence that DNA damage repair is also modulated by JAK/STAT signaling [20–24]. Further, inhibiting JAK/STAT pathways, e.g., by the JAK1/2 inhibitor ruxolitinib, impaired HR and NHEJ, and was accompanied by reduced expression of different proteins involved in DNA damage response [23]. To analyze the impact of different JAKi on DSB induction, we quantified γH2AX and 53BP1 foci 24 h after JAKi treatment. Additionally, we measured residual γH2AX and 53BP1 foci in unstimulated lymphocytes 24 h after irradiation with 2 Gy in the presence of increasing JAKi concentrations, to investigate their impact on DNA repair. A significant increase of both DSB markers in non-irradiated and irradiated samples was determined in PBMCs after incubation with 10 µM filgotinib. Further, a dose-dependent accumulation of residual γH2AX-foci 24 h after radiation was observed in samples treated with pan-JAKi tofacitinib or baricitinib, whereas upadacitinib and MTX did not lead to enhanced levels of DBS foci.

Microscopic quantification of γH2AX foci represents the most sensitive approach when samples with low γH2AX levels were investigated. In contrast, flow cytometric measurement of intracellular γH2AX intensity is more suitable in samples with high γH2AX expression, where individual foci cannot be distinguished properly. Furthermore, flow cytometry offers the advantage of simultaneous DNA content analysis, since γH2AX levels differ depending on the cell cycle phase. DNA and histone content and intrinsic γH2AX expression increase as cells progressing from G_1 to S, G_2, and M phase [51]. Therefore, it is recommended to combine γH2AX quantification of proliferating cells with cell cycle analysis.

In the present study, DSB analysis had to be restricted to resting PBMCs since difficulties were encountered quantifying the γH2AX level in PHA-stimulated lymphocytes. The vast majority of isolated lymphocytes are in a resting state (G_0) exhibiting only a low baseline γH2AX level. Activation by antigen or mitogen stimulus induces chromatin remodeling and transcriptional activation. Thus, transition of lymphocytes from G_0 to G_1 phase also involves a strong endogenous induction of γH2AX [52]. In contrast to cells in S and G_2/M, G_1 cells cannot be differentiated from the G_0 phase by DNA content analysis. Preliminary data of flow cytometric γH2AX measurements combined with cell cycle staining based on DNA content revealed a reduction of γH2AX positive cells with increasing JAKi concentration, while a dose of 10 µM again induced a small rise in γH2AX intensity. Since cell proliferation and thereby high expression of intrinsic γH2AX in activated lymphocytes was inhibited with increasing concentrations of JAKi, this method was not sufficient to distinguish JAKi induced DNA damage or modulated DNA repair from endogenous γH2AX expression, which varied depending on activation status and cell cycle phase. Therefore, we discontinued this analysis of stimulated PBMCs. In future studies, modified protocols need to be established including additional proliferation markers, such as Ki67 [53]. Furthermore, precise differentiation of cells regarding their cell cycle phase will also allow one to analyze the influence of JAKi on proteins critical for HR, such as RAD51, which is primarily active in the S/G_2 cell cycle phase.

Although preclinical analysis applying multiple standardized genotoxicity assays did not reveal an enhanced DNA damaging potential of approved JAKi, there is increasing evidence that JAK/STAT signaling is involved in DNA damage repair and modulates chemo- and radiosensitivity. As reviewed in detail elsewhere, various in vivo and in vitro data demonstrated hyperactivation of JAK/STAT signaling, especially STAT3, in cancer cells contributing to cancer progression and radio- and chemoresistance [24,54–56]. STAT3 activation induced upregulation of DNA repair molecules, while STAT3 deficiency induced downregulation of proteins especially involved in DSB sensing and repair through HR, e.g., RAD51 [20,24,56]. Furthermore, the application of JAK inhibitor ruxolitinib downregulated key proteins of HR and NHEJ, thereby reducing DNA repair activity [22,23]. Bonner et al. also reported enhanced radiosensitivity and reduced DNA DSB repair in irradiated head and neck cancer cells treated with radiosensitizer cetuximab in combination with a JAK1 inhibitor [21]. Furthermore, Maranto et al. reported JAK2/STAT5A/B-dependent expression of Rad51 and suppression of HR but not NHEJ when STAT5A/B was knocked down [57].

Although JAKis show differences in their JAK-isoform selectivity, high dosage can also induce inhibition of additional JAK isoforms and off-target effects [4]. Based on data from pharmacological reviews published by FDA and EMA, mean maximal plasma concentrations (c_{max}) in human subjects treated with tofacitinib (5 mg/twice a day), baricitinib (4 mg/day), or upadacitinib (15 mg/day) reach values of approximately 0.15 µM [58–63]. A mean maximal plasma concentrations between 4 and 6.1 µM was reported after application of filgotinib (200 mg/day) [64,65]. Regarding published IC_{50} values obtained by cell-free enzymatic assays (summarized in Table S1), reported c_{max} exceed IC_{50} values of multiple JAK isoforms. With respect to doses used in our in vitro study, reported c_{max} of tofacitinib, baricitinib, and upadacitinib are multiple folds below concentrations associated with significant increases of apoptosis or γH2AX foci, whereas published cmax of filgotinib is in a magnitude comparable with the highest concentration (10 μM) applied. As JAKis show distinct pharmacokinetic profiles, e.g., hours per day above IC_{50} values and average daily STAT inhibition among different human leucocyte subpopulations need to be considered to evaluate particular safety and efficacy.

Such concentration-time profiles have been calculated for different JAKi by McInnes et al. [17] and Traves et al. [66]. Investigating cytokine-stimulated STAT activation authors reported similar daily average inhibition of JAK1-dependent signaling pathways. However, Travers et al. described highest JAK-1 selectivity of filgotinib, showing the least inhibition of JAK2- and JAK3-associated pathways when compared with tofacitinib, baricitinib, and upadacitinib and the least inhibition of JAK1/JAK3-related cytokines, such as IL-2, IL-15, or IL-21 [66].

Of note, IL-15 and IL-21 mediate proliferation and function of natural killer (NK) cells, which are essential for clearance of virus-infected and tumorigenic cells. JAKi treatment with tofacitinib and upadacitinib [17,67–71], but not with baricitinib or filgotinib [35,72,73], was accompanied with mild to moderate decrease of circulating NK cell number and impaired NK cell function. Although, these effects were not associated with an increased risk of infectious diseases or lymphoma. Investigating the effect of JAKi ruxolitinib in a murine breast cancer model Bottos et al. showed a JAKi-induced impairment of NK cell-mediated tumor immunosurveillance and enhanced metastasis formation, which were overcome by immunostimulation with IL-15 [74]. Until now, clinical relevance of JAKi-induced NK cell inhibition in RA treatment remains unclear [17,67,69]. Though, especially in regard with potentially affected DNA damage repair, this aspect also needs to be further investigated in long-term studies.

Cancer cells often exhibit dysregulations in DNA repair mechanisms. However, several studies also indicated enhanced DNA damage and DNA repair deficiencies in lymphocytes from RA patients [75–78]. In addition to studies investigating the role of different JAK inhibitors on DNA damage response pathways in primary cells from healthy donors or cancer cell lines, future trials also need to address the impact of JAKi on lymphocytes from patients with RA.

5. Conclusions

In conclusion, our study confirmed a comparable, dose-dependent inhibition of lymphocyte activation and proliferation in PBMCs treated with tofacitinib, baricitinib, and upadacitinib, independent of JAK selectivity. In line with reported IC_{50} values regarding JAK1-enzymatic activity and administered dosage in vivo concentrations of filgotinib had to be approximately two orders of magnitude higher to induce significant immunomodulatory effects. Furthermore, antiproliferating properties especially of JAK1-selective inhibitors may at least partially be caused by cytotoxicity, since high doses also affected cell viability. For the first time the effect of tofacitinib, baricitinib, upadacitinib, and filgotinib on DNA DSB induction and repair of radiation-induced DNA damage was investigated by applying γH2AX and 53BP1 foci analysis. Our results provide first evidence for a significant increase in DNA DSB markers after exposure to 10 μM filgotinib and a dose-dependent enrichment of residual γH2AX foci in irradiated samples incubated with pan-JAKi tofacitinib and baricitinib, possibly indicating attenuated DNA damage repair. Although these in vitro results do not necessarily represent behavior in vivo, additional studies need to be performed further investigating the impact of approved JAK inhibition on DNA damage response and their potential long-term effects in vitro and in vivo, also comprising analysis of RA patients. Since JAKi are also administered in combination with MTX, the impact of combined treatment additionally needs to be addressed in future trials, especially as MTX itself demonstrated JAK/STAT pathway inhibiting properties [79,80].

Supplementary Materials: The following are available online at https://www.mdpi.com/article/10.3390/jcm10071431/s1, Table S1: Summary of mean half-maximal inhibitory concentrations (IC_{50}) obtained by enzymatic assays with indicated ATP concentration (c_{ATP}) for different JAKi, Figure S1: Proliferation analysis by ^{3}H-thymidine incorporation assay 72 h after PHA-stimulation of PBMCs treated with indicated concentrations of methotrexate (MTX) either (a) immediately after activation or (b) 48 h after PHA-stimulation.

Author Contributions: Conceptualization: D.R. (Dirk Reinhold) and E.F.; methodology, A.R., L.V., K.G. and D.R. (Dirk Roggenbuck); validation, A.R., D.R. (Dirk Reinhold) and E.F.; formal analysis, A.R.; investigation, A.R., L.V., K.G.; resources, D.R. (Dirk Reinhold), E.F. and D.R. (Dirk Roggenbuck); data curation, A.R.; writing—original draft preparation, A.R., D.R. (Dirk Reinhold) and E.F.; writing—review and editing, L.V., K.G. and D.R. (Dirk Roggenbuck); visualization, A.R.; supervision, D.R. (Dirk Reinhold) and E.F.; project administration, D.R. (Dirk Reinhold) and E.F.; funding acquisition, D.R. (Dirk Reinhold) and E.F. All authors have read and agreed to the published version of the manuscript.

Funding: The project was supported by grants from the European Union Program Regional Development Fund of the Ministry of Economy, Science and Digitalisation in Saxony-Anhalt within the research alliance "Autonomy in Old Age".

Institutional Review Board Statement: The study was conducted according to the guidelines of the Declaration of Helsinki, and approved by the Ethics Committee of the Otto-von-Guericke-University Magdeburg (183/2020).

Informed Consent Statement: Informed consent was obtained from all subjects involved in the study.

Conflicts of Interest: Eugen Feist received honoraria for lectures and consultation from Lilly, Pfizer, Abbvie and Gilead. All other authors declare no conflict of interest. Dirk Roggenbuck is an employee of GA Generic Assays and Medipan and owns stocks and shares of both companies.

References

1. Smolen, J.S.; Aletaha, D.; Barton, A.; Burmester, G.R.; Emery, P.; Firestein, G.S.; Kavanaugh, A.; McInnes, I.B.; Solomon, D.H.; Strand, V.; et al. Rheumatoid arthritis. *Nat. Rev. Dis. Prim.* **2018**, *4*, 1–23. [CrossRef] [PubMed]
2. Semerano, L.; Decker, P.; Clavel, G.; Boissier, M.C. Developments with investigational Janus kinase inhibitors for rheumatoid arthritis. *Expert Opin. Investig. Drugs* **2016**, *25*, 1355–1359. [CrossRef]
3. Burmester, G.R.; Bijlsma, J.W.J.; Cutolo, M.; McInnes, I.B. Managing rheumatic and musculoskeletal diseases-past, present and future. *Nat. Rev. Rheumatol.* **2017**, *13*, 443–448. [CrossRef]
4. Bechman, K.; Yates, M.; Galloway, J.B. The new entries in the therapeutic armamentarium: The small molecule JAK inhibitors. *Pharmacol. Res.* **2019**, *147*, 104392. [CrossRef]
5. Krüger, K. Role of janus kinase inhibitors in the treatment of rheumatic diseases. *Internist* **2019**, *60*, 1215–1220. [CrossRef] [PubMed]
6. Winthrop, K.L. The emerging safety profile of JAK inhibitors in rheumatic disease. *Nat. Rev. Rheumatol.* **2017**, *13*, 234–243. [CrossRef] [PubMed]
7. Damsky, W.; Peterson, D.; Ramseier, J.; Al-Bawardy, B.; Chun, H.; Proctor, D.; Strand, V.; Flavell, R.A.; King, B. The emerging role of Janus kinase inhibitors in the treatment of autoimmune and inflammatory diseases. *J. Allergy Clin. Immunol.* **2020**. [CrossRef] [PubMed]
8. Menet, C.J.; Van Rompaey, L.; Geney, R. Advances in the Discovery of Selective JAK Inhibitors. *Prog. Med. Chem.* **2013**, *52*, 153–223. [PubMed]
9. Salas, A.; Hernandez-Rocha, C.; Duijvestein, M.; Faubion, W.; McGovern, D.; Vermeire, S.; Vetrano, S.; Vande Casteele, N. JAK–STAT pathway targeting for the treatment of inflammatory bowel disease. *Nat. Rev. Gastroenterol. Hepatol.* **2020**, *17*, 323–337. [CrossRef]
10. Schwartz, D.M.; Kanno, Y.; Villarino, A.; Ward, M.; Gadina, M.; O'Shea, J.J. JAK inhibition as a therapeutic strategy for immune and inflammatory diseases. *Nat. Rev. Drug Discov.* **2017**, *16*, 843–862. [CrossRef]
11. O'Shea, J.J.; Plenge, R. JAKs and STATs in Immunoregulation and Immune-Mediated Disease. *Immunity* **2013**, *36*, 542–550. [CrossRef] [PubMed]
12. Villarino, A.V.; Kanno, Y.; O'Shea, J.J. Mechanisms and consequences of Jak-STAT signaling in the immune system. *Nat. Immunol.* **2017**, *18*, 374–384. [CrossRef] [PubMed]
13. Harrington, R.; Al Nokhatha, S.A.; Conway, R. Jak inhibitors in rheumatoid arthritis: An evidence-based review on the emerging clinical data. *J. Inflamm. Res.* **2020**, *13*, 519–531. [CrossRef]
14. Dhillon, S.; Keam, S.J. Filgotinib: First Approval. *Drugs* **2020**, *80*, 1987–1997. [CrossRef] [PubMed]
15. O'Shea, J.J.; Gadina, M. Selective Janus kinase inhibitors come of age. *Nat. Rev. Rheumatol.* **2019**, *15*, 74–75. [CrossRef] [PubMed]

16. Choy, E.H. Clinical significance of Janus Kinase inhibitor selectivity. *Rheumatology* **2019**, *58*, 953–962. [CrossRef]
17. McInnes, I.B.; Byers, N.L.; Higgs, R.E.; Lee, J.; Macias, W.L.; Na, S.; Ortmann, R.A.; Rocha, G.; Rooney, T.P.; Wehrman, T.; et al. Comparison of baricitinib, upadacitinib, and tofacitinib mediated regulation of cytokine signaling in human leukocyte subpopulations. *Arthritis Res. Ther.* **2019**, *21*, 1–10. [CrossRef]
18. Russell, A.S. Activated lymphocytes in the peripheral blood of patients with rheumatoid arthritis. *J. Rheumatol.* **1990**, *17*, 589–596.
19. Kitanaga, Y.; Imamura, E.; Nakahara, Y.; Fukahori, H.; Fujii, Y.; Kubo, S.; Nakayamada, S.; Tanaka, Y. In vitro pharmacological effects of peficitinib on lymphocyte activation: A potential treatment for systemic sclerosis with JAK inhibitors. *Rheumatology* **2020**, *59*, 1957–1968. [CrossRef]
20. Barry, S.P.; Townsend, P.A.; Knight, R.A.; Scarabelli, T.M.; Latchman, D.S.; Stephanou, A. STAT3 modulates the DNA damage response pathway. *Int. J. Exp. Pathol.* **2010**, *91*, 506–514. [CrossRef]
21. Bonner, J.A.; Trummell, H.Q.; Bonner, A.B.; Willey, C.D.; Bredel, M.; Yang, E.S. Enhancement of Cetuximab-Induced Radiosensitization by JAK-1 Inhibition. *BMC Cancer* **2015**, *15*, 1–12. [CrossRef]
22. Gupta, P.; Sharma, Y.; Viswanathan, P.; Gupta, S. Cellular cytokine receptor signaling and ATM pathway intersections affect hepatic DNA repair. *Cytokine* **2020**, *127*, 154946. [CrossRef] [PubMed]
23. Nieborowska-Skorska, M.; Maifrede, S.; Dasgupta, Y.; Sullivan, K.; Flis, S.; Le, B.V.; Solecka, M.; Belyaeva, E.A.; Kubovcakova, L.; Nawrocki, M.; et al. Ruxolitinib-induced defects in DNA repair cause sensitivity to PARP inhibitors in myeloproliferative neoplasms. *Blood* **2017**, *130*, 2848–2859. [CrossRef] [PubMed]
24. Yang, P.L.; Liu, L.X.; Li, E.M.; Xu, L.Y. Stat3, the challenge for chemotherapeutic and radiotherapeutic efficacy. *Cancers* **2020**, *12*, 2459. [CrossRef]
25. Bonner, W.M.; Redon, C.E.; Dickey, J.S.; Nakamura, A.J.; Sedelnikova, O.A.; Solier, S.; Pommier, Y. GammaH2AX and cancer. *Nat. Rev. Cancer* **2008**, *8*, 957–967. [CrossRef]
26. Marková, E.; Schultz, N.; Belyaev, I.Y. Kinetics and dose-response of residual 53BP1/γ-H2AX foci: Co-localization, relationship with DSB repair and clonogenic survival. *Int. J. Radiat. Biol.* **2007**, *83*, 319–329. [CrossRef]
27. Rothkamm, K.; Barnard, S.; Moquet, J.; Ellender, M.; Rana, Z.; Burdak-Rothkamm, S. DNA damage foci: Meaning and significance. *Environ. Mol. Mutagen.* **2015**, *56*, 491–504. [CrossRef] [PubMed]
28. Reddig, A.; Roggenbuck, D.; Reinhold, D. Comparison of different immunoassays for γH2AX quantification. *J. Lab. Precis. Med.* **2018**, *3*, 80. [CrossRef]
29. Willitzki, A.; Lorenz, S.; Hiemann, R.; Guttek, K.; Goihl, A.; Hartig, R.; Conrad, K.; Feist, E.; Sack, U.; Schierack, P.; et al. Fully automated analysis of chemically induced γH2AX foci in human peripheral blood mononuclear cells by indirect immunofluorescence. *Cytom. A* **2013**, *83*, 1017–1026. [CrossRef]
30. Wöltgens, J.H.M.; Lyaruu, D.M.; Bronckers, A.L.J.J.; Van Duin, M.A.; Bervoets, T.J.M. Effect of methotrexate on cell proliferation in developing hamster molar tooth germs in vitro. *Eur. J. Oral Sci.* **1998**, *106*, 156–159. [CrossRef]
31. Lefevre, P.L.C.; Vande Casteele, N. Clinical Pharmacology of Janus Kinase Inhibitors in Inflammatory Bowel Disease. *J. Crohns. Colitis* **2020**, *14*, S725–S736. [CrossRef]
32. Angelini, J.; Talotta, R.; Roncato, R.; Fornasier, G.; Barbiero, G.; Cin, L.D.; Brancati, S.; Scaglione, F. JAK-inhibitors for the treatment of rheumatoid arthritis: A focus on the present and an outlook on the future. *Biomolecules* **2020**, *10*, 1002. [CrossRef]
33. Gilead Sciences Gilead Receives Complete Response Letter for Filgotinib for the Treatment of Moderately to Severely Active Rheumatoid Arthritis. Available online: https://www.businesswire.com/news/home/20200818005811/en/ (accessed on 30 December 2020).
34. Markham, A.; Keam, S.J. Peficitinib: First Global Approval. *Drugs* **2019**, *79*, 887–891. [CrossRef]
35. Tanaka, Y.; Izutsu, H. Peficitinib for the treatment of rheumatoid arthritis: An overview from clinical trials. *Expert Opin. Pharmacother.* **2020**, *21*, 1015–1025. [CrossRef]
36. Pope, J.; Sawant, R.; Tundia, N.; Du, E.X.; Qi, C.Z.; Song, Y.; Tang, P.; Betts, K.A. Comparative Efficacy of JAK Inhibitors for Moderate-To-Severe Rheumatoid Arthritis: A Network Meta-Analysis. *Adv. Ther.* **2020**, *37*, 2356–2372. [CrossRef]
37. Lee, Y.H.; Song, G.G. Comparative efficacy and safety of tofacitinib, baricitinib, upadacitinib, and filgotinib in active rheumatoid arthritis refractory to biologic disease-modifying antirheumatic drugs. *Z. Rheumatol.* **2020**. [CrossRef]
38. Dowty, M.E.; Lin, T.H.; Jesson, M.I.; Hegen, M.; Martin, D.A.; Katkade, V.; Menon, S.; Telliez, J.B. Janus kinase inhibitors for the treatment of rheumatoid arthritis demonstrate similar profiles of in vitro cytokine receptor inhibition. *Pharmacol. Res. Perspect.* **2019**, *7*, 1–11. [CrossRef] [PubMed]
39. Damoiseaux, J. The IL-2—IL-2 receptor pathway in health and disease: The role of the soluble IL-2 receptor. *Clin. Immunol.* **2020**, *218*, 108515. [CrossRef] [PubMed]
40. Shatrova, A.N.; Mityushova, E.V.; Vassilieva, I.O.; Aksenov, N.D.; Zenin, V.V.; Nikolsky, N.N.; Marakhova, I.I. Time-dependent regulation of IL-2R α-chain (CD25) expression by TCR signal strength and IL-2-induced STAT5 signaling in activated human blood T lymphocytes. *PLoS ONE* **2016**, *11*, e167215. [CrossRef] [PubMed]
41. Nakajima, H.; Liu, X.W.; Wynshaw-Boris, A.; Rosenthal, L.A.; Imada, K.; Finbloom, D.S.; Hennighausen, L.; Leonard, W.J. An indirect effect of Stat5a in IL-2-induced proliferation: A critical role for stat5a in IL-2-mediated IL-2 receptor α chain induction. *Immunity* **1997**, *7*, 691–701. [CrossRef]

42. Parampalli Yajnanarayana, S.; Stübig, T.; Cornez, I.; Alchalby, H.; Schönberg, K.; Rudolph, J.; Triviai, I.; Wolschke, C.; Heine, A.; Brossart, P.; et al. JAK1/2 inhibition impairs T cell function in vitro and in patients with myeloproliferative neoplasms. *Br. J. Haematol.* **2015**, *169*, 824–833. [CrossRef] [PubMed]
43. Nesher, G.; Moore, T.L. The in vitro effects of methotrexate on peripheral blood mononuclear cells: Modulation by methyl donors and spermidine. *Arthritis Rheum.* **1990**, *33*, 954–959. [CrossRef] [PubMed]
44. Genestier, L.; Paillot, R.; Fournel, S.; Ferraro, C.; Miossec, P.; Revillard, J.P. Immunosuppressive properties of methotrexate: Apoptosis and clonal deletion of activated peripheral T cells. *J. Clin. Investig.* **1998**, *102*, 322–328. [CrossRef] [PubMed]
45. Fairbanks, L.D.; Rückemann, K.; Qiu, Y.; Hawrylowicz, C.M.; Richards, D.F.; Swaminathan, R.; Kirschbaum, B.; Simmonds, H.A. Methotrexate inhibits the first committed step of purine biosynthesis in mitogen-stimulated human T-lymphocytes: A metabolic basis for efficacy in rheumatoid arthritis? *Biochem. J.* **1999**, *342*, 143–152. [CrossRef]
46. Herman, S.; Zurgil, N.; Deutsch, M. Low dose methotrexate induces apoptosis with reactive oxygen species involvement in T lymphocytic cell lines to a greater extent than in monocytic lines. *Inflamm. Res.* **2005**, *54*, 273–280. [CrossRef] [PubMed]
47. Romão, V.C.; Lima, A.; Bernardes, M.; Canhão, H.; Fonseca, J.E. Three decades of low-dose methotrexate in rheumatoid arthritis: Can we predict toxicity? *Immunol. Res.* **2014**, *60*, 289–310. [CrossRef]
48. Bedoui, Y.; Guillot, X.; Sélambarom, J.; Guiraud, P.; Giry, C.; Jaffar-Bandjee, M.C.; Ralandison, S.; Gasque, P. Methotrexate an old drug with new tricks. *Int. J. Mol. Sci.* **2019**, *20*, 5023. [CrossRef]
49. Vítor, A.C.; Huertas, P.; Legube, G.; de Almeida, S.F. Studying DNA Double-Strand Break Repair: An Ever-Growing Toolbox. *Front. Mol. Biosci.* **2020**, *7*, 24. [CrossRef]
50. Jeggo, P.A.; Löbrich, M. How cancer cells hijack DNA double-strand break repair pathways to gain genomic instability. *Biochem. J.* **2015**, *471*, 1–11. [CrossRef]
51. Turinetto, V.; Giachino, C. Survey and summary multiple facets of histone variant H2AX: A DNA double-strand-break marker with several biological functions. *Nucleic Acids Res.* **2015**, *43*, 2489–2498. [CrossRef]
52. Tanaka, T.; Kajstura, M.; Halicka, H.D.; Traganos, F.; Darzynkiewicz, Z. Constitutive histone H2AX phosphorylation and ATM activation are strongly amplified during mitogenic stimulation of lymphocytes. *Cell Prolif.* **2007**, *40*, 1–13. [CrossRef] [PubMed]
53. Vignon, C.; Debeissat, C.; Georget, M.T.; Bouscary, D.; Gyan, E.; Rosset, P.; Herault, O. Flow Cytometric Quantification of All Phases of the Cell Cycle and Apoptosis in a Two-Color Fluorescence Plot. *PLoS ONE* **2013**, *8*, e68425. [CrossRef] [PubMed]
54. Hall, W.A.; Sabharwal, L.; Udhane, V.; Maranto, C.; Nevalainen, M.T. Cytokines, JAK-STAT Signaling and Radiation-Induced DNA Repair in Solid Tumors: Novel Opportunities for Radiation Therapy. *Int. J. Biochem. Cell Biol.* **2020**, *127*, 105827. [CrossRef] [PubMed]
55. Spitzner, M.; Ebner, R.; Wolff, H.A.; Michael Ghadimi, B.; Wienands, J.; Grade, M. STAT3: A novel molecular mediator of resistance to chemoradiotherapy. *Cancers* **2014**, *6*, 1986–2011. [CrossRef]
56. Wang, X.; Zhang, X.; Qiu, C.; Yang, N. STAT3 Contributes to Radioresistance in Cancer. *Front. Oncol.* **2020**, *10*, 1–8. [CrossRef] [PubMed]
57. Maranto, C.; Udhane, V.; Hoang, D.T.; Gu, L.; Alexeev, V.; Malas, K.; Cardenas, K.; Brody, J.R.; Rodeck, U.; Bergom, C.; et al. STAT5A/B Blockade Sensitizes Prostate Cancer to Radiation through Inhibition of RAD51 and DNA Repair. *Clin. Cancer Res.* **2018**, *24*, 1917–1931. [CrossRef]
58. Pharmacology Review NDAReference ID: 3205502. Available online: https://www.accessdata.fda.gov/drugsatfda_docs/nda/2012/203214Orig1s000PharmR.pdf (accessed on 18 March 2021).
59. Pharmacology Review NDAReference ID: 4261989. Available online: https://www.accessdata.fda.gov/drugsatfda_docs/nda/2018/207924Orig1s000PharmR.pdf (accessed on 18 March 2021).
60. Clinical Pharmacology and Biopharmaceutics Review NDAReference ID: 4435111. Available online: https://www.accessdata.fda.gov/drugsatfda_docs/nda/2019/211675Orig1s000ClinPharmR.pdf (accessed on 18 March 2021).
61. Assessment Report EMA/CHMP/853224/2016. Available online: https://www.ema.europa.eu/en/documents/assessment-report/xeljanz-epar-public-assessment-report_en.pdf (accessed on 18 March 2021).
62. Assessment Report EMA/520470/2020. Available online: https://www.ema.europa.eu/en/documents/variation-report/olumiant-h-c-4085-ii-0016-epar-assessment-report-variation_en.pdf (accessed on 18 March 2021).
63. Assessment Report EMA/608624/2019. Available online: https://www.ema.europa.eu/en/documents/assessment-report/rinvoq-epar-public-assessment-report_en.pdf (accessed on 18 March 2021).
64. Assessment Report EMA/424374/2020. Available online: https://www.ema.europa.eu/en/documents/assessment-report/jyseleca-epar-public-assessment-report_en.pdf (accessed on 18 March 2021).
65. Vanhoutte, F.; Mazur, M.; Voloshyn, O.; Stanislavchuk, M.; Van der Aa, A.; Namour, F.; Galien, R.; Meuleners, L.; van 't Klooster, G. Efficacy, Safety, Pharmacokinetics, and Pharmacodynamics of Filgotinib, a Selective JAK-1 Inhibitor, After Short-Term Treatment of Rheumatoid Arthritis: Results of Two Randomized Phase IIa Trials. *Arthritis Rheumatol.* **2017**, *69*, 1949–1959. [CrossRef]
66. Traves, P.G.; Murray, B.; Campigotto, F.; Galien, R.; Meng, A.; Di Paolo, J.A. JAK selectivity and the implications for clinical inhibition of pharmacodynamic cytokine signalling by filgotinib, upadacitinib, tofacitinib and baricitinib. *Ann. Rheum. Dis.* **2021**. [CrossRef]
67. Kameda, H.; Takeuchi, T.; Yamaoka, K.; Oribe, M.; Kawano, M.; Zhou, Y.; Othman, A.A.; Pangan, A.L.; Kitamura, S.; Meerwein, S.; et al. Efficacy and safety of upadacitinib in Japanese patients with rheumatoid arthritis (SELECT-SUNRISE): A placebo-controlled phase IIb/III study. *Rheumatology* **2020**, *59*, 3303–3313. [CrossRef]

68. Weinhold, K.J.; Bukowski, J.F.; Brennan, T.V.; Noveck, R.J.; Staats, J.S.; Lin, L.; Stempora, L.; Hammond, C.; Wouters, A.; Mojcik, C.F.; et al. Reversibility of peripheral blood leukocyte phenotypic and functional changes after exposure to and withdrawal from tofacitinib, a Janus kinase inhibitor, in healthy volunteers. *Clin. Immunol.* **2018**, *191*, 10–20. [CrossRef]
69. Nocturne, G.; Pascaud, J.; Ly, B.; Tahmasebi, F.; Mariette, X. JAK inhibitors alter NK cell functions and may impair immunosurveillance against lymphomagenesis. *Cell. Mol. Immunol.* **2020**, *17*, 552–553. [CrossRef]
70. Parmentier, J.M.; Voss, J.; Graff, C.; Schwartz, A.; Argiriadi, M.; Friedman, M.; Camp, H.S.; Padley, R.J.; George, J.S.; Hyland, D.; et al. In vitro and in vivo characterization of the JAK1 selectivity of upadacitinib (ABT-494). *BMC Rheumatol.* **2018**, *2*, 1–11. [CrossRef]
71. Genovese, M.C.; Smolen, J.S.; Weinblatt, M.E.; Burmester, G.R.; Meerwein, S.; Camp, H.S.; Wang, L.; Othman, A.A.; Khan, N.; Pangan, A.L.; et al. Efficacy and Safety of ABT-494, a Selective JAK-1 Inhibitor, in a Phase IIb Study in Patients With Rheumatoid Arthritis and an Inadequate Response to Methotrexate. *Arthritis Rheumatol.* **2016**, *68*, 2857–2866. [CrossRef]
72. Tarrant, J.M.; Galien, R.; Li, W.; Goyal, L.; Pan, Y.; Hawtin, R.; Zhang, W.; Van der Aa, A.; Taylor, P.C. Filgotinib, a JAK1 Inhibitor, Modulates Disease-Related Biomarkers in Rheumatoid Arthritis: Results from Two Randomized, Controlled Phase 2b Trials. *Rheumatol. Ther.* **2020**, *7*, 173–190. [CrossRef] [PubMed]
73. Galien, R.; Brys, R.; Van Der Aa, A.; Harrison, P.; Tasset, C. Absence of effects of filgotinib on erythrocytes, CD8+ and NK cells in rheumatoid arthritis patients brings further evidence for the JAK1 selectivity of filgotinib. *Arthritis Rheumatol.* **2015**, *67*, 3–4.
74. Bottos, A.; Gotthardt, D.; Gill, J.W.; Gattelli, A.; Frei, A.; Tzankov, A.; Sexl, V.; Wodnar-Filipowicz, A.; Hynes, N.E. Decreased NK-cell tumour immunosurveillance consequent to JAK inhibition enhances metastasis in breast cancer models. *Nat. Commun.* **2016**, *7*, 1–12. [CrossRef] [PubMed]
75. Galita, G.; Brzezińska, O.; Gulbas, I.; Sarnik, J.; Poplawska, M.; Makowska, J.; Poplawski, T. Increased Sensitivity of PBMCs Isolated from Patients with Rheumatoid Arthritis to DNA Damaging Agents Is Connected with Inefficient DNA Repair. *J. Clin. Med.* **2020**, *9*, 988. [CrossRef] [PubMed]
76. Souliotis, V.L.; Vlachogiannis, N.I.; Pappa, M.; Argyriou, A.; Sfikakis, P.P. DNA damage accumulation, defective chromatin organization and deficient DNA repair capacity in patients with rheumatoid arthritis. *Clin. Immunol.* **2019**, *203*, 28–36. [CrossRef]
77. Shao, L. Dna damage response signals transduce stress from rheumatoid arthritis risk factors into t cell dysfunction. *Front. Immunol.* **2018**, *9*, 1–8. [CrossRef]
78. Li, Y.; Goronzy, J.J.; Weyand, C.M. DNA damage, metabolism and aging in pro-inflammatory T cells: Rheumatoid arthritis as a model system. *Exp. Gerontol.* **2018**, *105*, 118–127. [CrossRef]
79. Gremese, E.; Alivernini, S.; Tolusso, B.; Zeidler, M.P.; Ferraccioli, G. JAK inhibition by methotrexate (and csDMARDs) may explain clinical efficacy as monotherapy and combination therapy. *J. Leukoc. Biol.* **2019**, *106*, 1063–1068. [CrossRef] [PubMed]
80. Thomas, S.; Fisher, K.H.; Snowden, J.A.; Danson, S.J.; Brown, S.P. Methotrexate is a JAK/STAT pathway inhibitor. *PLoS ONE* **2015**, *10*, e130078. [CrossRef]

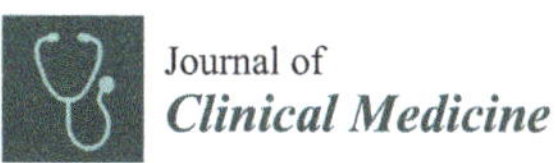
Journal of
Clinical Medicine

MDPI

Article

COVID-19 in Autoinflammatory Diseases with Immunosuppressive Treatment

Tatjana Welzel [1,2], Samuel Dembi Samba [1], Reinhild Klein [3], Johannes N. van den Anker [2,4,†] and Jasmin B. Kuemmerle-Deschner [1,*,†]

1 Pediatric Rheumatology and Autoinflammation Reference Center Tuebingen (arcT), University Children's Hospital Tuebingen, 72076 Tuebingen, Germany; tatjana.welzel@med.uni-tuebingen.de or tatjana.welzel@ukbb.ch (T.W.); Dembi.Samba@med.uni-tuebingen.de (S.D.S.)
2 Pediatric Pharmacology and Pharmacometrics, University Children's Hospital Basel (UKBB), University of Basel, 4056 Basel, Switzerland; JohannesN.vandenAnker@ukbb.ch or JVandena@childrensnational.org
3 Department of Internal Medicine II, Immunopathological Laboratory, 72076 Tuebingen, Germany; Reinhild.Klein@med.uni-tuebingen.de
4 Divison of Clinical Pharmacology, Children's National Hospital, 111 Michigan Avenue, NW, Washington, DC 20010, USA
* Correspondence: jasmin.kuemmerle-deschner@med.uni-tuebingen.de or kuemmerle.deschner@uni-tuebingen.de
† The authors contributed equally.

Abstract: COVID-19 disease increases interleukin (IL)-1β release. Anti-IL-1-treatment is effective in IL-1-mediated autoinflammatory diseases (AID). This case series presents COVID-19 in patients with IL-1-mediated and unclassified AID with immunosuppressive therapy (IT). Patient 1 is a 34-year-old woman with an unclassified AID and methotrexate. Patients 2 and 3 (14-year-old girl and 12-year-old boy, respectively) have a Cryopyrin-Associated Periodic Syndrome (*NLRP3 p.Q703K* heterozygous, CAPS) treated with canakinumab 150 mg/month since three and five years, respectively. Patient 4 is a 15-year-old girl who has had familial Mediterranean fever (*MEFV* p.*M694V* homozygous) for 3 years treated with canakinumab 150 mg/month and colchicine. All patients had a mild acute COVID-19 course, particularly the adolescent patients. A few weeks after COVID-19 recovery, both CAPS patients developed increased AID activity, necessitating anti-IL-1-treatment intensification in one patient. At day 100, one out of four patients (25%) showed positive antibody response to SARS-CoV-2. This is one of the first reports providing follow-up data about COVID-19 in AID. The risk for severe acute COVID-19 disease was mild/moderate, but increased AID activity post-COVID-19 was detected. Follow-up data and data combination are needed to expand understanding of COVID-19 and SARS-CoV-2 immunity in AID and the role of IT.

Keywords: Interleukin-1; autoinflammatory diseases; CAPS; FMF; coronavirus; SARS-CoV-2 antibody response

Citation: Welzel, T.; Samba, S.D.; Klein, R.; van den Anker, J.N.; Kuemmerle-Deschner, J.B. COVID-19 in Autoinflammatory Diseases with Immunosuppressive Treatment. *J. Clin. Med.* **2021**, *10*, 605. https://doi.org/10.3390/jcm10040605

Academic Editor: Eugen Feist, Eugen Feist and Erkan Demirkaya
Received: 27 November 2020
Accepted: 2 February 2021
Published: 5 February 2021

1. Introduction

Autoinflammatory diseases (AID) are rare, potentially life-threatening conditions caused by pathogenic gene variants encoding for inflammasomes leading to excessive production of pro-inflammatory cytokines [1]. The NLRP3 inflammasome plays an important role in the pathogenesis of the Cryopyrin-Associated Periodic Syndrome (CAPS) activating caspase-1 (Figure 1). In the familial Mediterranean fever (FMF) pathologic pyrin variants can increase caspase-1 activation. FMF and CAPS are interleukin (IL)-1 mediated AID. IL-1β is one of the most prominent products of inflammasome activation and a key regulator of systemic inflammation (Figure 1); therefore, maintenance anti-IL-1 treatment plays a pivotal role, particularly in IL-1-mediated AID management [2–4]. The achievement of low or no disease activity is crucial to avoid morbidity and mortality caused by uncontrolled inflammation. Infections can trigger disease activity in AID. High disease activity results in disease flares with fevers, inflammation of joints, eyes, skin and serous membranes coupled with increased inflammatory markers, and may result in a macrophage activation syndrome, similar to cytokine storm syndrome (CSS) [5–9].

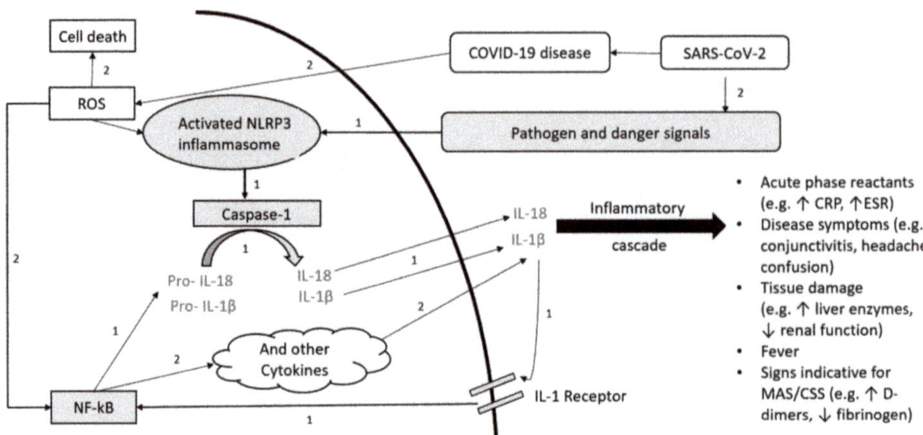

Figure 1. Schematic overview of the pathogenesis for IL-1-mediated autoimmune disease (AID) and COVID-19. (1.) Pathogenesis of NLRP3 Inflammasome associated AID (**gray**): Inflammasome formation is induced by a variety of triggers. Activated NLRP3 subsequently drives caspase-1 activation. Caspase-1 mediates transformation from pro-IL-1β and pro-IL-18 to active IL-1β and IL-18. The positive feedback loop stimulates NF-kB. (2.) SARS-CoV-2 pathogenesis (**white**): SARS-CoV-2 can stimulate a hyperinflammatory immune response with epithelial cell-mediated production of reactive oxygen species (ROS). ROS can stimulate NF-kB and NLRP3. Both pathways (1. and 2.) result in increased cytokine levels with laboratory signs and clinical symptoms associated with hypercytokinemia. Abbreviations: SARS-CoV-2: severe acute respiratory syndrome coronavirus 2; COVID-19: coronavirus disease 2019; ROS: reactive oxygen species; NLRP3: (NOD)-like receptor protein 3; NF-kB: nuclear factor kappa B; IL: interleukin; CRP: C-reactive protein, ESR: Erythrocyte sedimentation rate, MAS: macrophage activation syndrome; CSS: cytokine storm syndrome.

The coronavirus disease 2019 (COVID-19) is associated with cytokine dysregulation, increased IL-1β, tumor necrosis factor (TNF) and IL-6 release with hyperinflammation and risk of CSS (Figure 1) [10–14]. Poor COVID-19 outcome correlates with clinical and laboratory features of the CSS [5]. The avoidance of hypercytokinemia is a pivotal therapeutic aim in COVID-19, similar to AID, and cytokine targeting agents, such as anti-IL-1 treatment, anti-IL-6 treatment or Janus kinase inhibitors may be promising [12,13,15]. Whereas male sex, older age, smoking and comorbidities/underlying diseases, such as cardiovascular and respiratory diseases, diabetes mellitus or obesity seem to be related with higher risk for severe COVID-19 [16–19], children seem to be less severely affected compared to adults [20,21]. However, in the past months reports about a pediatric inflammatory multisystem syndrome temporally associated with COVID-19 (PIMS-TS)/multisystem inflammatory condition associated with COVID-19 (MIS-C) in children are emerging [22–24]. It is known that infection can trigger AID activity. Increased AID activity or AID flares are also associated with cytokine release and hypercytokinemia. Therefore, it might be possible that COVID-19 and the underlying AID may influence each other with increased risk for CSS. Several AID patients have maintenance immunosuppressive treatments (IT), which is also used in COVID-19 treatment. Patients receiving IT in general seem not to be at increased risk to develop COVID-19 or to show more severe disease courses [25–28]. Up to now, outcome data for patients with underlying AID and confirmed COVID-19 are scarce and particularly follow-up data addressing the underlying AID and its disease activity are missing. Furthermore, no data and follow-up data addressing seroconversion and antibody response to SARS-CoV-2 in AID patients with IT are available.

In this case series, we describe three patients with an IL-1-mediated AID and one patient with an unclassified AID. All patients are treated with maintenance IT and developed COVID-19. We describe: (i) the acute clinical COVID-19 course and furthermore we report follow-up data for the first 100 days after COVID-19 diagnosis addressing, (ii) the clinical course of the underlying disease, (iii) laboratory data, (iv) antibody response to SARS-CoV-2, and (v) IT modifications, where needed.

2. Methods and Patients

2.1. Study Design

This is an observational single center case series of four consecutive patients with AID, who were diagnosed or highly suspected for COVID-19 in March 2020. All IL-1-mediated AID patients were treated at the time of COVID-19 symptom onset with IT according to international recommendations [3,4]. The patients had a follow-up of 100 days. At the follow-up visits, therapy was adjusted according to established treat-to-target strategies if necessary [29]. The patients' data were captured in a standardized way in the designated institutional web-based Arthritis and Rheumatism Database and Information System (ARDIS) [30]. Individual patient's informed consent was obtained for data analysis and publication. A waiver of ethical approval was obtained from the University of Tuebingen Institutional Review Board (951/2020A).

2.2. Patients

2.2.1. Patient 1

Patient 1 is a 34-year-old woman diagnosed with an unclassified AID with undifferentiated arthritis. Disease symptoms within the last 12 years were recurrent fever of 1–2 days duration every 3 to 10 weeks including highly elevated inflammatory parameters during flares, abdominal pain with diarrhea, oral aphthosis, and arthritis, mainly affecting the palmar joints. A comprehensive work-up including clinical and laboratory examinations and imaging excluded malignancies, immunodeficiencies, autoimmune diseases and infections. The institutional genetic AID panel test for common AID (e.g., AID caused by (i) IL-1, (ii) interferon, (iii) nuclear factor kappa B (NF-kB) dysregulation in keratocytes, (iv) NF-kB also affecting interferon signaling, (v) NF-kB dysregulation and granulomatous diseases and (vi) systemic macrophage activation) was negative. Treatment for arthritis was started with sulfasalazine but without any improvement. Therefore, treatment was changed to adalimumab and later to etanercept. Both biological disease modifying antirheumatic drugs (bDMARDs) had to be stopped due to side effects. For the last nine years, she has been treated with subcutaneous methotrexate (MTX) with dose increases during recent years, finally up to 20 mg weekly, resulting in mild disease activity (physician global assessment (PGA) 2).

2.2.2. Patient 2

Patient 2 is a 14-year-old girl. She lives in the same household as patient 1, who is her mother, and was diagnosed at the age of 9 years with CAPS. Since her late infancy she experienced recurrent episodes of fever, musculoskeletal complaints, gastrointestinal symptoms and fatigue coupled with severely elevated C-reactive protein (CRP) and serum amyloid A (SAA) during disease flares. A comprehensive work-up excluded malignancies, immunodeficiencies, autoimmune diseases and infections. The institutional genetic AID test detected a heterozygous p.Q703K variant in the *NLRP3* gene. As this low-penetrance variant can be associated with fevers and gastrointestinal symptoms [31], the variant was postulated as being causative for her disease symptoms. Anakinra 2 mg/kg/day was started due to moderate to high disease activity, as partial to good response to anti-IL-1 treatment has been reported for these variants [31]. At the age of 11 years a switch to canakinumab 150 mg/every 4 weeks (q4w) was established, resulting in no to mild disease activity during the last three years (PGA $\leq$ 2).

2.2.3. Patient 3

Patient 3 is the 12-year-old brother of patient 2 and the son of patient 1. He was diagnosed with CAPS (heterozygous *NLRP3* p.Q703K variant) at the age of 7 years after exclusion of malignancies, immunodeficiencies, autoimmune diseases and infections. Since age 5, he had recurrent fevers with urticaria-like rashes, abdominal pain, arthralgia/arthritis and highly elevated inflammatory markers (SAA and CRP) during flares. Treatment was started immediately, after CAPS diagnosis, with anakinra 2 mg/kg/day resulting in prompt improvement of high disease activity. A switch to canakinumab injections at 4 mg/kg/q4w was performed for better compliance. During recent years he achieved a stable mild to moderate disease activity on canakinumab 150 mg s.c/q4w (PGA 1–3).

2.2.4. Patient 4

Patient 4 is a 15-year-old girl diagnosed with FMF (homozygous p.M694V variant in the *MEFV* gene) at four years of age. Treatment was started with colchicine 0.5 mg/day with a stepwise dose increase due to persistent high clinical and laboratory disease activity. As the patient showed colchicine resistance at 1.5 mg/day and intolerance at 2 mg/day colchicine, anti-IL-1 treatment was started at the age of six years according to recommendations for FMF [3]. Treatment response was achieved with anakinra 2 mg/kg/day combined with colchicine 1 mg/day. Daily injections were not well tolerated and therefore therapy was switched to canakinumab 2 mg/kg/q4w and later 150 mg/q4w. During the last three years she showed no to mild disease activity (PGA $\leq$ 2).

2.3. Monitoring and Follow-Up Visits

The patients' monitoring included physical examination, laboratory assessments and symptom diaries. The patients captured their daily AID symptoms in a diary similar to the Autoinflammatory Disease Activity Index (AIDAI) [32]. Disease activity was assessed for the underlying AID by the physician at each clinical visit. Disease activity was defined as physician global assessment (PGA), recorded on a 10 cm visual analog scale (VAS) with 0 representing no disease activity and 10 maximum disease activity. Furthermore, disease activity was assessed by the patients (PPGA) and recorded on a 10 cm VAS comparable to the PGA. Laboratory monitoring included the inflammatory markers CRP, SAA, S-100 proteins, and erythrocyte sedimentation rate (ESR). Additionally, blood count, liver enzymes and kidney function tests were performed. SARS-CoV-2 antibody-tests were performed for each patient during follow-up visits, if the patient and their parents agreed to the test. Antibodies were detected by ELISA with an in-house assay as published previously [33]. Briefly, microtiter plates were coated with the SARS-CoV-2 proteins nucleocapsid, spike 1 (both obtained from SinoBiological; Peking, China), and the RBD-spike 1 protein (GenScript; New Jersey, USA) at concentrations of 0.1 µg/mL, 0.2 µg/mL, and 0.3 µg/mL, respectively. Patients' sera were used at a dilution of 1:500 for the demonstration of IgG- and IgM-antibodies and 1:100 for the detection of IgA-antibodies. Bound antibodies were detected with peroxidase conjugated goat anti-human IgG-, IgM- and IgA-antibodies (DIANOVA, Hamburg, Germany) at dilutions of 1:3000, 1:2000, and 1:650, respectively. As substrate o-phenylendiamine was used. Reactivity was given as arbitrary units (AU). Optimal antigen- and serum dilutions have been evaluated by serial dilutions prior to analysis. In each assay four sera with defined AU (high, medium, low, and negative) were tested as standard sera. Applying all three antigens in parallel, sensitivity of the assay for the demonstration of anti-SARS-CoV-2-antibodies was 97% and specificity 99%.

3. Results

3.1. Acute COVID-19 Course

3.1.1. Patient 1

At day one of disease onset, patient 1 developed rhinitis, fever, headache, fatigue and cough (Figure 2). On day 10, she reported a loss of taste and additionally she complained about nausea, emesis and abdominal pain. On day 14, home oxygen was started due to respiratory insufficiency. On day 21, a computed tomography of the lungs was performed showing typical signs of ground-glass opacities. MTX was administered four days before symptom onset and was discontinued when first symptoms suggestive for COVID-19 appeared. During the acute episode, no laboratory work-up was performed.

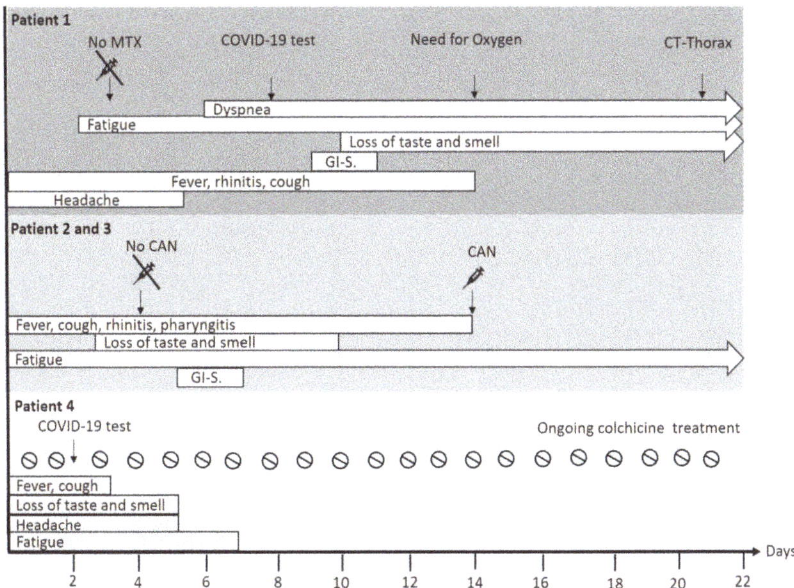

Figure 2. Overview of symptoms of the acute COVID-19 disease course in AID patients. Acute COVID-19 disease course was less severe in the three adolescent AID patients with canakinumab maintenance treatment as compared to the adult patient treated with methotrexate. Particularly patient 4, who was treated with daily colchicine and who had received canakinumab 150 mg s.c. 4 days before COVID-19 was confirmed, had a short and mild disease course. Abbreviations: CAN: Canakinumab; CT: Computed tomography; COVID-19: Coronavirus disease 2019; GI-S.: Gastrointestinal symptoms such as nausea, diarrhea, emesis, abdominal pain; MTX: Methotrexate. Legend: ⇨ongoing disease symptoms on day 22 after COVID-19 onset.

3.1.2. Patient 2 and 3

Disease courses in patients 2 and 3 were similar. They developed fever, cough, pharyngitis, fatigue and rhinitis ten days after first disease symptoms of patient 1 (Figure 2). Between day 3 and 13, both reported a loss of taste and smell. On day six, they complained about nausea and abdominal pain. Patient 2 additionally had diarrhea. At day 14 both siblings recovered and only persistent fatigue was reported. Canakinumab was administered at day 14 after symptom onset, with a total delay of 10 days compared to usual dosing regimen (Figure 2). No laboratory work-up was performed during the acute disease course.

3.1.3. Patient 4

Patient 4 developed fever, cough, loss of taste and smell, and headache four days after her last canakinumab injection (Figure 2). Cessation of cough and fever was reported two to three days after symptom onset. Disappearance of headache and normalized smell and taste was reported 5 days after the onset of COVID-19 symptoms. Fatigue was present until day 7. Recovery was reported since day 8. Canakinumab injections and also colchicine treatment were continued (Figure 2).

3.2. Follow-Up Visits

3.2.1. Patient 1

At first follow-up visit patient 1 still suffered from severe fatigue, loss of taste and smell, dyspnea and ongoing muscoloskeletal complaints with arthralgia (Table 1). PGA was estimated with 2. The ESR was mildly elevated but otherwise the laboratory results were normal (Table 2). MTX was restarted at day 90. At second follow-up taste and smell were normal, but fatigue and dyspnea during physical exercises were still present. Inflammatory parameters were no longer elevated and disease activity was stable (Tables 1 and 2).

3.2.2. Patient 2

Patient 2 reported ongoing mild to moderate fatigue and intermittent mild erythematous macular rash at the first follow-up visit. The PGA showed mild disease activity, whereas the patient estimated disease activity as moderate (Table 1). No ongoing inflammation was detected (Table 2). At second follow-up mild rash and fatigue persisted. One mild flare was reported. No inflammation was detected (Tables 1 and 2).

3.2.3. Patient 3

At the first follow-up patient 3 reported moderate erythematous macular rash, severe fatigue and arthralgia (Table 1). PGA and PPGA had increased to 4 and 7, respectively. However, laboratory results revealed no inflammation (Table 2). Between the first and second follow-up he showed typical signs of active CAPS with persistent urticarial-like rashes, conjunctivitis, sever fatigue, intermittent subfebrile temperatures and arthralgia. Additionally he complained about mild abdominal pain without signs of peritonitis, diarrhea or nausea. Vital signs, liver enzymes, kidney function tests, creatinine kinase, fibrinogen, ferritin, thrombocytes and hemoglobin were normal. The canakinumab dose was increased to 300 mg/q4w. At the second follow-up, symptoms were still present but milder (Table 1), and inflammatory markers could not be detected anymore (Table 2).

3.2.4. Patient 4

Patient 4 reported neither COVID-19 nor FMF symptoms at the first and second follow-up visits (Table 1). Laboratory parameters did not change during the follow-up period (Table 2).

3.3. Nasopharyngeal COVID-19 Tests and Antibody Response to SARS-CoV-2

Patient 1 was tested with nasopharyngeal COVID-19 test (RT-PCR) on day 8 after onset of COVID-19 symptoms and received a positive test result on day 11. Patient 2 and 3 were tested negative two days before their first COVID-19 symptoms occurred. After symptom onset, both were diagnosed clinically for COVID-19 due to suggestive symptoms and close contact to a person with confirmed COVID-19. Patient 4 was tested positive two days after onset of COVID-19 symptoms. At first follow-up visit, the antibody response to SARS-CoV-2 was tested in patient 2, confirming that she had COVID-19. At day 100 COVID-19 post-infection three out of four patients (75%) showed no antibody response to SARS-CoV-2 (Table 3).

Table 1. Clinical symptoms before and after COVID-19 symptom onset.

	PGA (0–10 cm)	PPGA (0–10 cm)	Flares/3 Months	Fever	Rash	Fatigue	Dyspnea	Arthralgia
Patient 1								
Before COVID-19	2	2	1	-	-	+	-	+
~Day 40 *	2	n.a.	n.a.	-	-	+++	++	+
~Day 100 *	2	n.a	n.a.	-	-	++	+	+
Patient 2								
Before COVID-19	≤2	≤2	0	-	-	-	-	-
Day 40 *	2	5	n.a	-	+	+/++	-	-
Day 100 *	2	2	1	-	+	+	-	-
Patient 3								
Before COVID-19	1–3	2	0	-	-	+	-	-
Day 40 *	4	7	n.a.	-	++	+++	-	+
Day 100 *,[1]	5	7	3	+/++	-	+++	-	++
Patient 4								
Before COVID-19	≤2	0	0	-	-	-	-	-
Day 40 *	2	n.a.	n.a.	-	-	-	-	+
Day 100 *	1	0	0	-	-	-	-	-

Abbreviations: PGA: physician global assessment recorded on a visual analog scale with 0= no disease activity and 10= maximum disease activity; PPGA: Disease activity estimated by the patient similar recorded to the PGA; n.a.: not available, Symptom severity: - absence, + mild, ++ moderate, +++ severe; * after COVID-19 onset; [1] five days after Canakinumab increase (300 mg/q4w).

Table 2. Laboratory results before and after COVID-19 symptom onset.

	Hb (g/dl)	Leuc (10S9/l)	Plt (10S9/l)	ESR (mm/h)	CRP (mg/dl)	IL-6 (ng/L)	S100A8/A9 (μg/mL)	sl-ILR2 (U/mL)	SAA (mg/L)
Patient 1									
Before COVID-19	11.8	5.52	197	8	0.34	<2.0	2.9	n.a.	2
~Day 40 *	12.4	5.30	256	22	0.72	3.0	16.4	267	4
~Day 100 *	11.6	5.92	231	13	1.54	n.a.	6.2	n.a.	6
Patient 2									
Before COVID-19	13.5	4.30	303	5	0.01	<2.0	11.3	n.a.	1
Day 40 *	14.3	5.09	239	n.a.	0.01	2.7	10.4	215	2
Day 100 *	13.9	5.38	301	2	0.01	n.a.	6.3	n.a.	1
Patient 3									
Before COVID-19	14.3	5.37	319	2	0.01	<2.0	3.2	n.a.	1
Day 40 *	15.0	5.63	305	4	0.02	2.7	6.9	164	2
Day 100 *,[1]	14.5	5.78	300	2	0.01	2.8	5.7	n.a.	2
Patient 4									
Before COVID-19	13.2	5.54	191	13	0.14	2.9	64.4	n.a.	19
Day 40 *	13.3	4.61	180	2	0.05	n.a.	n.a.	n.a.	10
Day 100 *	12.5	4.06	174	7	0.07	3.7	40.9	n.a	15

Abbreviations. Hb: Hemoglobin; Leuc: Leucocytes; Plt: Platelets; ESR: Erythrocyte sedimentation rate; CRP: C-reactive protein, IL-6: Interleukin-6; S100A8/A9: S100 protein A8/A9; sl-ILR2: soluble Interleukin Receptor 2; SAA: Serum Amyloid A; n.a.: not available; * after COVID-19 symptom onset; [1] five days after increased Canakinumab dose (300 mg/q4w).

Table 3. Test results for COVID-19/SARS-CoV-2 antibodies.

	COVID-19 Test (Nasopharyngeal)	SARS-CoV-2 Antibodies § (Serum)
Patient 1		
Day 8 *	Positive	n.a.
~Day 40 *	n.a.	n.a.
~Day 100 *	n.a.	Negative
Patient 2		
Day -2 (before COVID-19 symptom onset)	Negative	
Day 40 *	n.a.	Positive IgG (19.4 U/mL) and IgA (15.2 U/mL) SARS-CoV-2-nucleocapside, Positive IgG SARS-CoV-2-spike (18.3 U/mL), Positive IgG SARS-CoV-2-RBD (19.9 U/mL)
Day 100 *	n.a.	Negative
Patient 3		
Day -2 (before COVID-19 symptom onset)	Negative	n.a
Day 40 *	n.a.	n.a.
Day 100*,1	n.a.	Positive IgG (59.3 U/mL) and IgA (28.6 U/mL) SARS-CoV-2-nucleocapside
Patient 4		
Day 2*	Positive	n.a.
Day 40*	n.a.	n.a.
Day 100*	n.a.	Negative

Abbreviations: n.a.: not available; * after COVID-19 symptom onset; [1] five days after canakinumab increase (300 mg/q4w), § Antibody against SARS-CoV-2-spike, SARS-CoV-2-RBD, SARS-CoV-2-nucleocapside, Reference values: SARS-CoV-2-nucleocapside: IgG >11.0 U/mL, IgA >4.4 U/mL; SARS-CoV-2-spike: IgG >15.0 U/mL, IgA >6.0 U/mL, SARS-CoV-2-spike-RBD: IgG >15.0 U/mL, IgA >14.0 U/mL.

4. Discussion

This is one of the first case series illustrating the acute COVID-19 disease course and follow-up data in patients with IL-1-mediated and unclassified AID treated with IT. All patients had common COVID-19 symptoms and no one needed admission to the intensive care unit. The acute COVID-19 disease course was milder in the adolescent patients treated with maintenance anti-IL-1 treatment compared to the adult patient with maintenance MTX. Although all patients recovered, fatigue was a common long-lasting symptom reported by 75% of patients after acute COVID-19. One patient with CAPS experienced increased AID disease activity necessitating adjustment of anti-IL-1 treatment (canakinumab 300 mg/q4w) a few weeks after acute COVID-19 disease course. At day 100 post COVID-19-infection, in three out of four patients (75%), SARS-CoV-2 antibodies were undetectable.

4.1. COVID-19 Disease Course and AID

AID patients with IT and controlled AID activity can show typical COVID-19 symptoms, but seem not to be at increased risk for severe acute COVID-19. Typical COVID-19 symptoms are fever, respiratory symptoms (rhinitis, dyspnea, and coughing), sore throat, loss of taste/smell, muscle pain additionally headache, and gastrointestinal symptoms [34–38]. The patients in this case series showed common COVID-19 symptoms. All four patients had IT, but none had a severe disease course. These observations are in line with previous published data showing that patients with IT, particularly children, seem not to be at increased risk to develop (i) COVID-19 or (ii) a more severe disease course or (iii) an inferior outcome after being infected with COVID-19 in comparison with the general population [26–28,39–41].

Data for patients with AID are scarce. Haslak et al. studied 404 AID patients (90% FMF, 3.4% CAPS, 0.2% TRAPS, 6.1% others) with COVID-19 [25]. He reported six FMF patients with colchicine tested positive for COVID-19 and all recovered completely [25]. Additionally, he reported one asymptomatic CAPS patient with canakinumab, who was tested negative for COVID-19 although he had close contact to family members with confirmed COVID-19 [25]. Similarly, Koker et al. reported negative test results for an asymptomatic FMF patient and a CAPS patient suffering from arthralgia, both with maintenance anti-IL-1 treatment and close contact to family members with confirmed COVID-19 [27]. A 70-year-old CAPS patient treated with canakinumab 150 mg/q8w and confirmed COVID-19 showed a very mild clinical disease course with a soon recovery [42]. Usually, a 70-year-old patient would be regarded at high risk for experiencing a serious COVID-19 disease course. Therefore, the authors hypothesized that cytokine blockade may protect from cytokine storm and thus ameliorate the gravity of the clinical picture of COVID-19 [42]. COVID-19 seems to be associated with a massive inflammatory response that appears to occur via stimulation of the NLRP3 inflammasome [43]. The NLRP3 inflammasome plays also an important role in mediating systemic inflammation in CAPS (Figure 1). This raises the questions if (i) patients with NLRP3 inflammasome-associated cytokine release are at higher risk of hypercytokinemia and increased AID activity during or after acute COVID-19; and if (ii) maintenance anti-IL-1 treatment, applied in IL-1-mediated AID to avoid inflammasome activation and cytokine release, also reduces COVID-19-related cytokine dysregulation accounting for mild or asymptomatic COVID-19 disease courses in these patients. The three adolescent patients with IL-1-mediated AID and anti-IL-1 treatment in this case series had very mild COVID-19 symptoms. Whereas the FMF patient did not show any signs of increased AID activity, patient 2 reported mildly increased disease activity without need for therapy adjustment during follow-up. Patient 3 required dose increase of anti-IL-treatment (canakinumab 300 mg/q4w) a few weeks after acute COVID-19, due to moderate to severe AID activity compared to pre-COVID-19 era. Although canakinumab was administered with a delay of 10 days in patient 2 and 3 it can be expected that the IL-1β blocking effects were still present. Canakinumab has a long half-live ($t_{1/2}$) of 28 days, so that from a pharmacologic point of view 95–99% of the drug will be eliminated after 84–140 days. In comparison to the adolescent patients, patient 1 had a more severe COVID-19 disease course, which might have several reasons (e.g., age, other risk factors). In patient 1 maintenance MTX treatment was stopped with symptom occurrence. Despite the relatively short MTX plasma half-life, MTX can persist intracellularly in red blood cells as MTX polyglutamate (MTXGlu). The median half-life elimination of MTXGlu ranges from 1.2 to 4.3 weeks, resulting in a median time of 15 weeks after MTX cessation (range 3 to ≥32 weeks) to become undetectable [44]. This case series indicates that patients with IL-1-mediated or unclassified AID with maintenance IT can experience typical COVID-19 symptoms without AID flares during acute COVID-19 and seem not to be at an increased risk for a severe acute COVID-19 disease course. However, follow-up visits are important as similarly to other infections COVID-19 can increase the underlying AID activity a few weeks later with the need for therapy adjustment.

4.2. Antibody Response to SARS-CoV-2

In three out of four patients in this case series, no SARS-CoV-2 antibody response was detectable at day 100. There is evidence that most patients seroconvert to SARS-CoV-2 specific IgG antibodies within 2 to 4 weeks after symptom onset [45–47]. Murchu et al. reviewed 74 studies and reported, that IgG could be detected in all reviewed patients (N = 24) at 49–65 days and that neutralizing antibodies were detected in 92%–100% of patients up to 53 days [45]. SARS-CoV-2 antibody decline after COVID-19 is under current research. Decrease of COVID-19 immunity might be possible similar as seen in other coronaviridae [45,48]. Seow at al. detected high neutralizing antibody titers at >60 days in individuals with high peak infective doses, whereas patients with lower peaks returned to baseline over a relatively short period suggesting decrease of COVID-19 immunity [49].

To differentiate between re-infection and persistent viral shedding, To et al. performed a comparative genome virus analysis in a patient with a second episode of COVID-19 symptoms 142 days after the first confirmed COVID-19 episode and found a re-infection by a different strain [50]. Similarly, Tillett et al. detected genetically significant differences between virus variants in a patient tested positive in April and June for COVID-19 [51]. Whereas Tillett et al. reported that the second episode was symptomatically more severe than the first, Bentivegna et al. reported an asymptomatic female patient at her second COVID-19 episode [51,52]. Interestingly, she was tested positive for SARS-CoV-2-specific IgG (CLIA assay) after onset of COVID-19 symptoms [52]. Torres et al. reported an otherwise healthy female patient with COVID-19 reinfection 12 weeks after first confirmed COVID-19 [53]. At the first COVID-19 episode she was tested negative for IgG antibody response to SARS-CoV-2 at day 23, 33 and 67 [53]. Although Freeman at al. discovered that pediatric immunocompromised patients are capable of producing an antibody response to SARS-CoV-2, they reported that one out of two documented RT-PCR positive patients did not show any seroconversion [54].

At day 100, three out of four patients (75%) in our case series had no detectable antibody response. As one of these patients displayed SARS-CoV-2 antibodies at day 40, antibody loss can be postulated for this patient. For the two others patients, it cannot be determined if they (i) did not develop antibodies or (ii) had a loss of immunity. We were unable to find (i) any other follow-up data on antibody response to SARS-CoV-2 in patients with IT, immunosuppressive diseases or AID; (ii) data on COVID-19 reinfection in this particular patient group; or (iii) long-term follow-up data for antibody-responses in immunocompetent patients. Taken together, we can summarize that SARS-CoV-2 antibody decline is currently incompletely understood. The sparse data from this case series might raise the question of whether patients with IT might have a risk for no seroconversion or loss of antibody response to SARS-CoV-2. More research in this area is necessary and antibody monitoring in patients with IT might help to better understand their risk regarding COVID-19 reinfection. It is important to be aware of the possibility of COVID-19 re-infection in patients with IT.

4.3. Limitations

This case series has several limitations. First of all, the sample size is small. However, AID are orphan diseases and therefore, data of COVID-19 confirmed AID patients is rare. To our knowledge this is the first case series reporting follow-up data of COVID-19 in IL-1-mediated and undifferentiated AID patients. Moreover, particularly regarding laboratory values, there is missing data. All patients were diagnosed at the end of March through the first wave of the COVID-19 pandemic and the start of lockdown in several countries in Europe. March was a very challenging month for the health care systems in Europe as COVID-19 test resources were limited, SARS-CoV-2 antibody tests initially were not available and several university hospitals could not schedule regular visits for their chronically ill/immunosuppressed outpatients. Consequently, some diagnostic tests—now being well established—were not done regularly. In addition, some missing data can be explained as we report patients from a real-life cohort. However, standardized outcome evaluation of the included patients combined with advanced laboratory testing resulted in comparable high-quality data captured in ARDIS. Antibody response was only tested using ELISA for all patients at day 100 and only in patient 2 at day 40. Additional nasopharyngeal COVID-19 RT-PCR was not performed at day 40 and 100, due to the reasons explained above. Although data from this case series are not generalizable, due to small sample size, important insights can be gained which may be taken into account in case AID patients with and without IT develop COVID-19.

5. Conclusions

Patients with IL-1-mediated or unclassified AID and maintenance IT can experience typical COVID-19 symptoms, but seem not to be at an increased risk for severe acute

COVID-19 disease course. However, follow-up visits are important to monitor AID activity as COVID-19 may increase underlying AID activity a few weeks after acute infection, necessitating IT dose adjustments. In this case series, only one patient had detectable antibodies against SARS-CoV-2 at day 100. Therefore, AID patients with IT should be monitored carefully for new COVID-19 symptoms and should be re-tested if indicated. Data from international registries and follow-up data combination of COVID-19 in AID and monitoring of SARS-CoV-2 antibodies will help to better understand COVID-19 and SARS-CoV-2 immunity in AID and the role of IT.

Author Contributions: Conceptualization, T.W. and J.N.v.d.A.; data curation, T.W., S.D.S., R.K.; writing—original draft preparation, T.W.; patients care: S.D.S. and J.B.K.-D.; writing—review and editing, S.D.S., R.K., J.N.v.d.A. and J.B.K.-D.; supervision, J.N.v.d.A. and J.B.K.-D. All authors have read and agreed to the published version of the manuscript.

Funding: This research received no external funding.

Institutional Review Board Statement: A waiver of ethical approval was obtained from the University of Tuebingen Institutional Review Board (951/2020A).

Informed Consent Statement: Informed consent was obtained from all subjects involved in the study.

Data Availability Statement: Data is contained within the article.

Acknowledgments: We thank cand. med. Lea Oefelein, Christine Michler (arcT coordinator) and Susanne Sterz (arcT study nurse) for their support in administrative tasks. Furthermore, we are thankful to the patients for the informed consent provided to publish these data.

Conflicts of Interest: T.W., S.D.S., R.K. and J.N.v.d.A. declare no conflict of interest. J.B.K.-D. received grant support and speaker's fees from Novartis and SOBI. No external source had a role in the design of this article; in the collection, analyses, or interpretation of data; in the writing of the manuscript, or in the decision to publish this article.

References

1. Broderick, L.; De Nardo, D.; Franklin, B.S.; Hoffman, H.M.; Latz, E. The inflammasomes and autoinflammatory syndromes. *Annu. Rev. Pathol.* **2015**, *10*, 395–424. [CrossRef]
2. De Torre-Minguela, C.; Mesa Del Castillo, P.; Pelegrin, P. The NLRP3 and Pyrin Inflammasomes: Implications in the Pathophysiology of Autoinflammatory Diseases. *Front. Immunol.* **2017**, *8*, 43. [CrossRef] [PubMed]
3. Ozen, S.; Demirkaya, E.; Erer, B.; Livneh, A.; Ben-Chetrit, E.; Giancane, G.; Ozdogan, H.; Abu, I.; Gattorno, M.; Hawkins, P.N.; et al. EULAR recommendations for the management of familial Mediterranean fever. *Ann. Rheum. Dis.* **2016**, *75*, 644–651. [CrossRef] [PubMed]
4. Ter Haar, N.M.; Oswald, M.; Jeyaratnam, J.; Anton, J.; Barron, K.S.; Brogan, P.A.; Cantarini, L.; Galeotti, C.; Grateau, G.; Hentgen, V.; et al. Recommendations for the management of autoinflammatory diseases. *Ann. Rheum. Dis.* **2015**, *74*, 1636–1644. [CrossRef] [PubMed]
5. Henderson, L.A.; Canna, S.W.; Schulert, G.S.; Volpi, S.; Lee, P.Y.; Kernan, K.F.; Caricchio, R.; Mahmud, S.; Hazen, M.M.; Halyabar, O.; et al. On the alert for cytokine storm: Immunopathology in COVID-19. *Arthritis Rheumatol.* **2020**, *72*, 1059–1063. [CrossRef]
6. Rigante, D.; Emmi, G.; Fastiggi, M.; Silvestri, E.; Cantarini, L. Macrophage activation syndrome in the course of monogenic autoinflammatory disorders. *Clin. Rheumatol.* **2015**, *34*, 1333–1339. [CrossRef]
7. Horneff, G.; Rhouma, A.; Weber, C.; Lohse, P. Macrophage activation syndrome as the initial manifestation of tumour necrosis factor receptor 1-associated periodic syndrome (TRAPS). *Clin. Exp. Rheumatol.* **2013**, *31*, 99–102.
8. Rigante, D.; Capoluongo, E.; Bertoni, B.; Ansuini, V.; Chiaretti, A.; Piastra, M.; Pulitano, S.; Genovese, O.; Compagnone, A.; Stabile, A. First report of macrophage activation syndrome in hyperimmunoglobulinemia D with periodic fever syndrome. *Arthritis Rheumatol.* **2007**, *56*, 658–661. [CrossRef]
9. Lachmann, H.J. Periodic fever syndromes. *Best Pract. Res. Clin. Rheumatol.* **2017**, *31*, 596–609. [CrossRef]
10. Conti, P.; Ronconi, G.; Caraffa, A.; Gallenga, C.E.; Ross, R.; Frydas, I.; Kritas, S.K. Induction of pro-inflammatory cytokines (IL-1 and IL-6) and lung inflammation by Coronavirus-19 (COVI-19 or SARS-CoV-2): Anti-inflammatory strategies. *J. Biol. Regul. Homeost. Agents* **2020**, *34*, 327–331. [PubMed]
11. Ouedraogo, D.D.; Tiendrebeogo, W.J.S.; Kabore, F.; Ntsiba, H. COVID-19, chronic inflammatory rheumatic disease and anti-rheumatic treatments. *Clin. Rheumatol.* **2020**, *39*, 2069–2075. [CrossRef]
12. Zhang, C.; Wu, Z.; Li, J.W.; Zhao, H.; Wang, G.Q. Cytokine release syndrome in severe COVID-19: Interleukin-6 receptor antagonist tocilizumab may be the key to reduce mortality. *Int. J. Antimicrob. Agents* **2020**, *55*, 105954. [CrossRef] [PubMed]

13. Bhaskar, S.; Sinha, A.; Banach, M.; Mittoo, S.; Weissert, R.; Kass, J.S.; Rajagopal, S.; Pai, A.R.; Kutty, S. Cytokine Storm in COVID-19-Immunopathological Mechanisms, Clinical Considerations, and Therapeutic Approaches: The REPROGRAM Consortium Position Paper. *Front. Immunol.* **2020**, *11*, 1648. [CrossRef]
14. Qin, C.; Zhou, L.; Hu, Z.; Zhang, S.; Yang, S.; Tao, Y.; Xie, C.; Ma, K.; Shang, K.; Wang, W.; et al. Dysregulation of Immune Response in Patients With Coronavirus 2019 (COVID-19) in Wuhan, China. *Clin. Infect. Dis.* **2020**, *71*, 762–768. [CrossRef]
15. Fajgenbaum, D.C.; June, C.H. Cytokine Storm. *New Engl. J. Med.* **2020**, *383*, 2255–2273. [CrossRef] [PubMed]
16. Li, X.; Xu, S.; Yu, M.; Wang, K.; Tao, Y.; Zhou, Y.; Shi, J.; Zhou, M.; Wu, B.; Yang, Z.; et al. Risk factors for severity and mortality in adult COVID-19 inpatients in Wuhan. *J. Allergy Clin. Immunol.* **2020**, *146*, 110–118. [CrossRef]
17. Zhou, F.; Yu, T.; Du, R.; Fan, G.; Liu, Y.; Liu, Z.; Xiang, J.; Wang, Y.; Song, B.; Gu, X.; et al. Clinical course and risk factors for mortality of adult inpatients with COVID-19 in Wuhan, China: A retrospective cohort study. *Lancet* **2020**, *395*, 1054–1062. [CrossRef]
18. Richardson, S.; Hirsch, J.S.; Narasimhan, M.; Crawford, J.M.; McGinn, T.; Davidson, K.W.; Northwell, C.-R.C.; Barnaby, D.P.; Becker, L.B.; Chelico, J.D.; et al. Presenting Characteristics, Comorbidities, and Outcomes Among 5700 Patients Hospitalized With COVID-19 in the New York City Area. *JAMA* **2020**, *323*, 2052–2059. [CrossRef]
19. Zheng, Z.; Peng, F.; Xu, B.; Zhao, J.; Liu, H.; Peng, J.; Li, Q.; Jiang, C.; Zhou, Y.; Liu, S.; et al. Risk factors of critical & mortal COVID-19 cases: A systematic literature review and meta-analysis. *J. Infect.* **2020**, *81*, e16–e25.
20. Lu, X.; Zhang, L.; Du, H.; Zhang, J.; Li, Y.Y.; Qu, J.; Zhang, W.; Wang, Y.; Bao, S.; Li, Y.; et al. SARS-CoV-2 Infection in Children. *New Engl. J. Med.* **2020**, *382*, 1663–1665. [CrossRef]
21. Dong, Y.; Mo, X.; Hu, Y.; Qi, X.; Jiang, F.; Jiang, Z.; Tong, S. Epidemiology of COVID-19 Among Children in China. *Pediatrics* **2020**, *145*, e20200702. [CrossRef] [PubMed]
22. Belhadjer, Z.; Meot, M.; Bajolle, F.; Khraiche, D.; Legendre, A.; Abakka, S.; Auriau, J.; Grimaud, M.; Oualha, M.; Beghetti, M.; et al. Acute Heart Failure in Multisystem Inflammatory Syndrome in Children in the Context of Global SARS-CoV-2 Pandemic. *Circulation* **2020**, *142*, 429–436. [CrossRef] [PubMed]
23. Whittaker, E.; Bamford, A.; Kenny, J.; Kaforou, M.; Jones, C.E.; Shah, P.; Ramnarayan, P.; Fraisse, A.; Miller, O.; Davies, P.; et al. Clinical Characteristics of 58 Children With a Pediatric Inflammatory Multisystem Syndrome Temporally Associated With SARS-CoV-2. *JAMA* **2020**, *324*, 259–269. [CrossRef]
24. Riphagen, S.; Gomez, X.; Gonzalez-Martinez, C.; Wilkinson, N.; Theocharis, P. Hyperinflammatory shock in children during COVID-19 pandemic. *Lancet* **2020**, *395*, 1607–1608. [CrossRef]
25. Haslak, F.; Yildiz, M.; Adrovic, A.; Sahin, S.; Koker, O.; Aliyeva, A.; Barut, K.; Kasapcopur, O. Management of childhood-onset autoinflammatory diseases during the COVID-19 pandemic. *Rheumatol. Int.* **2020**, *40*, 1423–1431. [CrossRef] [PubMed]
26. Filocamo, G.; Minoia, F.; Carbogno, S.; Costi, S.; Romano, M.; Cimaz, R. Pediatric Rheumatology Group of the Milan A: Absence of severe complications from SARS-CoV-2 infection in children with rheumatic diseases treated with biologic drugs. *J. Rheumatol.* **2020**. [CrossRef]
27. Koker, O.; Demirkan, F.G.; Kayaalp, G.; Cakmak, F.; Tanatar, A.; Karadag, S.G.; Sonmez, H.E.; Omeroglu, R.; Aktay Ayaz, N. Does immunosuppressive treatment entail an additional risk for children with rheumatic diseases? A survey-based study in the era of COVID-19. *Rheumatol. Int.* **2020**, *40*, 1613–1623. [CrossRef] [PubMed]
28. Favalli, E.G.; Monti, S.; Ingegnoli, F.; Balduzzi, S.; Caporali, R.; Montecucco, C. Incidence of COVID-19 in Patients With Rheumatic Diseases Treated With Targeted Immunosuppressive Drugs: What Can We Learn From Observational Data? *Arthritis Rheumatol.* **2020**, *72*, 1600–1606. [CrossRef]
29. Hansmann, S.; Lainka, E.; Horneff, G.; Holzinger, D.; Rieber, N.; Jansson, A.F.; Rosen-Wolff, A.; Erbis, G.; Prelog, M.; Brunner, J.; et al. Consensus protocols for the diagnosis and management of the hereditary autoinflammatory syndromes CAPS, TRAPS and MKD/HIDS: A German PRO-KIND initiative. *Pediatr. Rheumatol. Online J.* **2020**, *18*, 17. [CrossRef]
30. Kuemmerle-Deschner, J.; Ihle, J.; Orlikowski, T.; Dannecker, G.E. ARDIS-Arthritis and Rheumatism Database and Information System. *Arthritis Rheum.* **1999**, *42*, S327.
31. Kuemmerle-Deschner, J.B.; Verma, D.; Endres, T.; Broderick, L.; de Jesus, A.A.; Hofer, F.; Blank, N.; Krause, K.; Rietschel, C.; Horneff, G.; et al. Clinical and Molecular Phenotypes of Low-Penetrance Variants of NLRP3: Diagnostic and Therapeutic Challenges. *Arthritis Rheumatol.* **2017**, *69*, 2233–2240. [CrossRef] [PubMed]
32. Piram, M.; Frenkel, J.; Gattorno, M.; Ozen, S.; Lachmann, H.J.; Goldbach-Mansky, R.; Hentgen, V.; Neven, B.; Stojanovic, K.S.; Simon, A.; et al. A preliminary score for the assessment of disease activity in hereditary recurrent fevers: Results from the AIDAI (Auto-Inflammatory Diseases Activity Index) Consensus Conference. *Ann. Rheum. Dis.* **2011**, *70*, 309–314. [CrossRef] [PubMed]
33. Glaeser, L.; Henes, J.; Kotter, I.; Vogel, W.; Kanz, L.; Klein, R. Molecular recognition patterns of anti-topoisomerase I-antibodies in patients with systemic sclerosis before and after autologous stem cell transplantation. *Clin. Exp. Rheumatol.* **2018**, *36*, 28–35.
34. Paderno, A.; Schreiber, A.; Grammatica, A.; Raffetti, E.; Tomasoni, M.; Gualtieri, T.; Taboni, S.; Zorzi, S.; Lombardi, D.; Deganello, A.; et al. Smell and taste alterations in COVID-19: A cross-sectional analysis of different cohorts. *Int. Forum Allergy Rhinol.* **2020**, *10*, 955–962. [CrossRef] [PubMed]
35. Baj, J.; Karakula-Juchnowicz, H.; Teresinski, G.; Buszewicz, G.; Ciesielka, M.; Sitarz, E.; Forma, A.; Karakula, K.; Flieger, W.; Portincasa, P.; et al. COVID-19: Specific and Non-Specific Clinical Manifestations and Symptoms: The Current State of Knowledge. *J. Clin. Med.* **2020**, *9*, 1753. [CrossRef]

36. Yang, W.; Cao, Q.; Qin, L.; Wang, X.; Cheng, Z.; Pan, A.; Dai, J.; Sun, Q.; Zhao, F.; Qu, J.; et al. Clinical characteristics and imaging manifestations of the 2019 novel coronavirus disease (COVID-19): A multi-center study in Wenzhou city, Zhejiang, China. *J. Infect.* **2020**, *80*, 388–393. [CrossRef] [PubMed]
37. Cui, X.; Zhao, Z.; Zhang, T.; Guo, W.; Guo, W.; Zheng, J.; Zhang, J.; Dong, C.; Na, R.; Zheng, L.; et al. A systematic review and meta-analysis of children with coronavirus disease 2019 (COVID-19). *J. Med. Virol.* **2021**, *93*, 1057–1069. [CrossRef]
38. Zhang, C.; Gu, J.; Chen, Q.; Deng, N.; Li, J.; Huang, L.; Zhou, X. Clinical and epidemiological characteristics of pediatric SARS-CoV-2 infections in China: A multicenter case series. *PLoS Med.* **2020**, *17*, e1003130. [CrossRef]
39. Perez-Martinez, A.; Guerra-Garcia, P.; Melgosa, M.; Frauca, E.; Fernandez-Camblor, C.; Remesal, A.; Calvo, C. Clinical outcome of SARS-CoV-2 infection in immunosuppressed children in Spain. *Eur. J. Pediatr.* **2020**, *12*, 1–5. [CrossRef]
40. Gerussi, A.; Rigamonti, C.; Elia, C.; Cazzagon, N.; Floreani, A.; Pozzi, R.; Pozzoni, P.; Claar, E.; Pasulo, L.; Fagiuoli, S.; et al. Coronavirus Disease 2019 (COVID-19) in autoimmune hepatitis: A lesson from immunosuppressed patients. *Hepatol. Commun.* **2020**, *4*, 1257–1262. [CrossRef]
41. Kainth, M.K.; Goenka, P.K.; Williamson, K.A.; Fishbein, J.S.; Subramony, A.; Barone, S.; Belfer, J.A.; Feld, L.M.; Krief, W.I.; Palumbo, N.; et al. Early Experience of COVID-19 in a US Children's Hospital. *Pediatrics* **2020**, *146*, e2020003186. [CrossRef]
42. Moutsopoulos, H.M. Anti-inflammatory therapy may ameliorate the clinical picture of COVID-19. *Ann. Rheum. Dis.* **2020**, *79*, 1253–1254. [CrossRef]
43. Freeman, T.L.; Swartz, T.H. Targeting the NLRP3 Inflammasome in Severe COVID-19. *Front. Immunol.* **2020**, *11*, 1518. [CrossRef] [PubMed]
44. Dalrymple, J.M.; Stamp, L.K.; O'Donnell, J.L.; Chapman, P.T.; Zhang, M.; Barclay, M.L. Pharmacokinetics of oral methotrexate in patients with rheumatoid arthritis. *Arthritis Rheum.* **2008**, *58*, 3299–3308. [CrossRef] [PubMed]
45. Murchu, E.O.; Byrne, P.; Walsh, K.A.; Carty, P.G.; Connolly, M.; De Gascun, C.; Jordan, K.; Keoghan, M.; O'Brien, K.K.; O'Neill, M.; et al. Immune response following infection with SARS-CoV-2 and other coronaviruses: A rapid review. *Rev. Med. Virol.* **2020**, e2162. [CrossRef]
46. Kellam, P.; Barclay, W. The dynamics of humoral immune responses following SARS-CoV-2 infection and the potential for reinfection. *J. Gen. Virol.* **2020**, *101*, 791–797. [CrossRef] [PubMed]
47. Long, Q.X.; Liu, B.Z.; Deng, H.J.; Wu, G.C.; Deng, K.; Chen, Y.K.; Liao, P.; Qiu, J.F.; Lin, Y.; Cai, X.F.; et al. Antibody responses to SARS-CoV-2 in patients with COVID-19. *Nat. Med.* **2020**, *26*, 845–848. [CrossRef]
48. Callow, K.A.; Parry, H.F.; Sergeant, M.; Tyrrell, D.A. The time course of the immune response to experimental coronavirus infection of man. *Epidemiol. Infect.* **1990**, *105*, 435–446. [CrossRef] [PubMed]
49. Seow, J.; Graham, C.; Merrick, B.; Acors, S.; Pickering, S.; Steel, K.J.A.; Hemmings, O.; O'Byrne, A.; Kouphou, N.; Galao, R.P.; et al. Longitudinal observation and decline of neutralizing antibody responses in the three months following SARS-CoV-2 infection in humans. *Nat. Microbiol.* **2020**, *5*, 1598–1607. [CrossRef]
50. To, K.K.; Hung, I.F.; Ip, J.D.; Chu, A.W.; Chan, W.M.; Tam, A.R.; Fong, C.H.; Yuan, S.; Tsoi, H.W.; Ng, A.C.; et al. COVID-19 re-infection by a phylogenetically distinct SARS-coronavirus-2 strain confirmed by whole genome sequencing. *Clin. Infect. Dis.* **2020**. [CrossRef]
51. Tillett, R.L.; Sevinsky, J.R.; Hartley, P.D.; Kerwin, H.; Crawford, N.; Gorzalski, A.; Laverdure, C.; Verma, S.C.; Rossetto, C.C.; Jackson, D.; et al. Genomic evidence for reinfection with SARS-CoV-2: A case study. *Lancet Infect. Dis.* **2021**, *21*, 52–58. [CrossRef]
52. Bentivegna, E.; Sentimentale, A.; Luciani, M.; Speranza, M.L.; Guerritore, L.; Martelletti, P. New IgM seroconversion and positive RT-PCR test after exposure to the virus in recovered COVID-19 patient. *J. Med. Virol.* **2020**. [CrossRef]
53. Torres, D.A.; Ribeiro, L.; Riello, A.; Horovitz, D.D.G.; Pinto, L.F.R.; Croda, J. Reinfection of COVID-19 after 3 months with a distinct and more aggressive clinical presentation: Case report. *J. Med. Virol.* **2020**. [CrossRef] [PubMed]
54. Freeman, M.C.; Rapsinski, G.J.; Zilla, M.L.; Wheeler, S.E. Immunocompromised Seroprevalence and Course of Illness of SARS-CoV-2 in One Pediatric Quaternary Care Center. *J. Pediatric Infect. Dis. Soc.* **2020**. [CrossRef] [PubMed]

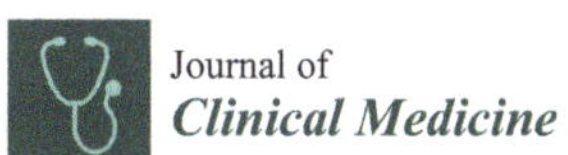
Journal of
Clinical Medicine

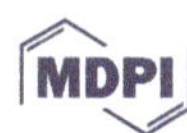

Article

Tumor Necrosis Factor Receptor-Associated Periodic Syndrome (TRAPS) with a New Pathogenic Variant in *TNFRSF1A* Gene in a Family of the Adult Male with Renal AA Amyloidosis—Diagnostic and Therapeutic Challenge for Clinicians

Jolanta Zegarska [1,†], Ewa Wiesik-Szewczyk [2,†], Ewa Hryniewiecka [1], Beata Wolska-Kusnierz [3], Dariusz Soldacki [2,4], Magdalena Kacprzak [5], Agnieszka Sobczynska-Tomaszewska [5], Kamila Czerska [5], Pawel Siedlecki [6,7], Karina Jahnz-Rozyk [2], Ewa Bernatowska [3], Radoslaw Zagozdzon [1,4,6,*] and Leszek Paczek [1,6,*]

1. Department of Immunology, Transplant Medicine and Internal Diseases, Medical University of Warsaw, 59 Nowogrodzka St., 02-006 Warsaw, Poland; jzegarska@wum.edu.pl (J.Z.); elhryniewiecka@gmail.com (E.H.)
2. Department of Internal Medicine, Pulmonology, Allergy and Clinical Immunology, Central Clinical Hospital of the Ministry of National Defense, Military Institute of Medicine in Warsaw, 128 Szaserów St., 04-141 Warsaw, Poland; ewa.w.szewczyk@gmail.com (E.W.-S.); dariusz.soldacki@gmail.com (D.S.); kjrozyk@wim.mil.pl (K.J.-R.)
3. Department of Immunology, Children's Memorial Health Institute, 20 Dzieci Polskich Ave., 04-730 Warsaw, Poland; bwolska@interia.pl (B.W.-K.); ewa.bernatowska@gmail.com (E.B.)
4. Department of Clinical Immunology, Medical University of Warsaw, 59 Nowogrodzka St., 02-006 Warsaw, Poland
5. MEDGEN Medical Centre, 9a Wiktorii Wiedenskiej St., 02-954 Warsaw, Poland; mk@medgen.pl (M.K.); agnieszka.sobczynska@medgen.pl (A.S.-T.); kamila.czerska@medgen.pl (K.C.)
6. Department of Bioinformatics, Institute of Biochemistry and Biophysics, Polish Academy of Sciences, 5a Adolfa Pawinskiego St., 02-106 Warsaw, Poland; psiedlecki@gmail.com
7. Department of Systems Biology, University of Warsaw, 1 Miecznikowa 1., 02-096 Warsaw, Poland

* Correspondence: radoslaw.zagozdzon@wum.edu.pl (R.Z.); leszek.paczek@wum.edu.pl (L.P.); Tel.: +48-22-502-14-72 (R.Z.); +48-22-502-16-41 (L.P.); Fax: +48-22-502-21-59 (R.Z.); +48-22-502-21-27 (L.P.)

† These authors contributed equally to this work.

Citation: Zegarska, J.; Wiesik-Szewczyk, E.; Hryniewiecka, E.; Wolska-Kusnierz, B.; Soldacki, D.; Kacprzak, M.; Sobczynska-Tomaszewska, A.; Czerska, K.; Siedlecki, P.; Jahnz-Rozyk, K.; et al. Tumor Necrosis Factor Receptor-Associated Periodic Syndrome (TRAPS) with a New Pathogenic Variant in *TNFRSF1A* Gene in a Family of the Adult Male with Renal AA Amyloidosis—Diagnostic and Therapeutic Challenge for Clinicians. *J. Clin. Med.* **2021**, *10*, 465. https://doi.org/10.3390/jcm10030465

Academic Editor: Eugen Feist

Received: 30 December 2020
Accepted: 19 January 2021
Published: 26 January 2021

Publisher's Note: MDPI stays neutral with regard to jurisdictional claims in published maps and institutional affiliations.

Abstract: Tumor necrosis factor receptor-associated periodic syndrome (TRAPS) belongs to systemic autoinflammatory diseases (AIDs). Many of these syndromes are genetically conditioned and can be inherited. Diagnosis relies on clinical symptoms and should be confirmed by genetic testing. One of the most serious complications is AA amyloidosis. We present the diagnostic route of a 33-year-old male with AA amyloidosis and his children, leading to diagnosis of monogenic autoinflammatory syndrome, confirmed by genetic analysis. A novel variant of the in-frame insertion type in one allele of *TNFRSF1A* gene was found by whole exome sequencing and confirmed by Sanger sequencing, which allowed a diagnosis of TRAPS. Three-dimensional modeling was used to assess the structural changes introduced into TNFR1 molecule by the insertion. The analysis of the 3D model revealed that accommodation of the 4AA insert induces misalignment of three cysteine bridges (especially the C70-C96 bridge) in the extracellular domain, leading to putatively misfolded and improperly functioning TNFR1. Three of the patient's daughters inherited the same variant of the *TNFRSF1A* gene and presented TRAPS symptoms. TRAPS is a very rare disease, but in the presence of suggestive symptoms the genetic diagnostic workout should be undertaken. Early diagnosis followed by appropriate clinical management can prevent irreversible complications.

Keywords: new genetic variant; monogenic autoinflammatory syndrome; diagnostic delay; anakinra; damage index; genetic inheritance; personalized therapy

1. Introduction

Monogenic autoinflammatory diseases (AIDs) cover a spectrum of syndromes, which lead to chronic or recurrent inflammation caused by activation of the innate immune system, typically in the absence of high autoantibody titers [1]. The four most common monogenic AIDs are: NLRP3-associated autoinflammatory disease (NLRP3-AID), familial Mediterranean fever (FMF), mevalonate kinase deficiency (MKD), and tumor necrosis factor receptor-associated periodic fever syndrome (TRAPS).

TRAPS is an autosomal dominant disease, caused by mutations in *TNFRSF1A* gene which encodes the protein named tumor necrosis factor receptor 1 (TNFR1), which plays a crucial role in the inflammation and apoptosis [1]. The estimated prevalence of TRAPS is one per million. Symptoms include recurrent episodes of fever, lasting about 3 weeks, abdominal, chest, and muscle pains, skin rash, typically found on the limbs, periorbital edema, and joint pain [2]. Inflammatory markers are always elevated during acute episodes. The onset of the disease may occur at any age, from infancy to late adulthood, but most patients have their first episode in childhood. In most cases, relatives are affected, and positive family history strongly supports the diagnosis. AA amyloidosis is the main long-term complication of TRAPS. Depending on the genetic variant, it is estimated that 2–24% of untreated patients with TRAPS would develop AA amyloidosis [2–5], usually in mid-adulthood, but the risk of this complication has significantly been decreased by modern anti-inflammatory therapies [6]. The evaluation of patient with systemic AA amyloidosis, in whom an obvious cause cannot be identified, is a challenge in clinical practice, as there are over 100 diseases associated with AA amyloidosis. Among them, strong association is reported for AIDs. The correlation is not unexpected, because autoinflammatory syndromes often cause the long-standing inflammation [7]. However, due to low awareness and heterogenous presentation, especially in sporadic cases, the diagnosis of AIDs might be overlooked. Indeed, long diagnostic delay is usually reported. Importantly, the proper diagnosis allows for avoiding the complications and progressive, irreversible organ damage. Moreover, worse prognosis and unfavorable outcomes of renal transplantation is reported in AA amyloidosis in the course of AIDs [8].

The therapies include corticosteroid therapy, non-steroidal anti-inflammatory drugs (NSAIDs) during flares or a treatment based on biological agents, depending on the requirements of the particular patient and disease severity [9,10]. Targeted anti-inflammatory treatment is the only option in preventing further systemic deposition of amyloid and recurrence of amyloidosis in transplanted organ.

The aim of the study was the identification of molecular basis and inheritance pattern of disease in an adult male with AA amyloidosis and episodes of fever suspected of AID, as well as in the members of his family.

2. Materials and Methods

2.1. Patients

4 patients were included in the study—proband and all his 3 children (daughters). At the admission, the proband was 33-year-old Caucasian male, who was referred for nephrology consultation because of proteinuria, chronic renal failure with estimated glomerular filtration rate (eGFR) 69 mL/min./1.73 m^2, and biopsy-proven kidney AA amyloidosis.

2.2. Methods of Molecular Analysis

Next-generation sequencing (NGS). Whole exome sequencing (WES) was performed. Patient's genomic DNA was extracted from the whole blood sample, and sequencing library was prepared according to Agilent Sure-Select Human All Exon V5 protocol. The enriched DNA libraries were sequenced by the Illumina HiSeq4000 instrument (Illumina, Inc., Sand Diego, CA, USA). All procedures for exome sequencing were conducted by Macrogen (Seoul, Korea). Raw sequencing reads were mapped to the reference genome using BWA [11]. Duplicates were removed using Picard software (Broad Institute, Cambridge, MA, USA), and variants were named using Samtools software (SourceForge, San

Diego, CA, USA). Variants in 289 genes connected with autoinflammatory diseases were analyzed (the list of genes [12] is presented in Supplementary Table S1). The following in silico prediction software programs were used to assist with interpretation of pathogenicity of detected variant: Alamut visual v 2.9.0 (Interactive biosoftware, SOPHiAGENETICS, CH-1025 Saint Sulpice, Switzerland). The presence of the variant in control populations was checked in 1000Genomes [13], the Exome Variant Server [14], and the Exome Aggregation Consortium (Broad Institute) and gnomAD (Broad Institute).

2.3. 3D Protein Modeling

The newly identified AHRH insertion was manually introduced into the structure of TNFR1 (Tumor necrosis factor receptor superfamily member 1A; PDB:1FT4) with the MAV (Multalign Viewer) module of UCSF (University of California San Francisco, CA, USA) Chimera software (v 1.14) [15]. Next, the Modeler software [16] was used to generate 5 different models of the modified structure. The resulting models were validated with zDOPE (Discrete Optimized Protein Energy score [17]). Final model was subjected to a short minimization procedure (MMTK—Molecular Modelling Toolkit, Center for Molecular Biophysics, CNRS-Orleans, France) with Amber ff14SB force field, 100 steps of steepest descent and 10 steps conjugate gradient) to lessen the sterical constraints introduced by the modeling procedure.

3. Results

3.1. Patients

3.1.1. Patient 1—Proband

33-year-old Caucasian male was referred for nephrology consultation because of proteinuria 3.2–5.7 g/day; chronic renal failure with estimated glomerular filtration rate (eGFR) 69 mL/min./1.73 m^2 and biopsy-proven kidney AA amyloidosis. On admission, he complained of chronic fatigue; otherwise, he denied any other symptoms. His family medical history was reported as irrelevant. His comorbidities were as follows: arterial hypertension, hypercholesterolemia, normocytic anemia. There were no clinically relevant findings during physical examination, except for the post-appendicitis scar in right lower quadrant of the abdomen.

In routine laboratory tests, the erythrocyte sedimentation rate (ESR) was 47 mm/h (reference range: 0–12 mm/h), and serum concentration of C-reactive protein (CRP) 61.17 mg/L (reference range: up to 9 mg/L), serum amyloid A (SAA) 60.9 mg/L (reference range: up to 6.4 mg/L). Laboratory work-up for anti nuclear (ANA), anti-neutrophil cytoplasmic (ANCA) antibodies and rheumatoid factor were negative. Blood and urine cultures were also negative.

Detailed analysis of his past medical history revealed that from the age of 7 the patient reported recurrent episodes of abdominal pain with fever up to 40 °C, upper respiratory tract symptoms (pharyngitis, tonsillitis), arthralgia of elbow, knee, and wrists and elevated inflammatory parameters. These episodes were recurring irregularly, at least twice a year, with fever lasting 7–10 days and abdominal pain lasting 10–14 days. He was repeatedly hospitalized and suspected of infections (at the age of 7), chronic endocarditis (aged 14), lambliasis with cholangitis (aged 13), or connective tissue diseases. Episodes of abdominal pain were the rationale for appendectomy (age 14). Inflammatory bowel disease and chronic pancreatitis were excluded. Despite extensive research, the reason for recurrent fevers was not identified. During adolescence, recurrent acute episodes stopped, but chronic low-grade fever and fatigue persisted. At the age of 28, the patient was diagnosed with proteinuria, kidney function impairment, and arterial hypertension. Kidney biopsy specimen revealed AA amyloidosis.

Based on the medical history, AIDs were included as a potential cause for AA amyloidosis. Initial suspicion of FMF was made and treatment with colchicine 0.5 mg/day twice a day was ordered, with short-time improvement of ESR and CRP. An attempt to increase colchicine dosage to 0.5 mg three times a day was unsuccessful due to diarrhea. Moreover, genetic tests for FMF did not reveal any known pathogenic variants in exons 2, 3, and 10 of *MEFV* gene. Due to unsatisfactory effectiveness of the treatment and sustained suspicion of AID as the cause of AA amyloidosis, the genetic diagnostic work-up was continued by next-generation sequencing (NGS).

3.1.2. Remaining Patients

Patient 2

At the age of 7, Patient 1's daughter had been referred for consultation due to episodes of fever up to 39 °C lasting for 6–10 days accompanied by severe abdominal pain, lymphadenopathy (cervical, inguinal) and recurrent pharyngitis. Flares have been occurring irregularly 4–5 times a year since the age of 2. Her physical examination between episodes was normal. She had constantly elevated SAA during and between febrile flares (67–813 mg/dL). Until the diagnosis of the father, her symptoms were treated as typical childhood infections.

Patient 3

At the age of 9, the second daughter had presented fever episodes. Her symptoms have been sporadic and mild, and lasted approx. 10 days. She responded well to antipyretic treatment. Her acute inflammatory reactants were high during flares (CRP up to 6.0 mg/dL), and between episodes were within the reference range (SAA 3.7 mg/dL).

Patient 4

At the age of 17, the oldest daughter presented with severe abdominal pain, low-grade fever 37.5 °C. No abnormalities were found on additional investigation except for abnormal inflammatory markers (CRP 8.2 mg/dL). Symptoms persisted for 3 weeks, without response on NSAID and resolved spontaneously. Otherwise, her medical history was unremarkable. Her acute inflammatory reactants between episodes were within the reference range (SAA 0.8 mg/dL, CRP 0.2 mg/dL).

3.2. Genetic Results

Genetic Variant Identification

As the result of WES analysis of Patient 1, the novel variant of the insertion type: c.362_363insTGCAAGACACAG in one allele of *TNFRSF1A* gene was identified (Supplementary Figure S1). Then, the NM_001065.5:c.362_363insTGCAAGACACAG/p.(Arg121_Asp122insAlaArgHisArg) variant was confirmed by Sanger sequencing (Figure 1).

Because the NM_001065.5:p.(Arg121_Asp122insAlaArgHisArg) insert has been identified in the TNFR1 protein for the first time, we decided to assess the potential effects of this insertion on the protein structure by 3D modeling (Figure 2). The acquired 3D model suggested that the insert may influence three cysteine bridges, with the C70–C96 being the crucial one for correctly orienting CRD2 and CRD3 domains. Accommodation of the 4AA insert leads to misalignment cysteine bridges leading to putatively misfolded and improperly functioning TNFR1. Therefore, the NM_001065.5:p.(Arg121_Asp122insAlaArgHisArg) insert should be considered pathogenic. This notion warrants further investigations on the potential phenotypic changes induced by this novel TNFR1 variant under experimental conditions, preferably by comparison with some previously identified pathogenic variants, as exemplified in [18,19].

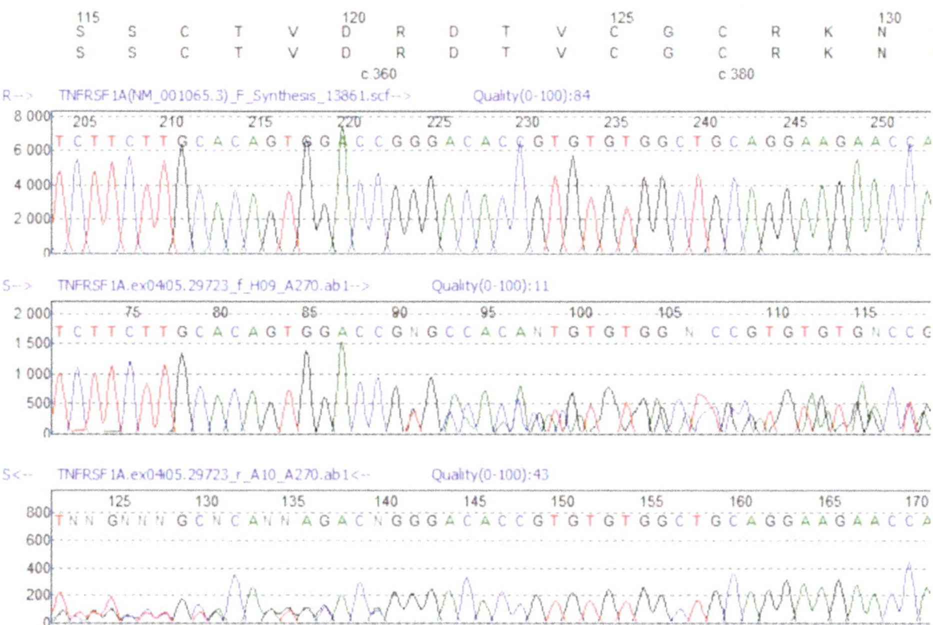

Figure 1. Sanger sequencing of NM_001065.5:c.362_363insTGCAAGACACAG variant. The alignment to wild sample sequence is visualized using Mutation Surveyor Software, v.4.0.7 (Softgenetics, State College, PA 16803, USA). The upper panel represents the reference sequence, underneath—Sanger sequencing of mutated sample—from forward (middle panel) and from reverse (bottom panel) primers.

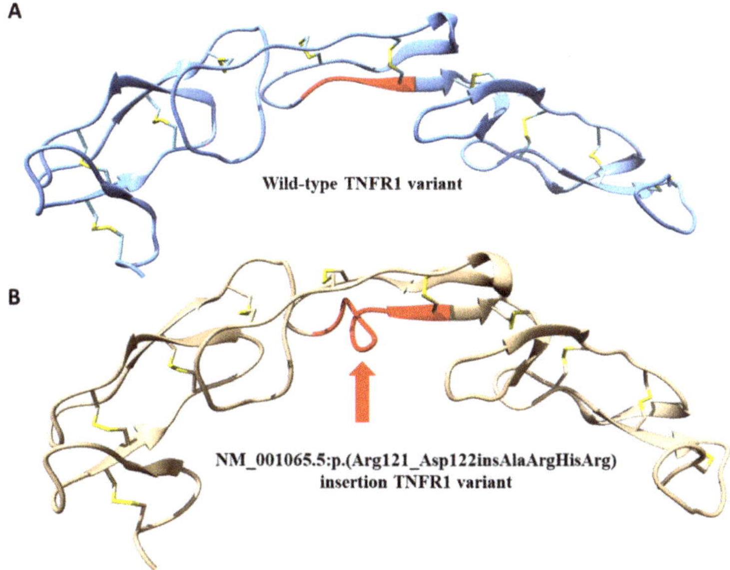

Figure 2. (**A**,**B**) Comparison between the structure of wild-type variant of TNFR1 protein (**A**) and modeling of the predicted misfolding (red arrow) resulting from the NM_001065.5: p.(Arg121_Asp122insAlaArgHisArg) insertion in the pathogenic variant of TNFR1 (**B**).

3.3. Management

From 19 December 2017, when biologic treatment for AIDs got reimbursement in Poland, Patient 1 started treatment with an interleukin 1 inhibitor—anakinra, 100 mg subcutaneously/day, as home therapy. At the beginning, he was taking the medication irregularly due to moderate local side effects (rush, skin burning). Patient 1 was re-educated about the aim of treatment, mode of application, and then continued the treatment regularly. After 3 months of follow-up, local side effects completely disappeared. In parallel, low-grade fever and fatigue resolved. Inflammatory parameters normalized: CRP to 0.1 mg/dL (reference range: 0.8 mg/dL), SAA to 0.6 mg/dL (reference range: to 0.64 mg/dL) and stay within reference range after 24 months treatment. His kidney function and proteinuria are stable (creatinine level 1.7 mg/dL, proteinuria 2.0 g/day).

From the patient's perspective: during the 2-year follow-up despite initial doubts related to local reactions after administration of the preparation, we observed a very good compliance with the treatment principles. The applied targeted therapy not only resulted in the normalization of inflammatory parameters, but also eliminated the troublesome symptoms of excessive fatigue and the patient returned to his work on the farm. Currently, he feels free from burden of symptoms and from his point of view can give financial and personal support for his family members.

Patient 2 has started the treatment with IL-1 blocker (anakinra). Rapid response was observed with remission of symptoms within 2 days and normalization of lab results after 7 days (CRP 0.8 mg/dL; SAA 7.3 mg/dL). There were no flares during next 18 months of follow-up.

Patient 3 and Patient 4 remain asymptomatic and have currently normal laboratory results. They do not need chronic pharmacological treatment at present and are under thorough medical control.

4. Discussion

We present results of diagnostics that included NGS sequencing in a patient with kidney AA amyloidosis and all his children. The clinical presentation of the adult male patient was suggestive for AIDs, but not specific for a particular type of AID, including TRAPS, according to the clinical criteria acknowledged at the time of patient's admission [20]. Predominant clinical symptoms were episodes of fever and severe abdominal pain in childhood, arthralgia and fatigue in adulthood, and AA amyloidosis as a long-term complication. Patient's family history was negative, as well as the medical history in respect of migratory rash and periorbital edema—the more specific indicators for TRAPS [21]. According to the literature, the experts asked to indicate signs and symptoms regarded the most helpful in their practice for the diagnostics of TRAPS cited the following: recurrent long-lasting fever episodes, positive family history, periorbital edema, abdominal pain, myalgia, cutaneous rash, arthralgia, and monocytic fasciitis [22]. The onset of the disease in the reported male patient, as in most cases of TRAPS, was in his childhood, but at the time of diagnosis he presented the pattern typical for a chronic disease without inflammatory, acute flares. Notably, in his case it took approx. 29 years from the onset of the disease till the confirmation of diagnosis. Moreover, the proband developed AA amyloidosis and kidney failure, but it occurred quite early, in his twenties, while Lachman et al. found that the median age of developing of amyloidosis in TRAPS population was 43 years [5].

In clinical practice, there is a challenge to appropriately qualify the sporadic cases of AA amyloidosis for further genetic evaluation. Generally, when the clinical symptoms presented by the given patient are adherent with the diagnostic criteria for a specific AID (e.g., TRAPS), the genetic method of choice should be a targeted sequencing of the respective gene by the Sanger method. In the adult patient with AA amyloidosis reported hereby, an initial attempt was made of a targeted sequencing of selected exons of the *MEFV* gene, which proved unsuccessful. In the last decade, due to application of the next-generation sequencing (NGS), the genetic diagnosis in patients with AIDs has greatly improved and remarkable progress has been made in the genetic characterization of the undiagnosed patients and the sporadic cases [23]. Importantly, TRAPS is genetically heterogeneous. More than 140 *TNFRSF1A* variants have been recognized up to date [24]. *TNFRSF1A* gene comprises 10 exons. Most of the variants are single-nucleotide substitutions (95%), but deletions and insertions have also been reported. Most sequence variants lie within exons 2 to 4 and result in amino acid substitutions which disrupt important cysteine-cysteine disulfide bonds within the extracellular domain (cysteine-rich domains, CRDs). A single splicing mutation also perturbs the first CRD due to the insertion of 4 amino acids. The most common are low-penetrance variants R92Q and P46L. Another common variant is T50M. Generally, mutations that result in cysteine substitutions lead to higher penetrance of the clinical phenotype (93% versus 82% for non-cysteine residue substitutions), and increase the probability of developing amyloidosis (24% versus 2% for no cysteine residue substitutions) [2].

Hereby, to establish the diagnosis, we performed WES with subsequent analysis of genes connected with autoinflammatory diseases. As a result, we identified a novel *TNFRSF1A* variant of in-frame insertion type that putatively influences three cysteine bridges and the structure of TNFR1 protein leading to its dysfunction or loss of function. The variant was confirmed by Sanger analysis. To the best of our knowledge, this variant has not been reported up to date. Thus, the important question is whether this novel genetic variant is pathogenic. Notably, it was found in one allele, which corresponds to the fact that TRAPS is an autosomal dominant disease. Clinical arguments for its pathogenicity are that the same genetic variant was found in three symptomatic relatives (i.e., daughters). However, clinical spectrum varies among family members and leads to personalized management. Therefore, further research laboratory tests, e.g., in the cell culture models, are necessary to respond the question of pathogenicity with acceptable precision.

Management of TRAPS should be adjusted case by case. It can involve corticosteroid therapy, NSAIDs during flares or a treatment based on biological agents, mainly TNF receptor-IgG1 Fc fusion protein etanercept [25] or interleukin 1 inhibitors [9]. Current data indicate that anti-IL-1 compounds are the most effective drugs in patients with pathogenic variants [26]. Such treatment eliminates the clinical symptoms and inhibits progression of AA amyloidosis. Indeed, the efficiency of anti-IL-1 agents in TRAPS treatment has been proved. Anakinra, a recombinant and slightly modified version of the human interleukin 1 receptor antagonist protein or canakinumab, a human monoclonal antibody targeted at interleukin-1 beta can be used. In 47 TRAPS patients from the US, the European Union, and the eastern Mediterranean, treatment with anakinra versus anti-TNF agents as the first biologic therapy led to significantly higher clinical and biochemical responses [27]. In one adult with amyloidosis-related renal failure, anakinra led to the disappearance of manifestations of TRAPS and decrease of laboratory abnormalities, including proteinuria [28]. Moreover, this treatment is considered safe, as in the presented case the side effects were local and self-limiting. Canakinumab was effective in controlling and preventing fever flares in patients with TRAPS, colchicine-resistant FMF, and MKD [29,30]. In contrast to anakinra, which is administered daily, canakinumab can be given every 4–8 weeks. The limitation of its use is the high cost, and that at present time it is not reimbursed in Poland.

As mentioned above, management of TRAPS and qualification for biologic treatment should be personalized. In this study, three additional family members of the patient are symptomatic and have undergone diagnostic workout, but based on their symptoms and the estimated risk of end-organ damage, the goals and manners of management differ. The father (proband) is treated continuously with anakinra to stop the AA amyloidosis progression. His 7-year-old daughter received anakinra treatment before any damage accrual occurred, and in future it may be possible to pause the medication. Finally, two daughters are covered by watch-and-wait strategy, as flares were sporadic, and inflammatory markers are within reference range between attacks.

Our study has some limitations. We did not perform the functional studies on the newly identified variant. Moreover, the pathogenicity of the variant could be further supported by the assessment (e.g., by flow cytometry) of TNFR1 presence on the respective cells, and the serum concentrations of soluble TNFR1, TNF-α, and perhaps other proinflammatory cytokines. However, none these tests are routinely performed in the medical centers involved in the current study. Furthermore, given the information collected in this report, it would be preliminary to speculate what would be the pathophysiological and/or molecular mechanism(s) responsible for the pathogenicity of the newly identified variant. In theory, such effects may rely on the exaggerated activation of NF-κB pathway [18] and/or hyperresponsiveness to the proinflammatory stimuli [19], and then induction of subsequent inflammatory cascading. As mentioned, this should be further investigated in properly designed functional studies. Despite its limitations, our study supports the notion that in cases of AA amyloidosis of unknown origin, the monogenic AID, including TRAPS, should be considered.

5. Conclusions

TRAPS is a very rare disease and can be overlooked in differential diagnosis, especially if clinical picture is not specific. The diagnosis is usually delayed leading to organ damage with the most serious complications, i.e., the development of secondary inflammatory amyloidosis and kidney failure. In diagnosis, the crucial role is played by the genetic testing, preferably by NGS. Hereby, in an adult male with AA amyloidosis and his family members we identified a novel in-frame insertion-type pathogenic variant in one allele of *TNFRSF1A* gene that caused TRAPS. Setting up the correct diagnosis of TRAPS allows for the choice of a suitable treatment. Indeed, anti-IL-1 agents provide efficient and safe therapy that eliminates clinical symptoms and prevents the patients from the organ damage, which is exemplified in the current report.

Supplementary Materials: The following are available online at https://www.mdpi.com/2077-0383/10/3/465/s1, Figure S1: Next-generation (whole exome) sequencing and alignment visualization using Integrative Genomics Viewer (IGV), Table S1: Genes connected with inborn errors of immune system analyzed by NGS in 33-years-old man with AA renal amyloidosis.

Author Contributions: Conceptualization, J.Z., E.W.-S. and R.Z.; methodology, K.C.; software, A.S.-T. and P.S.; validation, M.K.; formal analysis, K.C. and B.W.-K.; investigation, B.W.-K. and E.H.; resources, P.S. and D.S.; data curation, K.C. and P.S.; writing—original draft preparation, J.Z. and E.W.-S.; writing—review and editing, R.Z.; visualization, K.C. and P.S.; supervision, L.P., K.J.-R. and E.B.; project administration, E.H. and D.S.; funding acquisition, R.Z and L.P. All authors have read and agreed to the published version of the manuscript.

Funding: This research received no external funding.

Institutional Review Board Statement: The local Bioethics Committee of the Medical University of Warsaw waived the requirement for ethical permission due to the retrospective character of this noninvasive follow-up observation study (waiver No. AKBE/339/2019, 2 December 2019). All routine diagnostic and therapeutic procedures described within the study were carried out after obtaining a written informed consent from the patient.

Informed Consent Statement: We obtained a written informed consent from the patients/representativ for the publication of this report.

Data Availability Statement: The novel molecular variant was 184 submitted to the ClinVar database (http://www.ncbi.nlm.nih.gov/clinvar; Submission ID: SUB6616942).

Conflicts of Interest: The authors declare no conflict of interest.

References

1. McDermott, M.F.; Aksentijevich, I.; Galon, J.; McDermott, E.M.; Ogunkolade, B.W.; Centola, M.; Mansfield, E.; Gadina, M.; Karenko, L.; Pettersson, T.; et al. Germline mutations in the extracellular domains of the 55 kDa TNF receptor, TNFR1, define a family of dominantly inherited autoinflammatory syndromes. *Cell* **1999**, *97*, 133–144. [CrossRef]
2. Hull, K.M.; Drewe, E.; Aksentijevich, I.; Singh, H.K.; Wong, K.; McDermott, E.M.; Dean, J.; Powell, R.J.; Kastner, D.L. The TNF receptor-associated periodic syndrome (TRAPS): Emerging concepts of an autoinflammatory disorder. *Medicine (Baltimore)* **2002**, *81*, 349–368. [CrossRef] [PubMed]

3. Aksentijevich, I.; Galon, J.; Soares, M.; Mansfield, E.; Hull, K.; Oh, H.H.; Goldbach-Mansky, R.; Dean, J.; Athreya, B.; Reginato, A.J.; et al. The tumor-necrosis-factor receptor-associated periodic syndrome: New mutations in TNFRSF1A, ancestral origins, genotype-phenotype studies, and evidence for further genetic heterogeneity of periodic fevers. *Am. J. Hum. Genet.* **2001**, *69*, 301–314. [CrossRef] [PubMed]
4. Toro, J.R.; Aksentijevich, I.; Hull, K.; Dean, J.; Kastner, D.L. Tumor necrosis factor receptor-associated periodic syndrome: A novel syndrome with cutaneous manifestations. *Arch. Dermatol.* **2000**, *136*, 1487–1494. [CrossRef] [PubMed]
5. Lachmann, H.J.; Papa, R.; Gerhold, K.; Obici, L.; Touitou, I.; Cantarini, L.; Frenkel, J.; Anton, J.; Kone-Paut, I.; Cattalini, M.; et al. The phenotype of TNF receptor-associated autoinflammatory syndrome (TRAPS) at presentation: A series of 158 cases from the Eurofever/EUROTRAPS international registry. *Ann. Rheum. Dis.* **2014**, *73*, 2160–2167. [CrossRef]
6. Cudrici, C.; Deuitch, N.; Aksentijevich, I. Revisiting TNF Receptor-Associated Periodic Syndrome (TRAPS): Current Perspectives. *Int. J. Mol. Sci.* **2020**, *21*, 3263. [CrossRef]
7. Brunger, A.F.; Nienhuis, H.L.A.; Bijzet, J.; Hazenberg, B.P.C. Causes of AA amyloidosis: A systematic review. *Amyloid* **2020**, *27*, 1–12. [CrossRef]
8. Sarihan, I.; Caliskan, Y.; Mirioglu, S.; Ozluk, Y.; Senates, B.; Seyahi, N.; Basturk, T.; Yildiz, A.; Kilicaslan, I.; Sever, M.S. Amyloid A Amyloidosis After Renal Transplantation: An Important Cause of Mortality. *Transplantation* **2020**, *104*, 1703–1711. [CrossRef]
9. Ter Haar, N.; Lachmann, H.; Ozen, S.; Woo, P.; Uziel, Y.; Modesto, C.; Kone-Paut, I.; Cantarini, L.; Insalaco, A.; Neven, B.; et al. Treatment of autoinflammatory diseases: Results from the Eurofever Registry and a literature review. *Ann. Rheum. Dis.* **2013**, *72*, 678–685. [CrossRef]
10. Ozen, S.; Demir, S. Monogenic Periodic Fever Syndromes: Treatment Options for the Pediatric Patient. *Paediatr. Drugs* **2017**, *19*, 303–311. [CrossRef]
11. Li, H.; Durbin, R. Fast and accurate long-read alignment with Burrows-Wheeler transform. *Bioinformatics* **2010**, *26*, 589–595. [CrossRef] [PubMed]
12. Bousfiha, A.; Jeddane, L.; Al-Herz, W.; Ailal, F.; Casanova, J.L.; Chatila, T.; Conley, M.E.; Cunningham-Rundles, C.; Etzioni, A.; Franco, J.L.; et al. The 2015 IUIS Phenotypic Classification for Primary Immunodeficiencies. *J. Clin. Immunol.* **2015**, *35*, 727–738. [CrossRef] [PubMed]
13. 1000Genomes. Available online: http://www.1000genomes.org (accessed on 19 October 2016).
14. Exome Variant Server. Available online: http://evs.gs.washington.edu/EVS (accessed on 19 October 2016).
15. Pettersen, E.F.; Goddard, T.D.; Huang, C.C.; Couch, G.S.; Greenblatt, D.M.; Meng, E.C.; Ferrin, T.E. UCSF Chimera—A visualization system for exploratory research and analysis. *J. Comput. Chem.* **2004**, *25*, 1605–1612. [CrossRef] [PubMed]
16. Sali, A.; Blundell, T.L. Comparative protein modelling by satisfaction of spatial restraints. *J. Mol. Biol.* **1993**, *234*, 779–815. [CrossRef] [PubMed]
17. Shen, M.Y.; Sali, A. Statistical potential for assessment and prediction of protein structures. *Protein Sci.* **2006**, *15*, 2507–2524. [CrossRef]
18. Greco, E.; Aita, A.; Galozzi, P.; Gava, A.; Sfriso, P.; Negm, O.H.; Tighe, P.; Caso, F.; Navaglia, F.; Dazzo, E.; et al. The novel S59P mutation in the TNFRSF1A gene identified in an adult onset TNF receptor associated periodic syndrome (TRAPS) constitutively activates NF-kappaB pathway. *Arthritis Res. Ther.* **2015**, *17*, 93. [CrossRef]
19. Tsuji, S.; Matsuzaki, H.; Iseki, M.; Nagasu, A.; Hirano, H.; Ishihara, K.; Ueda, N.; Honda, Y.; Horiuchi, T.; Nishikomori, R.; et al. Functional analysis of a novel G87V TNFRSF1A mutation in patients with TNF receptor-associated periodic syndrome. *Clin. Exp. Immunol.* **2019**, *198*, 416–429. [CrossRef]
20. Federici, S.; Sormani, M.P.; Ozen, S.; Lachmann, H.J.; Amaryan, G.; Woo, P.; Kone-Paut, I.; Dewarrat, N.; Cantarini, L.; Insalaco, A.; et al. Evidence-based provisional clinical classification criteria for autoinflammatory periodic fevers. *Ann. Rheum. Dis.* **2015**, *74*, 799–805. [CrossRef]
21. Gattorno, M.; Hofer, M.; Federici, S.; Vanoni, F.; Bovis, F.; Aksentijevich, I.; Anton, J.; Arostegui, J.I.; Barron, K.; Ben-Cherit, E.; et al. Classification criteria for autoinflammatory recurrent fevers. *Ann. Rheum. Dis.* **2019**, *78*, 1025–1032. [CrossRef]
22. Federici, S.; Vanoni, F.; Ben-Chetrit, E.; Cantarini, L.; Frenkel, J.; Goldbach-Mansky, R.; Gul, A.; Hoffman, H.; Kone-Paut, I.; Kuemmerle-Deschner, J.; et al. An International Delphi Survey for the Definition of New Classification Criteria for Familial Mediterranean Fever, Mevalonate Kinase Deficiency, TNF Receptor-associated Periodic Fever Syndromes, and Cryopyrin-associated Periodic Syndrome. *J. Rheumatol.* **2019**, *46*, 429–436. [CrossRef]
23. Rowczenio, D.M.; Lachmann, H.J. How to prescribe a genetic test for the diagnosis of autoinflammatory diseases? *Presse Med.* **2019**, *48*, e49. [CrossRef] [PubMed]
24. Rigante, D.; Frediani, B.; Cantarini, L. A Comprehensive Overview of the Hereditary Periodic Fever Syndromes. *Clin. Rev. Allergy Immunol.* **2018**, *54*, 446–453. [CrossRef] [PubMed]
25. Drewe, E.; McDermott, E.M.; Powell, R.J. Treatment of the nephrotic syndrome with etanercept in patients with the tumor necrosis factor receptor-associated periodic syndrome. *N. Engl. J. Med.* **2000**, *343*, 1044–1045. [CrossRef] [PubMed]
26. Papa, R.; Lane, T.; Minden, K.; Touitou, I.; Cantarini, L.; Cattalini, M.; Obici, L.; Jansson, A.F.; Belot, A.; Frenkel, J.; et al. INSAID Variant Classification and Eurofever Criteria Guide Optimal Treatment Strategy in Patients with TRAPS: Data from the Eurofever Registry. *J. Allergy Clin. Immunol. Pract.* **2020**. [CrossRef] [PubMed]

27. Ozen, S.; Kuemmerle-Deschner, J.B.; Cimaz, R.; Livneh, A.; Quartier, P.; Kone-Paut, I.; Zeft, A.; Spalding, S.; Gul, A.; Hentgen, V.; et al. International Retrospective Chart Review of Treatment Patterns in Severe Familial Mediterranean Fever, Tumor Necrosis Factor Receptor-Associated Periodic Syndrome, and Mevalonate Kinase Deficiency/Hyperimmunoglobulinemia D Syndrome. *Arthritis Care Res. (Hoboken)* **2017**, *69*, 578–586. [CrossRef]
28. Gentileschi, S.; Rigante, D.; Vitale, A.; Sota, J.; Frediani, B.; Galeazzi, M.; Cantarini, L. Efficacy and safety of anakinra in tumor necrosis factor receptor-associated periodic syndrome (TRAPS) complicated by severe renal failure: A report after long-term follow-up and review of the literature. *Clin. Rheumatol.* **2017**, *36*, 1687–1690. [CrossRef]
29. La Torre, F.; Caparello, M.C.; Cimaz, R. Canakinumab for the treatment of TNF-receptor associated periodic syndrome. *Expert Rev. Clin. Immunol.* **2017**, *13*, 513–523. [CrossRef]
30. De Benedetti, F.; Gattorno, M.; Anton, J.; Ben-Chetrit, E.; Frenkel, J.; Hoffman, H.M.; Kone-Paut, I.; Lachmann, H.J.; Ozen, S.; Simon, A.; et al. Canakinumab for the Treatment of Autoinflammatory Recurrent Fever Syndromes. *N. Engl. J. Med.* **2018**, *378*, 1908–1919. [CrossRef]

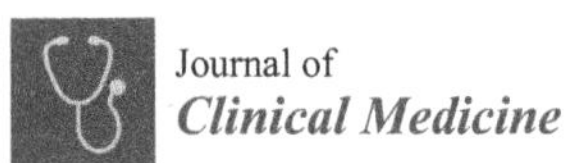
Journal of
Clinical Medicine

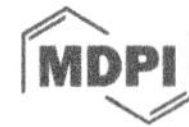

Article

Evaluate the Differences in CT Features and Serum IgG4 Levels between Lymphoma and Immunoglobulin G4-Related Disease of the Orbit

Wei-Hsin Yuan [1,2,3,*], Anna Fen-Yau Li [3,4], Shu-Yi Yu [2,3], Ying-Yuan Chen [3,5], Chia-Hung Wu [2,3], Hui-Chen Hsu [6], Jiing-Feng Lirng [2,3] and Wan-You Guo [2,3]

1 Division of Radiology, Taipei Municipal Gan-Dau Hospital (Managed by Taipei Veterans General Hospital), Taipei 11260, Taiwan
2 Department of Radiology, Taipei Veterans General Hospital, Taipei 11217, Taiwan; frankfbo@gmail.com (S.-Y.Y.); chwu16@vghtpe.gov.tw (C.-H.W.); jflirng@vghtpe.gov.tw (J.-F.L.); wyguo@vghtpe.gov.tw (W.-Y.G.)
3 School of Medicine, National Yang-Ming University, Taipei 10556, Taiwan; Fyli@vghtpe.gov.tw (A.F.-Y.L.); yychen354@gmail.com (Y.-Y.C.)
4 Department of Pathology, Taipei Veterans General Hospital, Taipei 11217, Taiwan
5 Division of Radiology, National Yang-Ming University Hospital, Yilan City 26058, Taiwan
6 Department of Medical Imaging, Taiwan Adventist Hospital, Taipei 10556, Taiwan; hueichenhsu@gmail.com
* Correspondence: williamyuan.tw@gmail.com

Received: 14 June 2020; Accepted: 27 July 2020; Published: 29 July 2020

Abstract: Background: Benign immunoglobulin G4 (IgG4)-related orbital disease (IgG4-ROD)—characterized as tumors mimicking malignant orbital lymphoma (OL)—responds well to steroids, instead of chemotherapy, radiotherapy and/or surgery of OL. The objective of this study was to report the differences in computed tomography (CT) features and- serum IgG4 levels of IgG4-ROD and OL. Methods: This study retrieved records for patients with OL and IgG4-ROD from a pathology database during an eight-year-and-five-month period. We assessed the differences between 16 OL patients with 27 lesions and nine IgG4-ROD patients with 20 lesions according to prebiopsy CT features of lesions and prebiopsy serum IgG4 levels and immunoglobulin G (IgG) levels This study also established the receiver-operating curves (ROC) of precontrast and postcontrast CT Hounsfield unit scales (CTHU), serum IgG4 levels, serum IgG levels and their ratios. Results: Significantly related to IgG4-ROD (all $p < 0.05$) were the presence of lesions with regular borders, presence of multiple lesions—involving both lacrimal glands on CT scans—higher median values of postcontrast CTHU, postcontrast CTHU/precontrast CTHU ratios, serum IgG4 levels and serum IgG4/IgG level ratios. Compared to postcontrast CTHU, serum IgG4 levels had a larger area under the ROC curve (0.847 [95% confidence interval (CI): 0.674–1.000, $p = 0.005$] vs. 0.766 [95% CI: 0.615–0.917, $p = 0.002$]), higher sensitivity (0.889 [95% CI: 0.518–0.997] vs. 0.75 [95% CI: 0.509–0.913]), higher specificity (0.813 [95% CI: 0.544–0.960] vs. 0.778 [95% CI: 0.578–0.914]) and a higher cutoff value (≥132.5 mg/dL [milligrams per deciliter] vs. ≥89.5). Conclusions: IgG4-ROD showed distinct CT features and elevated serum IgG4 (≥132.5 mg/dL), which could help distinguish IgG4-ROD from OL.

Keywords: immunoglobulin G4-related orbital disease (IgG4-ROD); orbital lymphoma (OL); computed tomography (CT); Hounsfield unit

---

1. Introduction

Orbital space-occupying lesions comprise a wide range of benign and malignant masses [1]. The top eight ocular adnexal lesions include lymphoid tumors, inflammatory disease, cavernous hemangioma, lymphangioma, meningioma, optic nerve glioma, metastatic breast cancer and capillary hemangioma [2]. Several studies indicate that ocular adnexal lymphomas almost account for up to half of all malignant orbital lesions in adults [2–4].

Immunoglobulin G4–related disease—which can involve any organs including orbital structures—is a systemic fibroinflammatory condition due to tissue infiltration by immunoglobulin G4 (IgG4) plasma cells [5]. IgG4-related disease in orbit tends to form tumor-like lesions, which are difficult to differentiate from intraorbital lymphoma because both are tumors rich in lymphoplasmacytic infiltration [6]. Lymphoma, one of the most common orbital malignancies in adults [3,4], needs radiotherapy, systemic chemotherapy and/or surgery [7,8]. In contrast, approximately 90% of patients with IgG4-related orbital disease (IgG4-ROD) respond well to steroid therapy [5] Therefore, rapid and accurate diagnosis of IgG4-ROD to help patients receive early steroid treatment is critical.

IgG4-related disease diagnostic criteria commonly follow: a serum IgG4 concentration higher than 135 mg/dL (milligrams per deciliter) [9], the ratio of IgG4-positive/immunoglobulin G (IgG)-positive plasma cell (IgG4+/IgG+ ratio) is >40% or IgG4+ cells > 10/high-powered field of biopsy sample [9]. However, up to 40% of patients with IgG4-related disease may have serum IgG4 levels within the normal range [10]. Pathology and immunohistochemistry remain the gold standard for accurate diagnosis of IgG4-related disease [5,11].

Furthermore, orbital neoplasm rupture via biopsy may lead to tumor seeding and poor prognosis [12]. Integrating clinical findings, serologic data and radiological features is important to establish the prebiopsy diagnosis of IgG4-ROD [12]. Computed tomography (CT) scans provide rapid high-resolution images of orbits for radiological feature extraction [13]. As such, this study integrates CT qualitative and quantitative (Hounsfield unit density) features, serum IgG, and IgG4 levels to differentiate IgG4-ROD from orbital lymphoma (OL).

2. Material and Methods

2.1. Patients

The Institutional Review Board of Taipei Veterans General Hospital (TVGH) approved this study to waive informed consent because of the retrospective nature of the research.

A doctor (SYY) blinded from the research hypothesis searched pathologic results from the pathology database at TVGH using the keywords "orbit" or "orbital" for cases from 1 January 2010, to 31 May 2018.

The research returned 178 patients with orbital lesions and pathologic results. Thirteen (7%) of 178 patients had multiple orbital lesions (≥2): one (7.7%) of the thirteen patients with lung carcinoid tumors and multiple metastases in the right orbital cavity and 12 (92.3%) patients with lymphoplasmacyte-rich lesions (5 patients with orbital lymphoma; 7 patients with IgG4-ROD). The other 165 (93%) of the 178 patients showed only one lesion in the orbital cavity or eyelid. Sixteen (9%) of the 178 patients had orbital lymphoma (OL) and 9 (5%) patients had IgG4-related orbital disease (IgG4-ROD).

Among these patients, this study only considered patients who had OL or IgG4-ROD with prebiopsy precontrast and postcontrast orbital CT scans, serum IgG4 levels and serum IgG levels and excluded those were younger than 20 years of age or pregnant cases or those lacked prebiopsy CT and serologic data.

As a result, 25 patients pathologically diagnosed as OL (16 patients) or IgG4-ROD (9 patients) met the inclusion criteria and had prebiopsy orbital CT scans, serum IgG4 levels and serum IgG levels. All patients met the eligibility criteria. We enrolled 25 patients to collect and analyze demographic data, symptoms and signs, past medical histories, CT qualitative and quantitative (Hounsfield unit density) features of orbital lesions, serum IgG levels and serum IgG4 levels of patients with IgG4-ROD from those of patients with OL.

2.2. CT Imaging Techniques

This study examined orbital CT images taken by a multiple-detector computed tomography (MDCT) scanner for the selected 25 patients. MDCT scanners of orbit or face included iCT 256 (256-slice, n = 5), Philips Healthcare, Cleveland, OH, USA, Somatom Sensation 16 (16-slice, n = 4), Siemens Healthcare, Forchheim, Germany, ECLOS Hitachi Medical Corporation (16-slice, n = 1), Tokyo, Japan, and Aquilion 64, Toshiba Medical Systems (64-slice, n = 15), Tochigi, Japan. Orbital CT scans were obtained with or without an intravenous contrast medium, which included iobitridol (Xenetix 350; Guerbet, Rue Jean Chaptal, Aulnary-sous-Bios, France, 350 mg I [Iodine]/mL [milliliter]) and iohexol (Omnipaque 350; GE healthcare, Carrigtohill, Co., Cork, Ireland, 350 mg I/mL). The data records showed that twenty-five patients underwent an intravenous power injection as a bolus of 1.2-mL/kg (kilogram) iodine-based contrast medium at 1 mL/second (s). Postcontrast CT images were performed after the complete injection of contrast medium. The axial sections of precontrast and postcontrast orbital CT images scanned along the transaxial direction with the sections parallel to the optic nerve along a line from the inferior border of the maxillary sinus to the middle part of the frontal region. A Hitachi CT scanner took the slice thickness for image viewing of axial images at 1.25 mm (mm) and other MDCT scanners at 2–4 mm. The coronal and sagittal sections of postcontrast orbital CT images were reformatted with 2–4 mm in slice thickness. The reconstruction matrix for MDCT scans of orbit was 512 × 512.

2.3. Analysis of Images and Pathologic Diagnosis

Two experienced radiologists (CHW and YYC) reanalyzed orbital lesions of the 25 patients on orbital CT images with axial, sagittal and/or coronal images together without knowledge of pathologic diagnosis of orbital tumors. The consensus from the two radiologists served as the final interpretation of images. If the two radiologists could not reach an agreement on any features from orbital CT scans, a third experienced radiologist (HCH) mediated the disagreement.

This study analyzed the following orbital CT features of each lesion or of each patient: maximum diameter of a lesion, lesion borders, homogeneity of CT density, a lesion involving extraocular muscle tendons, the lacrimal sac, lacrimal gland, preseptal space, extraconal, conal or intraconal orbital compartments, the optic nerve, infraorbital nerve, presence or absence of bone remodeling, single tumor or multiple lesions and single or bilateral orbital involvement, single or bilateral lacrimal gland involvement. This study also measured the mean values of the precontrast and postcontrast CT Hounsfield unit scales (CTHU) of each orbital lesion among the 25 patients.

A regular border of an orbital tumor on CT scans indicated the contour of a lesion from the surrounding tissue was smooth for more than 75% of the lesion. An irregular border of a lesion showed microlobulated, microangulated or indistinct contour from the surrounding tissue with ≥25% of the lesion. Lesion involvement indicated lesion infiltration, invasion or encasement on orbital CT scans.

This study measured CTHU for all 47 orbital lesions of 25 patients on both pre and postcontrast prebiopsy CT scans. The region of interest (ROI) maker in an oval shape was placed in the center of each lesion to cover 50% of the largest tumor area on CT axial images, avoiding the inclusion of bone and blood vessels (Figure 1). This study also calculated postcontrast CTHU divided by precontrast CTHU.

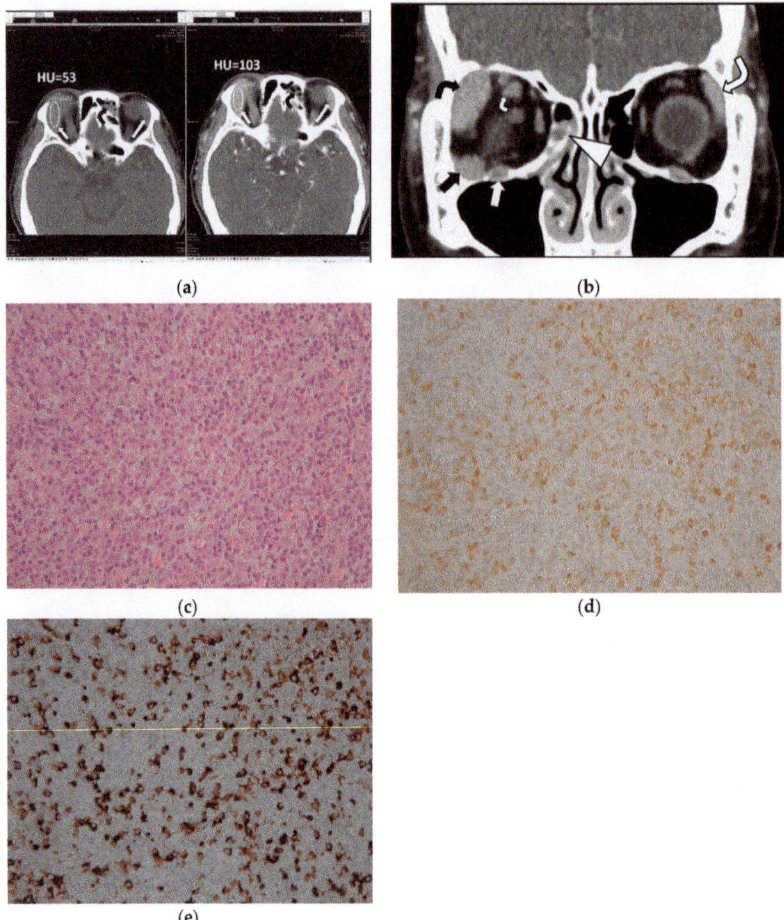

Figure 1. A 68-year-old man with immunoglobulin G4 (IgG4)-related orbital disease (IgG4-ROD) shows multiple tumors in bilateral orbital cavities. (**a**) Axial computed tomography (CT) scans show masses in bilateral lacrimal glands (short and large arrows). The mean value of CT Hounsfield unit scale (CTHU) is measured at the enlarged right lacrimal gland (short arrows) on a picture archiving and communication system monitor. The region of interest (ROI) marker in an oval shape is placed in the center of the mass (short arrows) to cover 50% of the largest tumor area. The mean value of precontrast CTHU is 53 and that of postcontrast CTHU is 103. Sinusitis is found in the left frontal sinus with mucus retention (black curved arrows); (**b**) Coronal postcontrast CT scan shows multiple masses or enlargement in various ophthalmic tissues with regular borders and homogeneous contrast enhancement in bilateral orbital cavities as follows: a mass at the extraconal compartment of the right orbital cavity (black arrow),the right lacrimal gland (black curved arrow), the left lacrimal gland (large white curve arrow), the right superior rectus muscle belly (small white curve arrow) and the right infraorbital nerve (white arrow). Sinusitis is noted in the right ethmoid sinus with mucus retention (arrowhead); (**c**) Pathologic specimen shows infiltration of many lymphoplasma cells and mild fibrosis (hematoxylin–eosin stain, original magnification ×200); (**d**) Immunostaining for immunoglobulin G (IgG)-expression shows many plasma cells are positive for IgG stains (original magnification ×200); (**e**) Immunostaining for IgG4-expression shows abundant IgG4-positive plasma cells have infiltrated the lesion. IgG4-postive/IgG-positive plasma cell ratio is more than 40%. There are more than 100 IgG4-positive plasma cells in one high-powered field (>100/HPF) (original magnification ×200).

An experienced pathologist (AFYL) with 29 years of experience in pathology diagnosis reviewed the pathologic and immunohistochemical sections of the specimens of the 25 patients to confirm pathologic results of OL and IgG4-ROD. The two main pathologic criteria of IgG4-ROD included (1) IgG4+/IgG+ ratio > 40%, and/or (2) IgG4+ cells > 10/high-powered field (HPF) in histopathologic examination [5,9,14].

The radiologist (WHY) integrated demographic data, patient symptoms, signs and past histories, prebiopsy serum IgG4 levels and IgG levels and CT imaging interpretations and the mean values of CTHU measurement results of the 25 patients to evaluate the differences in CT qualitative and quantitative features, serum IgG and IgG4 levels between OL and IgG4-ROD.

2.4. Statistical Analysis

This study used SPSS version 19.0 software (SPSS, Inc., Chicago, IL, USA) for data analysis. Specially, we applied the Mann–Whitney U test to compare continuous variables because of the small sample size and the $\chi 2$ or Fisher's exact test for categorical variables at the level of significance of $p < 0.05$. Receiver operating characteristic (ROC) curve analysis calculated the area under the ROC curve to identify diagnostic values of CTHU, serum IgG4 levels and serum IgG levels of IgG4-ROD. This study assessed the findings based on sensitivity, specificity and accuracy with a 95% confidence interval (95% CI).

3. Results

The median age (mean ± standard deviation [SD], range) of the selected 25 patients was 59 (58.20 ± 10.61, 32–78). The median age (mean ± SD, range) of 16 patients with OL was 60.5 (59.31 ± 9.20, 41–78) and that of 9 patients with IgG4-ROD was 58 (56.22 ± 13.11, 32–69) ($p = 0.934$, Mann–Whitney U test). Of the 25 patients, 17 (68%) were male and 8 (32%) were female. Twelve (12 or 71%) of the 17 male patients were OL and 5 (29%) were IgG4-ROD; four (50%) of 8 females were OL patients and 4 (50%) were IgG4-ROD ($p = 0.3942$, Fisher's exact test).

The 25 patients showed proptosis, palpable mass and/or eyelid swelling—none of the 25 patients suffered from orbital pain or tender palpable mass. Six (6 or 24%) of the 25 patients had malignancy histories. Five (83%) of the 6 patients with malignant histories had OL: one with renal cell carcinoma, one with prostatic cancer and soft palate follicular lymphoma, one with squamous cell carcinoma of the tongue, one with follicular lymphoma involving lung, neck lymph nodes and bone marrow and one with chronic lymphocytic leukemia. Only one (17%) of the 6 patients with malignant history was an IgG4-ROD patient who had ovarian cancer. Patient malignant histories of the two groups had no significant difference ($p = 0.3644$, Fisher's exact test).

A pathologist (AFYL) reviewed the pathologic sections of the 25 patients. The pathologic review concluded 13 patients with extranodal marginal zone lymphoma of mucosa-associated lymphoid tissue (MALT lymphoma), 1 with low-grade B cell lymphoma with plasmacytic differentiation, 1 with diffuse large B cell lymphoma, 1 with follicular lymphoma and 9 with IgG4-ROD. The histopathologic findings of the 9 patients with IgG4-ROD showed diffuse lymphoplasmacytic infiltration, IgG4-positive (IgG4+) plasma cells, IgG-positive (IgG+) plasma cells and various degree fibrosis. Seven (78%) of the nine IgG4-ROD patients showed IgG4+ cells > 100 cells/HPF and IgG4+/IgG+ ratio > 40% (Figure 1). Another 2 of the 9 IgG4-ROD patients (22%) had IgG4+ plasma cell < 50 cells/HPF and IgG4+/IgG+ ratio > 40%.

Furthermore, CT images indicated a total of 47 orbital tumors among the 25 patients: 27 lesions were OL and 20 lesions were IgG4-ROD. Of 47 orbital tumors, none appeared inside the eyeball.

Tables 1 and 2 summarize CT features of 47 tumors among the 25 patients, of which 16 had orbital lymphoma and 9 had IgG4-ROD.

Table 1. Computed tomography (CT) features of 47 tumors among the 25 patients with orbital lymphoma or immunoglobulin G4-related orbital disease (IgG4-ROD) on prebiopsy orbital CT scans.

Orbital CT Scans	Orbital Lymphoma *n* (%)	IgG4-ROD *n* (%)	*p*
Tumor Size, median (mean ± SD, range)	2.58 (2.62 ± 1.149, 0.98–5.16)	3.17 (2.70 ± 1.233, 0.66–5.1)	0.667 @
Lesion border			0.0069 #
Regular	10 (38)	16 (62)	
Irregular	17 (81)	4 (19)	
Precontrast CT density			1 #
Homogeneous	26 (57)	20 (43)	
Heterogeneous	1 (100)	0 (0)	
Postcontrast CT contrast-enhancement			1 #
Homogeneous	26 (57)	20 (43)	
Heterogeneous	1 (100)	0 (0)	
Extraocular muscle tendon involvement			0.1138 #
Presence	10 (77)	3 (23)	
Absence	17 (50)	17 (50)	
Lacrimal sac involvement			1 #
Presence	3 (60)	2 (40)	
Absence	24 (57)	18 (43)	
Preseptal space involvement			1 #
Presence	8 (62)	5 (38)	
Absence	19 (56)	15 (44)	
Lacrimal gland involvement			0.0085 #
Presence	8 (36)	14 (64)	
Absence	19 (76)	6 (24)	
Orbital compartment involvement			0.4813 #
Extraconal or/and conal	20 (53)	17 (47)	
Intraconal	7 (78)	3 (22)	
Optic nerve involvement			1 #
Presence	5 (63)	3 (37)	
Absence	22 (56)	17 (44)	
Infraorbital nerve involvement			1 #
Presence	1 (50)	1 (50)	
Absence	26 (58)	19 (42)	
Bone remodeling			0.2507 #
Presence	3 (100)	0 (0)	
Absence	24 (55)	20 (45)	

n (%)—number (percentage); SD—standard deviation; @—Mann–Whitney U test; #—Fisher's exact test.

Table 2. CT features of the 25 patients with orbital lymphoma or immunoglobulin G4-related orbital disease (IgG4-ROD) on prebiopsy orbital CT scans.

Orbital CT Scans	Orbital Lymphoma *n* (%)	IgG4-ROD *n* (%)	*p*
Tumor number			0.0414 #
Single	11 (85)	2 (15)	
Multiple (≥2)	5 (42)	7 (58)	
Orbital involvement			0.0168 #
One side	12 (86)	2 (14)	
Bilateral	4 (36)	7 (64)	
Bilateral lacrimal gland involvement			0.0022 #
Presence	2 (22)	7 (78)	
Absence	14 (88)	2 (12)	
Sinusitis			0.6882 #
Presence	7 (58)	5 (42)	
Absence	9 (69)	4 (31)	

n (%)—number (percentage); #—Fisher's exact test.

Specifically, of the 16 patients with OL, eleven (69%) had a solitary tumor in an orbital cavity or at eyelids, 1 (6%) had 2 tumors, 2 (13%) had 3 and 2 (13%) had 4. The other 9 out of the 25 patients had IgG4-ROD: 2 (22%) with 1 tumor; 5 (56%) with 2 tumors, 1 (11%) with 3 tumors and 1 (11%) with 5 tumors. CT features statistically significantly associated with IgG4-ROD included lesions with regular borders ($p = 0.0069$), multiple tumors ($p = 0.0414$), lacrimal gland involvement ($p = 0.0085$), lesions involving bilateral lacrimal glands and bilateral orbital cavities ($p = 0.0022$ and $p = 0.0168$, respectively, Figure 1).

In contrast, tumors involving the extraconal, conal or intraconal space, lacrimal sac, optic nerve, extraocular muscle tendon, infraorbital nerve, preseptal space and presence of sinusitis and bone remodeling were ineffectual to differentiate IgG4-ROD from orbital lymphoma (Figures 1 and 2; all $p > 0.05$, Fisher's exact test). Two IgG4-ROD patients and 6 OL patients had a solitary tumor involving the preseptal space (Figure 2).

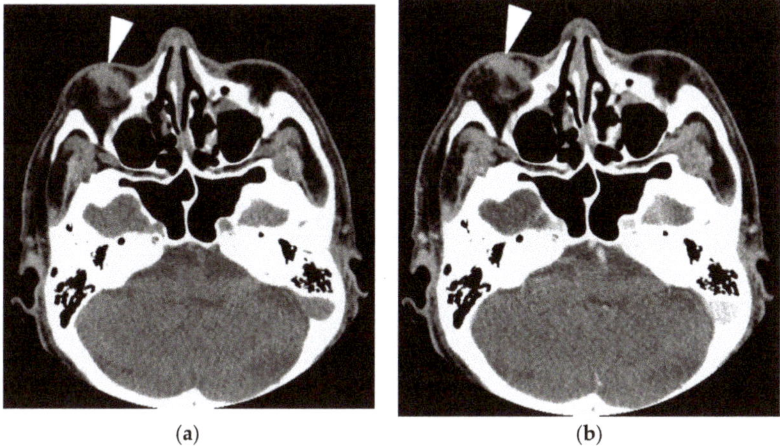

(a) (b)

Figure 2. A 66-year-old man with orbital lymphoma shows a painless solitary lesion at the right lower eyelid. (**a**) Axial precontrast CT image shows a small nodule with an irregular border and homogeneous density involves the preseptal space of the right lower eyelid (arrowhead). Precontrast CT Hounsfield unit scale (CTHU) of the nodule is 57; (**b**) Axial postcontrast CT image shows the nodule demonstrates homogeneous enhancement (arrowhead). Postcontrast CTHU of the nodule is 68. Serum IgG4 level of the patient is 44.3 mg/dL.

Table 3 shows the descriptive statistical prebiopsy values of precontrast CT Hounsfield unit scales (CTHU), postcontrast CTHU and postcontrast CTHU/precontrast CTHU ratios of 27 tumors of OL and 20 tumors of IgG4-ROD on prebiopsy CT scans.

Table 4 demonstrates descriptive statistical prebiopsy values of serum IgG4 levels, serum IgG levels and the ratios of serum IgG4 level/serum IgG level of the 16 patients with OL and the 9 patients with IgG4-ROD.

Table 3. Descriptive statistical prebiopsy values of precontrast CT Hounsfield unit scales (Pre HU), postcontrast CTHU (Post HU) and postcontrast CTHU/precontrast CTHU ratios (Post HU/Pre HU) of 27 tumors of orbital lymphoma and 20 tumors of IgG4-related orbital disease (IgG4-ROD) on prebiopsy orbital CT scans.

	Orbital Lymphoma $n = 27$			IgG4-ROD $n = 20$		
Parameter	**Pre HU**	**Post HU**	**Post HU/Pre HU**	**Pre HU**	**Post HU**	**Post HU/Pre HU**
Median	49	80	1.51	51	93.5	1.8
Mean	51.8	78.9	1.55	54.1	93.8	1.77
SD	10.28	13.58	0.27	10.69	19.02	0.42
Quartile 1	45	68	1.37	45.5	87	1.41
Quartile 3	57	89	1.76	61.25	103	2.08
minimum	36	56	1.17	40	51	1.06
Maximum	76	102	2.31	77	125	2.49
Outlier 1	76		2.31		51	
Outlier 2					59	

n—number; SD—standard deviation.

Table 4. The descriptive statistical prebiopsy values of serum IgG4 levels (serum IgG4), serum immunoglobulin G (IgG) levels (serum IgG) and the ratios of serum IgG4 level/serum IgG level (serum IgG4/IgG) of the 16 patients with orbital lymphoma and the 9 patients with IgG4-ROD.

	Orbital Lymphoma $n = 16$			IgG4-ROD $n = 9$		
Parameter (mg/dL)	**Serum IgG4**	**Serum IgG**	**Serum IgG4/IgG**	**Serum IgG4**	**Serum IgG**	**Serum IgG4/IgG**
Median	57.65	1345	0.042	675	1560	0.241
Mean	135.73	1307.94	0.106	756.49	2108.56	0.32
SD	199.82	332.42	0.1502	733.78	1326.07	0.2325
Quartile 1	28.23	979	0.022	142	1232	0.107
Quartile 3	125.4	1594.5	0.123	1140	3080	0.563
minimum	8.1	725	0.011	28.9	1110	0.026
Maximum	780	1915	0.524	2297.9	4645	0.59
Outlier 1	339.5		0.404		4112	
Outlier 2	780		0.524		4645	

n—number; mg/dL—milligram/deciliter; SD—standard deviation.

Figures 3 and 4 show the differences in postcontrast CTHU, postcontrast CTHU/precontrast CTHU ratios, serum IgG4 levels and serum IgG4 level/serum IgG level ratios were statistically significant between the two groups (all $p < 0.05$, Mann–Whitney U test).

Figure 3 shows that the areas under the ROC curve (AUC) of precontrast CTHU, postcontrast CTHU and the ratios of postcontrast CTHU/precontrast CTHU were 0.56 (95% CI: 0.393–0.727, $p = 0.484$), 0.766 (95% CI: 0.615–0.917, $p = 0.002$) and 0.670 (95% CI: 0.498–0.842, $p = 0.048$). According to Figure 4, the AUC for serum IgG4 levels, serum IgG levels and the ratios of serum IgG4/serum IgG were 0.847 (95% CI: 0.674–1.000, $p = 0.005$), 0.684 (95% CI: 0.455–0.913, $p = 0.134$) and 0.819 (95% CI: 0.639–1.000, $p = 0.009$), respectively.

Compared with above data, the AUC using postcontrast CTHU (= 0.766) and serum IgG4 levels (= 0.847) was moderately accurate for the diagnostic yield of IgG4-ROD because both AUC measures fell between 0.7 and 0.9. The largest Jordon index 0.528 [(sensitivity−[1−specificity] = 0.528)] suggested a cutoff value of postcontrast CTHU equal to 89.5. The sensitivity and specificity were 0.75 (95% CI: 0.509–0.913) and 0.778 (95% CI: 0.578–0.914), respectively. As to serum IgG4 level, the largest Jordon index (0.701) suggested a cutoff value equal to 132.5 mg/dL, which resulted in sensitivity of 0.889 (95% CI: 0.518–0.997) and specificity of 0.813 (95% CI: 0.544–0.960), respectively.

For patients with postcontrast CTHU ≥ 89.5 in at least one orbital nodule in the two groups, 7 (58%) were IgG4-ROD patients and 5 (42%) were OL patients ($p = 0.0414$, Fisher's exact test). For serum IgG4 levels ≥ 132.5 mg/dL, 8 (73%) were IgG4-ROD patients and 3 (27%) OL ($p = 0.0021$).

The postcontrast CTHU and serum IgG4 levels for patients with a solitary orbital tumor in the two groups of OL and IgG4-ROD patients were as follows: higher postcontrast CTHU (≥89.5) in 3 OL patients and 1 IgG4-ROD case; lower postcontrast CTHU (<89.5) in 8 OL and 1 IgG4-ROD; and lower serum IgG4 levels (<132.5) in all 11 OL patients and 1 IgG4-ROD case with higher CTHU. In addition, one IgG4-ROD patient with a lower postcontrast CTHU showed a higher serum IgG4 level ≥ 132.5.

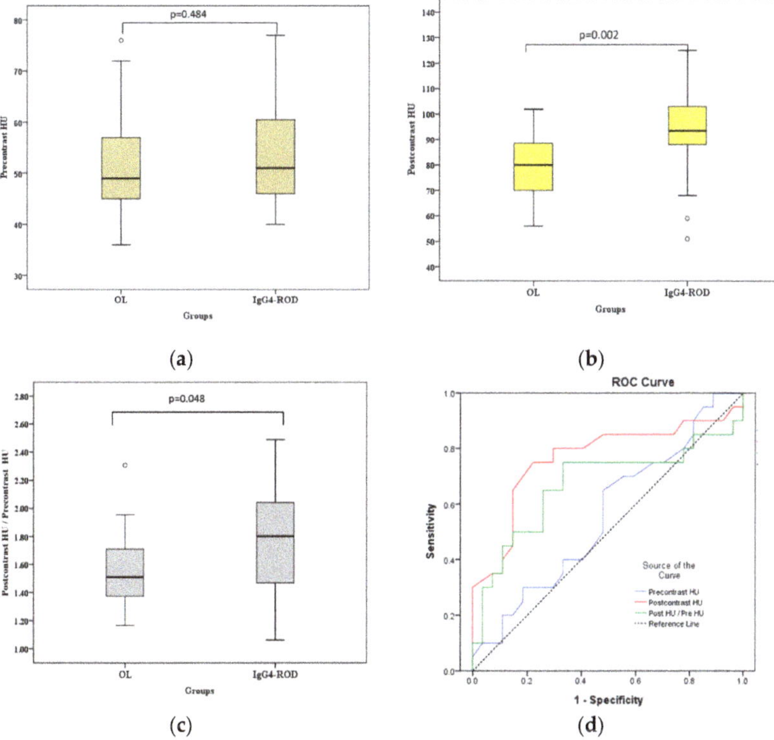

(a) (b) (c) (d)

Figure 3. Box-and-whisker plots and receiver operating characteristic (ROC) curve analysis of precontrast computed tomography (CT) Hounsfield unit scale (CTHU), postcontrast CTHU, postcontrast CTHU/precontrast CTHU ratios between orbital lymphoma (OL) and immunoglobulin G4-related orbital disease (IgG4-ROD). Bars = medians. (**a**) Precontrast CTHU (precontrast HU) shows a nonsignificant difference between the two groups ($p = 0.484$, Mann–Whitney U test); (**b**) Postcontrast CTHU (postcontrast HU) shows a significant difference between the two groups ($p = 0.002$, Mann–Whitney U test); (**c**) Postcontrast CTHU/precontrast CTHU ratios (postcontrast HU/precontrast HU) show a significant difference between the two groups ($p = 0.048$, Mann–Whitney U test); (**d**) Areas under the ROC curve (AUC) of precontrast CTHU (precontrast HU), postcontast CTHU (postcontrast HU) and postcontrast CTHU/precontrast CTHU ratios (postcontrast HU/precontrast HU) are 0.56 (95% CI: 0.393–0.727, $p = 0.484$), 0.766 (95% CI: 0.615–0.917, $p = 0.002$) and 0.670 (95% CI: 0.498–0.842, $p = 0.048$), respectively. ○—an outlier.

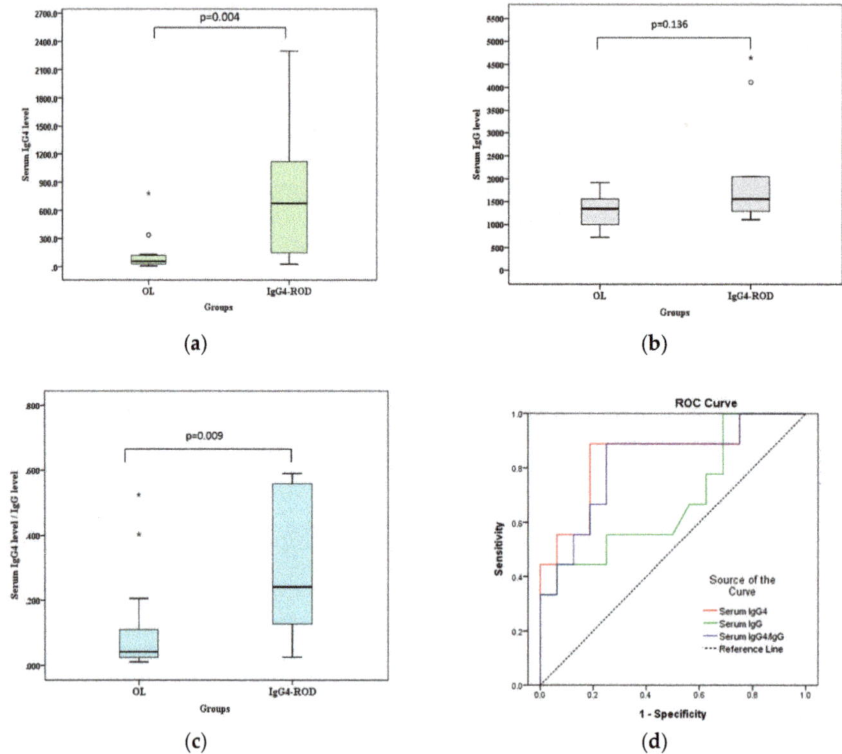

Figure 4. Box-and-whisker plots and receiver operating characteristic curve (ROC) analysis of serum immunoglobulin G4 (IgG4) levels, serum immunoglobulin G (IgG) levels and serum IgG4 level/serum IgG level ratios between orbital lymphoma (OL) and IgG4-related orbital disease (IgG4-ROD). Bars = medians. (**a**) Serum IgG4-levels demonstrate a significant difference between the two groups (p = 0.004, Mann–Whitney U test); (**b**) Serum IgG levels demonstrate a nonsignificant difference between the two groups (p = 0.136, Mann–Whitney U test); (**c**) Serum IgG4 level/IgG level ratios (serum IgG4 level/IgG level) demonstrate a significant difference between the two groups (p = 0.009, Mann–Whitney U test); (**d**) The areas under the ROC curve of serum IgG4 level (serum IgG4), serum IgG level (serum IgG) and serum IgG4 level/IgG level ratio (serum IgG4/IgG) are 0.847 (95% CI: 0.674 to 1.000, p = 0.005), 0.684 (95% CI: 0.455 to 0.913, p = 0.134) and 0.819 (95% CI: 0.639 to 1.000, p = 0.009), respectively. * and ○—outliers.

The postcontrast CTHU and serum IgG4 level for patients with multiple orbital lesions in the two groups were as follows: lower postcontrast CTHU (<89.5) were noted in 3 OL patients and in 1 IgG4-ROD case; higher postcontrast CTHU (≥89.5) were found in 2 OL patients and in 6 IgG4-ROD cases; higher serum IgG4 levels (≥132.5 mg/dL) were found in 3 OL patients and in 7 IgG4-ROD cases; lower serum IgG4 levels (<132.5 mg/dL) appeared in 2 OL patients. Two of the three OL patients with lower postcontrast CTHU showed OL involving bilateral lacrimal glands, who had different serum IgG4 levels: 51.3 and 339.5, respectively. Concurrent higher postcontrast CTHU and a higher serum IgG4 level were found in 1 OL patient (1/5, 20%) with multiple tumors in the left orbital cavity and in 6 IgG4-ROD cases with tumors involving bilateral lacrimal glands. Lower postcontrast CTHU and higher serum IgG4 level were noted in only one IgG4-ROD (1/7, 14%) case, who showed tumors mainly in intraconal spaces of bilateral orbits.

If this study used "lesions with bilateral lacrimal gland involvement" (the most significant qualitative CT feature in statistics, p = 0.0022), "bilateral lacrimal gland involvement and a higher serum IgG4 level (≥132.5 mg/dL) ($p = 0.0005$)" or "bilateral lacrimal gland involvement and higher postcontrast CTHU (≥89.5, quantitative CT feature) ($p = 0.00047$)" or "higher postcontrast CTHU and a higher serum IgG4 level" ($p = 0.0029$) as helpful test tools for diagnosis of IgG4-ROD (Table 5), sensitivity, specificity and accuracy of the first test (Test 1), the second (Test 2), the third (Test 3) and the latest one (Test 4) were as follows (Table 5): 0.78 (95% CI: 0.3999–0.972), 0.88 (95% CI: 0.617–0.985) and 0.84 (95% CI: 0.639–0.955) for Test 1; 0.78 (95% CI: 0.3999–0.972), 0.94 (95% CI: 0.698–0.998) and 0.88 (95% CI: 0.688–0.975) for Test 2; 0.67 (95% CI: 0.299–0.925), 1 (95% CI: 0.794–1) and 0.88 (95% CI: 0.688–0.975) for Test 3; 0.67 (95% CI: 0.299–0.925), 0.94 (95% CI: 0.698–0.998) and 0.84 (95% CI: 0.639–0.955) for Test 4. In Table 5, Test 3 had 100% of positive predictive value (PPV). Test 1 & Test 2 had the highest negative predictive value (NPV) 0.88.

Table 5. Contingency table of four helpful testing tools for diagnosis of IgG4-related orbital disease (IgG4-ROD).

	Test 1	Test 2	Test 3	Test 4
True positive, n	7	7	6	6
False negative, n	2	2	3	3
False positive, n	2	1	0	1
True negative, n	14	15	16	15
Sensitivity	0.78	0.78	0.67	0.67
(95% CI)	(0.40–0.972)	(0.40–0.972)	(0.299–0.925)	(0.299–0.925)
Specificity	0.88	0.94	1.0	0.94
(95% CI)	(0.617–0.985)	(0.698–0.998)	(0.794–1.0)	(0.698–0.998)
PPV	0.78	0.88	1.0	0.86
(95% CI)	(0.478–0.931)	(0.504–0.98)	(*)	(0.460–0.977)
NPV	0.88	0.88	0.84	0.83
(95% CI)	(0.670–0.960)	(0.687–0.962)	(0.679–0.931)	(0.663–0.927)
Accuracy	0.84	0.88	0.88	0.84
(95% CI)	(0.639–0.955)	(0.688–0.975)	(0.688–0.975)	(0.639–0.955)

n, patient number; Test 1 to Test 4 represent four helpful tools for diagnosis of IgG4-ROD; Test 1, orbital lesions with bilateral lacrimal gland involvement on CT scans; Test 2, orbital lesions with bilateral lacrimal gland involvement on CT scans and a higher serum IgG4 level (≥132.5 mg/dL [milligrams per deciliter]); Test 3, orbital lesions with bilateral lacrimal gland involvement and higher postcontrast CTHU (CT Hounsfield unit scales ≥ 89.5) on CT scans; Test 4, orbital lesions with higher postcontrast CTHU (≥89.5) and a higher serum IgG4 level (≥132.5 mg/dL); (95% CI), (95% confidence interval); *—not shown in the statistics operation; PPV—positive predictive value—NPV—negative predictive value.

4. Discussion

The IgG4-related disease can result in fibroinflammatory lesions at nearly any anatomic site [14]. OL is malignant and needs radiotherapy, chemotherapy and/or operation [4,7,8]. IgG4-ROD is benign and approximately 90% of patients respond well to steroid treatment [5]. Both of malignant OL and benign IgG4-ROD are lymphoplasmacytic infiltrated mass-like lesions, which make clinicians difficult to differentiate from each other [6]. This study showed that lesions with regular borders, multiple tumors, lacrimal gland involvement, simultaneous involvement of bilateral lacrimal glands and bilateral orbital cavities and higher medians of postcontrast CTHU and serum IgG4 levels were significantly related to IgG4-ROD (all $p < 0.05$). Postcontrast CTHU ≥ 89.5 showed 0.75 sensitivity and 0.778 specificity with the AUC = 0.766 (95% CI: 0.615–0.917, $p = 0.002$); serum IgG4 levels ≥ 132.5 mg/dL had 0.889 sensitivity and 0.813 specificity, with the AUC = 0.847 (95% CI: 0.674–1.000, $p = 0.005$, Figures 3 and 4). A lesion with regular borders is most likely to be a slow growing benign mass or less likely to be an indolent malignant tumor [1]. IgG4-ROD being benign usually presented as lesions with regular borders in this study.

Serum IgG4 levels account for 3% to 6% total amount of serum IgG levels [15]. Hamano et al. [16] reported a cutoff value of 135 mg/dL to differentiate autoimmune pancreatitis from pancreatic cancer with a high sensitivity (95%), specificity (97%) and accuracy (97%). This study identified a cutoff value

132.5 mg/dL (close to 135 mg/dL) to distinguish IgG4-ROD from OL at diagnostic accuracy (AUC) of 84.7% with 88.9% sensitivity and 81.3% specificity.

However, approximately 40–50% of patients with biopsy-proven IgG4-related disease have normal serum IgG4 concentrations [10,14,17]. In our study, normal serum IgG4 (<132.5 mg/dL) occurred in 13 (81%) of 16 OL patients and one IgG4-ROD patient (1/9, 11%), who had a solitary orbital lesion. There may be several reasons to explain why in our study there was a lower percentage of IgG4-ROD with normal serum IgG4 levels: first, our study was a small sample research, which may have selection bias; second, serum IgG4 levels may vary according to the specific organ involved [10]; finally, elevated serum IgG4 levels represent a subtype of IgG4-related disease with more inflammatory features and worsening disease activity [17]. Our IgG4-ROD patients (8/9, 89%) could be developing an active IgG4-related disease with elevated serum IgG4 concentrations.

Patient's age, standard imaging features and localizing orbital lesions to intraconal, conal or extraconal compartments help limit the differential diagnosis [18]. Our study showed no significant difference in median ages between patients with OL and IgG4-ROD (p = 0.934, Mann–Whitney U test). Lesions with regular borders, multiple orbital tumors, lacrimal gland involvement, lesions simultaneously involving bilateral lacrimal glands and bilateral orbital cavities and higher postcontrast CTHU (≥89.5) on orbital CT scans were significantly associated with IgG4-ROD (all $p < 0.05$). The difference in extraconal, conal and intraconal compartments of orbital lesions between OL and IgG4-ROD groups was not statistically significant (p = 0.4813). In addition to CT, magnetic resonance imaging (MRI) also helps in further diagnostic workup of orbital tumors and provides ocular anatomy for lesions involvement, perineural spread and intracranial extension [12]. Both retinoblastomas typically found in children and uveal melanomas in adults appear in the globe. Retinoblastoma is slightly hyperintense on T1 weighted MRI (T1WI) and very hypointense relative to vitreous on T2-weighted MRI (T2WI) and well contrast enhancement on postcontrast CT and contrast-enhanced (CE) MRI [12,18]. Ninety percent of retinoblastomas demonstrate calcifications on precontrast CT scans [18]. Melanomas with melanin show characteristic hyperintensity on T1WI and hypointensity on T2WI [12,18]. For intraconal orbital tumors, gliomas common among children result in fusiform enlargement of the optic nerve on axial CT and MRI [12,18]. In contrast, meningiomas, commonly seen in the 5th decade of life, classically show the contrast-enhancing tumor with a "tram-tract" configuration alongside the optic nerve on axial postcontrast CT or CE MRI [12]. The most common benign orbital tumor in adults is a cavernous hemangioma, which typically demonstrates a well-defined dense unilateral orbital intraconal mass with intra-tumoral calcifications on precontrast CT scans and MRI. The enhancement spread pattern on a dynamic postcontrast CT and dynamic CE T1WI can help to distinguish between cavernous hemangioma and schwannoma [18,19]. Cavernous hemangiomas show initial patchy enhancement on arterial phase, but schwannomas start a wide area of enhancement. The most common congenital orbital nodules are dermoids, which usually show a well outlined round or oval tumor with a capsule and low density or fat contents in the extraconal space on CT scans or MRI [18]. Due to fat contents, dermoids typically show hyperintensity on T1WI, hyperintensity on T2WI and hypointensity on short tau inversion recovery MRI (STIR) [18]. Benign mixed tumor of lacrimal gland usually seen in middle-aged patients demonstrates a well-circumscribed round or oval tumor with homogeneous enhancement on postcontrast CT and CE MRI [12]. Malignant epithelial lacrimal gland tumors show a mass with a well- or poor-defined margin with associated bony remodeling or destruction in 70% cases on CT scans [18].

Multiple or multicompartmental orbital masses include venolymphatic malformations (VLM), rhabdomyosarcoma (RMS), plexiform neurofibroma, thyroid ophthalmopathy (TO), orbital pseudotumor (OP), lymphoma, metastases and IgG4-ROD [18]. The first three types of masses are common among children; the last five, among adults [3,5,18]. VLM usually appears poorly defined, lobulated and multiloculated lesions with various signal intensity on T1WI and T2WI [18]. VLM may demonstrate fluid–fluid level on MRI, which is highly suggestive of the diagnosis of VLM [12]. VLM, RMS and plexiform neurofibroma may have similar findings on CT and MRI [18]. TO causes enlarged bilateral myositis of the extraocular muscles, often involves medial and inferior rectus muscles with sparing tendinous insertions on CT and MRI [12] and is related to elevated thyroid-stimulating hormone level [18]. OP, IgG4-ROD and OL show similar MRI features on conventional sequences, which are hypointense on T1WI and T2WI and well contrast enhancement on postcontrast T1WI. Furthermore, diffusion-weighted imaging (DWI) with apparent diffusion coefficient (ADC) mapping can help to differentiate between benign and malignant orbital lesions [1,18]. Sepahdari et al. have reported that an ADC value < 1.0×10^{-3} mm^2/ sec and an ADC ratio < 1.2 are optimal for predicting orbital malignant tumors [1,18]. Prior studies used ADC value < 1.0×10^{-3} mm^2/ sec and ADC ratio < 1.2 to differentiate orbital lymphoma from benign OP and IgG4-ROD with more than 95% accuracy [1,18]. However, ADC values and ratios cannot differentiate OP from IgG4-ROD because the two disease have similar these values [1,18]. OP manifests with the most common acute unilateral painful mass in adults, which assist in differentiating OP from TO, OL and IgG4-ROD. Pain is uncommon in TO, OL and IgG4-ROD [12,18]. None of 25 patients in this study suffered from orbital pain or tender palpable mass, either. Consistent with the result of our research, Fujita et al. have reported that IgG4-ROD commonly presents involving bilateral lacrimal glands [15], which can distinguish OL and OP from IgG4-ROD. A clinician can suggest the diagnosis of orbital metastasis only when clinically primary malignancy is known [18].

An effective clinical diagnosis or appropriate disease classification for IgG4-related disease needs the integration of clinical findings, radiological features and serologic or pathologic data [12]. None of our 25 patients suffered from painful orbital lesions. Four tests for IgG4-ROD diagnosis used in this study included serologic serum IgG4 levels, radiological CT qualitative (lesions with bilateral lacrimal gland involvement) and/or quantitative features (postcontrast CTHU ≥ 89.5). Of the four tests, Test 2 (lesions with bilateral lacrimal gland involvement and a higher serum IgG4 level [≥132.5 mg/dL]) with the highest sensitivity (78%), a higher specificity (94%), a higher PPV (88%), the highest NPV (88%) and the highest accuracy (88%) could be the better prebiopsy test to distinguish IgG4-ROD from OL.

This study had only two IgG4-ROD patients with a solitary tumor, which was a small sample and lacked specific CT features. Prebiopsy diagnosis of a solitary IgG4-ROD could depend on a painless orbital mass, postcontrast CTHU ≥ 89.5 and serum IgG4 level ≥ 132.5 mg/dL. Tissue proof is an ultimate diagnostic way. However, biopsy is not always suitable for orbital lesions. The best medical option for a benign mixed tumor or malignant mass of the lacrimal gland may be excision en bloc without biopsy once clinical and imaging diagnosis. However, incomplete excision or ruptures of neoplasms via biopsy may result in tumor recurrence, malignant transformation of a mixed tumor and poor prognosis [12]. In clinical practice, some IgG4-ROD patients may be at high risk for biopsy and/or refuse biopsy. However, once these patients meet possible diagnosis of IgG4-ROD [20], systemic steroid treatment may be a good alternative. The criteria for possible IgG4-ROD diagnosis include elevated serum IgG4 (≥135 mg/dL), enlargement of the lacrimal gland or masses, enlargement or hypertrophic lesions in various orbital tissues [20]. Clinicians could forgo further biopsy if such patients respond well to glucocorticoids within weeks, such as reductions in the size of tumors, improvements of symptoms and a significant decrease in serum IgG4 [20]. Alternative non-vital organ or lip biopsy may be an acceptable option [21].

Sato et al. [22] reported that 17 (81%) of 21 patients with IgG4-ROD had involvement of the lacrimal glands and 13 (70.6%) of 17 cases showed bilateral lacrimal gland swellings. Our study also showed that seven (78%) of nine patients with IgG4-ROD had bilateral lacrimal gland involvement, which could distinguish IgG4-ROD from OL (p = 0.0022). Neither Sato et al. nor this study had patients with IgG4-ROD originating from conjunctival or subconjunctival tissue. However, prior research suggested that IgG4-ROD can also develop at conjunctival tissue [23,24].

This study has several limitations. First, this retrospective research had a small sample of patients. Second, the patients in this study received different brands of contrast agents and CT machine, which could produce potential bias in measurement of CTHU. Last, incomplete data records ruled out the possibility of deciphering a detailed correlation between CT features and clinical presentations of OL and IgG4 ROD.

5. Conclusions

This study compared prebiopsy precontrast and postcontrast CT features, serum IgG4 and serum IgG levels of IgG4-ROD with those of OL. The key findings showed that IgG4-ROD had high correlation with the presence of lesions with regular borders, presence of multiple lesions, lesions involving the lacrimal gland, both lacrimal glands and bilateral orbital cavities on CT scans, higher values of postcontrast CTHU, postcontrast CTHU/precontrast CTHU ratios, serum IgG4 levels and serum IgG4/IgG level ratios (all $p < 0.05$). For diagnosis of IgG4-ROD, postcontrast CTHU ≥ 89.5 and serum IgG4 level ≥ 132.5 mg/dL provided moderate diagnostic accuracy, AUC = 0.776 and 0.847, respectively, which were higher than those of postcontrast HU/precontrast HU and serum IgG4/IgG level ratio. The special CT features and elevated serum IgG4 levels could help differentiate IgG4-ROD from OL. Prebiopsy diagnosis of the uncommon solitary type of IgG4-ROD could also depend on a painless orbital mass and elevated CTHU ≥ 89.5 and serum IgG4 level ≥ 132.5 mg/dL.

Author Contributions: Conceptualization, W.-H.Y. and A.F.-Y.L.; methodology, W.-H.Y. and A.F.-Y.L.; software, W.-H.Y.; validation, W.-H.Y. and A.F.-Y.L.; formal analysis, Y.-Y.C., C.-H.W., H.-C.H., A.F.-Y.L.; investigation, Y.-Y.C., C.-H.W., H.-C.H., A.F.-Y.L.; resources, S.-Y.Y.; data curation, S.-Y.Y., W.-H.Y.; writing—original draft preparation, W.-H.Y.; writing—review and editing, W.-H.Y.; visualization, W.-Y.G.; supervision, J.-F.L. and W.-Y.G.; project administration, W.-H.Y.; funding acquisition, W.-H.Y. All authors have read and agreed to the published version of the manuscript.

Funding: This research received no external funding.

Acknowledgments: We thank May Yuan for English language editing.

Conflicts of Interest: The authors declare no conflict of interests.

References

1. Sepahdari, A.R.; Aakalu, V.K.; Setabutr, P.; Shiehmorteza, M.; Naheedy, J.H.; Mafee, M.F. Indeterminate orbital masses: Restricted diffusion at MR imaging with echo-planar diffusion-weighted imaging predicts malignancy. *Radiology* **2010**, *256*, 554–564. [CrossRef]
2. Shields, J.A.; Shields, C.L.; Scartozzi, R. Survey of 1264 patients with orbital tumors and simulating lesions: The 2002 Montgomery Lecture, part 1. *Ophthalmology* **2004**, *111*, 997–1008. [CrossRef]
3. Politi, L.S.; Forghani, R.; Godi, C.; Resti, A.G.; Ponzoni, M.; Bianchi, S.; Iadanza, A.; Ambrosi, A.; Falini, A.; Ferreri, A.J.; et al. Ocular adnexal lymphoma: Diffusion-weighted mr imaging for differential diagnosis and therapeutic monitoring. *Radiology* **2010**, *256*, 565–574. [CrossRef] [PubMed]
4. Sjo, L.D. Ophthalmic lymphoma: Epidemiology and pathogenesis. *Acta Ophthalmol.* **2009**, *87*, 1–20. [CrossRef] [PubMed]
5. Detiger, S.E.; Karim, A.F.; Verdijk, R.M.; van Hagen, P.M.; van Laar, J.A.M.; Paridaens, D. The treatment outcomes in IgG4-related orbital disease: A systematic review of the literature. *Acta Ophthalmol.* **2019**, *97*, 451–459. [CrossRef]
6. Hiwatashi, A.; Yoshiura, T.; Togao, O.; Yamashita, K.; Kikuchi, K.; Fujita, Y.; Yoshikawa, H.; Koga, T.; Obara, M.; Honda, H. Diffusivity of intraorbital lymphoma vs. IgG4-related DISEASE: 3D turbo field echo with diffusion-sensitised driven-equilibrium preparation technique. *Eur. Radiol.* **2014**, *24*, 581–586.
7. Damato, B.; Bever, G.J.; Kim, D.J.; Afshar, A.R.; Rubenstein, J.L. An audit of retinal lymphoma treatment at the University of California San Francisco. *Eye* **2019**, *34*, 515–522. [CrossRef] [PubMed]
8. Lee, J.; Yoon, J.S.; Kim, J.S.; Koom, W.S.; Cho, J.; Suh, C.O. Long-term outcome, relapse patterns, and toxicity after radiotherapy for orbital mucosa-associated lymphoid tissue lymphoma: Implications for radiotherapy optimization. *Jpn. J. Clin. Oncol.* **2019**, *49*, 664–670. [CrossRef] [PubMed]
9. Toyoda, K.; Oba, H.; Kutomi, K.; Furui, S.; Oohara, A.; Mori, H.; Sakurai, K.; Tsuchiya, K.; Kan, S.; Numaguchi, Y. MR imaging of IgG4-related disease in the head and neck and brain. *AJNR Am. J. Neuroradiol.* **2012**, *33*, 2136–2139. [CrossRef]

10. Ginat, D.T.; Freitag, S.K.; Kieff, D.; Grove, A.; Fay, A.; Cunnane, M.; Moonis, G. Radiographic patterns of orbital involvement in IgG4-related disease. *Ophthalmic Plast. Reconstr. Surg.* **2013**, *29*, 261–266. [CrossRef]
11. Khosroshahi, A.; Cheryk, L.A.; Carruthers, M.N.; Edwards, J.A.; Bloch, D.B.; Stone, J.H. Brief Report: Spuriously low serum IgG4 concentrations caused by the prozone phenomenon in patients with IgG4-related disease. *Arthritis Rheumatol.* **2014**, *66*, 213–217. [CrossRef] [PubMed]
12. Tailor, T.D.; Gupta, D.; Dalley, R.W.; Keene, C.D.; Anzai, Y. Orbital neoplasms in adults: Clinical, radiologic, and pathologic review. *Radiographics* **2013**, *33*, 1739–1758. [CrossRef] [PubMed]
13. Yuan, W.H.; Hsu, H.C.; Cheng, H.C.; Guo, W.Y.; Teng, M.M.; Chen, S.J.; Lin, T.C. CT of globe rupture: Analysis and frequency of findings. *AJR Am. J. Roentgenol.* **2014**, *202*, 1100–1107. [CrossRef] [PubMed]
14. Wallace, Z.S.; Naden, R.P.; Chari, S.; Choi, H.K. The 2019 American College of Rheumatology/European League Against Rheumatism classification criteria for IgG4-related disease. *Arthritis Rheumatol.* **2020**, *72*, 7–19. [CrossRef] [PubMed]
15. Fujita, A.; Sakai, O.; Chapman, M.N.; Sugimoto, H. IgG4-related disease of the head and neck: CT and MR imaging manifestations. *Radiographics* **2012**, *32*, 1945–1958. [CrossRef] [PubMed]
16. Hamano, H.; Kawa, S.; Horiuchi, A.; Unno, H.; Furuya, N.; Akamatsu, T.; Fukushima, M.; Nikaido, T.; Nakayama, K.; Usuda, N.; et al. High serum IgG4 concentrations in patients with sclerosing pancreatitis. *N. Engl. J. Med.* **2001**, *344*, 732–738. [CrossRef]
17. Wallace, Z.S.; Deshpande, V.; Mattoo, H.; Mahajan, V.S.; Kulikova, M.; Pillai, S.; Stone, J.H. IgG4-Related Disease: Clinical and Laboratory Features in One Hundred Twenty-Five Patients. *Arthritis Rheumatol.* **2015**, *67*, 2466–2475. [CrossRef]
18. Purohit, B.S.; Vargas, M.I.; Ailianou, A.; Merlini, L.; Poletti, P.A.; Platon, A.; Delattre, B.M.; Rager, O.; Burkhardt, K.; Becker, M. Orbital tumours and tumour-like lesions: Exploring the armamentarium of multiparametric imaging. *Insights Imaging* **2016**, *7*, 43–68. [CrossRef]
19. Tanaka, A.; Mihara, F.; Yoshiura, T.; Togao, O.; Kuwabara, Y.; Natori, Y.; Sasaki, T.; Honda, H. Differentiation of cavernous hemangioma from schwannoma of the orbit: A dynamic MRI study. *AJR Am. J. Roentgenol.* **2004**, *183*, 1799–1804. [CrossRef]
20. Yu, W.K.; Tsai, C.C.; Kao, S.C.; Liu, C.J. Immunoglobulin G4-related ophthalmic disease. *Taiwan J. Ophthalmol.* **2018**, *8*, 9–14. [CrossRef]
21. Akiyama, M.; Kaneko, Y.; Hayashi, Y.; Takeuchi, T. IgG4-related disease involving vital organs diagnosed with lip biopsy: A case report and literature review. *Medicine* **2016**, *95*, e3970. [CrossRef] [PubMed]
22. Sato, Y.; Ohshima, K.; Ichimura, K.; Sato, M.; Yamadori, I.; Tanaka, T.; Takata, K.; Morito, T.; Kondo, E.; Yoshino, T. Ocular adnexal IgG4-related disease has uniform clinicopathology. *Pathol. Int.* **2008**, *58*, 465–470. [CrossRef] [PubMed]
23. da Fonseca, F.L.; Ramos Rde, I.; de Lima, P.P.; Nogueira, A.B.; Matayoshi, S. Unilateral eyelid mass as an unusual presentation of ocular adnexal IgG4-related inflammation. *Cornea* **2013**, *32*, 517–519. [CrossRef] [PubMed]
24. Lee, H.S.; Choi, W.; Kim, G.E.; Yoon, K.C. Case of Primary Isolated Subconjunctival IgG4-Related Disease. *Cornea* **2018**, *37*, 926–928. [CrossRef] [PubMed]

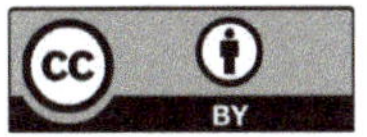

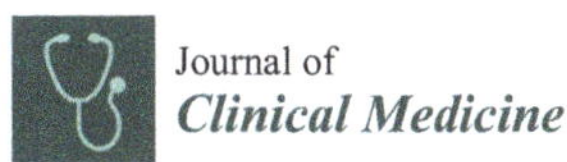

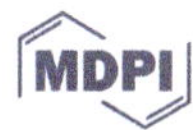

Article

Combined Use of Febuxostat and Colchicine Does Not Increase Acute Hepatotoxicity in Patients with Gout: A Retrospective Study

Yoon-Jeong Oh and Ki Won Moon *

Division of Rheumatology, Department of Internal Medicine, Kangwon National University School of Medicine, Chuncheon 24289, Korea; yjgark640@gmail.com

* Correspondence: kiwonmoon@kangwon.ac.kr; Tel.: +82-33-258-9470; Fax: +82-33-258-2455

Received: 5 April 2020; Accepted: 12 May 2020; Published: 15 May 2020

Abstract: Colchicine has been effectively used to prevent acute flares in patients with gout, but drug-related adverse events have frequently occurred. We investigated whether colchicine therapy with febuxostat is associated with hepatotoxicity in gout patients. Gout patients treated with (n = 121) or without (n = 57) colchicine were enrolled upon initiating febuxostat as a urate-lowering treatment, and clinical and laboratory data at diagnosis were compared. Logistic regression analysis was performed to evaluate the risk factors related to hepatotoxicity. Median age of the with-colchicine and without-colchicine groups was 51.0 (37.0–62.0) and 56.0 (43.5–68.5) years, respectively. During the three months of febuxostat prescription, the prevalence of hepatotoxicity was 13/121 (10.9%) in the with-colchicine group and 4/57 (7.0%) in the without-colchicine group, without statistical significance. The rate of colchicine use was not different between the study subjects with or without hepatotoxicity (76.5% vs. 67.1%, p = 0.587). Pre-existing liver disease was significantly associated with increased risk of hepatotoxicity after febuxostat treatment (odds ratio, 4.083; 95% confidence interval, 1.326–12.577; p = 0.014). Colchicine may be safely used as a prophylactic agent for gout patients with febuxostat. However, upon initiating febuxostat, it is recommended to monitor the development of acute liver injury in gout patients with underlying liver disease.

Keywords: gout; febuxostat; colchicine; hepatotoxicity; prophylaxis

---

1. Introduction

Gout is a common and treatable form of inflammatory arthritis resulting from the chronic deposition of monosodium urate crystals, which form in the presence of increased urate concentrations [1]. Recent studies have reported that incidence and prevalence rates of gout are rapidly increasing in many countries due to various factors, such as change of dietary habits and comorbid conditions [2,3]. Previous studies have also reported that gout is associated with a number of comorbidities, including cardiovascular disease (CVD), type II diabetes, obesity, dyslipidemia, chronic kidney disease (CKD), nonalcoholic fatty liver disease, and metabolic syndrome [4]. These comorbidities play an important role in determining the medication for treatment options in patients with gout.

Early episodes of acute gouty attack resolve spontaneously within several days or weeks, but repeated acute flares can lead to chronic arthritis with the formation of tophi and joint damage, which contribute to disability and decreased quality of life. Therefore, uric acid-lowering therapy (ULT) as well as prophylaxis of acute attack is one of the treatment goals of gout [5]. A recent guideline for gout management has recommended that when initiating ULT, prophylactic treatment with anti-inflammatory drugs for at least 6 months reduces the frequency of gout flares [6].

Colchicine is a systemic anti-inflammatory agent, and has been regarded as a first line prophylactic drug to prevent gout flare. However, it also has many side effects, such as gastrointestinal symptoms (including diarrhea), muscle pain or weakness, drug-to-drug interactions, renal impairment, and abnormal liver function tests [7]. Therefore, before colchicine treatment, it is necessary to consider the underlying diseases and concomitant medications.

A previous study has shown that colchicine is associated with a risk of hepatotoxicity in gout patients prescribed febuxostat [8], which has also been reported to induce acute liver injury [9]. However, there are few studies regarding hepatic safety of colchicine as a prophylactic therapy in gout patients treated with febuxostat. We investigated whether the concomitant use of colchicine and febuxostat increases hepatotoxicity in gout patients, and evaluated the factors associated with hepatotoxicity in gout patients treated with febuxostat.

2. Materials and Methods

2.1. Study Subjects

A total of 319 patients initially diagnosed with gout at Kangwon National University Hospital from January 2012 to December 2018 were included. Exclusion criteria were as follows: age at the time of diagnosis <18 years, patients who used uric acid-lowering agents in asymptomatic hyperuricemia, and patients whose follow-up period was less than 3 months. Patients who had a history of allopurinol use were also excluded. A total of 178 gout patients treated with febuxostat were included. The study was approved by the Institutional Review Board of Kangwon National University Hospital and conducted in accordance with the Declaration of Helsinki (IRB protocol number: 2019-12-009).

2.2. Data Collection

All data were retrieved from electronic medical records of Kangwon National University Hospital. Demographic data, including age, gender, concomitant medications (uric acid-lowering agents, colchicine, aspirin, diuretics including furosemide, and thiazide), and comorbidities data (hypertension, diabetes mellitus, CVD, heart failure, dyslipidemia, liver cirrhosis, fatty liver, CKD, and dementia), were collected. Liver disease (as defined as liver cirrhosis or fatty liver) was diagnosed by abdominal ultrasound or abdominal computed tomography. We also collected the following biochemical laboratory data: uric acid, aspartate aminotransferase (AST), alanine aminotransferase (ALT), blood urea nitrogen (BUN), creatinine (Cr), total cholesterol, triglyceride, low-density lipoprotein (LDL) and high-density lipoprotein (HDL), at time of diagnosis. In addition, uric acid, AST, ALT, BUN, and Cr were obtained one and three months after initiating febuxostat.

2.3. Definition of Hepatotoxicity

Hepatotoxicity was defined as more than three times the upper normal limit when the baseline AST/ALT was normal, and double the baseline AST/ALT when the baseline was abnormally elevated [10].

2.4. Statistical Analysis

Continuous variables were expressed as the mean ± standard deviation (SD) or as the median (interquartile range, IQR), while categorical variables were expressed as number percentages (%). The Chi-square test was used to compare the categorical data between the colchicine users and nonusers. Continuous values were compared using the Student's t-test for parametric data or the Mann–Whitney U test for nonparametric data. Multivariate logistic regression analysis was performed to estimate the relative risk of hepatotoxicity in the study subjects. Age, dosage of febuxostat, ALT, hyperlipidemia, and liver disease identified by univariate analysis as significant predictors of hepatotoxicity (with a p-value < 0.2) were included in the multivariate model. Subgroup analysis was also performed; patients with liver cirrhosis were excluded. All statistical analyses were performed using SPSS (version 23.0, Chicago, IL, USA). A p-value less than 0.05 was considered statistically significant.

3. Results

3.1. Baseline Characteristics of Gout Patients with or without Colchicine

The baseline characteristics of the study patients (n = 178) with or without prophylactic colchicine are shown in Table 1. Of the 178 patients, 121 (69.7%) used prophylactic colchicine with febuxostat. The median age (IQR) of colchicine users was 51.0 (37.0–62.0) years, and those without colchicine was 56.0 (43.5–68.5) years, which was not significantly different. The two groups did not differ in terms of disease duration, symptom duration, duration of febuxostat use, dosage of febuxostat, baseline laboratory findings (including uric acid, AST, ALT, and lipid profile), and comorbidities (CVD, dyslipidemia, liver disease, and dementia). There was no difference in the hepatotoxicity between the febuxostat with and without colchicine groups (13/121 [10.7%] vs. 4/57 [7.0%], p = 0.587) (Figure 1). Subgroup analysis according to diabetes or CVD revealed no statistically significant differences in the development of hepatotoxicity between the patients with and without colchicine.

Table 1. Comparison of baseline characteristics according to the use of colchicine.

	Colchicine User (N = 121)	Colchicine No-User (N = 57)	p Value
Age, years	51.0 (37.0–62.0)	56.0 (43.5–68.5)	0.203
Male	119 (98.3)	49 (86.0)	0.002
Disease duration, months	26.6 (15.4–61.7)	23.9 (16.4–41.6)	0.748
Symptom duration, months	36.1 (5.2–73.3)	13.6 (0.8–55.2)	0.134
Duration of febuxostat use, months	17.6 (10.3–27.7)	20.8 (14.5–31.0)	0.165
Dosage of febuxostat, mg/day	59.2 ± 21.5	56.8 ± 19.9	0.491
Duration of colchicine use, months	13.3 (6.9–21.5)		
Dosage of colchicine, mg/day	0.6 ± 0.2		
Presence of tophi	24 (19.8)	9 (15.8)	0.680
Renal stone	9 (7.4)	5 (8.8)	1.0
Family history	9 (7.4)	4 (7.0)	1.0
Previous history of cancer	8 (6.6)	4 (7.0)	1.0
Gout flares within 3 months	14/113 (12.4)	24/51 (47.1)	<0.001
Comorbidities			
Hypertension	46 (38.0)	34 (59.6)	0.010
Diabetes mellitus	10 (8.3)	14 (24.6)	0.005
Cerebrovascular disease	15 (12.4)	14 (24.6)	0.051
Heart failure	1 (0.8)	4 (7.0)	0.037
Dyslipidemia	31 (25.6)	14 (24.6)	1.0
Hypertriglyceridemia	56 (46.3)	23 (40.4)	0.589
Liver disease	24 (19.8)	13 (22.8)	0.694
Chronic kidney disease (eGFR < 60 mL/min/1.73 m^2)	8 (6.6)	19 (33.3)	<0.001
Dementia	1 (0.8)	1 (1.8)	0.539
Laboratory findings			
Uric acid (mg/dL)	8.6 (7.0–9.9)	8.4 (6.9–9.8)	0.618
AST (IU/L)	29.0 (23.0–36.0)	26.5 (23.0–37.8)	0.163
ALT (IU/L)	31.5 (22.0–44.3)	27.5 (19.0–43.0)	0.465
BUN (mg/dL)	15.3 (12.9–19.3)	18.9 (13.3–27.1)	0.139
Cr (mg/dL)	1.0 (0.8–1.1)	1.1 (0.9–1.8)	0.006
eGFR (mL/min/1.73 m^2)	89.0 (75.0–104.5)	70.0 (34.0–96.5)	0.020
Total cholesterol (mg/dL)	190.0 (154.0–216.0)	171.5 (146.5–203.8)	0.078
Triglyceride (mg/dL)	207.0 (123.0–292.0)	199.5 (129.0–260.5)	0.897
LDL (mg/dL)	112.5 (86.3–135.0)	106.0 (82.0–128.0)	0.268
HDL (mg/dL)	46.0 (40.0–51.0)	43.0 (37.3–54.0)	0.508
Medications			
Aspirin	14 (11.6)	13 (22.8)	0.072
Diuretics	8 (6.6)	15 (26.3)	0.001

Results are expressed as the mean ± SD, as the median (interquartile range, IQR), or as number (%). AST, aspartate aminotransferase; ALT, alanine aminotransferase; BUN, blood urea nitrogen; Cr, creatinine; eGFR, estimated glomerular filtration rate; LDL, low-density lipoprotein; HDL, high-density lipoprotein.

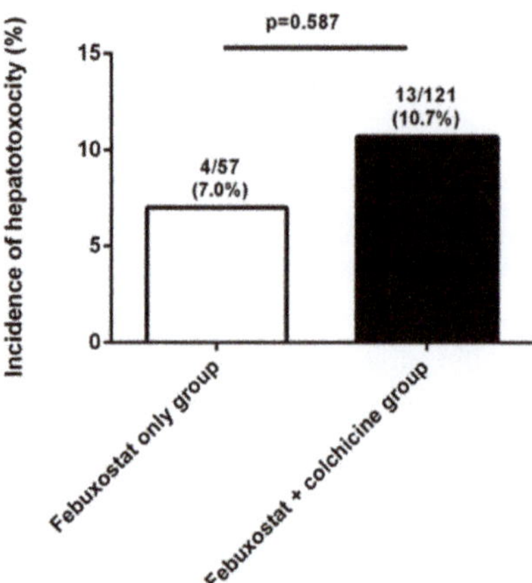

Figure 1. Incidence of hepatotoxicity between the groups with or without colchicine in patients with gout treated febuxostat.

However, the laboratory results indicating renal function were significantly worse in patients without colchicine than those with colchicine. In addition, the use of colchicine was significantly less in patients with hypertension, diabetes mellitus, heart failure, and CKD. When initiating ULT, gout flares occurred more frequently in patients without colchicine than those with colchicine (47.1% [24/51] vs. 12.4% [14/113], $p < 0.001$). Diuretics were more frequently used in patients without colchicine than those with colchicine (26.3% vs. 6.6%, $p = 0.001$). Among the 37 patients with liver disease, 30 were diagnosed with alcoholic or nonalcoholic fatty liver and seven were diagnosed with liver cirrhosis. No patients presented with viral hepatitis.

3.2. Comparison of Baseline Characteristics According to Hepatotoxicity in Gout Patients on Febuxostat

Among the 178 patients, 17 subjects (9.6%) developed hepatotoxicity within three months after initiating febuxostat treatment. The baseline characteristics of gout patients with or without hepatotoxicity are shown in Table 2. The two groups did not differ in age, sex, disease duration, symptom duration, duration of febuxostat use, dosage of febuxostat or colchicine, and use of concomitant medications (aspirin or diuretics). The rate of colchicine use was not different between the groups with or without hepatotoxicity. In addition, the two groups did not differ in comorbidities except for liver disease. Strikingly, only pre-existing liver disease was significantly higher in patients with hepatotoxicity than in those without hepatotoxicity (8 [47.1%] vs. 29 [18%], $p = 0.01$). Incidence of hepatotoxicity was significantly more frequent in study subjects with liver disease than those without liver disease (Figure 2A). With the exception of cirrhotic patients, the incidence of hepatotoxicity was also high in patients with a fatty liver (Figure 2B). Baseline laboratory parameters, including uric acid, AST, and ALT, were similar between the two groups. However, LDL levels at the time of the gout diagnosis were significantly higher in the hepatotoxicity group than those in the no-hepatotoxicity group (142.0 [119.0–165.0] vs. 108.0 [82.0–129.0], $p = 0.01$).

Table 2. Comparison of baseline characteristics according to hepatotoxicity in gout patients with febuxostat.

	Hepatotoxicity ($N = 17$)	No Hepatotoxicity ($N = 161$)	p Value
Age, years	38.0 (34.0–60.0)	54.0 (39.0–64.0)	0.166
Male	17 (100.0)	151 (93.8)	0.601
Disease duration, months	24.3 (17.8–91.1)	26.1 (15.4–47.5)	1.0
Symptom duration, months	18.2 (0.8–90.2)	25.1 (3.9–67.9)	0.793
Duration of febuxostat use, months	17.5 (6.6–27.0)	19.2 (11.7–29.0)	0.645
Dosage of febuxostat, mg/day	50.6 ± 20.1	59.3 ± 21.0	0.109
Use of colchicine	13 (76.5)	108 (67.1)	0.587

Table 2. *Cont.*

	Hepatotoxicity (N = 17)	No Hepatotoxicity (N = 161)	p Value
Duration of colchicine use, months	7.0 (3.9–25.3)	13.4 (7.4–21.5)	0.975
Dosage of colchicine, mg/day	0.6 ± 0.2	0.6 ± 0.2	0.858
Presence of tophi	3 (17.6)	30 (18.6)	1.0
Gout flares	2 (11.8)	39 (24.2)	0.365
Comorbidities			
Hypertension	6 (35.3)	74 (46.0)	0.452
Diabetes mellitus	3 (17.6)	21 (13.0)	0.706
Cerebrovascular disease	2 (11.8)	27 (16.8)	1.0
Heart failure	1 (5.9)	4 (2.5)	0.398
Dyslipidemia	7 (41.2)	38 (23.6)	0.142
Hypertriglyceridemia	7 (41.2)	70 (43.4)	1.0
Liver disease	8 (47.1)	29 (18.0)	0.010
Chronic kidney disease (eGFR < 60 mL/min/1.73 m^2)	1 (5.9)	26 (16.1)	0.476
Dementia	1 (5.9)	1 (0.6)	0.182
Laboratory findings			
Uric acid (mg/dL)	8.6 (7.0–9.8)	8.5 (6.9–9.8)	1.0
AST (IU/L)	30.0 (26.5–44.8)	28.0 (23.0–35.3)	0.402
ALT (IU/L)	42.5 (20.0–76.3)	29.0 (21.0–41.3)	0.755
BUN (mg/dL)	13.3 (10.1–19.3)	15.9 (13.2–22.4)	0.793
Cr (mg/dL)	1.0 (0.8–1.2)	1.0 (0.9–1.2)	0.925
eGFR (mL/min/1.73 m^2)	84.0 (78.3–103.0)	85.5 (63.8–104.0)	0.8
Total cholesterol (mg/dL)	195.0 (157.0–230.0)	176.5 (151.0–210.3)	0.1
Triglyceride (mg/dL)	215.5 (137.8–282.8)	199.0 (123.0–292.0)	0.784
LDL (mg/dL)	142.0 (119.0–165.0)	108.0 (82.0–129.0)	0.01
HDL (mg/dL)	44.0 (40.0–51.0)	46.0 (39.0–52.0)	0.982
Medications			
Aspirin	3 (17.6)	24 (14.9)	0.726
Diuretics	1 (5.9)	22 (13.7)	0.702

Results are expressed as the mean ± SD, as the median (interquartile range, IQR), or as number (%). AST, aspartate aminotransferase; ALT, alanine aminotransferase; BUN, blood urea nitrogen; Cr, creatinine; eGFR, estimated glomerular filtration rate; LDL, low-density lipoprotein; HDL, high-density lipoprotein.

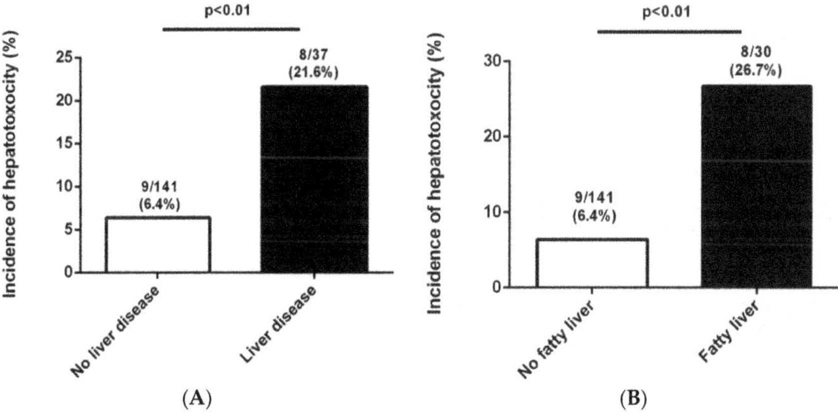

Figure 2. (**A**) Incidence of hepatotoxicity between the groups with or without liver disease in patients with gout treated febuxostat. (**B**) Incidence of hepatotoxicity between the groups with or without fatty liver in patients with gout treated febuxostat.

3.3. Logistic Regression Analysis for Hepatotoxicity in Gout Patients on Febuxostat

Univariate logistic regression analysis revealed that pre-existing liver disease was significantly associated with an increased risk of hepatotoxicity (odds ration [OR], 4.046; 95% confidence interval

[CI], 1.439–11.375; $p = 0.008$). After adjusting for age, febuxostat dosage, ALT, and hyperlipidemia, underlying liver disease was independently associated with a 4.1-fold increase in the risk of developing hepatotoxicity (OR, 4.083; 95% CI, 1.326–12.577; $p = 0.014$) (Table 3). A subgroup analysis excluding liver cirrhosis revealed that fatty liver was also an independent risk factor for the development of hepatotoxicity after febuxostat usage (OR, 2.353; 95% CI, 1.320–4.197; $p = 0.004$).

Table 3. Risk factors for hepatotoxicity in gout patients on febuxostat.

Baseline Variables	Univariate		Multivariate	
	OR (95% CI)	*p*	**OR (95% CI)**	*p*
Age	0.975 (0.946–1.006)	0.114	0.976 (0.941–1.013)	0.198
Duration of febuxostat use	0.990 (0.956–1.025)	0.573		
Febuxostat dosage	0.978 (0.952–1.005)	0.113	0.976 (0.946–1.006)	0.120
Colchicine use	1.595 (0.496–5.128)	0.433		
Duration of colchicine use	0.998 (0.954–1.043)	0.917		
Colchicine dosage	0.700 (0.015–32.928)	0.856		
ALT	1.016 (0.998–1.034)	0.082	1.010 (0.987–1.033)	0.415
LDL	1.0 (0.997–1.003)	0.821		
Hyperlipidemia	2.266 (0.807–6.360)	0.120	1.855 (0.581–5.920)	0.296
Chronic kidney disease	0.325 (0.041–2.555)	0.285		
Liver disease	4.046 (1.439–11.375)	0.008	4.083 (1.326–12.577)	0.014

Adjusted for age, febuxostat dose, ALT, hyperlipidemia and liver disease. OR, odds ratio; CI, confidence interval; ALT, alanine aminotransferase; LDL, low-density lipoprotein.

3.4. Side Effects of Colchicine

Thirteen (10.7%) of 121 patients treated with colchicine and febuxostat had acute liver injury, two (1.6%) patients had diarrhea, and one (0.8%) patient had a skin rash within three months after colchicine treatment. Meanwhile, of the 57 patients treated with febuxostat, four (7.0%) presented with only an acute liver injury [7.0% (febuxostat monotherapy group) vs. 10.7% (colchicine and febuxostat combination therapy group), $p = 0.587$] and two presented with diarrhea [3.5% (febuxostat monotherapy group) vs. 1.6% (colchicine and febuxostat combination therapy group), $p = 0.594$]; no patient developed a skin rash (0% vs. 0.8%, $p = 1.0$). There were no patients with muscle pain, muscle weakness, or neurotoxicity. Of the 13 patients who developed hepatotoxicity, nine continued to receive colchicine treatment, while four discontinued it. Ten patients (76.9%) used hepatotonics. In all patients with hepatotoxicity, liver function parameters recovered to their normal ranges or remained stable compared to their previous levels.

4. Discussion

In the present study, prophylactic colchicine did not increase the risk of acute hepatotoxicity in gout patients on febuxostat. However, in these patients, pre-existing liver disease may be associated with an increased risk of hepatotoxicity.

Gout is a common chronic inflammatory arthritis [1]. Recently, the incidence of younger gout patients has been increasing faster than older patients [2,11]. Therefore, gout is considered an important public healthcare issue. The goal of long-term treatments of gout is to reduce the levels of serum urate, subsequently avoiding acute gout attacks and inhibiting progression to chronic arthropathy. A uric acid-lowering agent is effective for lowering serum urate levels, and reduces the rate of gout flares and tophus burden [12]. However, during the initial use of ULT, rapid reduction in serum uric acid levels can often cause flares of gout, especially in the situation of in-patients, diuretics use, surgery, and overhydration [13–15]. Acute gout flare is a clinically evident episode of articular or periarticular inflammation induced by monosodium urate crystals [16], causing severe pain and disability of the articular joint. Therefore, gout flare is one of the most important concerns for patients as it can also affect their quality of life [17,18]. The European League Against Rheumatism (EULAR) recommendations have suggested that anti-inflammatory agents, such as low-dose colchicine or nonsteroidal anti-inflammatory drugs, should be used for at least six months when initiating ULT [6]. Previous studies reported that prophylactic treatment longer than six months is associated with fewer gout flares after initiating ULT [19,20].

Colchicine is an anti-inflammatory agent that has long been used to relieve pain and inflammation in acute gout attacks [21]. It inhibits the release of crystal-induced chemotactic factors from neutrophil lysosomes, blocks neutrophil adhesion to the endothelium, and reduces monosodium urate crystal-induced production of superoxide anions from neutrophils [22,23]. Therefore, colchicine effectively controls and prevents acute gout flare. However, it has also several toxicities, including gastrointestinal, renal, neuromuscular, hepatic, and cerebral toxicity, and bone marrow suppression [24–26].

When initiating colchicine in patients with gout, it is necessary to carefully check their comorbidities, and concomitant medications. There is a controversy around hepatotoxicity after colchicine treatment. Experimental studies have shown that colchicine causes hepatotoxicity, including acute hepatic necrosis and steatosis in animals [9,27]. Guo X. et al. reported that CYP3A inhibition was associated with colchicine-induced hepatotoxicity in animals [28]. However, a meta-analysis study demonstrated that adverse liver events did not increase in gout patients with colchicine use [29]. The present study also revealed that the number of patients with hepatotoxicity was not significantly higher in colchicine users than non-users. In addition, colchicine in patients with febuxostat did not increase their other side effects. Based on a previous meta-analysis and the present study results, colchicine can be safely used to prevent acute flares in gout patients on febuxostat.

Recent studies have shown that gout and hyperuricemia are significantly associated with metabolic syndrome [4]. Especially, hepatic steatosis and non-alcoholic fatty liver disease in younger gout patients have increased due to prevalent obesity and western dietary habits. Therefore, when treating hyperuricemia, hepatotoxicity has caused problems in these patients. A previous report demonstrated that febuxostat is associated with low risk of hepatotoxicity in Korean gout patients [8]. However, a recent randomized-controlled study from Huang et al. revealed that liver function abnormality was the most common adverse side-effect in gout patients treated with 80mg of febuxostat; febuxostat was discontinued in about 10% of the patients due to liver dysfunction [30]. Therefore, when initiating febuxostat therapy in patients with gout, it is important to identify the risk factors for development of hepatotoxicity in these patients. Our study demonstrated that febuxostat can increase the liver enzyme levels in patients with underlying liver diseases (such as fatty liver or liver cirrhosis). Therefore, we suggest the careful monitoring of liver function tests in patients with underlying liver disease after initiation of ULT.

There are several limitations to this study. First, the present study is a retrospective cohort design and the study populations were composed of a single medical center. Therefore, the number of study patients was relatively small and could introduce selection bias. Second, the liver diseases, including liver cirrhosis and fatty liver, were not confirmed by liver biopsy but rather diagnosed by imaging studies. Third, since hepatic side effects were defined by laboratory results, we could not exclude other causes of hepatotoxicity. Finally, it is possible that the adverse events of colchicine and gout flares may have been underestimated due to the retrospective design.

5. Conclusions

In conclusion, colchicine as a prophylactic therapy was not associated with acute hepatotoxicity in gout patients initiating febuxostat. Therefore, colchicine can be safely combined with febuxostat in gout patients without fatty liver or liver cirrhosis. However, attention needs to be paid to use of febuxostat in patients with pre-existing liver diseases.

Author Contributions: Conceptualization, Y.-J.O. and K.W.M.; Data curation, Y.-J.O.; Formal analysis, Y.-J.O.; Methodology, Y.-J.O. and K.W.M.; Writing—original draft, Y.-J.O.; Writing—review and editing, K.W.M. All authors have read and agreed to the published version of the manuscript.

Funding: This research received no external funding.

Acknowledgments: This study is supported by 2019 Kangwon National University Hospital Grant.

Conflicts of Interest: The authors declare no conflict of interest.

References

1. Dalbeth, N.; Merriman, T.R.; Stamp, L.K. Gout. *Lancet* **2016**, *388*, 2039–2052. [CrossRef]
2. Kim, J.W.; Kwak, S.G.; Lee, H.; Kim, S.K.; Choe, J.Y.; Park, S.H. Prevalence and incidence of gout in korea: Data from the national health claims database 2007–2015. *Rheumatol. Int.* **2017**, *37*, 1499–1506. [CrossRef] [PubMed]
3. Choi, H.K.; Atkinson, K.; Karlson, E.W.; Willett, W.; Curhan, G. Purine-rich foods, dairy and protein intake, and the risk of gout in men. *N. Engl. J. Med.* **2004**, *350*, 1093–1103. [CrossRef] [PubMed]
4. Thottam, G.E.; Krasnokutsky, S.; Pillinger, M.H. Gout and metabolic syndrome: A tangled web. *Curr. Rheumatol. Rep.* **2017**, *19*, 60. [CrossRef] [PubMed]
5. Khanna, D.; Fitzgerald, J.D.; Khanna, P.P.; Bae, S.; Singh, M.K.; Neogi, T.; Pillinger, M.H.; Merill, J.; Lee, S.; Prakash, S.; et al. 2012 american college of rheumatology guidelines for management of gout. Part 1: Systematic nonpharmacologic and pharmacologic therapeutic approaches to hyperuricemia. *Arthritis Care Res.* **2012**, *64*, 1431–1446. [CrossRef]
6. Richette, P.; Doherty, M.; Pascual, E.; Barskova, V.; Becce, F.; Castaneda-Sanabria, J.; Coyfish, M.; Guillo, S.; Jansen, T.L.; Janssens, H.; et al. 2016 updated eular evidence-based recommendations for the management of gout. *Ann. Rheum. Dis.* **2017**, *76*, 29–42. [CrossRef]
7. Todd, B.A.; Billups, S.J.; Delate, T.; Canty, K.E.; Kauffman, A.B.; Rawlings, J.E.; Wagner, T.M. Assessment of the association between colchicine therapy and serious adverse events. *Pharmacotherapy* **2012**, *32*, 974–980. [CrossRef]
8. Lee, J.S.; Won, J.; Kwon, O.C.; Lee, S.S.; Oh, J.S.; Kim, Y.G.; Lee, C.K.; Yoo, B.; Hong, S. Hepatic safety of febuxostat compared with allopurinol in gout patients with fatty liver disease. *J. Rheumatol.* **2019**, *46*, 527–531. [CrossRef]
9. Abbott, C.E.; Xu, R.; Sigal, S.H. Colchicine-induced hepatotoxicity. *ACG Case Rep. J.* **2017**, *4*, e120. [CrossRef]
10. Sharma, P.; Tyagi, P.; Singla, V.; Bansal, N.; Kumar, A.; Arora, A. Clinical and biochemical profile of tuberculosis in patients with liver cirrhosis. *J. Clin. Exp. Hepatol.* **2015**, *5*, 8–13. [CrossRef]
11. Kuo, C.F.; Grainge, M.J.; Zhang, W.; Doherty, M. Global epidemiology of gout: Prevalence, incidence and risk factors. *Nat. Rev. Rheumatol.* **2015**, *11*, 649–662. [CrossRef] [PubMed]
12. Frampton, J.E. Febuxostat: A review of its use in the treatment of hyperuricaemia in patients with gout. *Drugs* **2015**, *75*, 427–438. [CrossRef]
13. Fisher, M.C.; Pillinger, M.H.; Keenan, R.T. Inpatient gout: A review. *Curr. Rheumatol. Rep.* **2014**, *16*, 458. [CrossRef] [PubMed]
14. Kang, E.H.; Lee, E.Y.; Lee, Y.J.; Song, Y.W.; Lee, E.B. Clinical features and risk factors of postsurgical gout. *Ann. Rheum. Dis.* **2008**, *67*, 1271–1275. [CrossRef] [PubMed]
15. Janssen, C.A.; Oude Voshaar, M.A.H.; Ten Klooster, P.M.; Vonkeman, H.E.; van de Laar, M. Prognostic factors associated with early gout flare recurrence in patients initiating urate-lowering therapy during an acute gout flare. *Clin. Rheumatol.* **2019**, *38*, 2233–2239. [CrossRef]
16. Bursill, D.; Taylor, W.J.; Terkeltaub, R.; Abhishek, A.; So, A.K.; Vargas-Santos, A.B.; Gaffo, A.L.; Rosenthal, A.; Tausche, A.K.; Reginato, A.; et al. Gout, hyperuricaemia and crystal-associated disease network (g-can) consensus statement regarding labels and definitions of disease states of gout. *Ann. Rheum. Dis.* **2019**, *78*, 1592–1600. [CrossRef]
17. Tatlock, S.; Rudell, K.; Panter, C.; Arbuckle, R.; Harrold, L.R.; Taylor, W.J.; Symonds, T. What outcomes are important for gout patients? In-depth qualitative research into the gout patient experience to determine optimal endpoints for evaluating therapeutic interventions. *Patient* **2017**, *10*, 65–79. [CrossRef]
18. Lindsay, K.; Gow, P.; Vanderpyl, J.; Logo, P.; Dalbeth, N. The experience and impact of living with gout: A study of men with chronic gout using a qualitative grounded theory approach. *J. Clin. Rheumatol. Pract. Rep. Rheum. Musculoskelet. Dis.* **2011**, *17*, 1–6. [CrossRef]
19. Choi, H.J.; Lee, C.H.; Lee, J.H.; Yoon, B.Y.; Kim, H.A.; Suh, C.H.; Choi, S.T.; Song, J.S.; Joo, H.Y.; Choi, S.J.; et al. Current gout treatment and flare in south korea: Prophylactic duration associated with fewer gout flares. *Int. J. Rheum. Dis.* **2017**, *20*, 497–503. [CrossRef]

20. Feng, X.; Li, Y.; Gao, W. Prophylaxis on gout flares after the initiation of urate-lowering therapy: A retrospective research. *Int. J. Clin. Exp. Med.* **2015**, *8*, 21460–21465.
21. Dalbeth, N.; Lauterio, T.J.; Wolfe, H.R. Mechanism of action of colchicine in the treatment of gout. *Clin. Ther.* **2014**, *36*, 1465–1479. [CrossRef]
22. Nuki, G. Colchicine: Its mechanism of action and efficacy in crystal-induced inflammation. *Curr. Rheumatol. Rep.* **2008**, *10*, 218–227. [CrossRef] [PubMed]
23. Leung, Y.Y.; Yao Hui, L.L.; Kraus, V.B. Colchicine–update on mechanisms of action and therapeutic uses. *Semin. Arthritis Rheum.* **2015**, *45*, 341–350. [CrossRef] [PubMed]
24. Alayli, G.; Cengiz, K.; Canturk, F.; Durmus, D.; Akyol, Y.; Menekse, E.B. Acute myopathy in a patient with concomitant use of pravastatin and colchicine. *Ann. Pharmacother.* **2005**, *39*, 1358–1361. [CrossRef] [PubMed]
25. Yoon, K.H. Colchicine induced toxicity and pancytopenia at usual doses and treatment with granulocyte colony-stimulating factor. *J. Rheumatol.* **2001**, *28*, 1199–1200. [PubMed]
26. Terkeltaub, R.A.; Furst, D.E.; Digiacinto, J.L.; Kook, K.A.; Davis, M.W. Novel evidence-based colchicine dose-reduction algorithm to predict and prevent colchicine toxicity in the presence of cytochrome p450 3a4/p-glycoprotein inhibitors. *Arthritis Rheum.* **2011**, *63*, 2226–2237. [CrossRef] [PubMed]
27. Guo, X.; Lin, D.; Li, W.; Wang, K.; Peng, Y.; Zheng, J. Electrophilicities and protein covalent binding of demethylation metabolites of colchicine. *Chem. Res. Toxicol.* **2016**, *29*, 296–302. [CrossRef] [PubMed]
28. Guo, X.; Chen, Y.; Li, Q.; Yang, X.; Zhao, G.; Peng, Y.; Zheng, J. Studies on hepatotoxicity and toxicokinetics of colchicine. *J. Biochem. Mol. Toxicol.* **2019**, *33*, e22366. [CrossRef]
29. Stewart, S.; Yang, K.C.K.; Atkins, K.; Dalbeth, N.; Robinson, P.C. Adverse events during oral colchicine use: A systematic review and meta-analysis of randomised controlled trials. *Arthritis Res. Ther.* **2020**, *22*, 28. [CrossRef]
30. Huang, Y.Y.; Ye, Z.; Gu, S.W.; Jiang, Z.Y.; Zhao, L. The efficacy and tolerability of febuxostat treatment in a cohort of chinese han population with history of gout. *J. Int. Med Res.* **2020**, *48*, 300060520902950. [CrossRef]

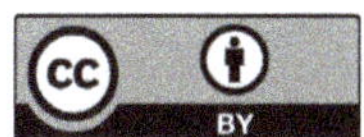

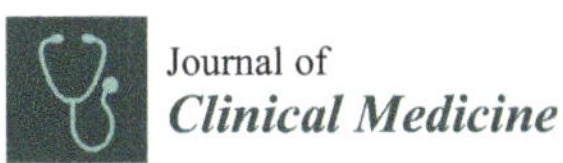

Journal of
Clinical Medicine

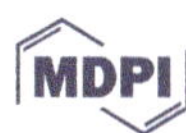

Review

Syndrome of Undifferentiated Recurrent Fever (SURF): An Emerging Group of Autoinflammatory Recurrent Fevers

Riccardo Papa, Federica Penco, Stefano Volpi, Diana Sutera, Roberta Caorsi and Marco Gattorno *

Center for Autoinflammatory Diseases and Immunodeficiencies, IRCCS Istituto Giannina Gaslini, 16147 Genoa, Italy; riccardopapa@gaslini.org (R.P.); federicapenco@gaslini.org (F.P.); stefanovolpi@gaslini.org (S.V.); dianasutera@icloud.com (D.S.); robertacaorsi@gaslini.org (R.C.)
* Correspondence: marcogattorno@gaslini.org; Tel.: +39-0105-6361

Abstract: Syndrome of undifferentiated recurrent fever (SURF) is a heterogeneous group of autoinflammatory diseases (AID) characterized by self-limiting episodes of systemic inflammation without a confirmed molecular diagnosis, not fulfilling the criteria for periodic fever, aphthous stomatitis, pharyngitis and adenopathy (PFAPA) syndrome. In this review, we focused on the studies enrolling patients suspected of AID and genotyped them with next generation sequencing technologies in order to describe the clinical manifestations and treatment response of published cohorts of patients with SURF. We also propose a preliminary set of indications for the clinical suspicion of SURF that could help in everyday clinical practice.

Keywords: autoinflammatory diseases; NGS; SURF; FMF; colchicine; anakinra

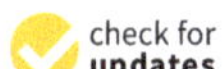

Citation: Papa, R.; Penco, F.; Volpi, S.; Sutera, D.; Caorsi, R.; Gattorno, M. Syndrome of Undifferentiated Recurrent Fever (SURF): An Emerging Group of Autoinflammatory Recurrent Fevers. *J. Clin. Med.* **2021**, *10*, 1963. https://doi.org/10.3390/jcm10091963

Academic Editor: Eugen Feist

Received: 28 February 2021
Accepted: 28 April 2021
Published: 3 May 2021

1. Introduction

Syndrome of undifferentiated recurrent fever (SURF) is a heterogeneous group of autoinflammatory diseases (AID) characterized by self-limiting episodes of systemic inflammation without a confirmed molecular diagnosis. First defined by Broderick et al., [1] SURF is increasingly diagnosed in patients with recurrent fever after exclusion of the main hereditary recurrent fevers (HRF) and periodic fever, aphthous stomatitis, pharyngitis and adenopathy (PFAPA) syndrome [2]. Recent evidence suggests the presence of a multi-organ presentation in SURF and, in a relevant percentage of the patients, a complete or at least partial response to colchicine, usually not observed with the same high frequency in PFAPA syndrome [3]. It is possible that omics-based technologies will provide a relevant opportunity to analyse the functional characteristics of immune cells in SURF patients, highlighting the pathological relevance of possible novel genes and supporting the development of new diagnostic tests. On the other hand, the response to colchicine suggests a possible crucial role of cytoskeleton and related proteins, as observed in the other form of HRF responding to this drug, namely the familial Mediterranean fever (FMF) [4]. In this systematic literature review, we will (1) identify a subgroup of patients with SURF among cohorts of patients with suspected AID undergoing next generation sequencing (NGS); (2) describe the clinical manifestations and therapeutic responses of these patients; (3) propose a set of indications for the clinical suspicion of SURF, with the aim of supporting the diagnostic approach in everyday life.

2. Materials and Methods

All the original English studies found in the PubMed database (https://pubmed.ncbi.nlm.nih.gov; accessed on 2 February 2020) with the queries: "periodic/recurrent fever/s" AND "NGS/Sanger"; "undefined/undifferentiated" AND "autoinflammatory"; "NGS/Sanger" AND "autoinflammatory", were included in this review (Figure 1). Excel software was used for the analysis. A descriptive statistical analysis was performed using frequencies and percentages for categorical variables; median and range for numerical variables.

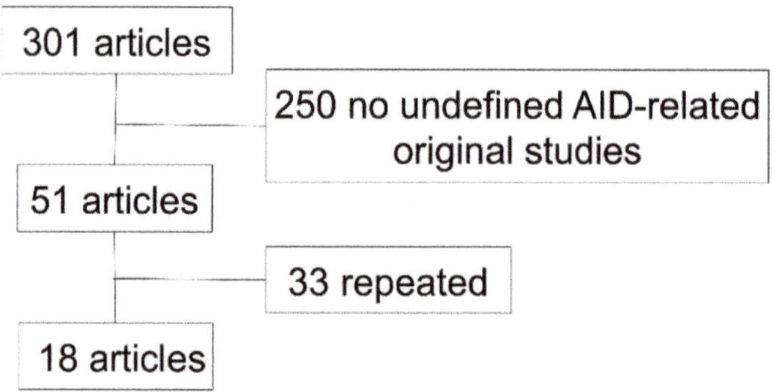

Figure 1. Original English studies found in the PubMed database (https://pubmed.ncbi.nlm.nih.gov; accessed on 2 February 2020) with the queries: "periodic/recurrent fever/s" AND "NGS/Sanger"; "undefined/undifferentiated" AND "autoinflammatory"; "NGS/Sanger" AND "autoinflammatory". AID, autoinflammatory diseases.

3. Results

3.1. Studies Selection and Main Characteristics

The main characteristics of the 18 studies regarding the performance of NGS analysis in patients suspected of AID are reported in Table 1. The number of these studies is increased overtime (Figure 2). Recurrent fever has been included in the enrolment criteria by 6/18 (33%) studies. A total of 2179 patients suspected of AID have been genotyped by NGS since 2014. Studies enrolling a large amount of patients usually did not perform an analysis of many genes and vice versa (Figure 3). However, the number of analysed genes in the NGS panels used in the available studies that only referred to AID did not exceed 55. Analysed genes of each study are reported in the Supplementary Table S1. The major enrolled ethnic groups of patients were Caucasian, Middle Eastern and Asian. The exclusion criteria of a previous diagnosis of PFAPA or clinical FMF was informed by the modified Marshall's criteria and the Tel-Hashomer's criteria, respectively.

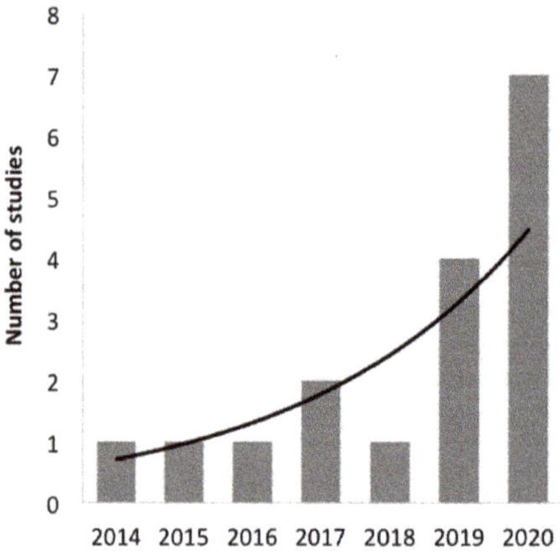

Figure 2. Trend line of studies in Table 1.

Table 1. Studies about the NGS analysis in patients suspected of AID.

N°	Study	Date	Enrollment Criteria	Pts	Ethnicity	Genes	MAF	Predictive in Silico Tools	Variant Classification Tools	Sanger Confirmation	Variants	Variants for Pts, Median (Range)	Pts with Clearly Pathogenic Variants	Pts with Likely Pathogenic Variants	Pts with VUS	Pts with Likely Benign or Benign Variants	Pts without Variants
1	Chandrakasan et al. [5]	2014	Periodic fever	66 *	Caucasian (14), African (7), others (5)°	7	ND	ND	Infevers	Yes	44	0.8 (0–4) *	25 (42)	0 (0)	6 (10)	0 (0)	28 (48)
2	De Pieri et al. [6]	2015	Periodic fever with negative or indefinite genetic analysis; PFAPA syndrome with very early onset and/or poor response to steroids or tonsillectomy	42	Caucasian	5	Any	SIFT, PP2, MT, MutationAssesor, HSF, NNSplice	EMGQN	Yes	38	0.9 (0–4)	0 (0)	0 (0)	24 (57)	5 (12)	13 (31)
3	Rusmini et al. [2]	2016	Systemic AID with at least one mutation in one AID-related gene by Sanger sequencing	50 **	Caucasian	10	<5%	SIFT, PP2	ND	Yes	254	5(ND)	23 (68)	7 (21)	4 (12)	0 (0)	0 (0)
4	Nakayama et al. [7]	2017	Clinical diagnosis of AID	108	Asian	12	<1%	ND	ND	Yes	27	0.25(ND)	ND	ND	ND	ND	ND
5	Omoyinmi et al. [8]	2017	Undiagnosed inflammatory diseases with clinician suspicion of a genetic cause and negative conventional genetic tests	50	Mixed	166	<1% ^	SIFT, PP2, MT	ACGS	Only VUS	325	6.5 (1–16)	6 (12)	11 (22)	31 (62)	0 (0)	2 (4)
6	Kostik et al. [9]	2018	Clinical suspicious of primary immunodeficiency with periodic fever	65	ND	302	<3%	SIFT, PP2, MT, CADD	ClinVar	ND	ND	ND	ND	ND	ND	ND	ND
7	Karacan et al. [10]	2019	Symptoms suggestive of a systemic AID; exclusion of typical FMF	196	Middle Eastern	15	<1%	ND	ClinVar, Infevers, HGMD	ND	ND	ND	14 (10)	27 (14)	97 (50) §	97 (50) §	58 (30)
8	Ozyilmaz et al. [11]	2019	Periodic fever	64	Middle Eastern	3	Any	ND	ClinVar	ND	13	0.2 (0–1)	4 (6)	0 (0)	3 (5)	6 (9)	51 (80)
9	Hua et al. [12]	2019	Chinese adults suspected of systemic AID	92	Asian	5	ND	ND	EMGQN, Infevers	ND	49	0.5 (0–4)	5 (5)	0 (0)	33 (36)	0 (0)	54 (59)
10	Boursier et al. [13]	2019	Suspected monogenic AID (except FMF, DADA2 and MKD after March 2018)	631	ND	55	ND	SIFT, PP2, MT, MES, HSF, NNSplice, SSF,	Infevers	ND	176	0.3 (ND)	44 (7)	50 (8)	63 (10)	0 (0)	474 (75)

Table 1. *Cont.*

N°	Study	Date	Enrollment Criteria	Pts	Ethnicity	Genes	MAF	Predictive in Silico Tools	Variant Classification Tools	Sanger Confirmation	Variants	Variants for Pts, Median (Range)	Pts with Clearly Pathogenic Variants	Pts with Likely Pathogenic Variants	Pts with VUS	Pts with Likely Benign or Benign Variants	Pts without Variants
11	Papa et al. [3]	2020	Pediatric onset systemic AID; exclusion of PFAPA syndrome and others etiologies; negative or not conclusive Sanger sequencing of suspected genes	50	Caucasian	41	<3%	SIFT, MT, FATHMM, MetaSVM, PROVEAN, CADD	ClinVar	Yes	100	2 (0–6)	3 (8)	3 (8)	25 (50)	10 (20)	9 (18)
12	Suspitsin et al. [14]	2020	Periodic fever	56	ND	354	ND	ND	ClinVar	Yes	ND	ND	9 (16) §	9 (16) §	7 (13)	40 (71) §	40 (71) §
13	Sözeri et al. [15]	2020	Symptoms suggestive of a systemic AID; exclusion of FMF, PFAPA syndrome and other common etiologies; positive Eurofever score for MKD, TRAPS and CAPS	71	Caucasian, Middle Eastern	16	<1%	SIFT, PP2, MT, GERP	EMGQN, ClinVar, HGMD, Eurofever criteria	ND	74	1 (0–3)	35 (49)	0 (0)	36 (51) §	36 (51) §	36 (51) §
14	Hidaka et al. [16]	2020	Unexplained fever	176	Asian	11	<1%	ND	ND	ND	ND	ND	29 (17)	0 (0)	53 (30)	0 (0)	94 (53)
15	Kosukcu et al. [17]	2020	Recurrent fever and high C-reactive protein along with clinical features of inflammation with a possible AID; infections excluded; negative analysis of 14 AID-related genes	11	Middle Eastern	WES	<1%	SIFT, PP2, MT, CADD, REVEL, VEST4	ND	ND	ND	ND	4 (36) §	4 (36) §	7 (64)	0 (0)	0 (0)
16	Wang et al. [18]	2020	Pediatric patients suspected of monogenic AID	288	Asian	3/347/WES	[illegible]	SIFT, PP2, MT, CADD, UMD-Predictor	ClinVar, Infevers, HGMD	Yes	ND	ND	79 (27)	ND	ND	ND	ND
17	Demir et al. [19]	2020	Symptoms suggestive of a systemic AID; exclusion of FMF, PFAPA syndrome, Blau syndrome, infantile sarcoidosis and other common etiologies; positive Eurofever score for MKD, TRAPS and CAPS	64	Caucasian, Middle Eastern	16	<1%	SIFT, PP2, MT, GERP	ClinVar, HGMD	Yes	ND	ND	15 (23)	21 (33) §	21 (33) §	28 (44) §	28 (44) §

Table 1. *Cont.*

N°	Study	Date	Enrollment Criteria	Pts	Ethnicity	Genes	MAF	Predictive in Silico Tools	Variant Classification Tools	Sanger Confirmation	Variants	Variants for Pts, Median (Range)	Pts with Clearly Pathogenic Variants	Pts with Likely Pathogenic Variants	Pts with VUS	Pts with Likely Benign or Benign Variants	Pts without Variants
18	Rama et al. [20]	2021	Symptoms of AID (>3 attacks, elevated CRP, age of onset <30 years); exclusion of Armenian, Turkish, Sephardic and Arabic when mentioned and other causes of inflammation	99	ND	55	<1%	SIFT, PP2, MT, MES, HSF, NNSplice, GVGD, Grantham score	Infevers	Yes	ND	ND	10 (10) §	10 (10) §	20 (20)	69 (70) §	69 (70) §

* seven patients were not analyzed; Hispanic, Vietnamese, Asian-Indian, Puerto Rican-Filipino-Mixed European; ** 16 patients were not classified; ^ except for the PRF1 p.A91V, TNFRSF1A p.R92Q, and NLRP3 p.V198M variants; § classification was not specified. Results are shown as numbers (%) unless stated otherwise. ND, not declared; NGS, next generation sequencing; MAF, minor allele frequency; AID, autoinflammatory diseases; FMF, familial Mediterranean fever; PFAPA, periodic fever, aphthous stomatitis, pharyngitis and adenopathy; MKD, mevalonate kinase deficiency; TRAPS, TNF receptor associated periodic syndrome; CAPS, cryopyrin-associated periodic syndrome; ACGS, Association for Clinical Genetics Society; EMGQN, European Molecular Genetics Quality Network; HGMD, Human Gene Mutation Database; CRP, C-reactive protein; VUS, variant of unknown significance; SIFT, Sorting Intolerant From Tolerant; PP2, Polymorphism Phenotyping version 2; MT, Mutation Taster; HSF, human splicing finder; NNSplice, Splice Site Prediction by Neural Network; CADD, Combined Annotation Dependent Depletion software; GERP, Genomic Evolutionary Rate Profiling; MES, Manufacturing Execution System; SSF, Splice Site Finder; FATHMM, Functional Analysis Through Hidden Markov Models; MetaSVM, Meta-analytic Support Vector Machine; PROVEAN, Protein Variation Effect Analyzer; REVEL, Rare Exome Variant Ensemble Learner; UMD, Universal Mutation Database; GVGD, Grantham Variation and Grantham Deviation.

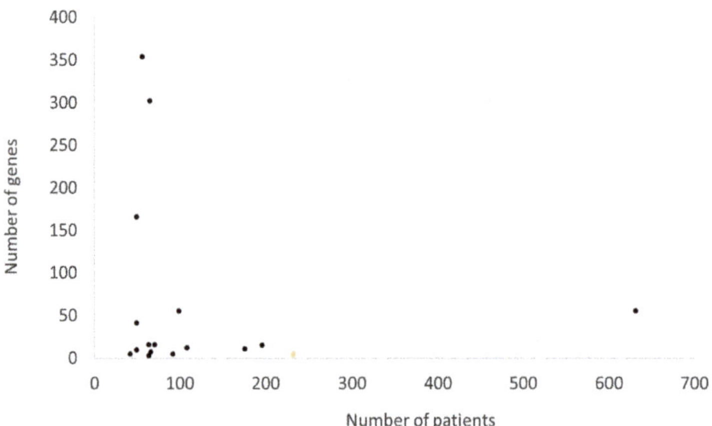

Figure 3. Correlation between the numbers of enrolled patients and analyzed genes of studies in Table 1 except the two using whole exome sequencing.

3.2. *Genotype-Phenotype Assessment*

All the analysed studies are reported in Table 1. The assessment of the pathogenicity of each identified variant was obtained by using the minor allele frequency (MAF), predictive software, classification tools and Sanger sequencing confirmation analysis in 12/18 (67%), 11/18 (61%), 14/18 (78%) and 10/18 (56%) studies, respectively. Some studies considered also the pattern of inheritance and available family data. For assessing the MAF, the 1000 Genome Project (http://www.1000genomes.org accessed on 2 February 2021), the Exome Variant Server (http://esv.gs.washington.edu/ESV/ accessed on 2 February 2021), the Exome Aggregation Consortium database (http://exac.broadinstitute.org/ accessed on 2 February 2021) and the Genome Aggregation database (https://gnomad.broadinstitute.org/ accessed on 2 February 2021) were used. Sorting Intolerant from Tolerant (SIFT; https://sift.bii.a-star.edu.sg/ accessed on 2 February 2021) is the most frequently used predictive in silico software (Figure 4), followed by the Polymorphism Phenotyping version 2 (PP2; http://genetics.bwh.harvard.edu/pph2/index.shtml accessed on 2 February 2021) and Mutation Taster (MT; http://www.mutationtaster.org/ accessed on 2 February 2021). Since its first description in 2014, the Combined Annotation Dependent Depletion software (CADD; https://cadd.gs.washington.edu/ accessed on 2 February 2021) is routinely implemented. The most used variant classification tools are ClinVar and the AID-focused website Infevers (https://infevers.umai-montpellier.fr/web/index.php accessed on 2 February 2021) that reports the International Study Group for Systemic Autoinflammatory Diseases (INSAID) variant classification (Figure 5).

3.3. *Variants Characteristics*

In total, more than 1100 variants were reported, ranging from 0.2 to 6.5 per patient. The median rate of detection of a pathogenic or likely pathogenic variant in an undefined AID patient was 20%, ranging from 0% to 89%. Thus, the number of undefined AID patients persists as quite high even if the NGS or the whole exome sequencing (WES) approach has been used (73% in Wang et al.). No studies using a whole genome sequencing approach in undefined AID patients have been published to date.

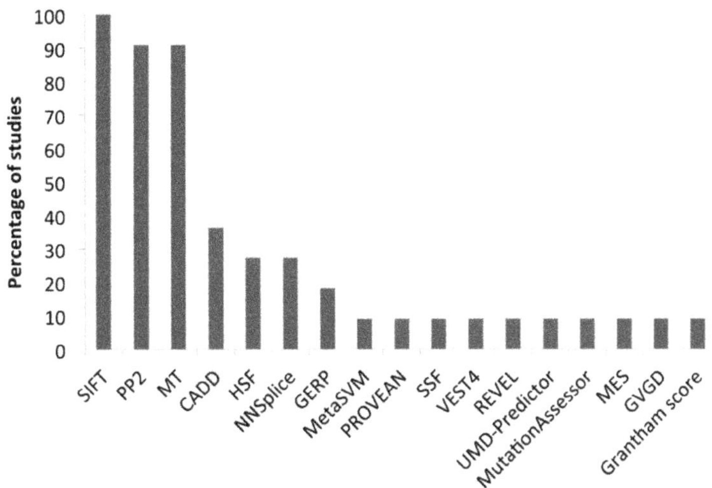

Figure 4. Predictive software of studies in Table 1. SIFT, Sorting Intolerant From Tolerant; PP2, Polymorphism Phenotyping version 2; MT, Mutation Taster; CADD, Combined Annotation Dependent Depletion software; HSF, human splicing finder; NNSplice, Splice Site Prediction by Neural Network; GERP, Genomic Evolutionary Rate Profiling; MetaSVM, Meta-analytic Support Vector Machine; PROVEAN, Protein Variation Effect Analyzer; SSF, Splice Site Finder; REVEL, Rare Exome Variant Ensemble Learner; UMD, Universal Mutation Database; MES, Manufacturing Execution System; GVGD, Grantham Variation and Grantham Deviation.

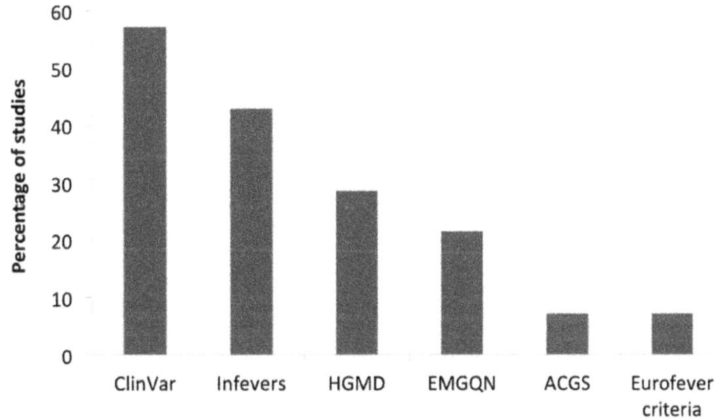

Figure 5. Classification tools of studies in Table 1. HGMD, Human Gene Mutation Database; EMGQN, European Molecular Genetics Quality Network; ACGS, Association for Clinical Genetics Society.

3.4. Clinical Manifestations

As reported in the Methods, patients with suspected AID and undefined recurrent fevers that did not reach a molecular diagnosis after NGS analysis were considered as SURF. Detailed clinical descriptions of 486 SURF patients were available in 5/18 (28%) studies reported in Table 1 and in an additional four specific studies found in the PubMed database.

Clinical features of these patients are reported in Table 2.

The larger cohorts of patients came from the international Eurofever registry, Japan and Middle East [16,19,21]. The median ages at the symptoms onset and patient enrollment are 13 (±13) and 25 (±18) years, respectively. In the four pediatric studies, the median diagnosis delay was 35 months (range 13–78) [5,19,22,23]. Males are 42% of the total. A positive family history ranged from 0% to 32%.

The median duration of inflammatory attacks was 4 ± 1 days with a monthly frequency (11 ± 2 attacks/years). The most frequently reported symptoms during fever attacks were fatigue and malaise (>70% of the patients; Figure 6). Arthralgia, abdominal pain, myalgia and eye manifestations were reported in >40% of the patients. Lymphadenopathy, rash/erythema and oral ulcers were less frequently reported (20–40% of the patients). Headache, pharyngitis, arthritis, nausea/vomiting, diarrhea and hepato/splenomegaly were reported in 10–20% of the patients, and chest pain and pericarditis in less than 10%. Sinusitis, urethritis/cystitis, genital ulcers, gonadal pain, neck stiffness, morning headache, febrile seizure, pleuritis, proteinuria, amyloidosis and sensorineural hearing loss were reported by only single studies.

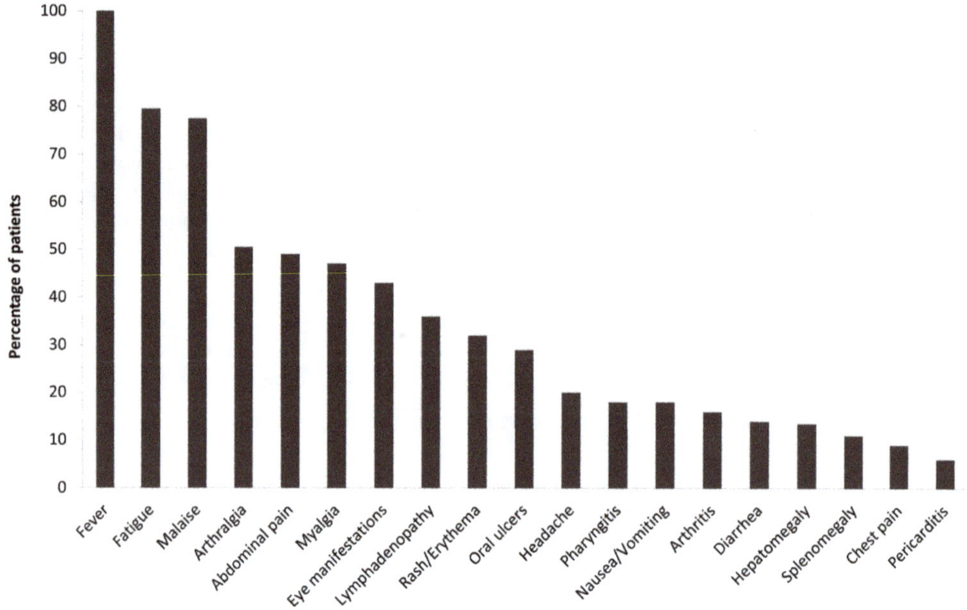

Figure 6. Clinical manifestations of SURF patients reported by at least two studies of Table 2. SURF, syndrome of undifferentiated recurrent fever.

3.5. Treatment Response

The effect of treatment was considered with different methods among the various studies and, herein, any judgement of an evident amelioration of the clinical manifestations after a given treatment. Only a few studies reported a difference between a partial and complete response, and not all authors carefully described the differences between these types of treatment response. Furthermore, on demand or continuous treatment was not always specified. Taking into account these general considerations, the efficacy rate of treatments used in SURF patients is shown in Figure 7. The most frequent treatments were steroids on demand (308 patients) with at least a partial efficacy described in >50% of patients, followed by continuous colchicine treatment (190 patients) and on demand non-steroidal anti-inflammatory drugs (NSAIDs) (127 patients) with a similar efficacy rate (56% and 65%, respectively). Anti-interleukin (IL)-1 treatment (mainly anakinra) was the most effective and frequently used biologic therapy, administered to 46 patients with an efficacy rate of 74%. DMARDs were less frequently used and less effective: 32 patients were treated with different drugs (methotrexate, ciclosporin, azathioprine, mycophenolate mofetil) with an efficacy rate of 48%. Adenoidectomy and tonsillectomy were performed in only 24 patients with a very low efficacy rate (9%).

Table 2. Characteristics of SURF patients published in the English literature.

Study	Chandrakasan et al. [5]	Harrison et al. [24]	De Pauli et al. [22]	Ozyilmaz et al. [11]	Ter Haar et al. [21]	Garg et al. [23]	Papa et al. [3]	Hidaka et al. [16]	Demir et al. [19]
Year	2014	2016	2018	2019	2019	2019	2020	2020	2020
Patients	25	11	23	9	180	22	34	133	49
Ethnicity (patients)	Caucasian (14), African (7), others (5)	Caucasian (10), Jewish (1)	Caucasian (20), Middle Eastern (2), others (1)	Middle Eastern	Mixed	Caucasian (11), Asian (5), Jewish (1), African (1), others (4)	Caucasian	Asian	Caucasian, Middle Eastern
Age at enrollment, median (range), years	2.5 (0–9)	ND	4.3 (2–9)	18 (1–47)	ND	ND	ND	39.9 (22–57)	5.9 (3–9)
Age at onset, median (range), years	1.4 (0–5)	35 (24–76)	0 (0–2)	ND	4.3 (1–12) **	0.61 (0–13.5)	ND	33.4 (13–53)	3 (1–6)
Adults onset	0 (0)	11 (100)	0 (0)	0 (0)	65 (35) **	0 (0)	ND	ND	ND
Gender, M:F	16:9	5:6	5:18	5:4	51:49 **	8:14	ND	66:67	34:15
Positive family history	0 (0)	0 (0)	ND	1 (11)	24 (13) **	7 (32)	ND	ND	12 (24)
Attacks/year, median (range)	8 (4–12)	ND	ND	ND	12 (5–14.5)	ND	12 (7–24)	ND ^	10 (6–12)
Attacks duration, median (range), days	4 (3–5)	ND	ND	ND	4 (3–7)	ND	5.9 (4.5–7.3)	ND ^	3 (2–4)
Clinical manifestations	25 (100)	11 (100)	23 (100)	9 (100)	180 (100)	22 (100)	34 (100)	133 (100)	49 (100)
Fever	25 (100)	11 (100)	ND	6 (67)	180 (100)	13 (59)	34 (100)	133 (100)	49 (100)
Abdominal pain	1 (4)	2 (18) ***	12 (52)	8 (89)	87 (48)	4 (18)	17 (50)	ND	31 (63)
Nausea/Vomiting	ND	2 (18) ***	ND	ND	44 (24)	5 (23)	3 (9)	ND	8 (16)
Diarrhea	2 (8)	2 (18) ***	ND	ND	30 (17)	3 (14)	3 (9)	40 (30)	5 (10)
Rash/Erythema	3 (12)	9 (82)	ND	ND	35 (20)	12 (55)	11 (32)	10 (8)	22 (45)
Genital ulcers	ND	1 (9)	ND	ND	ND	ND	ND	ND	ND
Oral ulcers	1 (4)	3 (27)	12 (52)	ND	53 (29)	ND	13 (38)	ND	14 (29)
Pharyngitis/Tonsillitis	1 (4)	ND	13 (57)	ND	47 (18)	ND	13 (38)	ND	5 (10)
Eye manifestations	ND	ND	ND	ND	ND	14 (64)	ND	ND	11 (22)
Arthritis	2 (8)	5 (46)	ND	1 (11)	12 (7)	12 (55)	7 (21)	ND	4 (8)
Arthralgia	ND	8 (72)	ND	ND	107 (59)	10 (46)	12 (35)	57 (43)	27 (55)
Myalgia	ND	8 (72)	15 (65)	ND	80 (44)	13 (59)	9 (27)	25 (19)	23 (47)
Headache	1 (4)	5 (46)	ND	1 (11)	67 (37)	1 (5)	7 (20)	ND	10 (20)
Morning headache	ND	ND	ND	ND	22 (12)	ND	ND	ND	ND
Fatigue	ND	11 (100) ***	ND	ND	106 (59)	ND	ND	ND	ND
Malaise	ND	11 (100) ***	ND	ND	99 (55)	ND	ND	ND	ND
Lymphadenopathy	1 (4)	4 (36)	ND	ND	76 (42)	12 (55)	6 (18)	ND	ND
Splenomegaly	ND	ND	ND	ND	20 (11)	ND	5 (15) ***	ND	1 (2)
Hepatomegaly	ND	ND	ND	ND	21 (12)	ND	5 (15) ***	ND	ND
Chest pain	ND	1 (9)	0 (0)	0 (0)	21 (12)	5 (23)	ND	17 (13)	4 (8)
Pericarditis	ND	2 (18)	ND	ND	10 (6)	ND	ND	ND	1 (2)
Urethritis/cystitis	ND	ND	ND	ND	6 (3)	ND	ND	ND	ND
Gonadal pain	ND	ND	ND	ND	3 (2)	ND	ND	ND	ND
Neck stiffness	1 (4)	ND	ND	ND	ND	ND	ND	ND	ND
Sinusitis	ND	6 (55)	ND	ND	ND	ND	ND	ND	ND

Table 2. *Cont.*

Study	Chandrakasan et al. [5]	Harrison et al. [24]	De Pauli et al. [22]	Ozyilmaz et al. [11]	Ter Haar et al. [21]	Garg et al. [23]	Papa et al. [3]	Hidaka et al. [16]	Demir et al. [19]
Febrile seizure	ND	ND	ND	ND	ND	ND	ND	ND	4 (8)
Pleuritis	ND	ND	ND	ND	ND	ND	ND	ND	1 (2)
Proteinuria	ND	ND	ND	ND	ND	ND	ND	ND	1 (2)
Amyloidosis	ND	ND	ND	ND	ND	ND	ND	ND	1 (2)
Sensorineural hearing loss	ND	ND	ND	0 (0)	ND	ND	ND	ND	0 (0)
Patients with information about the response to treatment	25 (100)	11 (100)	ND	ND	ND	22 (100)	18 (53)	133 (100)	49 (100)
On demand NSAIDs	ND	ND	ND	ND	80/105 (76%)	3/22 (14%)	ND	ND	ND
On demand steroids	ND	6/10 (60%)	16/21 (76%)	ND	85/104 (82%)	11/22 (50%)	17/18 (94%)	29/133 (22%)	ND
Colchicine	15/25 (60%)	0/3 (0)	6/13 (46%)	ND	29/49 (59%)	ND	14/18 (78%)	44/133 (33%)	31/49 (63%)
DMARDs	ND	0/10 (0)	ND	ND	7/10 (70%)	13/22 (59%)	ND	ND	ND
Anakinra	ND	10/11 (90%)	ND	ND	8/13 (62%)	16/22 (73%)	ND	ND	ND
Tonsillectomy/ Adenoidectomy	ND	ND	0/12 (0)	ND	2/12 (17%)	ND	ND	ND	ND

Hispanic, Vietnamese, Asian-Indian, Puerto Rican-Filipino-Mixed European; ** including seven patients with a chronic disease course; ^ 57.1% > 1 episodes/months and 54.9% ≤ 3 days; *** not specify. Results are shown as numbers (%) unless stated otherwise. ND, not declared; NSAIDs, non-steroidal anti-inflammatory drugs; DMARDs, disease-modifying anti-rheumatic drugs.

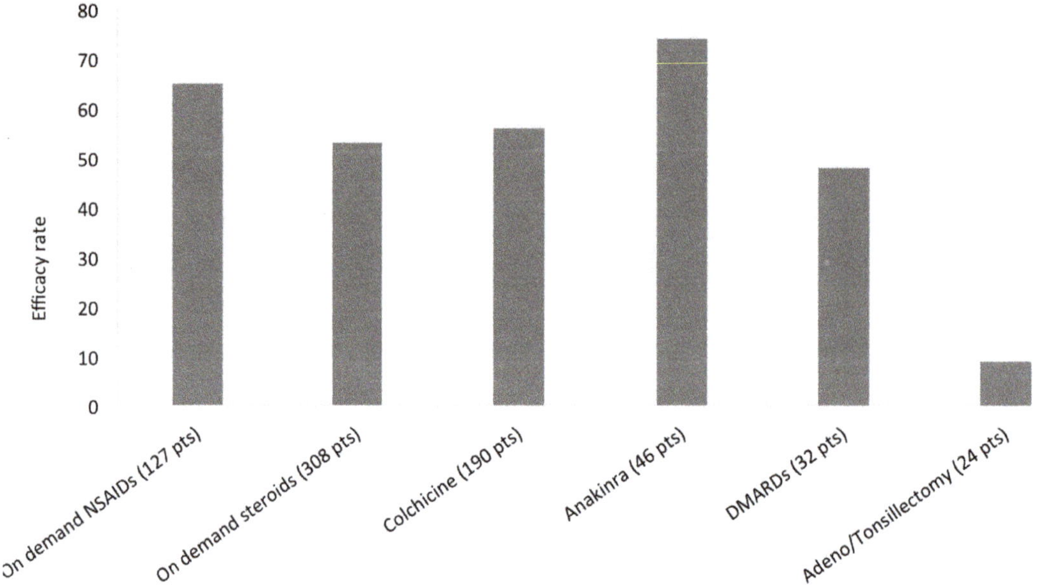

Figure 7. Treatment efficacy in SURF patients. SURF, syndrome of undifferentiated recurrent fever; NSAIDs, non-steroidal anti-inflammatory drugs; DMARDs, disease-modifying anti-rheumatic drug.

4. Discussion

In the present analysis, we systematically reviewed the papers enrolling patients with suspected AID who were extensively genotyped by NGS technology in order to define the clinical manifestations and response to treatment in patients with recurrence of undefined inflammatory attacks, not fulfilling any PFAPA criteria [25,26] and identified under the new term of SURF.

Inflammation is the first sign of immune system activation against pathogens and damage associated molecular patterns (DAMPS) in living organisms. In the case of the occurrence of inborn errors of immunity, the so-called *horror autoinflammaticus* may develop [27]. In the first conditions reported, the most characteristic clinical feature associated with AID was the recurrence of self-resolving fever attacks, namely HFR. However, a subclinical inflammation in affected patients may be associated with long term or life-threatening complications, such as amyloidosis, with an evident impact on quality of life and life expectation. An early diagnosis and a proper treatment may prevent a severe outcome.

Despite the fact that recurrence was implicit in the definition of the original group of HRF (FMF, MKD, TRAPS), the pathogenic mechanisms correlated with the alternation between flares of inflammation and periods of complete wellbeing still represent a dilemma. The existence is hypothesized of an unbalanced up-regulation of the inflammatory response to common hits, followed by a negative feedback able to down-modulate the primary cause of the immune system hyperactivation. This virtuous cycle prevents an early exitus in people with minor defects in the innate immune system that can cause milder AID phenotypes and allows these mutations to be inherited across future generations. The molecular definition of numerous monogenic AID during the last 20 years dramatically increased our knowledge of the pathways and proteins involved in the innate immune system [28]. However, the large amount of patients displaying undefined recurrent fevers even after NGS suggests a need for further discoveries in the field.

In this review, we define a subset of undefined AID patients with recurrent inflammatory attacks and systemic manifestations not fulfilling the typical features of PFAPA syndrome, that represents an homogeneous subgroup of patients with recurrent fevers characterized by the classical triad of pharyngitis, cervical lymph nodes enlargement and aphthosis [25]. Fever is the physiological reaction to an increased concentration of inflammatory cytokines in the blood during an inflammatory response. This systemic inflammation often requires systemic drugs, such as specific cytokine blockers or other therapies able to prevent the unbalanced inflammatory response.

Among these drugs, colchicine is an ancient and well known agent. Colchicine acts as a cytoskeleton stabilizer with an evident efficacy in some HRF, namely FMF [29]. A similar effect has been shown in the present review in the majority of SURF patients treated with this drug [9]. The clinical definition of SURF as a well-defined and homogeneous clinical entity may be useful to further investigate the molecular basis of the role of the cytoskeleton in the activation and regulation of the inflammatory response. Furthermore, future studies may delineate novel treatments able to control the clinical manifestations of SURF.

This literature review has a number of limitations. First, the variability of the inclusion criteria used in the different analysed studies is associated with a relevant heterogeneity of the studied populations. Notably, in some studies, the exclusion of non-autoinflammatory syndrome was not formally specified. Finally, the not-homogeneous distribution of genes included in the different NGS panels cannot exclude that some patients could harbour mutations of some genes related to AID not covered by the panel used for that study. It is worth noting, however, that in all the analysed studies, the NGS panel included at least the four genes most frequently associated with HRF, namely MEFV, MVK, TNFRSF1A and NLRP3.

In conclusion, we reviewed the literature data regarding an emerging group of patients with recurrent fevers distinct from HRF and PFAPA syndrome, now defined as SURF. According to the analysis of the literature, a set of the clinical variables that could help to distinguish SURF from PFAPA and HRF can be empirically proposed (Table 3). A proper statistical analysis comparing a homogeneous group of SURF patients with patients with HRF and PFAPA will allow the creation of evidence-based classification criteria for SURF, with the final aim of favoring the harmonization of future studies in the fascinating field of AID still without a precise clinical and molecular characterization.

Table 3. Proposed empirical indications for the clinical suspicion of SURF.

Mandatory features
Recurrent fever with elevated inflammatory markers [1]
Negative criteria for PFAPA [2]
Negative genotype for HRF [3]
Additional supporting features
Monthly attacks
Attacks duration of 3–5 days
Fatigue/malaise
Arthralgia/myalgia
Abdominal pain
Eye manifestations [4]
Continuous colchicine/anti-IL1 response [5]

[1] at least 3 similar episodes of fever of unknown origin in 6 months; [2] according to the modified Marshall's and/or Eurofever criteria. [3] not conclusive NGS and/or Sanger sequencing of at least the most commonly associated genes (MEFV, MVK, TNFRSF1A, NLRP3). [4] periorbital edema and/or corneal erythema. [5] amelioration of symptoms and/or acute phase reactants. PFAPA, periodic fever, aphthous stomatitis, pharyngitis and adenopathy; HRF, hereditary recurrent fever; IL, interleukin.

5. Footnote

The data in this study are derived from a personal interpretation of published data.

Supplementary Materials: The following are available online at https://www.mdpi.com/article/10.3390/jcm10091963/s1, Table S1: Analysed genes in the studies of the Table 1.

Author Contributions: Conceptualization, R.P. and M.G.; methodology, formal analysis, data curation, writing—original draft preparation, R.P.; validation, writing—review and editing, F.P., S.V., D.S., R.C. and M.G.; visualization, supervision, project administration, and funding acquisition, M.G. All authors have read and agreed to the published version of the manuscript.

Funding: Italian Ministry of Health.

Institutional Review Board Statement: Not applicable.

Informed Consent Statement: Not required.

Data Availability Statement: All the data of the present review derive from a personal interpretation of published data.

Acknowledgments: Several authors of this publication are members of the European Reference Network for Rare Immunodeficiency, Autoinflammatory and Autoimmune Diseases -Project ID No 739543.

Conflicts of Interest: The Authors declared no conflict of interest for this study.

References

1. Broderick, L.; Hoffman, H.M. Pediatric Recurrent Fever and Autoinflammation from the Perspective of an Allergist/Immunologist. *J. Allergy Clin. Immunol.* **2020**, *146*, 960–966.e2. [CrossRef]
2. Rusmini, M.; Federici, S.; Caroli, F.; Grossi, A.; Baldi, M.; Obici, L.; Insalaco, A.; Tommasini, A.; Caorsi, R.; Gallo, E.; et al. Next-Generation Sequencing and Its Initial Applications for Molecular Diagnosis of Systemic Auto-Inflammatory Diseases. *Ann. Rheum. Dis.* **2016**, *75*, 1550–1557. [CrossRef]
3. Papa, R.; Rusmini, M.; Volpi, S.; Caorsi, R.; Picco, P.; Grossi, A.; Caroli, F.; Bovis, F.; Musso, V.; Obici, L.; et al. Next Generation Sequencing Panel in Undifferentiated Autoinflammatory Diseases Identifies Patients with Colchicine-Responder Recurrent Fevers. *Rheumatology* **2020**, *59*, 344–360. [CrossRef]

4. Orange, D.E.; Yao, V.; Sawicka, K.; Fak, J.; Frank, M.O.; Parveen, S.; Blachere, N.E.; Hale, C.; Zhang, F.; Raychaudhuri, S.; et al. RNA Identification of PRIME Cells Predicting Rheumatoid Arthritis Flares. *N. Engl. J. Med.* **2020**, *383*, 218–228. [CrossRef]
5. Chandrakasan, S.; Chiwane, S.; Adams, M.; Fathalla, B.M. Clinical and Genetic Profile of Children with Periodic Fever Syndromes from a Single Medical Center in South East Michigan. *J. Clin. Immunol.* **2014**, *34*, 104–113. [CrossRef] [PubMed]
6. De Pieri, C.; Vuch, J.; De Martino, E.; Bianco, A.M.; Ronfani, L.; Athanasakis, E.; Bortot, B.; Crovella, S.; Taddio, A.; Severini, G.M.; et al. Genetic Profiling of Autoinflammatory Disorders in Patients with Periodic Fever: A Prospective Study. *Pediatr. Rheumatol. Online J.* **2015**, *13*, 11. [CrossRef]
7. Nakayama, M.; Oda, H.; Nakagawa, K.; Yasumi, T.; Kawai, T.; Izawa, K.; Nishikomori, R.; Heike, T.; Ohara, O. Accurate Clinical Genetic Testing for Autoinflammatory Diseases Using the Next-Generation Sequencing Platform MiSeq. *Biochem. Biophys. Rep.* **2017**, *9*, 146–152. [CrossRef] [PubMed]
8. Omoyinmi, E.; Standing, A.; Keylock, A.; Price-Kuehne, F.; Melo Gomes, S.; Rowczenio, D.; Nanthapisal, S.; Cullup, T.; Nyanhete, R.; Ashton, E.; et al. Clinical Impact of a Targeted Next-Generation Sequencing Gene Panel for Autoinflammation and Vasculitis. *PLoS ONE* **2017**, *12*, e0181874. [CrossRef]
9. Kostik, M.M.; Suspitsin, E.N.; Guseva, M.N.; Levina, A.S.; Kazantseva, A.Y.; Sokolenko, A.P.; Imyanitov, E.N. Multigene Sequencing Reveals Heterogeneity of NLRP12-Related Autoinflammatory Disorders. *Rheumatol. Int.* **2018**, *38*, 887–893. [CrossRef] [PubMed]
10. Karacan, İ.; Balamir, A.; Uğurlu, S.; Aydın, A.K.; Everest, E.; Zor, S.; Önen, M.Ö.; Daşdemir, S.; Özkaya, O.; Sözeri, B.; et al. Diagnostic Utility of a Targeted Next-Generation Sequencing Gene Panel in the Clinical Suspicion of Systemic Autoinflammatory Diseases: A Multi-Center Study. *Rheumatol. Int.* **2019**, *39*, 911–919. [CrossRef] [PubMed]
11. Ozyilmaz, B.; Kirbiyik, O.; Koc, A.; Ozdemir, T.R.; Kaya Ozer, O.; Kutbay, Y.B.; Erdogan, K.M.; Saka Guvenc, M.; Ozturk, C. Molecular Genetic Evaluation of NLRP3, MVK and TNFRSF1A Associated Periodic Fever Syndromes. *Int. J. Immunogenet.* **2019**, *46*, 232–240. [CrossRef]
12. Hua, Y.; Wu, D.; Shen, M.; Yu, K.; Zhang, W.; Zeng, X. Phenotypes and Genotypes of Chinese Adult Patients with Systemic Autoinflammatory Diseases. *Semin. Arthritis Rheum.* **2019**, *49*, 446–452. [CrossRef]
13. Boursier, G.; Rittore, C.; Georgin-Lavialle, S.; Belot, A.; Galeotti, C.; Hachulla, E.; Hentgen, V.; Rossi-Semerano, L.; Sarrabay, G.; Touitou, I. Positive Impact of Expert Reference Center Validation on Performance of Next-Generation Sequencing for Genetic Diagnosis of Autoinflammatory Diseases. *J. Clin. Med.* **2019**, *8*, 1729. [CrossRef]
14. Suspitsin, E.N.; Guseva, M.N.; Kostik, M.M.; Sokolenko, A.P.; Skripchenko, N.V.; Levina, A.S.; Goleva, O.V.; Dubko, M.F.; Tumakova, A.V.; Makhova, M.A.; et al. Next Generation Sequencing Analysis of Consecutive Russian Patients with Clinical Suspicion of Inborn Errors of Immunity. *Clin. Genet.* **2020**, *98*, 231–239. [CrossRef] [PubMed]
15. Sözeri, B.; Demir, F.; Sönmez, H.E.; Karadağ, Ş.G.; Demirkol, Y.K.; Doğan, Ö.A.; Doğanay, H.L.; Ayaz, N.A. Comparison of the Clinical Diagnostic Criteria and the Results of the Next-Generation Sequence Gene Panel in Patients with Monogenic Systemic Autoinflammatory Diseases. *Clin. Rheumatol.* **2020**. [CrossRef] [PubMed]
16. Hidaka, Y.; Fujimoto, K.; Matsuo, N.; Koga, T.; Kaieda, S.; Yamasaki, S.; Nakashima, M.; Migita, K.; Nakayama, M.; Ohara, O.; et al. Clinical Phenotypes and Genetic Analyses for Diagnosis of Systemic Autoinflammatory Diseases in Adult Patients with Unexplained Fever. *Mod. Rheumatol.* **2020**, 1–6. [CrossRef] [PubMed]
17. Kosukcu, C.; Taskiran, E.Z.; Batu, E.D.; Sag, E.; Bilginer, Y.; Alikasifoglu, M.; Ozen, S. Whole Exome Sequencing in Unclassified Autoinflammatory Diseases: More Monogenic Diseases in the Pipeline? *Rheumatology* **2020**. [CrossRef]
18. Wang, W.; Yu, Z.; Gou, L.; Zhong, L.; Li, J.; Ma, M.; Wang, C.; Zhou, Y.; Ru, Y.; Sun, Z.; et al. Single-Center Overview of Pediatric Monogenic Autoinflammatory Diseases in the Past Decade: A Summary and Beyond. *Front. Immunol.* **2020**, *11*. [CrossRef]
19. Demir, F.; Doğan, Ö.A.; Demirkol, Y.K.; Tekkuş, K.E.; Canbek, S.; Karadağ, Ş.G.; Sönmez, H.E.; Ayaz, N.A.; Doğanay, H.L.; Sözeri, B. Genetic Panel Screening in Patients with Clinically Unclassified Systemic Autoinflammatory Diseases. *Clin. Rheumatol.* **2020**, *39*, 3733–3745. [CrossRef] [PubMed]
20. Rama, M.; Mura, T.; Kone-Paut, I.; Boursier, G.; Aouinti, S.; Touitou, I.; Sarrabay, G. Is Gene Panel Sequencing More Efficient than Clinical-Based Gene Sequencing to Diagnose Autoinflammatory Diseases? A Randomized Study. *Clin. Exp. Immunol.* **2021**, *203*, 105–114. [CrossRef]
21. Ter Haar, N.M.; Eijkelboom, C.; Cantarini, L.; Papa, R.; Brogan, P.A.; Kone-Paut, I.; Modesto, C.; Hofer, M.; Iagaru, N.; Fingerhutová, S.; et al. Eurofever registry and the Pediatric Rheumatology International Trial Organization (PRINTO). Clinical Characteristics and Genetic Analyses of 187 Patients with Undefined Autoinflammatory Diseases. *Ann. Rheum. Dis.* **2019**, *78*, 1405–1411. [CrossRef] [PubMed]
22. De Pauli, S.; Lega, S.; Pastore, S.; Grasso, D.L.; Bianco, A.M.R.; Severini, G.M.; Tommasini, A.; Taddio, A. Neither Hereditary Periodic Fever nor Periodic Fever, Aphthae, Pharingitis, Adenitis: Undifferentiated Periodic Fever in a Tertiary Pediatric Center. *World J. Clin. Pediatr.* **2018**, *7*, 49–55. [CrossRef] [PubMed]
23. Garg, S.; Wynne, K.; Omoyinmi, E.; Eleftheriou, D.; Brogan, P. Efficacy and Safety of Anakinra for Undifferentiated Autoinflammatory Diseases in Children: A Retrospective Case Review. *Rheumatol. Adv. Pract.* **2019**, *3*, rkz004. [CrossRef]
24. Harrison, S.R.; McGonagle, D.; Nizam, S.; Jarrett, S.; van der Hilst, J.; McDermott, M.F.; Savic, S. Anakinra as a Diagnostic Challenge and Treatment Option for Systemic Autoinflammatory Disorders of Undefined Etiology. *JCI Insight* **2016**, *1*, e86336. [CrossRef] [PubMed]

25. Thomas, K.T.; Feder, H.M.; Lawton, A.R.; Edwards, K.M. Periodic Fever Syndrome in Children. *J. Pediatr.* **1999**, *135*, 15–21. [CrossRef]
26. Gattorno, M.; Hofer, M.; Federici, S.; Vanoni, F.; Bovis, F.; Aksentijevich, I.; Anton, J.; Arostegui, J.I.; Barron, K.; Ben-Cherit, E.; et al. Eurofever Registry and the Paediatric Rheumatology International Trials Organisation (PRINTO). Classification Criteria for Autoinflammatory Recurrent Fevers. *Ann. Rheum. Dis.* **2019**, *78*, 1025–1032. [CrossRef]
27. Masters, S.L.; Simon, A.; Aksentijevich, I.; Kastner, D.L. Horror Autoinflammaticus: The Molecular Pathophysiology of Autoinflammatory Disease (*). *Ann. Rev. Immunol.* **2009**, *27*, 621–668. [CrossRef]
28. Papa, R.; Picco, P.; Gattorno, M. The Expanding Pathways of Autoinflammation: A Lesson from the First 100 Genes Related to Autoinflammatory Manifestations. *Adv. Protein Chem. Struct. Biol.* **2020**, *120*, 1–44. [CrossRef]
29. Papa, R.; Penco, F.; Volpi, S.; Gattorno, M. Actin Remodeling Defects Leading to Autoinflammation and Immune Dysregulation. *Front. Immunol.* **2020**, *11*, 604206. [CrossRef] [PubMed]

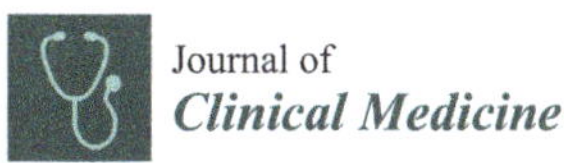
Journal of
Clinical Medicine

MDPI

Review

Autoinflammatory Features in Gouty Arthritis

Paola Galozzi, Sara Bindoli, Andrea Doria, Francesca Oliviero and Paolo Sfriso *

Rheumatology Unit, Department of Medicine—DIMED, University of Padova, 35128 Padova, Italy; paola.galozzi@unipd.it (P.G.); sara.bindoli@phd.unipd.it (S.B.); adoria@unipd.it (A.D.); Francesca.oliviero@unipd.it (F.O.)
* Correspondence: paolo.sfriso@unipd.it; Tel.: +39-049-821-2190

Abstract: In the panorama of inflammatory arthritis, gout is the most common and studied disease. It is known that hyperuricemia and monosodium urate (MSU) crystal-induced inflammation provoke crystal deposits in joints. However, since hyperuricemia alone is not sufficient to develop gout, molecular-genetic contributions are necessary to better clinically frame the disease. Herein, we review the autoinflammatory features of gout, from clinical challenges and differential diagnosis, to the autoinflammatory mechanisms, providing also emerging therapeutic options available for targeting the main inflammatory pathways involved in gout pathogenesis. This has important implication as treating the autoinflammatory aspects and not only the dysmetabolic side of gout may provide an effective and safer alternative for patients even in the prevention of possible gouty attacks.

Keywords: gout; autoinflammation; therapy; IL-1 inhibitors

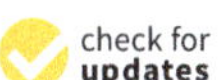

Citation: Galozzi, P.; Bindoli, S.; Doria, A.; Oliviero, F.; Sfriso, P. Autoinflammatory Features in Gouty Arthritis. *J. Clin. Med.* **2021**, *10*, 1880. https://doi.org/10.3390/jcm10091880

Academic Editor: Eugen Feist

Received: 12 March 2021
Accepted: 22 April 2021
Published: 26 April 2021

1. Introduction

The concept of autoinflammation resulted from the acknowledgment of monogenic diseases with seemingly unprovoked inflammation and without the high-titer autoantibodies or antigen-specific T cells seen in classic autoimmune diseases [1]. However, autoinflammation and autoimmunity are not sharply defined, as many diseases display features common to both conditions. This led to the concept of the immunological disease continuum, in which intermediate place was taken by polygenic diseases with prominent autoinflammatory and/or autoimmune components [2]. Gout is thus a multifactorial autoinflammatory disease.

Gout is the most common inflammatory arthritis with about 2–4% of prevalence worldwide, mainly in men over 40 and particularly in those with underlying comorbidities such as obesity, hypertension, coronary artery disease, diabetes, or metabolic diseases. The characteristic gouty flare has a distinctive clinical feature, achieving an acute painful synovitis caused by monosodium urate (MSU) crystals deposition in joints [3].

There has been an increasing amount of evidence about the autoinflammatory nature of gout. Similarly to autoinflammatory diseases, there is a malfunction of the innate immune system in gout. Indeed, hyperuricemia solely is not sufficient to induce gout; this strongly suggests further inflammatory and genetically determined elements contributing to the disease [4]. Further autoinflammatory aspects of gout are the typically self-limiting nature of acute flares and the central role of inflammatory cytokines, such as interleukin (IL)-1β, suggesting that pro- and anti-inflammatory regulatory pathways are involved in gout [5]. Recent and already consolidated autoinflammatory aspects of gout were reviewed in this work to provide important implications for treating challenging gouty inflammation.

2. Clinical Challenges and Differential Diagnosis

It is widely known that gout typically presents with an acute painful flare that can resolve spontaneously within a few days, with asymptomatic periods between attacks. It usually affects the first metatarsophalangeal joint, but large joints such as knee, wrist, and ankle may be involved as well, leading to a systemic acute inflammation [6].

Fever and fatigue are not uncommon symptoms during a gout attack, but have to be considered in the differential diagnostic process to infectious arthritis or, more severely, a systemic sepsis. Fever is also a prominent sign in many autoinflammatory diseases even though the fever patterns vary considerably (from episodic to continuous fever) [1]. In gout, fever can be present mostly when there is a polyarticular involvement, since the final production of IL-1β can be a possible trigger for fever in patients affected by crystal arthropathies. Although fever may be more prevalent in the case of calcium pyrophosphate crystal-induced arthritis than it is in gout, febrile systemic inflammatory diseases particularly in elderly people may be often caused by crystal-induced arthritis [7]. In general, the prevalence of fever in gout is driven by specific pyrogens (IL-1, IL-6, tumor necrosis factor (TNF)-α) with the inflammasome as a pivotal activator of the inflammatory cascade.

Cellulitis, a potentially serious skin infection caused by different types of bacteria (*β-hemolytic streptococci*, and generally group A streptococcus, i.e., *Streptococcus pyogenes*, followed by methicillin-sensitive *Staphylococcus aureus* [8]) may be clinically similar to a gouty attack, especially when involving lower limbs with concomitant redness and soft tissue swelling. In addition, it was observed that in patients with chronic gout, the polyarticular repeated attacks may induce a systemic inflammatory response syndrome (SIRS) without associated infections [9]. In addition, the uncommon axial involvement in polyarticular gout can induce a SIRS-like reaction mimicking a sepsis with the presence of a chronic crystal arthropathy [10].

Overall, distinguishing between an infection and an acute arthritis (septic or crystal-induced, like gouty arthritis) may be quite challenging. Ultrasound scans of the joints involved together with synovial fluid analysis remain the gold standard exams for the appropriate diagnosis; however, laboratory tests, including urate serum, inflammatory markers, and procalcitonin levels, and a primary immunological assessment (protein profile, immunoglobulins, etc.) should be performed to provide a global view of the patient.

3. Molecular Mechanisms of Gouty Inflammation

In gouty inflammation, different mediators are involved with distinct effects on the initiation, amplification, attenuation, and extinction of the acute flares (Figure 1). The core event in gouty inflammation remains the activation of leukocytes by MSU crystals, danger signals leading to the initiation of the inflammatory cascade [11]. The crystals are, indeed, the first endogenous activators of NLRP3 inflammasome, a large multiprotein complex implicated in the processing of IL-1β and IL-18 precursors into their active forms.

Inflammation in gout can be illustrated as a two-phase process, requiring separate and interacting signals [12]. Cell surface receptors such as Toll-like receptors (TLR) mediate the first signal, which provides upregulated expression of inflammasome components and of IL-1β and IL-18 precursors. In the context of gout, several endogenous molecules have been proposed to act as priming signals, including the complement protein C5a, the granulocyte-macrophage colony-stimulating factor GM-CSF, and the ligands of *TLR4* receptor S100A8/A9 [13]. Exogenous, dietary-induced first signal activators include long-chain saturated fatty acids such as palmitate. The synergy between long-chain free fatty acids, released after food intake, and MSU crystals for the release of IL-1β and induction of inflammation might represent the missing link between metabolic changes, inflammasome activation, and gout attacks [14].

This priming phase is necessary but cannot trigger the inflammasome assembly and activation without the contribution of a second, more specific, and MSU crystals-mediated phase.

The oligomerization of the NLRP3 inflammasome results in the recruitment of the adapter protein ASC and auto-activation of caspase-1, that catalyze in turns the cleavage of IL-1β and IL-18 precursors into the mature forms [15]. Then, IL-1β and IL-18 are secreted from the cells via secretory lysosomes or exosomes or via the gasdermin D channel. After neutrophils recruitment, a positive loop of inflammation can continue.

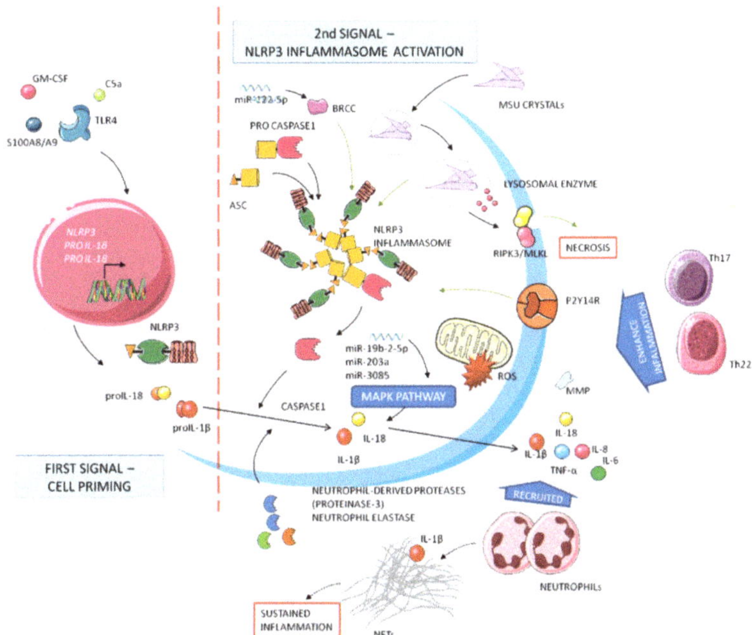

Figure 1. Complex network of molecular mechanisms implicated in gout. Inflammation has been defined by two stages: first signal (**left**) and second signal (**right**). Cell priming production of precursors of cytokines and inactive inflammasome molecules needs the subsequent activation step after Signal 2. IL-1β is critical to the upregulation of inflammatory processes.

During a gouty flare, MSU crystals phagocytosis induces degranulation, lysis of lysosomal and cell membranes, further recruitment of leukocytes, and release of inflammatory mediators; all of these processes contribute to the ongoing inflammation [16]. It has been recently observed that this process, notably known as pyroptosis, can be regulated by the P2Y14 receptor, linking intracellular cAMP and the gouty inflammatory cascade [17].

Neutrophils are recruited to the inflamed tissues by chemokines, such as MCP-1 and CXCL8/IL-8, and released cytokines, such as IL-1, IL-6, and TNF-α, as well as other mediators such as matrix metalloproteinases (MMP), prostaglandins, leukotrienes, ROS, and various lysosomal enzymes [18].

Inflammasome activation is surely an important, and possibly indispensable, pathway to induce inflammatory reactions in the joints. An inflammasome-independent mechanism can also activate IL-1β in gout. Neutrophil-derived proteases (proteinase-3) or elastase can indeed process the IL-1β precursor into its active form [19].

Recently, MSU crystals have been reported to be implicated in cell necrosis, mediated by the receptor-interacting protein (RIP) kinase-1, -3 and the pseudokinase mixed-lineage kinase domain-like (MLKL)-driven necroptosis pathways [20]. The complex RIPK3/MLKL can disrupt both plasma and mitochondrial membranes, leading to cell death.

MSU crystals are further implicated in the promotion of miRNAs, short non coding RNA molecules that can regulate gene expression subtly and with complexity. There are currently different miRNAs that have been found to play an activation role in acute gouty inflammation. miR-122-5p is reported to upregulate BRCC protein expression, activating the NLRP3 inflammasome [21]. Upregulation of miR-328-3p, miR-375-5p, and miR-299a positive regulates the apoptotic process by the p53 signaling pathway. Moreover, miR-203a, miR-3085, and miR-19b-2-5p regulate the MAPK signaling pathway to indirectly mediate the inflammatory response in gout [22].

While the activation of IL-1β and the role of NLRP3 in gout have been relatively well-established, the upstream pathways involved in MSU-triggered NLRP3 activation are not yet fully understood.

Considering the critical role of T cell subsets in modulating immune function, the relationship between T cell subsets and the underlying mechanisms of gouty arthritis has been increasingly considered. Enhanced immune responses mediated by Th1, Th17, or Th22 may bear a significant role in causing pro-inflammatory attacks during the development of gouty arthritis [23]. In contrast, regulatory T cell subsets such as Tregs and Th2 may inhibit the progression of gouty inflammation, carrying out an anti-inflammatory response.

Undoubtedly, IL-1β plays a pivotal role in gout; however, increasing evidence suggests other IL-1 family members can be involved in gout. IL-1α may be implicated in the local induction and amplification of gouty arthritis. IL-33, IL-37, and IL-38 have an inhibitory function in MSU crystal-induced inflammation. Furthermore, IL-37 regulates uric acid metabolism by affecting the protein level of PDZK1, a cytoskeletal controller of uric acid transport [24,25].

The importance of aberrant innate immune responses in the pathophysiology of gout is further supported by critical observations in over a decade of translational studies [26].

4. Resolution of Gouty Inflammation

After the protraction of the inflammatory cascade, a regulatory anti-inflammatory process attenuates gouty inflammation. It is indeed widely known that MSU-induced inflammation is characterized by spontaneous resolution [3]. Patients experiencing an acute attack improve within a few days and become chronic only if untreated. Masking MSU crystals and limiting the urate availability in circulation can help to remove the stimulatory trigger of a gout attack [27]. Known mechanisms associated with the resolution of gouty arthritis involve negative regulators of inflammasome and TLR signaling, regulators of pro-inflammatory cytokines, neutrophils, net-like structures, and pre-resolving mediators (Figure 2) [28]. Upon activation, macrophages up-regulate intracellular regulatory pathways, such as the SOCS3 pathway, believed to control the production of pro-inflammatory cytokines and for starting the production of anti-inflammatory cytokine (TGF-β1) and the secretion of soluble TNF-α receptors. TGF-β1 also reinforces the shutdown of inflammatory functions in macrophages and neutrophils, including inhibition of amplification of IL-1β signaling and downregulation of IL-1R expression [29,30].

Other anti-inflammatory cytokines (e.g., IL-10 and IL-37) have a key role in the resolution phase. IL-37, in particular, suppresses multiple innate inflammatory responses in vitro and in vivo, acting partially via inhibition of the NLRP3 inflammasome [27]. Other endogenous molecules involved in the disease self-limitation are lipoproteins ApoE and ApoB, a hormone receptor perixosome proliferator-activated receptor y (PPARy), a ketone body b-hydroxybutyrate (BHB), and an inhibitor of serine proteases α1-anti trypsin (AAT). Concerning lipoproteins, it has been reported that changes in the lipoproteins coating MSU crystals and their concentration in synovial fluid play an integral role in the self-limiting nature of an acute attack [31,32]. Both PPARy and BHB have been reported to reduce or inhibit the production of IL-1β [33,34]. It was also shown in a murine model that AAT blocked IL-1β production after MSU stimulation. Interestingly, AAT concentration and IL-1β production are linked to seasonality, since low AAT and high IL-1β levels are observed during gouty peaks in the spring and summer. Moreover, recent data demonstrate a rhythmic regulation of NLRP3 inflammasome expression and activation, linking the circadian clock to inflammatory resolution [35].

Other molecules might also contribute to the prompt resolution of inflammation in gout. The protein annexin A1 (AA1), a potential inhibitor of phospholipase A2, can decrease inflammation, thus promoting resolution in mouse models of gout [36]. In addition, miRNA 146a suppresses gouty inflammation via the downregulation of IL-1β, TNF, and NLRP3 levels by targeting TRAF6 and NF-kB signaling pathways [37]. Furthermore, exogenous substances, introduced with diet, can be involved in resolution of crystal-induced inflammation [38]. They can have immune, inflammatory, or regulatory properties. Among them, plant polyphenols are known to prevent hyperuricemia while short-chain fatty acids, such as butyrate, can suppress MSU-induced IL-1β production [39].

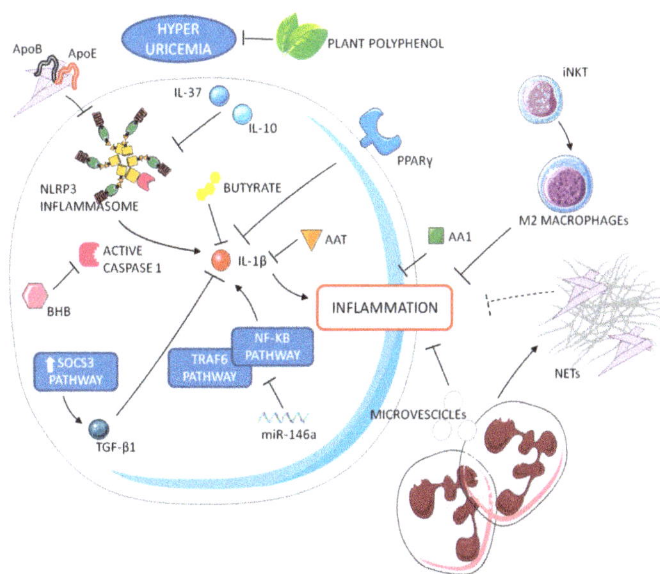

Figure 2. Resolution processes of gouty inflammation. Negative regulators of inflammasome and IL-1 operate in synergy with neutrophils and M2 macrophages to attenuate the inflammatory cascade.

An interesting mechanism of auto-regulation in gout, which is also associated to autoinflammatory syndromes self-resolution, is NETosis. MSU crystals are known to induce neutrophil extracellular traps (NETs), consisting of decondensed nuclear DNA coated with cell granule enzymes released to the extracellular space [40]. This process has been shown to be dependent, at least in part, on IL-1β [40] and independent from ROS [41]. NETs have been shown to have both inflammatory and anti-inflammatory effects. While NETosis has been supposed to facilitate crystal sequestration in aggregates within tissues, limiting the inflammatory response [42], these structures have also been associated to the formation of tophi and, consequently, to the chronic evolution of the disease [43]. Interestingly, Apostolidou et al. suggested that the inflammatory attacks of familial Mediterranean fever (FMF) can be regulated by NETs through the release of IL-1β. According to their study, in fact, neutrophils from FMF patients release NETs decorated with IL-1β during disease attacks but were resistant to the release of NETs under inflammatory stimuli during remission [44]. These observations might support a dual role for NET in crystal-induced IL-1ß production and, therefore, represents an interesting issue for future studies.

Neutrophils can further release phosphatidylserine positive microvescicles that suppress inflammasome activation and consequently inhibit IL-1β release in C5a primed macrophages [45].

A recent study supports the idea that T cells, specifically type 1 NKT cells or invariant NKT (iNKT) cells, can suppress the severity of gouty inflammation, promoting M2 polarization and thus contributing to immune homeostasis [46]. This data is consistent with our observation that macrophages polarization can address the ability of the macrophages to give an inflammatory (M1-related) or non-inflammatory (M2-related) response to pathogenic crystals [47], sustaining the role of a non-inflammatory phagocytosis of the crystals in the resolution of the process as already demonstrated by our group [48].

5. Genetics of Gout

The familial and hereditary nature of gout has long been recognized. However, it was only in the past decade that several genes involved in rare metabolic and kidney diseases were identified as being associated with the pathogenesis of gout. Many of the identified loci include genes encoding for urate transporter, and for urate metabolism [49]. Among these, solute carrier family 2 (*SLC2A9*) and ATP-binding cassette superfamily G member 2 (*ABCG2*) have multiple variants associated with serum urate levels and, overall, the increased risk of gout. Moreover, *ABCG2* has an established key role in the onset and in severity of gout [50].

In the last decade, advances in genotyping technologies have facilitated the identification of genes involved in initiating the inflammatory response to MSU crystals (Figure 3). These genetic associations yield additional findings on inflammatory regulation and shared pathways in the pathogenesis of gout. Furthermore, investigation on genes involved in autoinflammatory diseases, such as the *MEFV* gene of Familial Mediterranean fever, has obtained heterogeneous results of association with gouty inflammation [51,52].

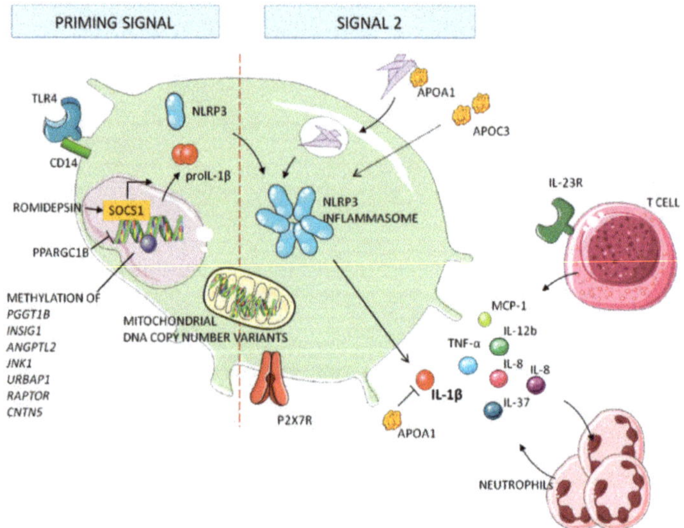

Figure 3. Genes involved in initiating the inflammatory response to MSU crystals. Many loci code for proteins involved in the inflammasome pathway; however, some mitochondrial and epigenetics factors have been reported to be associated with the inflammatory regulation of gouty arthritis.

5.1. Genes Involved in Processing NLRP3 Inflammasome

Many loci associated with gout are known to code for proteins directly involved in processing NLRP3 inflammasome, including membrane bound receptors, transcriptional regulators, ion channels, lipoproteins, and the inflammasome molecules (i.e., *APOA1, APOC3, CARD8, CD14, NLRP3, PPARGC1B, P2RX7*, and *TLR4*).

The *TLR4* gene, coding for a transmembrane pattern recognition receptor, an important mediator of gouty inflammation, is highly polymorphic. rs2149356 is the only variant currently associated with increased risk of gout in Han Chinese and European populations and may play a regulatory role of *TLR4* expression and IL-1 serum levels during flares [53]. These polymorphisms might affect the priming phase of the inflammatory process or might have a wider impact on the inflammatory response in these patients. The SNP rs25569190 in the *CD14* gene is reported to confer a gain-of-function to *CD14*, a co-receptor for the TLR2/4 receptor, possibly implicated in vitro in downstream inflammatory cytokine production [54]. A recent study, however, suggested an opposite role for *CD14* in self-limiting gout flares [55]. Various genetic variations in the *P2RX7* gene, coding for the P2X7 receptor implicated in inflammasome activation and probably a key regulator of IL-1β production by MSU crystals during acute gout flares, have been reported to be associated with gout: rs1653624, rs7958316, rs17525809, and rs3751142 [56]. Associated to the inflammatory signaling is also the *PPARGC1B* gene, encoding peroxisome proliferator-activated receptor γ (PPARγ) co-activator 1β. A linkage between gout incidence and polymorphisms has been reported in *PPARGC1B*, which increased NLRP3 and IL-1β expression [57]. Three SNPs were associated with gout: rs10491360, rs45520937, and rs7712296. Since PPARGC1B is known to regulate metabolism, these genetic variants might link metabolic deregulation with gouty inflammation.

Since lipoproteins can elicit inflammasome activation [31], genetic associations have been researched. rs670 in the *APOA1* gene increases the risk of gout and supports the APOA1 involvement in gouty inflammatory pathways [58]. APOA1 can bind MSU crystals and/or inhibit IL-1β production, having thus a role in initiation and/or resolution of gout attacks. The *APOC3* (rs5128) gene has a causal role in gout, decreasing the risk of gout and increasing expression of APOC3 [58]. Zewinger and colleagues, indeed, identified APOC3, a key player in triglyceride-rich lipoprotein metabolism, as a novel NLRP3 activator that promotes sterile inflammation and organ damage [59].

Along with its pathogenic role as a molecular mediator of inflammation, NLRP3's role is further established by its genetic association with gout. rs3806268 and rs10754558 variants were associated with increased risk of gout in Chinese cohorts [60]. The rs10754558 risk allele, associated with increased expression of NLRP3 during flares, may influence the regulation of NLRP3 expression. Functional variant rs2043211 in the gene encoding caspase recruitment domain-containing protein 8 (CARD8) demonstrated an association with gout in European and Chinese cohorts [61]. Since CARD8 negatively regulates the NLRP3 inflammasome, its genetic variant might raise inflammasome activity and contribute to the sustained NLRP3 engagement in gouty episodes.

5.2. Genes Involved in the Downstream Cascade of NLRP3 Inflammasome

Inflammatory cytokines and cytokine receptors, downstream products of the gouty inflammatory cascade, have also been studied for genetic association or susceptibility.

The first inflammatory modulating gene associated with gout was TNF-α in a Taiwanese cohort of patients [62]. TNF-α is a well-known proinflammatory cytokine with a major role in the pathogenesis of several diseases, including gout. The rs1800630 SNP was significantly associated with augmented risk of gout. rs114362 in the *IL-1B* gene, interacting with a *CARD8* variant (rs2043211), correlates with increased expression of IL-1β, IL-6, and gout risk [63]. This reinforces the central role of IL-1β in gouty inflammation. rs4073 in the *IL-8* gene and rs7517847 in the *IL-23* receptor gene conferred increased susceptibility to gout risk [64,65]. Klück V and colleagues recently provided genetic, mechanistic, and translational evidence that the anti-inflammatory cytokine IL-37 is implicated in the pathogenesis of gout [66]. IL-12b and MCP-1, two chemokines involved in the initiation and amplification of acute flares, presented, respectively, rs3212227 and rs1024611 variants associated with increased risk for the development of gout [64].

5.3. Mitochondrial and Epigenetic Factors in Gout

It has been proposed that mitochondrial function and epigenetics may be associated with gout, opening up another, mainly unexplored, source of genetic contributions to inflammation in gout. Mitochondrial DNA copy number variation was consistent with emerging research showing that mitochondria are important for the colocalization of the NLRP3 and ASC inflammasome subunits, a process essential for the generation of interleukin-1β in gout [67].

A recent promoter-wide methylation study evidenced aberrant methylation changes of *PGGT1B*, *INSIG1*, *ANGPTL2*, *JNK1*, *UBAP1*, *RAPTOR*, and *CNTN5* associated to gouty inflammation [68]. Epigenetic modifiers appear also to be linked to the MSU-induced inflammatory response in gout. Cleophas and colleagues showed that romidepsin, a histone deacetylase (HDAC) 1/2 inhibitor, controlled inflammation by increasing the expression of SOCS1 and decreasing cytokines production in response to MSU crystal stimulation [69].

6. Therapeutic Approaches

Gout pharmacological approaches are based both on the treatment of acute flares to control the hyperinflammation status and on the prevention of attacks using urate-lowering therapies such as xanthine oxidase inhibitors (allopurinol and febuxostat), uricosurics (probenecid, benzbromarone), and URAT1 inhibitors (lesinurad) [6]. Of course, when hyperuricemia occurs in a gouty patient, low serum urate maintenance is crucial to the avoidance of other acute attacks. Gout is considered not only a dysmetabolic disorder, but is classified as an inflammatory disease, for which the activation of the innate immune system, in particular the NLRP3 inflammasome pathway, plays a central role in its pathogenesis. For this reason, targeting inflammasome and IL-1β has become crucial in treating the inflammatory component of gout (Figure 4).

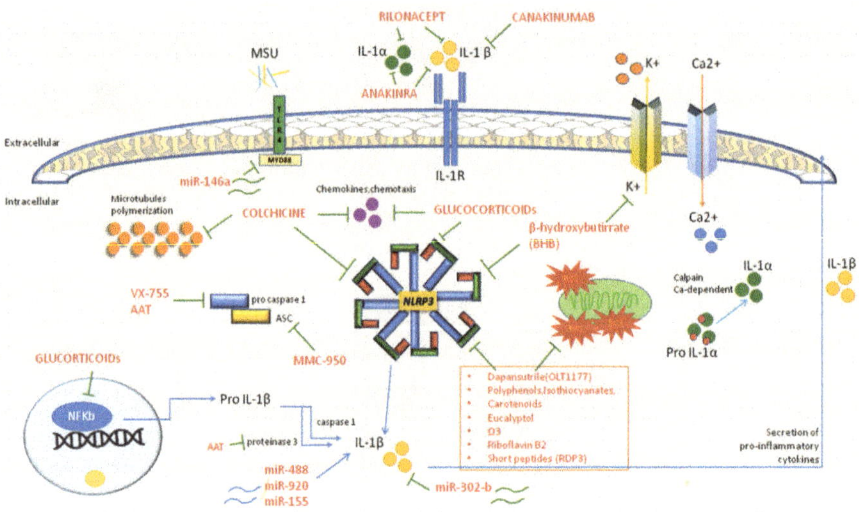

Figure 4. Inhibitory drugs (in **red**) of autoinflammatory mechanisms in gouty inflammation. Blue arrows indicate mechanisms of activation (i.e., maturation of IL-1α and IL-1β from precursors or the ability of miR-488 and miR-920 to induce the production of IL-1β). Green connectors identify inhibitory mechanisms towards NLRP3 or IL-1 processing.

6.1. *First Line Therapy: NSAIDs, Colchicine, and Glucocorticoids*

It is broadly recognized that therapy with monoclonal antibodies represents a second line choice when classical approaches are insufficient or contraindicated. The first line therapy for gouty attacks is represented by anti-inflammatory drugs (NSAIDs), colchicine and glucocorticoids, drugs recommended by ACR and EULAR guidelines as the primary approach [6,70]. Colchicine was the first drug approved for gout more than a decade ago by the FDA, and EULAR recommends it at the loading dose of 1 mg followed 1 h later by 0.5 mg on day one; the association with NSAIDs or glucocorticoids may curb the inflammatory status; however, it is mandatory to consider possible renal impairment, other drug interactions, and relevant comorbidities such as CVDs. In addition, low-dose colchicine or NSAIDs can be used in prophylaxis for at least 6 months or until 3 months after achieving the correct serum urate target. NSAIDs and glucocorticoids can be used as colchicine alternatives; however, particular attention should be paid in elderly people or those with multiple comorbidities, especially CVD and gastrointestinal bleeding for NSAIDs and hypertension and diabetes for glucocorticoids [6]. Colchicine is involved in the inflammasome-related anti-inflammatory mechanism. Indeed, colchicine acts on microtubule polymerization by binding both α- and β-tubulin to create a tubulin–colchicine complex that prevents the formation of microtubules in neutrophils and immune cells and in this way interfers with neutrophil adhesion and recruitment to inflamed tissues; moreover, the microtubule-disrupting effect hampers NLRP3 assembly and the subsequent release of IL-1β and oxygen-reactive species (ROS). In addition, the disarrangement of the microtubule structure may interfere with TNF-α release, with mast cell degranulation, and can reduce the discharge of other chemo-attractant mediators of the inflammatory response such as leukotriene B4 (LTB4) [71].

6.2. Second Line Therapy: IL-1 Inhibitors

The second line therapy provides for the use of IL-1 inhibitors and may be administered when patients are intolerant or refractory to traditional drugs (Table 1). To date, they include direct inhibitors of IL-1β (canakinumab and gevokizumab), selective inhibitor of the IL-1 receptor (anakinra), and a dimeric trap fusion protein (rilonacept) [7]. The efficacy of anakinra in gout was established in 2007 and despite there being no available randomized controlled trials (RCTs) to confirm the data, the drug seems to be effective in gouty patients. In particular, anakinra is adequate in patients with acute gouty arthritis unresponsive to the standard therapy and with a contraindication for NSAIDs, glucocorticoids, or colchicine [72,73]. The efficacy of rilonacept in gout has been investigated in one phase 3 RCT and in three RCTs in the prevention of flares during urate-lowering therapy [74]. The studies confirmed the efficacy of IL-1 inhibition in pain improvement and in a decrease of inflammation markers. Nevertheless, rilonacept is not currently approved by EMA nor FDA for gout. Canakinumab instead, was approved by EMA in 2013 for the treatment of gouty arthritis. The efficacy was investigated in RCTs [75], which showed a significant recovery in pain, swelling, and flare recurrence compared to that of patients taking only glucocorticoids. However, adverse events due to therapy should be considered, especially those related to infections of the upper respiratory tract, abscesses, and gastrointestinal disorders.

6.3. Novel Therapies Modulating Inflammatory Pathways

Recently, new treatments have been proposed to modulate and block the inflammatory pathways involved in gout pathogenesis (Table 1). Apart from colchicine, whose inhibition mechanism on NLRP3 has been aforementioned, other molecules able to hamper NLRP3 assembly should be considered. For example, beta-hydroxybutyrate, a ketone body produced in response to starvation, suppresses the potassium effluvium upstream of NLRP3, affecting the inflammasome assembly [81]; similarly, MMC-950 (also known as CP-456,773 or CRID3), a diarysolfonylurea-compound, can inhibit the NALP3-ASC oligomerization without affecting other inflammasome types [12]. Other inhibitors of inflammasome components include VX-765, also known as belnacasan, and α1 anti-trypsin (AAT), which are known to block Caspase I [78,79]. Dapansutrile, a novel β-sulfonyl nitrile compound, is an orally active small molecule that selectively inhibits NLRP3 in neutrophils and human monocyte-derived macrophages. An open-label phase IIa clinical trial (EU Clinical Trials Register, EudraCT 2016-000943-14) proved the efficacy of this molecule in reducing joint pain of gouty subjects and was well tolerated in terms of safety [80]. Another recent study [89] proved that beta-carotene (provitamin A) suppresses the NLRP3 inflammasome activation induced by MSU crystals in a mouse model. Indeed, molecular modeling and mutation assays revealed the interaction between β-carotene and the NLRP3 PYD; the oral administration of β-carotene in mice was proven to reduce the inflammation and to diminish IL-1β secretion from human synovial fluid cells isolated from gouty patients, demonstrating its inhibitory efficacy in human gout [82]. Procyanidin B2 (PCB2), a phenolic compound naturally present in grape seeds, apples, berry fruits, and tea [80], and eucalyptol [84] are known to have anti-inflammatory and antioxidant properties by suppressing NLRP3 activation in MSU-injected mice; other NLRP3 inhibitors with antioxidant properties include polydatin and resveratrol [90]; curcumin [83]; epigallocatechin gallate [12]; riboflavin (vitamin B2) [85]; and Omega-3 fatty acids (u-3 FAs) [86]. In addition, other new natural peptides are emerging as possible anti-gout treatments such as rice-derived-peptide-3 (RDP3), obtained from the water extract of shelled Oryza sativa fruits in China [87].

Table 1. Drugs and compounds proposed for gouty treatment targeting autoinflammatory mediators.

	Anti IL-1		
	Dosage	**Target**	**Reference**
Anakinra	100 mg daily	IL-1 receptor	[72]
Canakinumab	150 mg at baseline	IL-1β	[76]
Rilonacept (trap protein)	320 mg at baseline	Trap-fusion protein blocking both IL-α and Il-1β	[74]
lncRNA (miRNA-488, miRNA-920)	NA	IL-β	[77]
	IL-1β processing inhibitors		
	Dosage	**Target**	**Reference**
VX-765 (belnacasan)	NA	Caspase I	[78]
A1AT	NA	Caspase I	[79]
MMC-950 (CRID3)	NA	ASC complex	[37]
	NLRP3 inhibitors		
	Dosage	**Target**	**Reference**
Glucocorticoids	variable	NLRP3 (indirectly) NF-κB pathway	[6]
Colchicine	1 mg/day (followed by 0.5 mg after 30 min on day 1)	Microtubules polymerization, Chemokines, chemotaxis, NLRP3	[6]
Dapansutrile (OLT 1177)	100 mg/day, 300 mg/day, 1000 mg/day, or 2000 mg/day orally for 8 days	NLRP3	[80]
Beta-hydroxybutyrate (BHB)	NA	NLRP3, K+ channels	[81]
Polyphenols present in food (ProcyanidinB2, Curcumin, Epigallocatechingallate)	NA	NLRP3	[37,82,83]
Carotenoids (Beta-carotene) *Other compounds: Eucalyptol, Omega3 FAs, small peptides (RDP3), vitamins (riboflavin-B2)*	NA	NLRP3	[82,84–88]
	Receptor inhibitors		
	Dosage	**Target**	**Reference**
lncRNA (miRNA-146a)	NA	Myd88/*TLR4*	[47]

NA: not available.

Many other flavonoids are reported to exert anti-inflammatory effects on mouse models of gouty arthritis, inhibiting both stages of the NLRP3 inflammatory process. Overall, polyphenols (i.e., flavonoids, stilbenoids, and phenols), triterpenoids, isothiocyanates, and carotenoids play a pivotal role in many inflammatory conditions including gouty arthritis; therefore, different phytochemicals could represent a suitable pharmacological approach or, at least, a complementary treatment in addition to the standard therapy for the management of persistent inflammatory gout [88]. Finally, in recent years, expanding evidence has pointed out that long-noncoding RNAs (lncRNAs) and micro-RNAs (miRNAs) may be specifically expressed and involved in the regulation of inflammatory gouty arthritis. Studies from murine models observed that in miR-146a knockout mice, TNF receptor associated factor 6 (TRAF) and interleukin-1 receptor associated kinase (IRAK1) were upregulated; thus, it was supposed that miR-146a can downregulate the levels of pro-inflammatory cytokines in gout. Similarly, miR-302b is involved in a downregulatory pathway, while miR-155, miR-488 and miR-920 are known to induce the production of pro-inflammatory cytokines. Among lncRNAs, ANRIL upregulates NLRP3. Overall, lncRNAs and miRNAs, may function as regulators of the pathological processes of gout and might be used for diagnosis but also as therapeutic targeted for patients with gout. [22,91].

7. Future Perspectives

Increasing knowledge on the inflammatory mechanisms involved in gout in response to MSU crystals should aid in the development of new therapeutic compounds in the near future. Apart from anti-cytokines such as anti-IL-1, other new therapies should be identified to target the different components of the pathways involved in gout. Recently, new plant-derived natural compounds have been studied in murine models; however, the efficacy in gouty patients need to be confirmed. The therapeutic potential role of lnc-RNAs and miRNAs represents a new field of application; however, further studies are required to confirm their capability to curb or modify the inflammatory cascade involved in gout.

8. Concluding Remarks

Autoinflammation-related mechanisms contribute to diseases not usually considered primarily immune-mediated, including crystal-induced arthropathies. In recent years, the concept of gout moved from a purely metabolic disease to a more global autoinflammatory disease, leading to expanded treatment options targeting specific inflammatory mechanisms. Pursuing those types of therapies may provide more safe and effective alternatives for patients in the future, since gout represents the most prevalent destructive inflammatory joint disease.

Author Contributions: Writing—Original draft preparation, P.G., S.B., and P.S.; Review and editing, F.O., A.D. and P.S. All authors have read and agreed to the published version of the manuscript.

Funding: This work was funded by University of Padova, grant number DOR2033958/20 to P.S.

Institutional Review Board Statement: Not applicable.

Informed Consent Statement: Not applicable.

Data Availability Statement: Not applicable.

Conflicts of Interest: The authors declare no conflict of interest.

References

1. Kastner, D.L. Autoinflammation: Past, Present, and Future. In *Textbook of Autoinflammation*; Hashkes, P.J., Laxer, R.M., Simon, A., Eds.; Springer International Publishing: New York City, NY, USA, 2019; Volume 1, pp. 3–15.
2. McGonagle, D.; McDermott, M.F. A proposed classification of the immunological diseases. *PLoS Med.* **2006**, *3*, e297. [CrossRef] [PubMed]
3. Punzi, L.; Scanu, A.; Galozzi, P.; Luisetto, R.; Spinella, P.; Scirè, C.A.; Oliviero, F. One year in review 2020: Gout. *Clin. Exp. Rheumatol.* **2020**, *38*, 807–821. [PubMed]
4. Dalbeth, N.; Phipps-Green, A.; Frampton, C.; Neogi, T.; Taylor, W.J.; Merriman, T.R. Relationship between serum urate concentration and clinically evident incident gout: An individual participant data analysis. *Ann. Rheum. Dis.* **2018**, *77*, 1048–1052. [CrossRef] [PubMed]
5. Steiger, S.; Harper, J.L. Mechanisms of spontaneous resolution of acute gouty inflammation. *Curr. Rheumatol. Rep.* **2014**, *16*, 392. [CrossRef] [PubMed]
6. Dalbeth, N.; Merriman, T.R.; Stamp, L.K. Gout. *Lancet* **2016**, *388*, 2039–2052. [CrossRef]
7. Oliviero, F.; Bindoli, S.; Scanu, A.; Feist, E.; Doria, A.; Galozzi, P.; Sfriso, P. Autoinflammatory Mechanisms in Crystal-Induced Arthritis. *Front. Med.* **2020**, *7*. [CrossRef]
8. Bruun, T.; Rath, E.; Oppegaard, O.; Skrede, S. Beta-Hemolytic Streptococci and Necrotizing Soft Tissue Infections. *Adv. Exp. Med. Biol.* **2020**, *1294*, 73–86. [CrossRef]
9. Shah, D.; Mohan, G.; Flueckiger, P.; Corrigan, F.; Conn, D. Polyarticular Gout Flare Masquerading as Sepsis. *Am. J. Med.* **2015**, *128*, e11–e12. [CrossRef]
10. Goh, C.L.; Lai, F.Y.X.; Chee, A.; Junckerstorff, R. Back pain and fever: When the diagnosis becomes crystal clear. *Intern. Med. J.* **2018**, *48*, 480–481. [CrossRef]

11. Busso, N.; So, A. Mechanisms of inflammation in gout. *Arthritis Res. Ther.* **2010**, *12*, 206. [CrossRef]
12. So, A.K.; Martinon, F. Inflammation in gout: Mechanisms and therapeutic targets. *Nat. Rev. Rheumatol.* **2017**, *13*, 639–647. [CrossRef]
13. Terkeltaub, R. What makes gouty inflammation so variable? *BMC Med.* **2017**, *15*, 158. [CrossRef]
14. Joosten, L.A.; Netea, M.G.; Mylona, E.; Koenders, M.I.; Malireddi, R.K.; Oosting, M.; Stienstra, R.; van de Veerdonk, F.L.; Stalenhoef, A.F.; Giamarellos-Bourboulis, E.J.; et al. Engagement of fatty acids with Toll-like receptor 2 drives interleukin-1β production via the ASC/caspase 1 pathway in monosodium urate monohydrate crystal-induced gouty arthritis. *Arthritis Rheum.* **2010**, *62*, 3237–3248. [CrossRef]
15. Martinon, F.; Pétrilli, V.; Mayor, A.; Tardivel, A.; Tschopp, J. Gout-associated uric acid crystals activate the NALP3 inflammasome. *Nature* **2006**, *440*, 237–241. [CrossRef]
16. Dalbeth, N.; Haskard, D.O. Mechanisms of inflammation in gout. *Rheumatology* **2005**, *44*, 1090–1096. [CrossRef]
17. Li, H.; Jiang, W.; Ye, S.; Zhou, M.; Liu, C.; Yang, X.; Hao, K.; Hu, Q. P2Y (14) receptor has a critical role in acute gouty arthritis by regulating pyroptosis of macrophages. *Cell Death Dis.* **2020**, *11*, 394. [CrossRef] [PubMed]
18. Szekanecz, Z.; Szamosi, S.; Kovács, G.E.; Kocsis, E.; Benkő, S. The NLRP3 inflammasome—Interleukin 1 pathway as a therapeutic target in gout. *Arch. Biochem. Biophys.* **2019**, *670*, 82–93. [CrossRef] [PubMed]
19. Joosten, L.A.; Netea, M.G.; Fantuzzi, G.; Koenders, M.I.; Helsen, M.M.; Sparrer, H.; Pham, C.T.; van der Meer, J.W.; Dinarello, C.A.; van den Berg, W.B. Inflammatory arthritis in caspase 1 gene-deficient mice: Contribution of proteinase 3 to caspase 1-independent production of bioactive interleukin-1beta. *Arthritis Rheum.* **2009**, *60*, 3651–3662. [CrossRef] [PubMed]
20. Mulay, S.R.; Desai, J.; Kumar, S.V.; Eberhard, J.N.; Thomasova, D.; Romoli, S.; Grigorescu, M.; Kulkarni, O.P.; Popper, B.; Vielhauer, V.; et al. Cytotoxicity of crystals involves RIPK3-MLKL-mediated necroptosis. *Nat. Commun.* **2016**, *7*, 10274. [CrossRef] [PubMed]
21. Hu, J.; Wu, H.; Wang, D.; Yang, Z.; Dong, J. LncRNA ANRIL promotes NLRP3 inflammasome activation in uric acid nephropathy through miR-122-5p/BRCC3 axis. *Biochimie* **2019**, *157*, 102–110. [CrossRef] [PubMed]
22. Xu, Y.T.; Leng, Y.R.; Liu, M.M.; Dong, R.F.; Bian, J.; Yuan, L.L.; Zhang, J.G.; Xia, Y.Z.; Kong, L.Y. MicroRNA and long noncoding RNA involvement in gout and prospects for treatment. *Int. Immunopharmacol.* **2020**, *87*, 106842. [CrossRef]
23. Wang, B.; Chen, S.; Qian, H.; Zheng, Q.; Chen, R.; Liu, Y.; Shi, G. Role of T cells in the pathogenesis and treatment of gout. *Int. Immunopharmacol.* **2020**, *88*, 106877. [CrossRef] [PubMed]
24. Klück, V.; Liu, R.; Joosten, L.A.B. The role of interleukin-1 family members in hyperuricemia and gout. *Jt. Bone Spine* **2020**, *88*, 105092. [CrossRef]
25. Wan, W.; Shi, Y.; Ji, L.; Li, X.; Xu, X.; Zhao, D. Interleukin-37 contributes to the pathogenesis of gout by affecting PDZ domain-containing 1 protein through the nuclear factor-kappa B pathway. *J. Int. Med. Res.* **2020**, *48*, 300060520948717. [CrossRef]
26. Li, L.; Zhang, Y.; Zeng, C. Update on the epidemiology, genetics, and therapeutic options of hyperuricemia. *Am. J. Transl. Res.* **2020**, *12*, 3167–3181. [PubMed]
27. Stewart, S.; Tallon, A.; Taylor, W.J.; Gaffo, A.; Dalbeth, N. How flare prevention outcomes are reported in gout studies: A systematic review and content analysis of randomized controlled trials. *Semin. Arthritis Rheum.* **2020**, *50*, 303–313. [CrossRef]
28. Desai, J.; Steiger, S.; Anders, H.J. Molecular Pathophysiology of Gout. *Trends Mol. Med.* **2017**, *23*, 756–768. [CrossRef] [PubMed]
29. Dubois, C.M.; Ruscetti, F.W.; Palaszynski, E.W.; Falk, L.A.; Oppenheim, J.J.; Keller, J.R. Transforming growth factor beta is a potent inhibitor of interleukin 1 (IL-1) receptor expression: Proposed mechanism of inhibition of IL-1 action. *J. Exp. Med.* **1990**, *172*, 737–744. [CrossRef]
30. Chen, Y.H.; Hsieh, S.C.; Chen, W.Y.; Li, K.J.; Wu, C.H.; Wu, P.C.; Tsai, C.Y.; Yu, C.L. Spontaneous resolution of acute gouty arthritis is associated with rapid induction of the anti-inflammatory factors TGFβ1, IL-10 and soluble TNF receptors and the intracellular cytokine negative regulators CIS and SOCS3. *Ann. Rheum. Dis.* **2011**, *70*, 1655–1663. [CrossRef]
31. Scanu, A.; Oliviero, F.; Gruaz, L.; Sfriso, P.; Pozzuoli, A.; Frezzato, F.; Agostini, C.; Burger, D.; Punzi, L. High-density lipoproteins downregulate CCL2 production in human fibroblast-like synoviocytes stimulated by urate crystals. *Arthritis Res. Ther.* **2010**, *12*, R23. [CrossRef]
32. Ortiz-Bravo, E.; Sieck, M.S.; Schumacher, H.R., Jr. Changes in the proteins coating monosodium urate crystals during active and subsiding inflammation. Immunogold studies of synovial fluid from patients with gout and of fluid obtained using the rat subcutaneous air pouch model. *Arthritis Rheum.* **1993**, *36*, 1274–1285. [CrossRef]
33. Akahoshi, T.; Namai, R.; Murakami, Y.; Watanabe, M.; Matsui, T.; Nishimura, A.; Kitasato, H.; Kameya, T.; Kondo, H. Rapid induction of peroxisome proliferator-activated receptor gamma expression in human monocytes by monosodium urate monohydrate crystals. *Arthritis Rheum.* **2003**, *48*, 231–239. [CrossRef]
34. Youm, Y.H.; Nguyen, K.Y.; Grant, R.W.; Goldberg, E.L.; Bodogai, M.; Kim, D.; D'Agostino, D.; Planavsky, N.; Lupfer, C.; Kanneganti, T.D.; et al. The ketone metabolite β-hydroxybutyrate blocks NLRP3 inflammasome-mediated inflammatory disease. *Nat. Med.* **2015**, *21*, 263–269. [CrossRef] [PubMed]
35. Pourcet, B.; Duez, H. Circadian Control of Inflammasome Pathways: Implications for Circadian Medicine. *Front. Immunol.* **2020**, *11*, 1630. [CrossRef] [PubMed]
36. Galvão, I.; Vago, J.P.; Barroso, L.C.; Tavares, L.P.; Queiroz-Junior, C.M.; Costa, V.V.; Carneiro, F.S.; Ferreira, T.P.; Silva, P.M.; Amaral, F.A.; et al. Annexin A1 promotes timely resolution of inflammation in murine gout. *Eur. J. Immunol.* **2017**, *47*, 585–596. [CrossRef] [PubMed]

37. Dalbeth, N.; Pool, B.; Shaw, O.M.; Harper, J.L.; Tan, P.; Franklin, C.; House, M.E.; Cornish, J.; Naot, D. Role of miR-146a in regulation of the acute inflammatory response to monosodium urate crystals. *Ann. Rheum. Dis.* **2015**, *74*, 786–790. [CrossRef]
38. Oliviero, F.; Scanu, A. How Factors Involved in the Resolution of Crystal-Induced Inflammation Target IL-1β. *Front. Pharmacol.* **2017**, *8*, 164. [CrossRef]
39. Oliviero, F.; Scanu, A.; Zamudio-Cuevas, Y.; Punzi, L.; Spinella, P. Anti-inflammatory effects of polyphenols in arthritis. *J. Sci. Food Agric.* **2018**, *98*, 1653–1659. [CrossRef]
40. Mitroulis, I.; Kambas, K.; Chrysanthopoulou, A.; Skendros, P.; Apostolidou, E.; Kourtzelis, I.; Drosos, G.I.; Boumpas, D.T.; Ritis, K. Neutrophil extracellular trap formation is associated with IL-1β and autophagy-related signaling in gout. *PLoS ONE* **2011**, *6*, e29318. [CrossRef]
41. Davidsson, L.; Dahlstrand Rudin, A.; Sanchez Klose, F.P.; Buck, A.; Björkman, L.; Christenson, K.; Bylund, J. In Vivo Transmigrated Human Neutrophils Are Highly Primed for Intracellular Radical Production Induced by Monosodium Urate Crystals. *Int. J. Mol. Sci.* **2020**, *21*, 3750. [CrossRef]
42. Schauer, C.; Janko, C.; Munoz, L.E.; Zhao, Y.; Kienhöfer, D.; Frey, B.; Lell, M.; Manger, B.; Rech, J.; Naschberger, E.; et al. Aggregated neutrophil extracellular traps limit inflammation by degrading cytokines and chemokines. *Nat. Med.* **2014**, *20*, 511–517. [CrossRef]
43. Garcia-Gonzalez, E.; Gamberucci, A.; Lucherini, O.M.; Alì, A.; Simpatico, A.; Lorenzini, S.; Lazzerini, P.E.; Tripodi, S.; Frediani, B.; Selvi, E. Neutrophil extracellular traps release in gout and pseudogout depends on number of crystals regardless of leukocyte count. *Rheumatology* **2021**, keab087. [CrossRef] [PubMed]
44. Apostolidou, E.; Skendros, P.; Kambas, K.; Mitroulis, I.; Konstantinidis, T.; Chrysanthopoulou, A.; Nakos, K.; Tsironidou, V.; Koffa, M.; Boumpas, D.T.; et al. Neutrophil extracellular traps regulate IL-1β-mediated inflammation in familial Mediterranean fever. *Ann. Rheum. Dis.* **2016**, *75*, 269–277. [CrossRef]
45. Cumpelik, A.; Ankli, B.; Zecher, D.; Schifferli, J.A. Neutrophil microvesicles resolve gout by inhibiting C5a-mediated priming of the inflammasome. *Ann. Rheum. Dis.* **2016**, *75*, 1236–1245. [CrossRef]
46. Wang, J.; Yang, Q.; Zhang, Q.; Yin, C.; Zhou, L.; Zhou, J.; Wang, Y.; Mi, Q.S. Invariant Natural Killer T Cells Ameliorate Monosodium Urate Crystal-Induced Gouty Inflammation in Mice. *Front. Immunol.* **2017**, *8*, 1710. [CrossRef] [PubMed]
47. Galozzi, P.; Maschio, L.; Carraro, S.; Scanu, A.; Facco, M.; Oliviero, F. M2 macrophages as resolvers of crystal-induced inflammation. *Rheumatology* **2021**, keab122. [CrossRef]
48. Baggio, C.; Sfriso, P.; Cignarella, A.; Galozzi, P.; Scanu, A.; Mastrotto, F.; Favero, M.; Ramonda, R.; Oliviero, F. Phagocytosis and inflammation in crystal-induced arthritis: A synovial fluid and in vitro study. *Clin. Exp. Rheumatol.* **2020**, in press.
49. Tai, V.; Merriman, T.R.; Dalbeth, N. Genetic advances in gout: Potential applications in clinical practice. *Curr. Opin. Rheumatol.* **2019**, *31*, 144–151. [CrossRef] [PubMed]
50. Chen, C.J.; Tseng, C.C.; Yen, J.H.; Chang, J.G.; Chou, W.C.; Chu, H.W.; Chang, S.J.; Liao, W.T. ABCG2 contributes to the development of gout and hyperuricemia in a genome-wide association study. *Sci. Rep.* **2018**, *8*, 3137. [CrossRef]
51. Karaarslan, A.; Kobak, S.; Kaya, I.; Intepe, N.; Orman, M.; Berdelı, A. Prevalence and significance of MEFV gene mutations in patients with gouty arthritis. *Rheumatol. Int.* **2016**, *36*, 1585–1589. [CrossRef]
52. Salehzadeh, F.; Mohammadikebar, Y.; Haghi, R.N.; Asl, S.H.; Enteshary, A. Familial Mediterranean Fever Gene Mutations and Gout as an Auto-Inflammatory Arthropathy. *Med. Arch.* **2019**, *73*, 55–57. [CrossRef]
53. Qing, Y.F.; Zhou, J.G.; Zhang, Q.B.; Wang, D.S.; Li, M.; Yang, Q.B.; Huang, C.P.; Yin, L.; Pan, S.Y.; Xie, W.G.; et al. Association of *TLR4* Gene rs2149356 polymorphism with primary gouty arthritis in a case-control study. *PLoS ONE* **2013**, *8*, e64845. [CrossRef] [PubMed]
54. Scott, P.; Ma, H.; Viriyakosol, S.; Terkeltaub, R.; Liu-Bryan, R. Engagement of *CD14* mediates the inflammatory potential of monosodium urate crystals. *J. Immunol.* **2006**, *177*, 6370–6378. [CrossRef] [PubMed]
55. Duan, L.; Luo, J.; Fu, Q.; Shang, K.; Wei, Y.; Wang, Y.; Li, Y.; Chen, J. Decreased Expression of *CD14* in MSU-Mediated Inflammation May Be Associated with Spontaneous Remission of Acute Gout. *J. Immunol. Res.* **2019**, *2019*, 7143241. [CrossRef] [PubMed]
56. Tao, J.H.; Cheng, M.; Tang, J.P.; Dai, X.J.; Zhang, Y.; Li, X.P.; Liu, Q.; Wang, Y.L. Single nucleotide polymorphisms associated with P2X7R function regulate the onset of gouty arthritis. *PLoS ONE* **2017**, *12*, e0181685. [CrossRef]
57. Chang, W.C.; Jan Wu, Y.J.; Chung, W.H.; Lee, Y.S.; Chin, S.W.; Chen, T.J.; Chang, Y.S.; Chen, D.Y.; Hung, S.I. Genetic variants of PPAR-gamma coactivator 1B augment NLRP3-mediated inflammation in gouty arthritis. *Rheumatology* **2017**, *56*, 457–466. [CrossRef]
58. Rasheed, H.; Phipps-Green, A.J.; Topless, R.; Smith, M.D.; Hill, C.; Lester, S.; Rischmueller, M.; Janssen, M.; Jansen, T.L.; Joosten, L.A.; et al. Replication of association of the apolipoprotein A1-C3-A4 gene cluster with the risk of gout. *Rheumatology* **2016**, *55*, 1421–1430. [CrossRef] [PubMed]
59. Zewinger, S.; Reiser, J.; Jankowski, V.; Alansary, D.; Hahm, E.; Triem, S.; Klug, M.; Schunk, S.J.; Schmit, D.; Kramann, R.; et al. Apolipoprotein C3 induces inflammation and organ damage by alternative inflammasome activation. *Nat. Immunol.* **2020**, *21*, 30–41. [CrossRef] [PubMed]
60. Zhang, G.; Hu, C.; Luo, L.; Fang, F.; Chen, Y.; Li, J.; Peng, Z.; Pan, H. Clinical features and short-term outcomes of 221 patients with COVID-19 in Wuhan, China. *J. Clin. Virol.* **2020**, *127*, 104364. [CrossRef]
61. Chen, Y.; Ren, X.; Li, C.; Xing, S.; Fu, Z.; Yuan, Y.; Wang, R.; Wang, Y.; Lv, W. CARD8 rs2043211 polymorphism is associated with gout in a Chinese male population. *Cell. Physiol. Biochem.* **2015**, *35*, 1394–1400. [CrossRef]

62. Chang, S.J.; Tsai, P.C.; Chen, C.J.; Lai, H.M.; Ko, Y.C. The polymorphism -863C/A in tumour necrosis factor-alpha gene contributes an independent association to gout. *Rheumatology* **2007**, *46*, 1662–1666. [CrossRef]
63. McKinney, C.; Stamp, L.K.; Dalbeth, N.; Topless, R.K.; Day, R.O.; Kannangara, D.R.; Williams, K.M.; Janssen, M.; Jansen, T.L.; Joosten, L.A.; et al. Multiplicative interaction of functional inflammasome genetic variants in determining the risk of gout. *Arthritis Res. Ther.* **2015**, *17*, 288. [CrossRef]
64. Liu, S.; Yin, C.; Chu, N.; Han, L.; Li, C. IL-8 -251T/A and IL-12B 1188A/C polymorphisms are associated with gout in a Chinese male population. *Scand. J. Rheumatol.* **2013**, *42*, 150–158. [CrossRef]
65. Liu, S.; He, H.; Yu, R.; Han, L.; Wang, C.; Cui, Y.; Li, C. The rs7517847 polymorphism in the IL-23R gene is associated with gout in a Chinese Han male population. *Mod. Rheumatol.* **2015**, *25*, 449–452. [CrossRef] [PubMed]
66. Klück, V.; van Deuren, R.C.; Cavalli, G.; Shaukat, A.; Arts, P.; Cleophas, M.C.; Crişan, T.O.; Tausche, A.K.; Riches, P.; Dalbeth, N.; et al. Rare genetic variants in interleukin-37 link this anti-inflammatory cytokine to the pathogenesis and treatment of gout. *Ann. Rheum. Dis.* **2020**, *79*, 536–544. [CrossRef]
67. Gosling, A.L.; Boocock, J.; Dalbeth, N.; Harré Hindmarsh, J.; Stamp, L.K.; Stahl, E.A.; Choi, H.K.; Matisoo-Smith, E.A.; Merriman, T.R. Mitochondrial genetic variation and gout in Māori and Pacific people living in Aotearoa New Zealand. *Ann. Rheum. Dis.* **2018**, *77*, 571–578. [CrossRef]
68. Tseng, C.C.; Wong, M.C.; Liao, W.T.; Chen, C.J.; Lee, S.C.; Yen, J.H.; Chang, S.J. Systemic Investigation of Promoter-wide Methylome and Genome Variations in Gout. *Int. J. Mol. Sci.* **2020**, *21*, 4702. [CrossRef] [PubMed]
69. Cleophas, M.C.P.; Crişan, T.O.; Klück, V.; Hoogerbrugge, N.; Netea-Maier, R.T.; Dinarello, C.A.; Netea, M.G.; Joosten, L.A.B. Romidepsin suppresses monosodium urate crystal-induced cytokine production through upregulation of suppressor of cytokine signaling 1 expression. *Arthritis Res. Ther.* **2019**, *21*, 50. [CrossRef] [PubMed]
70. FitzGerald, J.D.; Dalbeth, N.; Mikuls, T.; Brignardello-Petersen, R.; Guyatt, G.; Abeles, A.M.; Gelber, A.C.; Harrold, L.R.; Khanna, D.; King, C.; et al. 2020 American College of Rheumatology Guideline for the Management of Gout. *Arthritis Care Res.* **2020**, *72*, 744–760. [CrossRef]
71. Dalbeth, N.; Lauterio, T.J.; Wolfe, H.R. Mechanism of action of colchicine in the treatment of gout. *Clin. Ther.* **2014**, *36*, 1465–1479. [CrossRef]
72. So, A.; De Smedt, T.; Revaz, S.; Tschopp, J. A pilot study of IL-1 inhibition by anakinra in acute gout. *Arthritis Res. Ther.* **2007**, *9*, R28. [CrossRef]
73. Chen, K.; Fields, T.; Mancuso, C.A.; Bass, A.R.; Vasanth, L. Anakinra's efficacy is variable in refractory gout: Report of ten cases. *Semin. Arthritis Rheum.* **2010**, *40*, 210–214. [CrossRef]
74. Terkeltaub, R.A.; Schumacher, H.R.; Carter, J.D.; Baraf, H.S.; Evans, R.R.; Wang, J.; King-Davis, S.; Weinstein, S.P. Rilonacept in the treatment of acute gouty arthritis: A randomized, controlled clinical trial using indomethacin as the active comparator. *Arthritis Res. Ther.* **2013**, *15*, R25. [CrossRef]
75. So, A.; De Meulemeester, M.; Pikhlak, A.; Yücel, A.E.; Richard, D.; Murphy, V.; Arulmani, U.; Sallstig, P.; Schlesinger, N. Canakinumab for the treatment of acute flares in difficult-to-treat gouty arthritis: Results of a multicenter, phase II, dose-ranging study. *Arthritis Rheum.* **2010**, *62*, 3064–3076. [CrossRef]
76. Schlesinger, N.; Alten, R.E.; Bardin, T.; Schumacher, H.R.; Bloch, M.; Gimona, A.; Krammer, G.; Murphy, V.; Richard, D.; So, A.K. Canakinumab for acute gouty arthritis in patients with limited treatment options: Results from two randomised, multicentre, active-controlled, double-blind trials and their initial extensions. *Ann. Rheum. Dis.* **2012**, *71*, 1839–1848. [CrossRef] [PubMed]
77. Zhou, W.; Wang, Y.; Wu, R.; He, Y.; Su, Q.; Shi, G. MicroRNA-488 and-920 regulate the production of proinflammatory cytokines in acute gouty arthritis. *Arthritis Res. Ther.* **2017**, *19*, 203. [CrossRef] [PubMed]
78. Xu, S.; Li, X.; Liu, Y.; Xia, Y.; Chang, R.; Zhang, C. Inflammasome inhibitors: Promising therapeutic approaches against cancer. *J. Hematol. Oncol.* **2019**, *12*, 64. [CrossRef] [PubMed]
79. Ebrahimi, T.; Rust, M.; Kaiser, S.N.; Slowik, A.; Beyer, C.; Koczulla, A.R.; Schulz, J.B.; Habib, P.; Bach, J.P. α1-antitrypsin mitigates NLRP3-inflammasome activation in amyloid β (1–42)-stimulated murine astrocytes. *J. Neuroinflamm.* **2018**, *15*, 282. [CrossRef]
80. Klück, V.; Jansen, T.; Janssen, M.; Comarniceanu, A.; Efdé, M.; Tengesdal, I.W.; Schraa, K.; Cleophas, M.C.P.; Scribner, C.L.; Skouras, D.B.; et al. Dapansutrile, an oral selective NLRP3 inflammasome inhibitor, for treatment of gout flares: An open-label, dose-adaptive, proof-of-concept, phase 2a trial. *Lancet Rheumatol.* **2020**, *2*, e270–e280. [CrossRef]
81. Goldberg, E.L.; Asher, J.L.; Molony, R.D.; Shaw, A.C.; Zeiss, C.J.; Wang, C.; Morozova-Roche, L.A.; Herzog, R.I.; Iwasaki, A.; Dixit, V.D. β-Hydroxybutyrate Deactivates Neutrophil NLRP3 Inflammasome to Relieve Gout Flares. *Cell Rep.* **2017**, *18*, 2077–2087. [CrossRef]
82. Qiao, C.Y.; Li, Y.; Shang, Y.; Jiang, M.; Liu, J.; Zhan, Z.Y.; Ye, H.; Lin, Y.C.; Jiao, J.Y.; Sun, R.H.; et al. Management of Gout-associated MSU crystals-induced NLRP3 inflammasome activation by procyanidin B2: Targeting IL-1β and Cathepsin B in macrophages. *Inflammopharmacology* **2020**, *28*, 1481–1493. [CrossRef] [PubMed]
83. Chen, B.; Li, H.; Ou, G.; Ren, L.; Yang, X.; Zeng, M. Curcumin attenuates MSU crystal-induced inflammation by inhibiting the degradation of IκBα and blocking mitochondrial damage. *Arthritis Res. Ther.* **2019**, *21*, 193. [CrossRef] [PubMed]
84. Yin, C.; Liu, B.; Wang, P.; Li, X.; Li, Y.; Zheng, X.; Tai, Y.; Wang, C.; Liu, B. Eucalyptol alleviates inflammation and pain responses in a mouse model of gout arthritis. *Br. J. Pharmacol.* **2020**, *177*, 2042–2057. [CrossRef] [PubMed]
85. Ahn, H.; Lee, G.S. Riboflavin, vitamin B2, attenuates NLRP3, NLRC4, AIM2, and non-canonical inflammasomes by the inhibition of caspase-1 activity. *Sci. Rep.* **2020**, *10*, 19091. [CrossRef]

86. Yan, Y.; Jiang, W.; Spinetti, T.; Tardivel, A.; Castillo, R.; Bourquin, C.; Guarda, G.; Tian, Z.; Tschopp, J.; Zhou, R. Omega-3 fatty acids prevent inflammation and metabolic disorder through inhibition of NLRP3 inflammasome activation. *Immunity* **2013**, *38*, 1154–1163. [CrossRef]
87. Liu, N.; Meng, B.; Zeng, L.; Yin, S.; Hu, Y.; Li, S.; Fu, Y.; Zhang, X.; Xie, C.; Shu, L.; et al. Discovery of a novel rice-derived peptide with significant anti-gout potency. *Food Funct.* **2020**, *11*, 10542–10553. [CrossRef]
88. Pellegrini, C.; Fornai, M.; Antonioli, L.; Blandizzi, C.; Calderone, V. Phytochemicals as Novel Therapeutic Strategies for NLRP3 Inflammasome-Related Neurological, Metabolic, and Inflammatory Diseases. *Int. J. Mol. Sci.* **2019**, *20*, 2876. [CrossRef]
89. Yang, G.; Lee, H.E.; Moon, S.J.; Ko, K.M.; Koh, J.H.; Seok, J.K.; Min, J.K.; Heo, T.H.; Kang, H.C.; Cho, Y.Y.; et al. Direct Binding to NLRP3 Pyrin Domain as a Novel Strategy to Prevent NLRP3-Driven Inflammation and Gouty Arthritis. *Arthritis Rheumatol.* **2020**, *72*, 1192–1202. [CrossRef] [PubMed]
90. Oliviero, F.; Zamudio-Cuevas, Y.; Belluzzi, E.; Andretto, L.; Scanu, A.; Favero, M.; Ramonda, R.; Ravagnan, G.; López-Reyes, A.; Spinella, P.; et al. Polydatin and Resveratrol Inhibit the Inflammatory Process Induced by Urate and Pyrophosphate Crystals in THP-1 Cells. *Foods* **2019**, *8*, 560. [CrossRef] [PubMed]
91. Li, X.; Pan, Y.; Li, W.; Guan, P.; You, C. The Role of Noncoding RNAs in Gout. *Endocrinology* **2020**, *161*. [CrossRef]

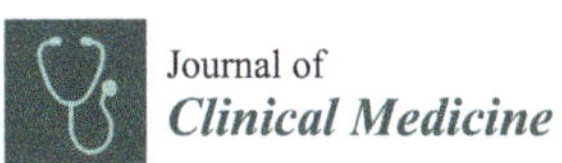

Journal of *Clinical Medicine*

MDPI

Review

Role of Proteasomes in Inflammation

Carl Christoph Goetzke [1,2,3,*], Frédéric Ebstein [4] and Tilmann Kallinich [1,2,3,5,*]

1 Charité–Universitätsmedizin Berlin, Corporate Member of Freie Universität Berlin, Humboldt-Universität zu Berlin, Department of Pediatrics, Division of Pulmonology, Immunology and Critical Care Medicine, Augustenburger Platz 1, 13353 Berlin, Germany
2 Berlin Institute of Health at Charité–Universitätsmedizin Berlin, Chariteplatz 1, 10117 Berlin, Germany
3 Deutsches Rheumaforschungszentrum, Chariteplatz 1, 10117 Berlin, Germany
4 Universitätsmedizin Greifswald, Institute of Medical Biochemistry and Molecular Biology, 7475 Greifswald, Germany; ebsteinf@uni-greifswald.de
5 Charité–Universitätsmedizin Berlin, Corporate Member of Freie Universität Berlin and Humboldt Universität zu Berlin, Center for Chronically Sick Children, Augustenburger Platz 1, 13353 Berlin, Germany
* Correspondence: carl-christoph.goetzke@charite.de (C.C.G.); tilmann.kallinich@charite.de (T.K.)

Abstract: The ubiquitin–proteasome system (UPS) is involved in multiple cellular functions including the regulation of protein homeostasis, major histocompatibility (MHC) class I antigen processing, cell cycle proliferation and signaling. In humans, proteasome loss-of-function mutations result in autoinflammation dominated by a prominent type I interferon (IFN) gene signature. These genomic alterations typically cause the development of proteasome-associated autoinflammatory syndromes (PRAAS) by impairing proteasome activity and perturbing protein homeostasis. However, an abnormal increased proteasomal activity can also be found in other human inflammatory diseases. In this review, we cast a light on the different clinical aspects of proteasomal activity in human disease and summarize the currently studied therapeutic approaches.

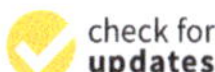

Keywords: proteasome; inflammation; autoinflammation; autoimmune; proteasome-associated autoinflammatory syndrome

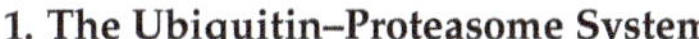

Citation: Goetzke, C.C.; Ebstein, F.; Kallinich, T. Role of Proteasomes in Inflammation. *J. Clin. Med.* **2021**, *10*, 1783. https://doi.org/10.3390/jcm10081783

Academic Editors: Eugen Feist and Burkhard Möller

Received: 14 March 2021
Accepted: 14 April 2021
Published: 20 April 2021

1. The Ubiquitin–Proteasome System

The ubiquitin–proteasome system (UPS) is the most important intracellular non-lysosomal pathway for protein breakdown in eukaryotic cells [1–3]. As such, it plays a critical role in preserving protein homeostasis and protecting the cells from harmful protein aggregation which would compromise cell integrity and function [4,5].

The UPS is a highly complex mechanism with well over 1000 different genes involved [6], about only 50 of which encode proteins serving proteasome function [7]. The vast majority of the remaining UPS genes encode components involved in the selective modification of intracellular substrates with the ubiquitin molecule for recognition and subsequent degradation by proteasomes [8,9]. The covalent attachment of ubiquitin to target proteins is mediated by a cascade reaction involving three enzymes. In the first step, an E1 ubiquitin-activating enzyme uses energy released by adenosine triphosphate (ATP) hydrolysis to form a covalent bond between a cysteine residue of its active site and the C-terminal glycine of ubiquitin [10,11]. The activated ubiquitin is then transferred onto an E2 ubiquitin-conjugating enzyme, which itself can bind to one of several E3 ubiquitin ligases. In the final step, E3 ubiquitin ligases mediate the transfer of ubiquitin to a lysine residue of target substrates [12] (Figure 1). Less frequently, ubiquitylation occurs on other acceptors sites including cysteine, threonine and serine residues as well as N-terminal methionine [12–15]. Remarkably, ubiquitin itself may be also subjected to ubiquitylation at either one of its seven lysine (K) residues (K6, K11, K27, K29, K33, K48 and K63) or its N-terminal methionine (M1—known as linear polyubiquitylation), thereby triggering the formation of poly-ubiquitin chains [16,17]. Depending on the K-linkage used for ubiquitylation, these poly-ubiquitin chains may decide different possible fates for the attached protein [18]. Among these ubiquitylation types, K48-linked poly-ubiquitin chains represent canonical signals for proteasome-mediated degradation [17,19], while K63-linked and linear (M1) polyubiquitylation may support non-proteolytic roles such as signaling [19–21]. Importantly, the process of ubiquitylation is counteracted by deubiquitinating enzymes (DUBs) [22], whose most prominent families include the ubiquitin-specific proteases (USPs) and the otubain proteases (OTUs) [23].

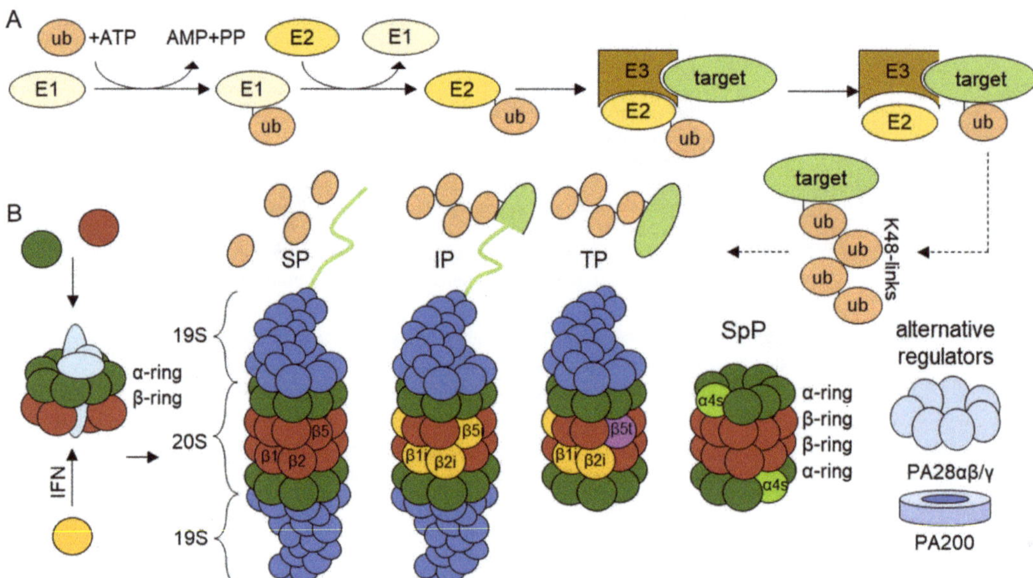

Figure 1. Schematic representation of ubiquitylation and proteasomal protein degradation. (**A**) Proteins destined for proteasomal degradation are conjugated with ubiquitin in a three-step cascade. First, E1-ubiquitin-activating enzymes bind to ubiquitin in an ATP-dependent reaction. This ubiquitin is transferred onto a E2-ubiquitin conjugating-enzyme. The E3-ubiquitin-ligase binds to both ubiquitin-conjugated E2-enzymes and target substrates which thereby undergo modification with ubiquitin. Ubiquitylated proteins can be polyubiquitylated. Depicted is a K48 linked polyubiquitylation, where ubiquitin is consecutively attached to the lysine 48 of the already bound ubiquitin. (**B**) The 20S proteasome core particle is made up of α- and β-subunits. The assembly to αββα asymmetric heptameric rings is guided by assembly chaperones. Each 20S core particle consists of two outer α-rings and two inner β-rings. In standard proteasomes (SPs), the catalytically active subunits are β1, β2 and β5. In immunoproteasomes (IPs), these subunits are replaced by the inducible subunits LMP2 (β1i), MECL1 (β2i) and LMP7 (β5i). IPs are preferentially incorporated to newly synthetized proteasomes in response to IFN, as indicated. Additional isotypes include the thymoproteasome (TP) which contains a unique β5t protease subunit and the spermatoproteasome (SpP) that incorporates a specific structural α4s subunit. The active sites of the catalytic subunits face the inside of the 20S barrel shape. Proteasomes can bind to different regulators on one or both sides. The 19S regulator has receptors for poly-ubiquitylated proteins and helps to unfold the proteins, remove ubiquitin from substrates and translocate them into the 20S for degradation. The regulators can attach to different isoforms on either or both sides. Additionally, combinations of the 19S regulator and PA28αβ/γ or PA200 regulators exist.

As alluded earlier, K48-linked ubiquitination is a prerequisite for the breakdown of intracellular proteins by 26S proteasome complexes, which themselves are made up of a 20S core particle (CP) and a 19S regulatory particle (RP) [24,25]. The 20S CP is a barrel-shaped multicatalytic protease consisting of four heptameric αββα rings. The outer two rings are each composed of seven different α-subunits, while the inner two rings each contain seven different β-subunits [26,27]. The catalytic activity of the 20S CP is driven by the β1, β2 and β5 subunits encoded by the *PSMB6*, *PSMB7* and *PSMB5* genes, respectively [28]. All three β-subunits carry N-terminal threonine active sites exposed to the inner chamber of the

20 CP and exhibit chymotrypsin-, trypsin and caspase-like activities [29]. The assembly of the 20S CP is a highly coordinated process guided by the proteasome-assembly chaperones (PAC)1-4 encoded by the *PSMG1-4* genes and the proteasome maturation protein (POMP) encoded by *POMP* [7,30,31].

Importantly, 20S CPs are usually capped by regulators at either one or both sides of the barrel-shaped structure. One prime example of such regulators is the 19S RP [32], a complex of approximately 20 subunits which is essential for the recognition of K48-linked polyubiquitinated proteins via the Rpn10 and Rpn13 subunits [33,34]. The 19S RP also ensures the ATP-dependent unfolding of substrates as well as the removal of the ubiquitin moieties before translocation into the 20S CP [35–37]. Other regulators include the proteasome activators (PA) 28-αβ, PA28-γ and PA200 [27]. The ability of the 20S CP to bind distinct regulators at both sides gives rise to multiple proteasome complexes whose respective biological relevance, however, remains to be better understood [38] (Figure 1). Degradation products produced by the UPS are usually 8–10 amino acid long-peptides [39]. Only a small fraction of them may enter the endoplasmic reticulum (ER) via transporter associated with antigen processing (TAP) and are presented onto major histocompatibility (MHC) class I molecules [40,41]. In this regard, the UPS is a major contributor to MHC class I antigen presentation. Conversely, the vast majority of proteasomal products are further degraded into amino acids by various peptidases.

1.1. Proteasome Isoforms

Besides the β1, β2 and β5 subunits traditionally referred to as standard subunits, proteasomes may incorporate alternative catalytic β-subunits including the inducible β1i (low molecular weight protein 2—LMP2), β2i (multicatalytic endopeptidase complex subunit 1—MECL1) and β5i (LMP7) to form so-called immunoproteasomes (IPs) [42–44]. While standard proteasomes (SPs) are found in virtually all tissues, IPs are predominantly expressed in immune cells or other cell types that have been exposed to type I and/or II interferons (IFN) [43,45].

It is believed that IPs are more effective than SPs at degrading substrates under stress conditions [46–49], thereby protecting the cells from the accumulation of insoluble ubiquitin-modified protein aggregates [4,43,50]. It is also understood that SPs and IPs differ in their cleavage rates [51], thereby modulating the supply of MHC class I-restricted peptide positively or negatively, depending on antigen primary structure [6]. Recently, IPs have also been shown to regulate inflammation, as discussed below. Apart from the standard and inducible subunits, 20S CPs may contain the β5t catalytic subunit (encoded by the *PSMB11* gene) which is exclusively expressed in thymus [52]. The assembly of β5t results in the formation of so-called thymus-proteasomes which participate in T-cell positive selection [52,53]. Another proteasome isoform is the spermatoproteasome which carries the α4s (encoded by *PSMA8*) alternative structural subunit, predominantly found in testis and involved in spermatogenesis [54] (Figure 1).

1.2. Proteasomes and Cellular Pro-Inflammatory-Pathways

Due to its ability to degrade multiple regulatory proteins, the UPS coordinates a myriad of cellular responses. Innate immunity is a prime example of such processes, whereby the UPS regulates key signaling cascades. For instance, activation of the NF-κB and MAPK pathways in response to pattern recognition receptors' (PRRs) engagement typically requires the generation of poly-ubiquitin chains at multiple levels. This is probably best depicted by the linear ubiquitin chain assembly complex (LUBAC) which contains the two E3 ubiquitin ligases HOIL-1L and HOIP [55]. By promoting the linear (M1-linked) ubiquitination of the IKK regulatory subunit NF-κB essential modulator (NEMO), LUBAC facilitates the phosphorylation of IκBα by IKK [55]. This phosphorylation serves as a signal for K48-linked poly-ubiquitylation and proteasomal degradation, thereby allowing the translocation of NF-κB into the nucleus for the transcription of genes encoding proinflammatory cytokines [56]. Further substrates of LUBAC include the receptor-interacting protein kinase

1 (RIPK1) involved in TNF signaling, which following linear ubiquitylation activates the proinflammatory NF-κB and MAPK pathways. The activation of RIPK1 is counterbalanced by the OTU DUB OTULIN, which is able to trim linear ubiquitin linkages [57]. In addition, K63-linked ubiquitin chains can result in the downstream activation of proinflammatory pathways, which is counteracted by the deubiquitinase A20 [58] (Figure 2).

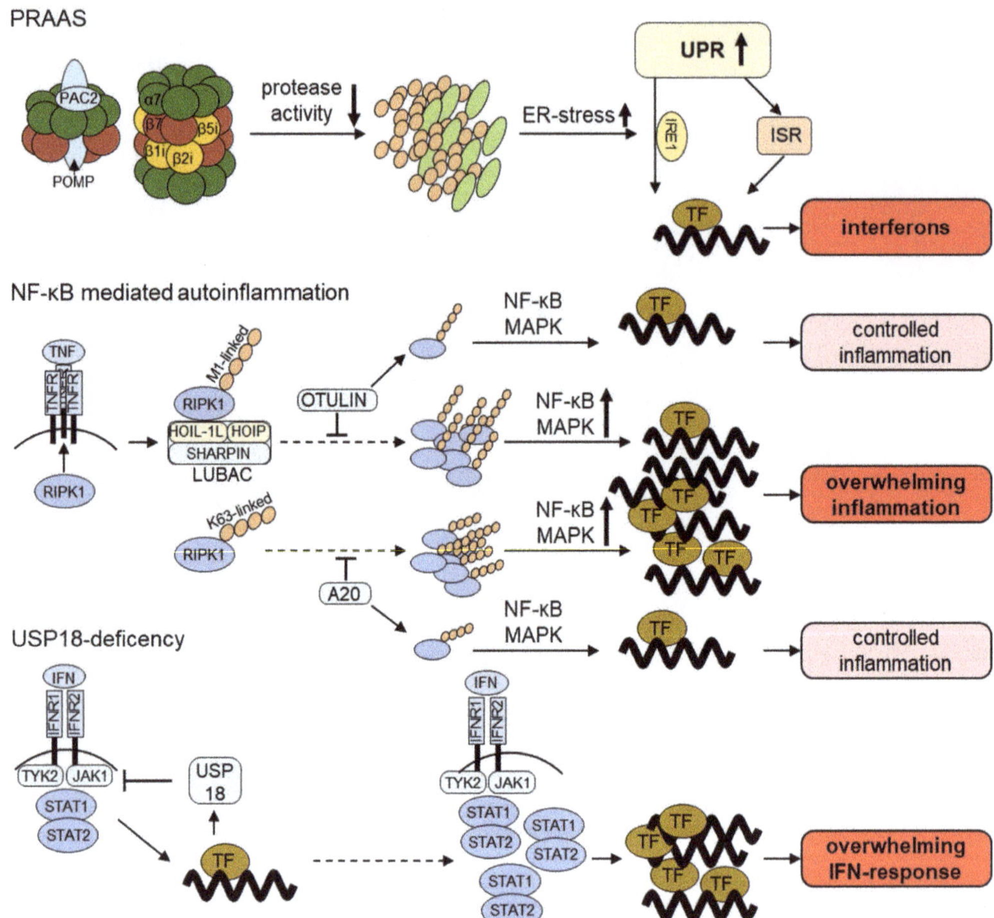

Figure 2. Current understanding of the pathogenesis of UPS dysfunction in autoinflammatory diseases. PRAAS (Proteasome-Associated Autoinflammatory Syndrome): proteasome loss-of-function mutations decrease proteasome proteolytic activity and result in intracellular accumulation of polyubiquitylated proteins. These proteotoxic aggregates induce ER-stress which initiates the unfolded protein response (UPR). The IRE1 (inositol-requiring enzyme 1) arm of the UPR has been shown to contribute to the transcription of IFN-stimulated genes (ISG). A possible involvement of the integrated stress response (ISR) in this process is also discussed. NF-κB-mediated autoinflammation: PPR and cytokine receptor activation requires ubiquitylation for the induction of pro-inflammatory signaling. Depicted is the activation of the TNF receptor 1 (TNFR). The receptor-interacting protein kinase 1 (RIPK1) binds to the activated TFNR and is ubiquitylated with linear (M1-linked) poly-ubiquitin chains by the LUBAC complex or with K63-linked polyubiquitin. Polyubiquitylation is counterbalanced by the deubiquitinating enzymes (DUB) OTULIN and A20 in order to control the activation of the NF-κB and MAPK pro-inflammatory pathways. USP18 deficiency: USP18 besides its DUB activity also directly regulates IFN signaling. It is upregulated following different pro-inflammatory stimuli and directly inhibits JAK1, thereby acting as a negative feedback loop. Disruption of this negative feedback leads to overwhelming inflammatory IFN response.

Overall, proinflammatory pathways have been shown to be dependent on both proteasomal activity and ubiquitylation [6]. Toll-like receptor (TLR) stimuli, for example, rely on active IPs for the full induction of proinflammatory cytokines via the MAPK pathway [59,60]. These studies were mainly performed in myeloid-derived immune cells, but lymphoid cells were affected as well [61]. Interestingly, IP activity was found to play a critical role in T-cell differentiation with inducible subunits favoring T helper (Th)1 and Th17 differentiation, while SPs promoted a regulatory T cell phenotype [60,62,63]. B cells, especially plasma cells (PC), have an increased sensitivity to proteotoxic stress and therefore, are extremely dependent on proper proteasome function for their survival [64–66]. The accumulation of protein aggregates that cannot be effectively degraded by proteasomes generally induces intracellular stress and activates the unfolded protein response (UPR). This, in turn, leads to compensatory mechanisms including the upregulation of proteasome isoforms to restore protein homeostasis [6,67].

2. Impaired Proteasomal Function—(Mono)genetic Defects in the Ubiquitin Proteasome-System in Autoinflammatory Disorders

2.1. Proteasome-Associated-Autoinflammatory-Syndrome (PRAAS)

A cause-and-effect relationship between proteasome dysfunction and chronic inflammation was first established in 2010, as loss-of-function mutations in the *PSMB8* gene were identified in patients suffering from autoinflammatory syndromes [68]. As disease manifestations included joint contractures, muscle atrophy, microcytic anemia and panniculitis-induced lipodystrophy, these syndromes were initially referred to as JMP syndromes. Shortly afterwards, further mutations in the very same *PSMB8* gene were found in patients presenting with similar autoinflammatory symptoms. Many different names have been proposed to describe these disorders, including Nakajo-Nishimura syndrome (NNS) [69], Japanese autoinflammatory syndrome with lipodystrophy (JASL) [70] and chronic atypical neutrophilic dermatosis with lipodystrophy and elevated temperature (CANDLE) syndrome [71]. As these syndromes share the same genetic etiology, these were subsequently brought together and referred to as proteasome-associated-autoinflammatory-syndromes (PRAAS) [72,73].

Disease starts usually in infancy up to early childhood and is characterized by arthritis, skin eruptions, lipodystrophy and myositis as well as muscle atrophy in all PRAAS forms. Recurring fever is also described in all syndromes but JMP. Further PRAAS hallmarks include basal ganglia calcifications and hepatosplenomegaly [68–70,73–75]. As for the skin lesions, they seem to slightly differ in presentation between syndromes, with CANDLE being associated with annular plaque and violaceous eyelids [74], while NNS and JASL mostly present with nodular erythema [69,70]. Additionally, lesions in JMP patients are described as erythematous macular/papular and nodules [68].

Laboratory findings are in line with the observed chronic inflammation, as elevated C-reactive protein levels and erythrocyte sedimentation rate are common in patients [72]. Unfortunately, beside genetic analysis, rapid diagnostic tests for PRAAS are not available so far. However, two biological traits highly specific to PRAAS may be used to help establish the presence of the disease. These include: (i) a typical type I IFN gene signature in the blood [7,75–77] and (ii) a ubiquitous proteasome loss of function. One way to detect type I IFN responses is to monitor the expression of IFN-stimulated genes (ISG) at the transcript level by qPCR and/or Nanostring technology [78,79] or at the protein level (i.e., SIGLEC1) using flow cytometry [80]. Impaired proteasomal function can be measured either directly using activity-based-probes showing cleavage capacity [68] or indirectly by assessing the content of ubiquitin-modified proteins by Western blotting [69].

Given that the first PRAAS genetic mutations were all identified within the *PSMB8* gene encoding the catalytic IP subunit β5i [71], it was initially assumed that these disorders were primarily caused by IP defects. This notion was, however, rapidly challenged by the fact that PRAAS patients may carry genomic alterations in other proteasome genes such as *PSMA3* [76], *PSMB4* [76], *PSMB9* [76], *POMP* [76,81], *PSMG2* [82] and *PSMB10* [83]. Surprisingly, a series of proteasome loss-of-function mutations affecting *PSMB1* [84], *PSMD12* [85] or *PSMC3* [86] were not associated with typical PRAAS phenotypes, as they were found in patients suffering from neurodevelopmental delay (NDD). While cognitive impairment is also detectable in PRAAS patients, NDD subjects fail to develop any clinical signs of autoinflammation. The reasons for these discrepancies are unclear and warrant further investigation.

Due to the inherent type I IFN gene signature, PRAAS may be placed into the category of interferonopathies. However, in contrast to other well-defined interferonopathies such as Aicardi–Goutières syndrome (AGS) or STING-associated vasculopathy with onset in infancy (SAVI), the molecular mechanisms leading to type I IFN production in PRAAS remain unclear. One particularly attractive hypothesis for the induction of sterile inflammation in PRAAS subjects is the propagation of ER stress. It is indeed well established that ER associated protein degradation (ERAD) function is compromised by proteasome defects, thereby resulting in the retention of misfolded proteins in the ER [87,88]. Perturbed protein homeostasis in the ER lumen is then sensed by the three ER-resident transmembrane receptors ATF6 (activating transcription factor 6), IRE1 (inositol-requiring enzyme 1) and PERK (protein kinase R (PKR)-like endoplasmic reticulum kinase) which in turn initiate the so-called unfolded protein response (UPR). This results in the activation of downstream transcriptions factors destined to upregulate ERAD component and/or chaperones [89]. Strikingly, it has been shown that sustained UPR activation may induce inflammation even in a pathogen-free context by various mechanisms [67,90]. For instance, the exposure of microglia to proteasome inhibitors leads to the production of inflammatory cytokines in an IRE1-dependent fashion [91]. The observation that PRAAS patients express typical ER stress markers [81], suggests that the UPR might be one the mechanisms underlying inflammation in these patients. Interestingly, the activation of the UPR also results in the transcription of genes encoding inhibitors of the mTORC1 signaling pathway [92–95]. A decreased activation of mTORC1 would result in decreased lipid biosynthesis and reduced amounts of cholesterol. The observation that cholesterol deficiency is a danger signal alerting the innate immune system [96] reinforces the notion that the UPR might play a key role in PRAAS pathogenesis.

Thus far, the therapeutic options for PRAAS are extremely limited. Subjects with PRAAS respond poorly to conventional or biologic disease-modifying antirheumatic drugs [76]. Recently, major advances have been made by introducing the JAK1/2 inhibitor baricitinib into the treatment protocols [97]. Baricitinib, which blocks inter alia IFN signaling, has shown promising effects in PRAAS patients, as it could reduce disease manifestation in 8 out of 10 patients and promote clinical/inflammatory remission in 5 out of 10 patients, even though one patient had to drop out because of an uncontrolled BK-virus infection [97]. Similarly, successful treatment of PRAAS with tofacitinib, a pan-JAK-inhibitor, was demonstrated in a case report [98].

2.2. *Further Genetic Inflammatory Diseases with a Link to the UPS*

Dysregulated ubiquitylation has recently been associated with NF-κB-related autoinflammatory diseases, also named relopathies [99]. Among them, three are currently associated with altered ubiquitylation patterns [100]. These include mutations within genes encoding LUBAC and the OTU-deubiquitinase OTULIN and A20.

Mutations in *RBCK*, encoding HOIL-1L [101], and *RNF31*, encoding HOIP [102], are found in patients suffering from autoinflammation and immunodeficiency. These are traditionally referred to as LUBAC-mutations, as they result in the impaired assembly of the LUBAC complex, thereby preventing the linear (M1) ubiquitylation of critical signal transducing proteins (for TNF-signaling RIPK1, as depicted in Figure 2). LUBAC deficiency induces cell-type specific and cytokine-specific down- but also upregulation of the NF-κB-pathway. Clinically, patients with mutations in either one of the LUBAC subunits present with multiorgan autoinflammation, recurring infections and intracellular muscular glycogen inclusions with consecutive (cardio-)myopathy (amylopectionsis) [101,102].

OUTLIN, which counteracts linear LUBAC ubiquitylation, may be subjected to several loss-of-function mutations in patients exhibiting enhanced NF-κB activation [57]. Consequently, this leads to increased secretion of pro-inflammatory cytokines due to unbalanced LUBAC-activity (Figure 2).The resulting disease is named otulipenia or otulin-related autoinflammatory syndrome (ORAS) [103], whereby patients suffer from recurring fevers, sterile neutrophilia, lipodystrophy, panniculitis and systemic inflammation with growth retardation [100].

Another DUB involved in a negative feedback regulation is A20, whose alterations are associated with severe autoinflammation. Heterozygous loss-of-function mutations in the gene *TNFAIP3* encoding A20 result in a Behçet-like disease named A20 haploinsufficiency [104,105]. Autoinflammation manifests early and is accompanied by bipolar oral and genital ulcers, inflammation of the eyes, exanthemas, and arthralgia/arthritis (ref). Furthermore, mutations within *TNFAIP3* have been found in autoimmune–lymphoproliferative syndrome (ALPS) [105]. In these diseases, autoinflammation is typically accompanied by immunodeficiency due to the severe dysregulation of the NF-κB-pathway [100] (Figure 2).

USP18 deficiency was recently described as a novel autoinflammatory disorder [106]. USP18 serves as a negative feedback for type I IFN-signaling besides its role as a DUB for the ubiquitin-like modifier ISG15 [107]. Genetic mutations resulting in USP18 loss-of-function of present with a pseudo-TORCH (toxoplasmosis, other [syphilis, varicella, mumps, parvovirus and HIV], rubella, cytomegalovirus, and herpes simplex) fetopathy due to the unmitigated IFN-induced inflammation [106]. Similarly, impaired trafficking of USP18 to the IFN receptor results in loss of USP18 activity and a phenocopy of USP18 deficiency [108]. Untreated USP18 deficiency results in neonatal death [106]. However, immediate treatment with JAK-inhibitors has been successful in a first case [109].

Most recently, mutations within the major E1 ubiquitin-activating enzyme ubiquitin-like modifier activating enzyme 1 (UBA1) have been associated with adult-onset autoinflammation [110,111]. In the affected patients, somatic mutations in peripheral blood myeloid cells in the X-chromosomal *UBA1* gene resulted in the expression of a catalytically impaired UBA1 isoform. Mechanistically the impaired ubiquitin-activating activity resulted in decreased polyubiquitylation and increased unfolded protein response. Thus, only males were found to be affected and somatic nature explains the late onset of inflammation. Clinical phenotypes can vary. Common inflammatory manifestations include relapsing perichondritis, Sweet's syndrome or vasculitis. Additionally, patients frequently present with hematological abnormalities including myelodysplastic syndrome. Due to the vacuoles found in myeloid precursor cells, the affected E1 enzyme on the X-chromosome, causing autoinflammation by a somatic the disease was named VEXAS [110].

3. Inflammation and Increased Proteasomal Activity

As the inducible β1i, β2i and β5i catalytic units are typically upregulated in response to inflammatory cytokines (as highlighted in the first chapter), the constitutive expression of IPs is a common hallmark of autoinflammatory diseases [112,113]. In this regard, other UPS-related biomarkers include proteasome-directed autoantibodies which were identified in multiple autoimmune diseases such as poly/dermatomyositis, systemic lupus erythematosus (SLE), Sjögren Syndrome (SjS) and multiple sclerosis (MS) [114–116]. Interestingly, these antibodies were capable of reducing proteasomal activation by PA28, at least in vitro [117]. Besides autoantibodies against proteasome subunits, circulating proteasomes were also found in various autoinflammatory diseases including SLE, rheumatoid arthritis (RA) or vasculitis [118]. Interestingly, the amounts of circulating proteasomes seemed to correlate with cellular damage, thereby making them good clinical markers for disease progression [119]. These findings led to multiple preclinical studies, investigating proteasomal activity in various autoinflammatory diseases and autoimmune diseases [59,60,120–125], as discussed below. Additionally, in autoimmune driven diseases further benefit from proteasome inhibition might be accounted to the specific proapoptotic effect on plasma cells [64,66,126,127].

3.1. Rheumatoid Arthritis

RA is a common autoimmune disease characterized by inflammation of the synovia and joints leading to cartilage and bone destruction [128]. It can be accompanied by systemic disorders, thereby potentially leading to high morbidity and increased mortality [128]. A key driver of RA pathogenesis is NF-κB [129], whose activation relies on proper proteasome function, as mentioned above. Hence, proteasome inhibition has proven clinically useful to reduce the production of interleukin (IL)-1β and IL-6 in T cells from RA patients [130]. In addition, blocking proteasome function by small molecule inhibitors has been shown to limit RA synovial cell proliferation by preventing the degradation of p53 [131]. Preclinical data from two mouse models of collagen antibody-induced arthritis and collagen-induced arthritis have also revealed that IP activity supports disease progression by promoting pro-inflammatory cytokine production and inflammatory joint infiltration [120].

3.2. Systemic Lupus Erythematosus

SLE is an autoimmune disease in which inflammation may target multiple organs, resulting in a very heterogeneous clinical manifestation with individual disease courses and various life-shortening and life-threatening complications [132]. Autoantibodies found in SLE target nuclear proteins are frequently produced by long-lived plasma cells (PC) that evade conventional B cell-targeted treatment [127]. However, due to their particularly high-rate production of secretory proteins, PCs generate large amounts of misfolded proteins in ER lumen that must be transported back to the cytosol by ERAD for subsequent degradation by proteasomes. For that reason, PCs are particularly sensitive to proteasome inhibition (as discussed below). A more direct involvement of proteasomes in SLE pathogenesis has been shown in mouse models in which specific IP inhibition was associated with reduced production of IFN-α [133], a critical disease marker [134]. Another hint for an active contribution of proteasomes to SLE comes from the observation that PA28γ is downregulated in lupus nephritis tissue [135]. Since PA28γ-capped proteasomes accelerate the turnover of phosphorylated STAT3 [135], it is highly likely that the decreased expression of PA28γ actively contributes to diseases pathogenesis. Interestingly, this notion seems to be specific to SLE, as the serum levels of circulating PA28γ in RA, SjS and other undifferentiated connective tissue diseases (CTDs) are increased and positively correlate with disease activity [136].

3.3. Sjögren Syndrome

Like RA and SLE, SjS is an autoimmune CTD. In SjS, autoimmunity leads to a chronic inflammation of salivatory and lacrimal glands [137]. It can manifest primarily or in combination with other autoimmune diseases and is the most frequent autoimmune CTD [137]. Besides the prevalence of anti-proteasome autoantibodies in SjS [138], the expression of the IP subunit LMP2 was significantly reduced in SjS salivatory glands [113,139]. The downregulation of LMP2 in SjS seems to occur as a consequence of increased protein turnover, as LMP2 mRNA were simultaneously upregulated. mRNA upregulation was most prominent in B cells and correlated with reduced susceptibility to proteasome inhibition [140]. However, proteasome inhibition in an animal model of SjS prevented disease development [141]. In this study, the beneficial effect of proteasome inhibitors was attributed to the prevention of Th17 differentiation and lymphocytic gland-infiltration. Furthermore, a variant of the *PSMB11* gene encoding the thymoproteasome specific β5t subunit was associated with the development SjS [142]. In this work, the introduction of this variant in mice resulted in impaired positive T-cell selection and an altered CD8+ T-cell receptor repertoire.

3.4. Inflammatory Bowel Disease

Besides CTD, it has been suspected that UPS dysfunction might be involved in the pathogenesis of other inflammatory diseases. For instance, it is thought that proteasomes participate in the progression of inflammatory bowel disease (IBD). The two main IBD forms are ulcerative colitis (UC) and Crohn's disease (CD), both of which presents with relapsing chronic inflammation of the gut and sustained activation of the NF-κB pathway [143]. Strikingly, the IP subunits β1i and β2i were found to be constitutively expressed in colons of patients with CD [144,145] and to a lesser extent in UC [145]. It has been proposed that the presence of IP in patients with IBD favors IκBα degradation, thereby promoting the excessive activation of NF-κB activation [146]. IP subunit expression and activity in CD might be involved in immunopathogenesis. However, a prominent role of IFN-γ (known to induce IP formation) in CD limits conclusions made from these ex vivo studies [144]. Preclinical studies have been carried out to investigate whether such differential expression of proteasome isoforms was disease-relevant. It could be confirmed that both proteasome pan- and IP-specific inhibitions reduced gut inflammation in mice [147,148]. For the targeted approach, a dual inhibition of at least two IP subunits was necessary [149].The protective mechanism was attributed to reduced NF-κB-signaling in all these studies.

3.5. Multiple Sclerosis

MS is an inflammatory disease of the central nervous system (CNS) resulting in demyelination and neuronal damage [150]. It is the most common CNS autoimmune disease whose molecular pathogenesis remains, however, poorly understood. It predominantly affects young adults and has a severe impact on the quality of life of these individuals [150]. Interestingly, LMP2 and PA28αβ were found to be enriched in immune cells and oligodendrocytes of MS lesions [151]. Further evidence for an involvement of IPs in MS pathogenesis was made by the identification of a *PSMB9* variant associated with a reduced risk of developing MS. It is understood that the beneficial effect of this variant is attributed to altered MHC class I-restricted myelin-derived peptides [151]. It was also shown that proteasome pan-inhibition could prevent the development of experimental autoimmune encephalitis (EAE, a mouse model of MS) in mice following the injection of antigens and/or antigen-specific CD4+ or CD8+ T cells [125,152,153]. Similar effects were observed by specifically inhibiting the two IP subunits LMP2 and LMP7 [125,149].

3.6. Further Inflammatory Diseases with a Link to the UPS

The critical role of the UPS in cytokine signaling, especially the NF-κB- and Th17 differentiation pathways makes it a good disease-causing candidate in many other inflammatory disorders. For example, in psoriasis, a chronic inflammatory skin disease, driven by both innate and adaptive immunity, genome wide association studies have shown a direct cause-and-effect relationship between UPS dysfunction and psoriasis [154,155]. A central role here is assigned to the IL-23/Th-17 axis and TNFα a cytokine upregulated by NF-κB [156]. Similarly, any UPS dysfunction might trigger auto-immune diseases because of inappropriate supply of MHC class I-restricted peptides. This view is supported by a genome wide association study in Behçet's disease [157].

4. The UPS as a Therapeutic Target

Bortezomib is the first proteasome inhibitor with FDA approval. It was initially described as an anti-inflammatory drug [158]. However, bortezomib and the second-generation proteasome inhibitor carfilzomib have only been clinically approved for treating malignancies such as multiple myeloma and mantle cell lymphoma so far [159–161]. Clinical data from a small study involving 12 patients with SLE [64] and a randomized double-blind controlled trial with 14 patients with SLE [162] have shown a beneficial effect of bortezomib on disease outcome. Similarly, in another study, bortezomib was shown to deplete PCs and reduce autoantibody production [127,163]. As discussed earlier, this effect can be easily explained by the fact that antigen-producing PCs need a high proteasomal capacity to degrade misfolded antibodies, which renders them susceptible to proteasome inhibition [127]. The perceived benefit of bortezomib is its proapoptotic effect on long-lived PCs. This effect is unfortunately not limited to pathogenic PCs but also depletes protective PCs [164]. Bortezomib has furthermore successfully been used in different cases of autoimmunity including autoimmune cytopenia, refractory primary SjS and encephalitis [165–168]. As all beneficial effects of bortezomib on the SLE disease course cannot be attributed to the reduction in autoantibodies [162], an additional anti-inflammatory effect is suspected. For instance, ex vitro stimulated T cells from healthy donors showed the reduced expression of inflammatory cytokines under proteasome inhibition by bortezomib [169]. A substantial part of the anti-inflammatory potential might also be attributed to overall cytotoxic effects on immune cells [170], which were most prominently observed in monocytes [124,170]. Similar effects on antibody formation has been observed in a small case series of anti-NMDA-receptor encephalitis [171], and a multicenter randomized controlled double-blinded study is currently recruiting patients [172] (ClinicalTrials identifier NCT03993262, https://clinicaltrials.gov/ct2/show/NCT03993262, accessed on 20 February 2021). However, a therapy with bortezomib is limited by the hematological and neurotoxic side effects [173]. The assumed effects are summarized in Figure 3.

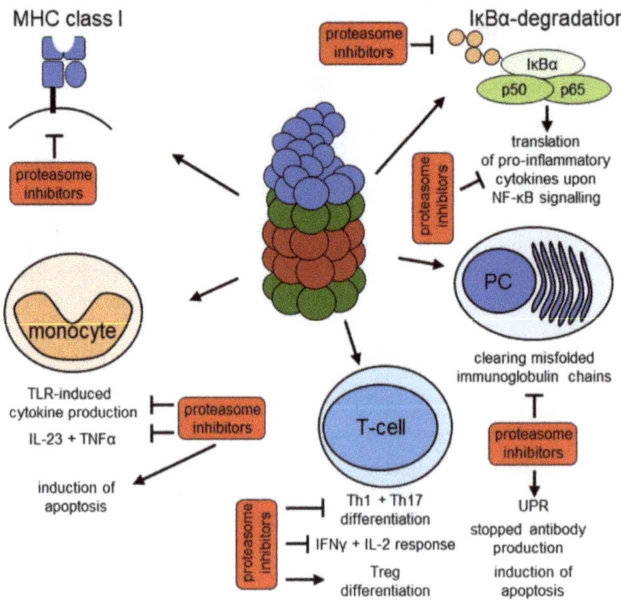

Figure 3. Overview of the potential anti-inflammatory mechanisms of proteasome inhibitors. Proteasome inhibitors including bortezomib, carfilzomib, ONX 0914 and KZR 616 were shown to exert anti-inflammatory effects via different mechanisms. These involve all cells: an influence on MHC class I antigen presentation (**top left**) and degradation of IκBα (**top right**), which results in NF-κB nuclear translocation and transcription of pro-inflammatory cytokines. Specific effects on cellular subsets include a targeted anti-inflammatory and proapoptotic effect on monocytes which results in a reduction in pro-inflammatory cytokine production upon TLR stimuli (**bottom left**). In T-cells, active IP are required for differentiation into Th1 and Th17 phenotypes (**bottom center**), whilst IP inhibition results in increased Treg differentiation and decreased IFN-γ production, as indicated. Plasma cells (PC) are especially sensitive to reduced proteasomal activity, which results in apoptosis most likely via activation of the UPR and in depletion of autoantibodies (**bottom right**).

Further proteasome inhibitors, particularly those only targeting the IP subunits, are currently under investigation [174], as they are thought to have fewer toxic side effects [175,176]. IP-specific inhibitors have been established in preclinical research [120,174] and have shown promising potential in multiple inflammatory disease models of various inflammatory and autoimmune disorders including experimental arthritis [120], sepsis-models [59], experimental autoimmune myocarditis [60] experimental autoimmune encephalomyelitis [125] and experimental colitis [121] inter alia [123,177–179].

For sufficient anti-inflammatory treatment, a co-inhibition of at least two IP catalytic subunits is necessary [149,179]. For immune cell depletion, including PC depletion, at least a partial added inhibitory effect on SPs is needed, as the catalytically active SP subunits β1, β2 and β5 are upregulated compensatory under highly specific IP inhibition in these cells [180]. The first human immunoproteasome inhibitor with such inhibitory capacity is KZR-616 [174]. It is currently in clinical phase 2 studies for treating systemic lupus erythematosus (ClinicalTrials identifier NCT03393013, https://www.clinicaltrials.gov/ct2/show/NCT03393013, accessed on 20 February 2021) and polymyositis/dermatomyositis (ClinicalTrials identifier NCT04033926, https://www.clinicaltrials.gov/ct2/show/NCT04033926, accessed on 20 February 2021).

Whilst proteasome inhibitors are well established, only limited data are currently available on the therapeutic potential of small molecule proteasome activators [181]. Examples of the very few substances capable of activating proteasomes include a MAPK inhibitor [181] and the protein kinase (PKA) activator Rolipram, which acts most likely by phosphorylating proteasomes [182]. Other substances increase proteasomal activity by the transcription of proteasome genes [183] or by the inhibition of DUBs [184] Clearly, further research is needed in this field, as increasing proteasome activity may provide treatment for patients with PRAAS or other diseases [181].

5. Conclusions

To summarize, the UPS is tightly involved in inflammation and (auto-)inflammatory diseases. It is involved in regulating pro-inflammatory pathways and is in turn upregulated during inflammation. Its exact role in the disease pathogenesis of inflammatory diseases is, however, still under investigation. Then again, impaired proteasomal activity is known to induce sterile inflammation, as observed in PRAAS patients. The exact mechanism is still not fully understood. Unravelling the pathogenesis of such diseases further will aid in better therapeutic approaches for PRAAS patients. For (auto-)inflammatory and auto-immune diseases, multiple mechanisms involved have been found. This resulted in successful initial clinical trials using the immunoproteasome as a therapeutic target. Larger studies with novel proteasome inhibitors with an optimized side-effect spectrum seem promising for larger randomized clinical trials.

Author Contributions: Literature research: C.C.G., F.E. and T.K.; writing—original draft preparation: C.C.G., F.E. and T.K.; writing—review and editing: C.C.G., F.E. and T.K.; visualization: C.C.G. All authors have read and agreed to the published version of the manuscript.

Funding: C.C.G. is a fellow in the BIH Charité Clinician Scientist Program funded by the Charité–Universitätsmedizin Berlin and the Berlin Institute of Health. The program was initiated and lead by Professor Duska Dragun to enable resident physicians to pursue a career in academic medicine. Professor Dragun passed away on 28 December of 2020. This publication is dedicated to her memory as a mentor, role model and stellar scientist. T.K. is a fellow of the BIH.

Institutional Review Board Statement: Not applicable.

Informed Consent Statement: Not applicable.

Acknowledgments: We acknowledge support from the German Research Foundation (DFG) and the Open Access Publication Fund of Charité—Universitätsmedizin Berlin.

Conflicts of Interest: The authors declare no conflict of interest.

References

1. Ciechanover, A. Intracellular protein degradation: From a vague idea thru the lysosome and the ubiquitin–proteasome system and onto human diseases and drug targeting. *Cell Death Differ.* **2005**, *12*, 1178–1190. [CrossRef] [PubMed]
2. Amm, I.; Sommer, T.; Wolf, D.H. Protein quality control and elimination of protein waste: The role of the ubiquitin–proteasome system. *Biochim. Biophys. Acta* **2014**, *1843*, 182–196. [CrossRef] [PubMed]

3. Pohl, C.; Dikic, I. Cellular quality control by the ubiquitin-proteasome system and autophagy. *Science* **2019**, *366*, 818–822. [CrossRef] [PubMed]
4. Warnatsch, A.; Bergann, T.; Krüger, E. Oxidation matters: The ubiquitin proteasome system connects innate immune mechanisms with MHC class I antigen presentation. *Mol. Immunol.* **2013**, *55*, 106–109. [CrossRef] [PubMed]
5. Zheng, C.; Geetha, T.; Babu, J.R. Failure of Ubiquitin Proteasome System: Risk for Neurodegenerative Diseases. *Neurodegener. Dis.* **2014**, *14*, 161–175. [CrossRef]
6. Çetin, G.; Klafack, S.; Studencka-Turski, M.; Krüger, E.; Ebstein, F. The Ubiquitin–Proteasome System in Immune Cells. *Biomolecules* **2021**, *11*, 60. [CrossRef]
7. Brehm, A.; Krüger, E. Dysfunction in protein clearance by the proteasome: Impact on autoinflammatory diseases. *Semin. Immunopathol.* **2015**, *37*, 323–333. [CrossRef]
8. Haas, A.L.; Siepmann, T.J. Pathways of ubiquitin conjugation. *FASEB J.* **1997**, *11*, 1257–1268. [CrossRef]
9. Pickart, C.M.; Eddins, M.J. Ubiquitin: Structures, functions, mechanisms. *Biochim. Biophys. Acta* **2004**, *1695*, 55–72. [CrossRef] [PubMed]
10. Pickart, C.M. Mechanisms Underlying Ubiquitination. *Annu. Rev. Biochem.* **2001**, *70*, 503–533. [CrossRef] [PubMed]
11. Pickart, C.M. Back to the Future with Ubiquitin. *Cell* **2004**, *116*, 181–190. [CrossRef]
12. Berndsen, C.; Wolberger, C. New insights into ubiquitin E3 ligase mechanism. *Nat. Struct. Mol. Biol.* **2014**, *21*, 301–307. [CrossRef]
13. McDowell, G.S.; Kucerova, R.; Philpott, A. Non-canonical ubiquitylation of the proneural protein Ngn2 occurs in both Xenopus embryos and mammalian cells. *Biochem. Biophys. Res. Commun.* **2010**, *400*, 655–660. [CrossRef] [PubMed]
14. Cadwell, K. Ubiquitination on Nonlysine Residues by a Viral E3 Ubiquitin Ligase. *Science* **2005**, *309*, 127–130. [CrossRef] [PubMed]
15. Vosper, J.M.; McDowell, G.S.; Hindley, C.J.; Fiore-Heriche, C.S.; Kucerova, R.; Horan, I.; Philpott, A. Ubiquitylation on Canonical and Non-canonical Sites Targets the Transcription Factor Neurogenin for Ubiquitin-mediated Proteolysis. *J. Biol. Chem.* **2009**, *284*, 15458–15468. [CrossRef] [PubMed]
16. Mallette, F.A.; Richard, S. K48-linked ubiquitination and protein degradation regulate 53BP1 recruitment at DNA damage sites. *Cell Res.* **2012**, *22*, 1221–1223. [CrossRef]
17. Pickart, C.M.; Fushman, D. Polyubiquitin chains: Polymeric protein signals. *Curr. Opin. Chem. Biol.* **2004**, *8*, 610–616. [CrossRef] [PubMed]
18. Akutsu, M.; Dikic, I.; Bremm, A. Ubiquitin chain diversity at a glance. *J. Cell Sci.* **2016**, *129*, 875–880. [CrossRef]
19. Grice, G.L.; Nathan, J.A. The recognition of ubiquitinated proteins by the proteasome. *Cell. Mol. Life Sci.* **2016**, *73*, 3497–3506. [CrossRef]
20. Sun, L.; Chen, Z.J. The novel functions of ubiquitination in signaling. *Curr. Opin. Cell Biol.* **2004**, *16*, 119–126. [CrossRef]
21. Grumati, P.; Dikic, I. Ubiquitin signaling and autophagy. *J. Biol. Chem.* **2018**, *293*, 5404–5413. [CrossRef]
22. Eletr, Z.M.; Wilkinson, K.D. Regulation of proteolysis by human deubiquitinating enzymes. *Biochim. Biophys. Acta* **2014**, *1843*, 114–128. [CrossRef] [PubMed]
23. Nijman, S.M.; Luna-Vargas, M.P.; Velds, A.; Brummelkamp, T.R.; Dirac, A.M.; Sixma, T.K.; Bernards, R. A Genomic and Functional Inventory of Deubiquitinating Enzymes. *Cell* **2005**, *123*, 773–786. [CrossRef] [PubMed]
24. Dahlmann, B. Proteasomes. *Essays Biochem.* **2005**, *41*, 31–48. [CrossRef]
25. Tanaka, K.; Mizushima, T.; Saeki, Y. The proteasome: Molecular machinery and pathophysiological roles. *Biol. Chem.* **2012**, *393*, 217–234. [CrossRef]
26. Bard, J.A.; Goodall, E.A.; Greene, E.R.; Jonsson, E.; Dong, K.C.; Martin, A. Structure and Function of the 26S Proteasome. *Annu. Rev. Biochem.* **2018**, *87*, 697–724. [CrossRef]
27. Budenholzer, L.; Cheng, C.L.; Li, Y.; Hochstrasser, M. Proteasome Structure and Assembly. *J. Mol. Biol.* **2017**, *429*, 3500–3524. [CrossRef]
28. Orlowski, M.; Wilk, S. Catalytic Activities of the 20 S Proteasome, a Multicatalytic Proteinase Complex. *Arch. Biochem. Biophys.* **2000**, *383*, 1–16. [CrossRef]
29. Kisselev, A.F.; Songyang, Z.; Goldberg, A.L. Why Does Threonine, and Not Serine, Function as the Active Site Nucleophile in Proteasomes? *J. Biol. Chem.* **2000**, *275*, 14831–14837. [CrossRef] [PubMed]
30. Rousseau, A.; Bertolotti, A. Regulation of proteasome assembly and activity in health and disease. *Nat. Rev. Mol. Cell Biol.* **2018**, *19*, 697–712. [CrossRef] [PubMed]
31. Bedford, L.; Paine, S.; Sheppard, P.W.; Mayer, R.J.; Roelofs, J. Assembly, structure, and function of the 26S proteasome. *Trends Cell Biol.* **2010**, *20*, 391–401. [CrossRef]
32. Liu, C.-W.; Jacobson, A.D. Functions of the 19S complex in proteasomal degradation. *Trends Biochem. Sci.* **2013**, *38*, 103–110. [CrossRef] [PubMed]
33. Deveraux, Q.; van Nocker, S.; Mahaffey, D.; Vierstra, R.; Rechsteiner, M. Inhibition of Ubiquitin-mediated Proteolysis by the Arabidopsis 26 S Protease Subunit S5a. *J. Biol. Chem.* **1995**, *270*, 29660–29663. [CrossRef] [PubMed]
34. Husnjak, K.; Elsasser, S.; Zhang, N.; Chen, X.; Randles, L.; Shi, Y.; Hofmann, K.; Walters, K.J.; Finley, D.; Dikic, I. Proteasome subunit Rpn13 is a novel ubiquitin receptor. *Nat. Cell Biol.* **2008**, *453*, 481–488. [CrossRef]
35. Smith, D.M.; Chang, S.-C.; Park, S.; Finley, D.; Cheng, Y.; Goldberg, A.L. Docking of the Proteasomal ATPases' Carboxyl Termini in the 20S Proteasome's α Ring Opens the Gate for Substrate Entry. *Mol. Cell* **2007**, *27*, 731–744. [CrossRef]
36. Finley, D. Recognition and Processing of Ubiquitin-Protein Conjugates by the Proteasome. *Annu. Rev. Biochem.* **2009**, *78*, 477–513. [CrossRef]
37. Shin, J.Y.; Muniyappan, S.; Tran, N.-N.; Park, H.; Lee, S.B.; Lee, B.-H. Deubiquitination Reactions on the Proteasome for Proteasome Versatility. *Int. J. Mol. Sci.* **2020**, *21*, 5312. [CrossRef] [PubMed]

38. Dahlmann, B. Mammalian proteasome subtypes: Their diversity in structure and function. *Arch. Biochem. Biophys.* **2016**, *591*, 132–140. [CrossRef] [PubMed]
39. Kloetzel, P.-M. The proteasome and MHC class I antigen processing. *Biochim. Biophys. Acta* **2004**, *1695*, 225–233. [CrossRef]
40. Seyffer, F.; Tampé, R. ABC transporters in adaptive immunity. *Biochim. Biophys. Acta Gen. Subj.* **2015**, *1850*, 449–460. [CrossRef] [PubMed]
41. Townsend, A.; Trowsdale, J. The transporters associated with antigen presentation. *Semin. Cell Biol.* **1993**, *4*, 53–61. [CrossRef] [PubMed]
42. Tanaka, K. Role of proteasomes modified by interferon-γ in antigen processing. *J. Leukoc. Biol.* **1994**, *56*, 571–575. [CrossRef]
43. Ebstein, F.; Kloetzel, P.-M.; Krüger, E.; Seifert, U.; Krueger, E. Emerging roles of immunoproteasomes beyond MHC class I antigen processing. *Cell. Mol. Life Sci.* **2012**, *69*, 2543–2558. [CrossRef]
44. Strehl, B.; Seifert, U.; Kruger, E.; Heink, S.; Kuckelkorn, U.; Kloetzel, P.-M.; Krueger, E. Interferon-gamma, the functional plasticity of the ubiquitin-proteasome system, and MHC class I antigen processing. *Immunol. Rev.* **2005**, *207*, 19–30. [CrossRef]
45. Aki, M.; Shimbara, N.; Takashina, M.; Akiyama, K.; Kagawa, S.; Tamura, T.; Tanahashi, N.; Yoshimura, T.; Tanaka, K.; Ichihara, A. Interferon-Gamma Induces Different Subunit Organizations and Functional Diversity of Proteasomes. *J. Biochem.* **1994**, *115*, 257–269. [CrossRef]
46. Seifert, U.; Bialy, L.P.; Ebstein, F.; Bech-Otschir, D.; Voigt, A.; Schröter, F.; Prozorovski, T.; Lange, N.; Steffen, J.; Rieger, M.; et al. Immunoproteasomes Preserve Protein Homeostasis upon Interferon-Induced Oxidative Stress. *Cell* **2010**, *142*, 613–624. [CrossRef] [PubMed]
47. Yun, Y.S.; Kim, K.H.; Tschida, B.; Sachs, Z.; Noble-Orcutt, K.E.; Moriarity, B.S.; Ai, T.; Ding, R.; Williams, J.; Chen, L.; et al. mTORC1 Coordinates Protein Synthesis and Immunoproteasome Formation via PRAS40 to Prevent Accumulation of Protein Stress. *Mol. Cell* **2016**, *61*, 625–639. [CrossRef] [PubMed]
48. Niewerth, D.; Kaspers, G.J.; Assaraf, Y.G.; Van Meerloo, J.; Kirk, C.J.; Anderl, J.; Blank, J.L.; Van De Ven, P.M.; Zweegman, S.; Jansen, G.; et al. Interferon-γ-induced upregulation of immunoproteasome subunit assembly overcomes bortezomib resistance in human hematological cell lines. *J. Hematol. Oncol.* **2014**, *7*, 7. [CrossRef] [PubMed]
49. Opitz, E.; Koch, A.; Klingel, K.; Schmidt, F.; Prokop, S.; Rahnefeld, A.; Sauter, M.; Heppner, F.L.; Völker, U.; Kandolf, R.; et al. Impairment of Immunoproteasome Function by β5i/LMP7 Subunit Deficiency Results in Severe Enterovirus Myocarditis. *PLoS Pathog.* **2011**, *7*, e1002233. [CrossRef] [PubMed]
50. Krüger, E.; Kloetzel, P.-M. Immunoproteasomes at the interface of innate and adaptive immune responses: Two faces of one enzyme. *Curr. Opin. Immunol.* **2012**, *24*, 77–83. [CrossRef] [PubMed]
51. Mishto, M.; Liepe, J.; Textoris-Taube, K.; Keller, C.; Henklein, P.; Weberruß, M.; Dahlmann, B.; Enenkel, C.; Voigt, A.; Kuckelkorn, U.; et al. Proteasome isoforms exhibit only quantitative differences in cleavage and epitope generation. *Eur. J. Immunol.* **2014**, *44*, 3508–3521. [CrossRef]
52. Murata, S.; Sasaki, K.; Kishimoto, T.; Niwa, S.-I.; Hayashi, H.; Takahama, Y.; Tanaka, K. Regulation of CD8+ T Cell Development by Thymus-Specific Proteasomes. *Science* **2007**, *316*, 1349–1353. [CrossRef]
53. Murata, S.; Takahama, Y.; Kasahara, M.; Tanaka, K. The immunoproteasome and thymoproteasome: Functions, evolution and human disease. *Nat. Immunol.* **2018**, *19*, 923–931. [CrossRef]
54. Kniepert, A.; Groettrup, M. The unique functions of tissue-specific proteasomes. *Trends Biochem. Sci.* **2014**, *39*, 17–24. [CrossRef]
55. Iwai, K.; Fujita, H.; Sasaki, Y. Linear ubiquitin chains: NF-κB signalling, cell death and beyond. *Nat. Rev. Mol. Cell Biol.* **2014**, *15*, 503–508. [CrossRef]
56. Alkalay, I.; Yaron, A.; Hatzubai, A.; Orian, A.; Ciechanover, A.; Ben-Neriah, Y. Stimulation-dependent I kappa B alpha phosphorylation marks the NF-kappa B inhibitor for degradation via the ubiquitin-proteasome pathway. *Proc. Natl. Acad. Sci. USA* **1995**, *92*, 10599–10603. [CrossRef]
57. Fiil, B.K.; Gyrd-Hansen, M. OTULIN deficiency causes auto-inflammatory syndrome. *Cell Res.* **2016**, *26*, 1176–1177. [CrossRef] [PubMed]
58. Wertz, I.E.; O'Rourke, K.M.; Zhou, H.; Eby, M.; Aravind, L.; Seshagiri, S.; Wu, P.; Wiesmann, C.; Baker, R.T.; Boone, D.L.; et al. De-ubiquitination and ubiquitin ligase domains of A20 downregulate NF-κB signalling. *Nat. Cell Biol.* **2004**, *430*, 694–699. [CrossRef] [PubMed]
59. Althof, N.; Goetzke, C.C.; Kespohl, M.; Voss, K.; Heuser, A.; Pinkert, S.; Kaya, Z.; Klingel, K.; Beling, A. The immunoproteasome-specific inhibitor ONX 0914 reverses susceptibility to acute viral myocarditis. *EMBO Mol. Med.* **2018**, *10*, 200–218. [CrossRef] [PubMed]
60. Bockstahler, M.; Fischer, A.; Goetzke, C.C.; Neumaier, H.L.; Sauter, M.; Kespohl, M.; Müller, A.-M.; Meckes, C.; Salbach, C.; Schenk, M.; et al. Heart-Specific Immune Responses in an Animal Model of Autoimmune-Related Myocarditis Mitigated by an Immunoproteasome Inhibitor and Genetic Ablation. *Circulation* **2020**, *141*, 1885–1902. [CrossRef]
61. Schmidt, C.; Berger, T.; Groettrup, M.; Basler, M. Immunoproteasome Inhibition Impairs T and B Cell Activation by Restraining ERK Signaling and Proteostasis. *Front. Immunol.* **2018**, *9*, 2386. [CrossRef]
62. Kalim, K.W.; Basler, M.; Kirk, C.J.; Groettrup, M. Immunoproteasome Subunit LMP7 Deficiency and Inhibition Suppresses Th1 and Th17 but Enhances Regulatory T Cell Differentiation. *J. Immunol.* **2012**, *189*, 4182–4193. [CrossRef]
63. Goetzke, C.C.; Althof, N.; Neumaier, H.L.; Heuser, A.; Kaya, Z.; Kespohl, M.; Klingel, K.; Beling, A. Mitigated viral myocarditis in A/J mice by the immunoproteasome inhibitor ONX 0914 depends on inhibition of systemic inflammatory responses in CoxsackievirusB3 infection. *Basic Res. Cardiol.* **2021**, *116*, 1–16. [CrossRef] [PubMed]
64. Alexander, T.; Sarfert, R.; Klotsche, J.; Kühl, A.; Rubbert-Roth, A.; Lorenz, H.-M.; Rech, J.; Hoyer, B.F.; Cheng, Q.; Waka, A.; et al. The proteasome inhibitior bortezomib depletes plasma cells and ameliorates clinical manifestations of refractory systemic lupus erythematosus. *Ann. Rheum. Dis.* **2015**, *74*, 1474–1478. [CrossRef]

65. Richardson, P.G.; Barlogie, B.; Berenson, J.; Singhal, S.; Jagannath, S.; Irwin, D.; Rajkumar, S.V.; Srkalovic, G.; Alsina, M.; Alexanian, R.; et al. A Phase 2 Study of Bortezomib in Relapsed, Refractory Myeloma. *N. Engl. J. Med.* **2003**, *348*, 2609–2617. [CrossRef] [PubMed]
66. Li, J.; Koerner, J.; Basler, M.; Brunner, T.; Kirk, C.J.; Groettrup, M. Immunoproteasome inhibition induces plasma cell apoptosis and preserves kidney allografts by activating the unfolded protein response and suppressing plasma cell survival factors. *Kidney Int.* **2019**, *95*, 611–623. [CrossRef]
67. Ebstein, F.; Harlowe, M.C.P.; Studencka-Turski, M.; Krüger, E. Contribution of the Unfolded Protein Response (UPR) to the Pathogenesis of Proteasome-Associated Autoinflammatory Syndromes (PRAAS). *Front. Immunol.* **2019**, *10*, 2756. [CrossRef] [PubMed]
68. Agarwal, A.K.; Xing, C.; DeMartino, G.N.; Mizrachi, D.; Hernandez, M.D.; Sousa, A.B.; De Villarreal, L.M.; Dos Santos, H.G.; Garg, A. PSMB8 Encoding the β5i Proteasome Subunit Is Mutated in Joint Contractures, Muscle Atrophy, Microcytic Anemia, and Panniculitis-Induced Lipodystrophy Syndrome. *Am. J. Hum. Genet.* **2010**, *87*, 866–872. [CrossRef] [PubMed]
69. Arima, K.; Kinoshita, A.; Mishima, H.; Kanazawa, N.; Kaneko, T.; Mizushima, T.; Ichinose, K.; Nakamura, H.; Tsujino, A.; Kawakami, A.; et al. Proteasome assembly defect due to a proteasome subunit beta type 8 (PSMB8) mutation causes the autoinflammatory disorder, Nakajo-Nishimura syndrome. *Proc. Natl. Acad. Sci. USA* **2011**, *108*, 14914–14919. [CrossRef]
70. Kitamura, A.; Maekawa, Y.; Uehara, H.; Izumi, K.; Kawachi, I.; Nishizawa, M.; Toyoshima, Y.; Takahashi, H.; Standley, D.M.; Tanaka, K.; et al. A mutation in the immunoproteasome subunit PSMB8 causes autoinflammation and lipodystrophy in humans. *J. Clin. Investig.* **2011**, *121*, 4150–4160. [CrossRef] [PubMed]
71. Liu, Y.; Ramot, Y.; Torrelo, A.; Paller, A.S.; Si, N.; Babay, S.; Kim, P.W.; Sheikh, A.; Lee, C.-C.R.; Chen, Y.; et al. Mutations in proteasome subunit β type 8 cause chronic atypical neutrophilic dermatosis with lipodystrophy and elevated temperature with evidence of genetic and phenotypic heterogeneity. *Arthritis Rheum.* **2011**, *64*, 895–907. [CrossRef]
72. McDermott, A.; Jacks, J.; Kessler, M.; Emanuel, P.D.; Gao, L. Proteasome-associated autoinflammatory syndromes: Advances in pathogeneses, clinical presentations, diagnosis, and management. *Int. J. Dermatol.* **2014**, *54*, 121–129. [CrossRef] [PubMed]
73. McDermott, A.; Jesus, A.A.; Liu, Y.; Kim, P.; Jacks, J.; Sanchez, G.A.M.; Chen, Y.; Kannan, A.; Schnebelen, A.; Emanuel, P.D.; et al. A case of proteasome-associated auto-inflammatory syndrome with compound heterozygous mutations. *J. Am. Acad. Dermatol.* **2013**, *69*, e29–e32. [CrossRef] [PubMed]
74. Torrelo, A.; Patel, S.; Colmenero, I.; Gurbindo, D.; Lendínez, F.; Hernández, A.; López-Robledillo, J.C.; Dadban, A.; Requena, L.; Paller, A.S. Chronic atypical neutrophilic dermatosis with lipodystrophy and elevated temperature (CANDLE) syndrome. *J. Am. Acad. Dermatol.* **2010**, *62*, 489–495. [CrossRef]
75. Feist, E.; Brehm, A.; Kallinich, T.; Krüger, E. Klinik und Genetik bei Proteasomen-assoziierten autoinflammatorischen Syndromen (PRAAS) Clinical aspects and genetics of proteasome-associated autoinflammatory syndromes (PRAAS). *Z. Rheumatol.* **2017**, *76*, 328–334. [CrossRef]
76. Brehm, A.; Liu, Y.; Sheikh, A.; Marrero, B.; Omoyinmi, E.; Zhou, Q.; Montealegre, G.; Biancotto, A.; Reinhardt, A.; De Jesus, A.A.; et al. Additive loss-of-function proteasome subunit mutations in CANDLE/PRAAS patients promote type I IFN production. *J. Clin. Investig.* **2015**, *125*, 4196–4211. [CrossRef] [PubMed]
77. Goldbach-Mansky, R. Immunology in clinic review series; focus on autoinflammatory diseases: Update on monogenic autoinflammatory diseases: The role of interleukin (IL)-1 and an emerging role for cytokines beyond IL-1. *Clin. Exp. Immunol.* **2012**, *167*, 391–404. [CrossRef]
78. Rice, G.I.; Melki, I.; Frémond, M.-L.; Briggs, T.A.; Rodero, M.P.; Kitabayashi, N.; Oojageer, A.; Bader-Meunier, B.; Belot, A.; Bodemer, C.; et al. Assessment of Type I Interferon Signaling in Pediatric Inflammatory Disease. *J. Clin. Immunol.* **2017**, *37*, 123–132. [CrossRef]
79. Kim, H.; De Jesus, A.A.; Brooks, S.R.; Liu, Y.; Huang, Y.; VanTries, R.; Sanchez, G.A.M.; Rotman, Y.; Gadina, M.; Goldbach-Mansky, R. Development of a Validated Interferon Score Using NanoString Technology. *J. Interf. Cytokine Res.* **2018**, *38*, 171–185. [CrossRef]
80. Orak, B.; Ngoumou, G.; Ebstein, F.; Zieba, B.; Goetzke, C.C.; Knierim, E.; Kaindl, A.M.; Panzer, A.; Theophil, M.; Berns, M.; et al. SIGLEC1 (CD169) as a potential diagnostical screening marker for monogenic interferonopathies. *Pediatr. Allergy Immunol.* **2021**, *32*, 621–625. [CrossRef]
81. Poli, M.C.; Ebstein, F.; Nicholas, S.K.; De Guzman, M.M.; Forbes, L.R.; Chinn, I.K.; Mace, E.M.; Vogel, T.P.; Carisey, A.F.; Benavides, F.; et al. Heterozygous Truncating Variants in POMP Escape Nonsense-Mediated Decay and Cause a Unique Immune Dysregulatory Syndrome. *Am. J. Hum. Genet.* **2018**, *102*, 1126–1142. [CrossRef]
82. De Jesus, A.A.; Brehm, A.; VanTries, R.; Pillet, P.; Parentelli, A.-S.; Sanchez, G.A.M.; Deng, Z.; Paut, I.K.; Goldbach-Mansky, R.; Krüger, E. Novel proteasome assembly chaperone mutations in PSMG2/PAC2 cause the autoinflammatory interferonopathy CANDLE/PRAAS4. *J. Allergy Clin. Immunol.* **2019**, *143*, 1939–1943.e8. [CrossRef] [PubMed]
83. Sarrabay, G.; Méchin, D.; Salhi, A.; Boursier, G.; Rittore, C.; Crow, Y.; Rice, G.; Tran, T.-A.; Cezar, R.; Duffy, D.; et al. PSMB10, the last immunoproteasome gene missing for PRAAS. *J. Allergy Clin. Immunol.* **2020**, *145*, 1015–1017.e6. [CrossRef]
84. Ansar, M.; Ebstein, F.; Özkoç, H.; Paracha, S.; Iwaszkiewicz, J.; Gesemann, M.; Zoete, V.; Ranza, E.; Santoni, F.; Sarwar, M.T.; et al. Biallelic variants in PSMB1 encoding the proteasome subunit β6 cause impairment of proteasome function, microcephaly, intellectual disability, developmental delay and short stature. *Hum. Mol. Genet.* **2020**, *29*, 1132–1143. [CrossRef] [PubMed]

85. Küry, S.; Besnard, T.; Ebstein, F.; Khan, T.N.; Gambin, T.; Douglas, J.; Bacino, C.A.; Sanders, S.J.; Lehmann, A.; Latypova, X.; et al. De Novo Disruption of the Proteasome Regulatory Subunit PSMD12 Causes a Syndromic Neurodevelopmental Disorder. *Am. J. Hum. Genet.* **2017**, *100*, 352–363. [CrossRef] [PubMed]
86. Kröll-Hermi, A.; Ebstein, F.; Stoetzel, C.; Geoffroy, V.; Schaefer, E.; Scheidecker, S.; Bär, S.; Takamiya, M.; Kawakami, K.; Zieba, B.; et al. Proteasome subunit PSMC3 variants cause neurosensory syndrome combining deafness and cataract due to proteotoxic stress. *EMBO Mol. Med.* **2020**, *12*, 11861. [CrossRef]
87. Nikesitch, N.; Tao, C.; Lai, K.; Killingsworth, M.; Bae, S.; Wang, M.; Harrison, S.; Roberts, T.L.; Ling, S.C.W. Predicting the response of multiple myeloma to the proteasome inhibitor Bortezomib by evaluation of the unfolded protein response. *Blood Cancer J.* **2016**, *6*, e432. [CrossRef]
88. Obeng, E.A.; Carlson, L.M.; Gutman, D.M.; Harrington, W.J., Jr.; Lee, K.P.; Boise, L.H. Proteasome inhibitors induce a terminal unfolded protein response in multiple myeloma cells. *Blood* **2006**, *107*, 4907–4916. [CrossRef]
89. Hetz, C.; Zhang, K.; Kaufman, R.J. Mechanisms, regulation and functions of the unfolded protein response. *Nat. Rev. Mol. Cell Biol.* **2020**, *21*, 421–438. [CrossRef]
90. Janssens, S.; Pulendran, B.; Lambrecht, B.N. Emerging functions of the unfolded protein response in immunity. *Nat. Immunol.* **2014**, *15*, 910–919. [CrossRef]
91. Studencka-Turski, M.; Çetin, G.; Junker, H.; Ebstein, F.; Krüger, E. Molecular Insight into the IRE1α-Mediated Type I Interferon Response Induced by Proteasome Impairment in Myeloid Cells of the Brain. *Front. Immunol.* **2019**, *10*, 2900. [CrossRef] [PubMed]
92. Mazor, K.M.; Stipanuk, M.H. GCN2- and eIF2α-phosphorylation-independent, but ATF4-dependent, induction of CARE-containing genes in methionine-deficient cells. *Amino Acids* **2016**, *48*, 2831–2842. [CrossRef] [PubMed]
93. Ye, J.; Palm, W.; Peng, M.; King, B.; Lindsten, T.; Li, M.O.; Koumenis, C.; Thompson, C.B. GCN2 sustains mTORC1 suppression upon amino acid deprivation by inducing Sestrin2. *Genes Dev.* **2015**, *29*, 2331–2336. [CrossRef] [PubMed]
94. Ohoka, N.; Yoshii, S.; Hattori, T.; Onozaki, K.; Hayashi, H. TRB3, a novel ER stress-inducible gene, is induced via ATF4–CHOP pathway and is involved in cell death. *EMBO J.* **2005**, *24*, 1243–1255. [CrossRef] [PubMed]
95. Kimball, S.R.; Jefferson, L.S. Induction of REDD1 gene expression in the liver in response to endoplasmic reticulum stress is mediated through a PERK, eIF2α phosphorylation, ATF4-dependent cascade. *Biochem. Biophys. Res. Commun.* **2012**, *427*, 485–489. [CrossRef]
96. York, A.G.; Williams, K.J.; Argus, J.P.; Zhou, Q.D.; Brar, G.; Vergnes, L.; Gray, E.E.; Zhen, A.; Wu, N.C.; Yamada, D.H.; et al. Limiting Cholesterol Biosynthetic Flux Spontaneously Engages Type I IFN Signaling. *Cell* **2015**, *163*, 1716–1729. [CrossRef] [PubMed]
97. Sanchez, G.A.M.; Reinhardt, A.; Ramsey, S.; Wittkowski, H.; Hashkes, P.J.; Berkun, Y.; Schalm, S.; Murias, S.; Dare, J.A.; Brown, D.; et al. JAK1/2 inhibition with baricitinib in the treatment of autoinflammatory interferonopathies. *J. Clin. Investig.* **2018**, *128*, 3041–3052. [CrossRef]
98. Patel, P.N.; Hunt, R.; Pettigrew, Z.J.; Shirley, J.B.; Vogel, T.P.; de Guzman, M.M. Successful treatment of chronic atypical neutrophilic dermatosis with lipodystrophy and elevated temperature (CANDLE) syndrome with tofacitinib. *Pediatr. Dermatol.* **2021**. [CrossRef] [PubMed]
99. Steiner, A.; Harapas, C.R.; Masters, S.L.; Davidson, S. An Update on Autoinflammatory Diseases: Relopathies. *Curr. Rheumatol. Rep.* **2018**, *20*, 39. [CrossRef]
100. Kallinich, T.; Hinze, C.; Wittkowski, H. Klassifikation autoinflammatorischer Erkrankungen anhand pathophysiologischer Mechanismen. *Z. Rheumatol.* **2020**, *79*, 624–638. [CrossRef]
101. Boisson, B.; Laplantine, E.; Prando, C.; Giliani, S.; Israelsson, E.; Xu, Z.; Abhyankar, A.; Israël, L.; Trevejo-Nunez, G.; Bogunovic, D.; et al. Immunodeficiency, autoinflammation and amylopectinosis in humans with inherited HOIL-1 and LUBAC deficiency. *Nat. Immunol.* **2012**, *13*, 1178–1186. [CrossRef] [PubMed]
102. Boisson, B.; Laplantine, E.; Dobbs, K.; Cobat, A.; Tarantino, N.; Hazen, M.; Lidov, H.G.; Hopkins, G.W.; Du, L.; Belkadi, A.; et al. Human HOIP and LUBAC deficiency underlies autoinflammation, immunodeficiency, amylopectinosis, and lymphangiectasia. *J. Exp. Med.* **2015**, *212*, 939–951. [CrossRef] [PubMed]
103. Zhou, Q.; Yu, X.; Demirkaya, E.; Deuitch, N.; Stone, D.; Tsai, W.L.; Kuehn, H.S.; Wang, H.; Yang, D.; Park, Y.H.; et al. Biallelic hypomorphic mutations in a linear deubiquitinase define otulipenia, an early-onset autoinflammatory disease. *Proc. Natl. Acad. Sci. USA* **2016**, *113*, 10127–10132. [CrossRef] [PubMed]
104. Zhou, Q.; Wang, H.; Schwartz, D.M.; Stoffels, M.; Park, Y.H.; Zhang, Y.; Yang, D.; Demirkaya, E.; Takeuchi, M.; Tsai, W.L.; et al. Loss-of-function mutations in TNFAIP3 leading to A20 haploinsufficiency cause an early-onset autoinflammatory disease. *Nat. Genet.* **2016**, *48*, 67–73. [CrossRef]
105. Takagi, M.; Ogata, S.; Ueno, H.; Yoshida, K.; Yeh, T.; Hoshino, A.; Piao, J.; Yamashita, M.; Nanya, M.; Okano, T.; et al. Haploinsufficiency of TNFAIP3 (A20) by germline mutation is involved in autoimmune lymphoproliferative syndrome. *J. Allergy Clin. Immunol.* **2017**, *139*, 1914–1922. [CrossRef]
106. Meuwissen, M.E.; Schot, R.; Buta, S.; Oudesluijs, G.; Tinschert, S.; Speer, S.D.; Li, Z.; Van Unen, L.; Heijsman, D.; Goldmann, T.; et al. Human USP18 deficiency underlies type 1 interferonopathy leading to severe pseudo-TORCH syndrome. *J. Exp. Med.* **2016**, *213*, 1163–1174. [CrossRef] [PubMed]
107. Basters, A.; Knobeloch, K.-P.; Fritz, G. USP18—A multifunctional component in the interferon response. *Biosci. Rep.* **2018**, *38*. [CrossRef]

108. Gruber, C.; Martin-Fernandez, M.; Ailal, F.; Qiu, X.; Taft, J.; Altman, J.; Rosain, J.; Buta, S.; Bousfiha, A.; Casanova, J.-L.; et al. Homozygous STAT2 gain-of-function mutation by loss of USP18 activity in a patient with type I interferonopathy. *J. Exp. Med.* **2020**, *217*. [CrossRef]
109. Alsohime, F.; Martin-Fernandez, M.; Temsah, M.-H.; Alabdulhafid, M.; Le Voyer, T.; Alghamdi, M.; Qiu, X.; Alotaibi, N.; Alkahtani, A.; Buta, S.; et al. JAK Inhibitor Therapy in a Child with Inherited USP18 Deficiency. *N. Engl. J. Med.* **2020**, *382*, 256–265. [CrossRef]
110. Beck, D.B.; Ferrada, M.A.; Sikora, K.A.; Ombrello, A.K.; Collins, J.C.; Pei, W.; Balanda, N.; Ross, D.L.; Cardona, D.O.; Wu, Z.; et al. Somatic Mutations in UBA1 and Severe Adult-Onset Autoinflammatory Disease. *N. Engl. J. Med.* **2020**, *383*, 2628–2638. [CrossRef]
111. Poulter, J.; Collins, J.C.; Cargo, C.; de Tute, R.M.; Evans, P.; Cardona, D.O.; Bowen, D.T.; Cunnington, J.R.; Baguley, E.; Quinn, M.; et al. Novel somatic mutations in UBA1 as a cause of VEXAS syndrome. *Blood* **2021**. [CrossRef] [PubMed]
112. Egerer, T.; Martínez-Gamboa, L.; Dankof, A.; Stuhlmüller, B.; Dorner, T.; Krenn, V.; Egerer, K.; Rudolph, P.E.; Burmester, G.-R.; Feist, E. Tissue-specific up-regulation of the proteasome subunit β5i (LMP7) in Sjögren's syndrome. *Arthritis Rheum.* **2006**, *54*, 1501–1508. [CrossRef]
113. Krause, S.; Kuckelkorn, U.; Dörner, T.; Burmester, G.-R.; Feist, E.; Kloetzel, P.-M. Immunoproteasome subunit LMP2 expression is deregulated in Sjogren's syndrome but not in other autoimmune disorders. *Ann. Rheum. Dis.* **2006**, *65*, 1021–1027. [CrossRef]
114. Feist, E.; Dörner, T.; Kuckelkorn, U.; Schmidtke, G.; Micheel, B.; Hiepe, F.; Burmester, G.R.; Kloetzel, P.M. Proteasome alpha-type subunit C9 is a primary target of autoantibodies in sera of patients with myositis and systemic lupus erythematosus. *J. Exp. Med.* **1996**, *184*, 1313–1318. [CrossRef]
115. Feist, E.; Kuckelkorn, U.; Dörner, T.; Dönitz, H.; Scheffler, S.; Hiepe, F.; Kloetzel, P.M.; Burmester, G.R. Autoantibodies in primary Sjögren's syndrome are directed against proteasomal subunits of the alpha and beta type. *Arthritis Rheum.* **1999**, *42*, 697–702. [CrossRef]
116. Mayo, I.; Arribas, J.; Villoslada, P.; Doforno, R.A.; Rodríguez-Vilariño, S.; Montalban, X.; de Sagarra, M.R.; Castaño, J.G. The proteasome is a major autoantigen in multiple sclerosis. *Brain* **2002**, *125*, 2658–2667. [CrossRef] [PubMed]
117. Brychcy, M.; Kuckelkorn, U.; Hausdorf, G.; Egerer, K.; Kloetzel, P.-M.; Burmester, G.-R.; Feist, E. Anti-20S proteasome autoantibodies inhibit proteasome stimulation by proteasome activator PA28. *Arthritis Rheum.* **2006**, *54*, 2175–2183. [CrossRef] [PubMed]
118. Egerer, K.; Kuckelkorn, U.; Rudolph, P.; Rückert, J.C.; Dörner, T.; Burmester, G.-R.; Kloetzel, P.-M.; Feist, E. Circulating proteasomes are markers of cell damage and immunologic activity in autoimmune diseases. *J. Rheumatol.* **2002**, *29*, 2045–2052.
119. Maruyama, H.; Hirayama, K.; Yamashita, M.; Ohgi, K.; Tsujimoto, R.; Takayasu, M.; Shimohata, H.; Kobayashi, M. Serum 20S proteasome levels are associated with disease activity in MPO-ANCA-associated microscopic polyangiitis. *BMC Rheumatol.* **2020**, *4*, 1–7. [CrossRef]
120. Muchamuel, T.; Basler, M.; Aujay, M.A.; Suzuki, E.; Kalim, K.W.; Lauer, C.; Sylvain, C.; Ring, E.R.; Shields, J.; Jiang, J.; et al. A selective inhibitor of the immunoproteasome subunit LMP7 blocks cytokine production and attenuates progression of experimental arthritis. *Nat. Med.* **2009**, *15*, 781–787. [CrossRef]
121. Basler, M.; Dajee, M.; Moll, C.; Groettrup, M.; Kirk, C.J. Prevention of Experimental Colitis by a Selective Inhibitor of the Immunoproteasome. *J. Immunol.* **2010**, *185*, 634–641. [CrossRef]
122. Schmidt, N.; Gonzalez, E.; Visekruna, A.; Kühl, A.; Loddenkemper, C.; Mollenkopf, H.; Kaufmann, S.H.; Steinhoff, U.; Joeris, T. Targeting the proteasome: Partial inhibition of the proteasome by bortezomib or deletion of the immunosubunit LMP7 attenuates experimental colitis. *Gut* **2010**, *59*, 896–906. [CrossRef] [PubMed]
123. Mundt, S.; Engelhardt, B.; Kirk, C.J.; Groettrup, M.; Basler, M. Inhibition and deficiency of the immunoproteasome subunit LMP7 attenuates LCMV-induced meningitis. *Eur. J. Immunol.* **2015**, *46*, 104–113. [CrossRef]
124. Basler, M.; Claus, M.; Klawitter, M.; Goebel, H.; Groettrup, M. Immunoproteasome Inhibition Selectively Kills Human CD14+ Monocytes and as a Result Dampens IL-23 Secretion. *J. Immunol.* **2019**, *203*, 1776–1785. [CrossRef] [PubMed]
125. Basler, M.; Mundt, S.; Muchamuel, T.; Moll, C.; Jiang, J.; Groettrup, M.; Kirk, C.J. Inhibition of the immunoproteasome ameliorates experimental autoimmune encephalomyelitis. *EMBO Mol. Med.* **2014**, *6*, 226–238. [CrossRef]
126. Feist, E.; Burmester, G.-R.; Krüger, E. The proteasome—Victim or culprit in autoimmunity. *Clin. Immunol.* **2016**, *172*, 83–89. [CrossRef] [PubMed]
127. Neubert, K.; Meister, S.; Moser, K.; Weisel, F.; Maseda, D.; Amann, K.; Wiethe, C.; Winkler, T.H.; Kalden, J.R.; Manz, R.; et al. The proteasome inhibitor bortezomib depletes plasma cells and protects mice with lupus-like disease from nephritis. *Nat. Med.* **2008**, *14*, 748–755. [CrossRef]
128. McInnes, I.B.; Schett, G. The Pathogenesis of Rheumatoid Arthritis. *N. Engl. J. Med.* **2011**, *365*, 2205–2219. [CrossRef] [PubMed]
129. Ilchovska, D.; Barrow, M. An Overview of the NF-kB mechanism of pathophysiology in rheumatoid arthritis, investigation of the NF-kB ligand RANKL and related nutritional interventions. *Autoimmun. Rev.* **2021**, *20*, 102741. [CrossRef] [PubMed]
130. van der Heijden, J.W.; Oerlemans, R.; Lems, W.F.; Scheper, R.J.; Dijkmans, B.A.; Jansen, G. The proteasome inhibitor bortezomib inhibits the release of NFkappaB-inducible cytokines and induces apoptosis of activated T cells from rheumatoid arthritis patients. *Clin. Exp. Rheumatol.* **2009**, *27*, 92–98.
131. Migita, K.; Tanaka, F.; Yamasaki, S.; Shibatomi, K.; Ida, H.; Kawakami, A.; Aoyagi, T.; Kawabe, Y.; Eguchi, K. Regulation of rheumatoid synoviocyte proliferation by endogenous p53 induction. *Clin. Exp. Immunol.* **2001**, *126*, 334–338. [CrossRef] [PubMed]
132. Dörner, T.; Furie, R. Novel paradigms in systemic lupus erythematosus. *Lancet* **2019**, *393*, 2344–2358. [CrossRef]

133. Ichikawa, H.T.; Conley, T.; Muchamuel, T.; Jiang, J.; Lee, S.; Owen, T.; Barnard, J.; Nevarez, S.; Goldman, B.I.; Kirk, C.J.; et al. Beneficial effect of novel proteasome inhibitors in murine lupus via dual inhibition of type I interferon and autoantibody-secreting cells. *Arthritis Rheum.* **2012**, *64*, 493–503. [CrossRef] [PubMed]
134. Rose, T.; Grützkau, A.; Hirseland, H.; Huscher, D.; Dähnrich, C.; Dzionek, A.; Ozimkowski, T.; Schlumberger, W.; Enghard, P.; Radbruch, A.; et al. IFNα and its response proteins, IP-10 and SIGLEC-1, are biomarkers of disease activity in systemic lupus erythematosus. *Ann. Rheum. Dis.* **2012**, *72*, 1639–1645. [CrossRef]
135. Yao, L.; Zhou, L.; Xuan, Y.; Zhang, P.; Wang, X.; Wang, T.; Meng, T.; Xue, Y.; Ma, X.; Shah, A.S.; et al. The proteasome activator REGγ counteracts immunoproteasome expression and autoimmunity. *J. Autoimmun.* **2019**, *103*, 102282. [CrossRef] [PubMed]
136. Gruner, M.; Moncsek, A.; Rödiger, S.; Kühnhardt, D.; Feist, E.; Stohwasser, R. Increased proteasome activator 28 gamma (PA28γ) levels are unspecific but correlate with disease activity in rheumatoid arthritis. *BMC Musculoskelet. Disord.* **2014**, *15*, 1–10. [CrossRef]
137. Witte, T. Sjögren-Syndrom. *Z. Rheumatol.* **2019**, *78*, 511–517. [CrossRef]
138. Feist, E.; Dörner, T.; Kuckelkorn, U.; Scheffler, S.; Burmester, G.-R.; Kloetzel, P.-M. Diagnostic importance of anti-proteasome antibodies. *Int. Arch. Allergy Immunol.* **2000**, *123*, 92–97. [CrossRef]
139. Morawietz, L.; Martinez-Gamboa, L.; Scheffler, S.; Hausdorf, G.; Dankof, A.; Kuckelkorn, U.; Doerner, T.; Egerer, K.; Burmester, G.-R.; Faustman, D.L.; et al. Expression of Proteasomal Immunosubunit ß1i Is Dysregulated in Inflammatory Infiltrates of Minor Salivary Glands in Sjögren's Syndrome. *J. Rheumatol.* **2009**, *36*, 2694–2703. [CrossRef]
140. Martinez-Gamboa, L.; Lesemann, K.; Kuckelkorn, U.; Scheffler, S.; Ghannam, K.; Hahne, M.; Gaber-Elsner, T.; Egerer, K.; Naumann, L.; Buttgereit, F.; et al. Gene Expression of Catalytic Proteasome Subunits and Resistance Toward Proteasome Inhibition of B Lymphocytes from Patients with Primary Sjögren Syndrome. *J. Rheumatol.* **2013**, *40*, 663–673. [CrossRef]
141. Xiaohui, W.; Lingyun, S.; Tian, J.; Wang, X.; Chen, Q.; Rui, K.; Ma, J.; Wang, S.; Wang, Q.; Wang, X.; et al. Proteasome inhibition suppresses Th17 cell generation and ameliorates autoimmune development in experimental Sjögren's syndrome. *Cell. Mol. Immunol.* **2017**, *14*, 924–934. [CrossRef] [PubMed]
142. Nitta, T.; Kochi, Y.; Muro, R.; Tomofuji, Y.; Okamura, T.; Murata, S.; Suzuki, H.; Sumida, T.; Yamamoto, K.; Takayanagi, H. Human thymoproteasome variations influence CD8 T cell selection. *Sci. Immunol.* **2017**, *2*, eaan5165. [CrossRef]
143. Schreiber, S.; Nikolaus, S.; Hampe, J. Activation of nuclear factor kappa B in inflammatory bowel disease. *Gut* **1998**, *42*, 477–484. [CrossRef] [PubMed]
144. Visekruna, A.; Slavova, N.; Dullat, S.; Gröne, J.; Kroesen, A.-J.; Ritz, J.-P.; Buhr, H.-J.; Steinhoff, U. Expression of catalytic proteasome subunits in the gut of patients with Crohn's disease. *Int. J. Color. Dis.* **2009**, *24*, 1133–1139. [CrossRef] [PubMed]
145. Visekruna, A.; Joeris, T.; Schmidt, N.; Lawrenz, M.; Ritz, J.-P.; Buhr, H.J.; Steinhoff, U. Comparative expression analysis and characterization of 20S proteasomes in human intestinal tissues. *Inflamm. Bowel Dis.* **2009**, *15*, 526–533. [CrossRef]
146. Visekruna, A.; Joeris, T.; Seidel, D.; Kroesen, A.; Loddenkemper, C.; Zeitz, M.; Kaufmann, S.H.; Schmidt-Ullrich, R.; Steinhoff, U. Proteasome-mediated degradation of IκBα and processing of p105 in Crohn disease and ulcerative colitis. *J. Clin. Investig.* **2006**, *116*, 3195–3203. [CrossRef]
147. Moallemian, R.; Rehman, A.U.; Zhao, N.; Wang, H.; Chen, H.; Lin, G.; Ma, X.; Yu, J. Immunoproteasome inhibitor DPLG3 attenuates experimental colitis by restraining NF-κB activation. *Biochem. Pharmacol.* **2020**, *177*, 113964. [CrossRef]
148. Vachharajani, N.; Joeris, T.; Luu, M.; Hartmann, S.; Pautz, S.; Jenike, E.; Pantazis, G.; Prinz, I.; Hofer, M.J.; Steinhoff, U.; et al. Prevention of colitis-associated cancer by selective targeting of immunoproteasome subunit LMP7. *Oncotarget* **2017**, *8*, 50447–50459. [CrossRef]
149. Basler, M.; Lindstrom, M.M.; LaStant, J.J.; Bradshaw, J.M.; Owens, T.D.; Schmidt, C.; Maurits, E.; Tsu, C.; Overkleeft, H.S.; Kirk, C.J.; et al. Co-inhibition of immunoproteasome subunits LMP2 and LMP7 is required to block autoimmunity. *EMBO Rep.* **2018**, *19*. [CrossRef]
150. Thompson, A.J.; Baranzini, S.; Geurts, J.; Hemmer, B.; Ciccarelli, O. Multiple sclerosis. *Lancet* **2018**, *391*, 1622–1636. [CrossRef]
151. Mishto, M.; Bellavista, E.; Ligorio, C.; Textoris-Taube, K.; Santoro, A.; Giordano, M.; D'Alfonso, S.; Listì, F.; Nacmias, B.; Cellini, E.; et al. Immunoproteasome LMP2 60HH Variant Alters MBP Epitope Generation and Reduces the Risk to Develop Multiple Sclerosis in Italian Female Population. *PLoS ONE* **2010**, *5*, e9287. [CrossRef]
152. VanderLugt, C.L.; Rahbe, S.M.; Elliott, P.J.; Canto, M.C.D.; Miller, S.D. Treatment of Established Relapsing Experimental Autoimmune Encephalomyelitis with the Proteasome Inhibitor PS-5191. *J. Autoimmun.* **2000**, *14*, 205–211. [CrossRef] [PubMed]
153. Hosseini, H.; André, P.; Lefevre, N.; Viala, L.; Walzer, T.; Peschanski, M.; Lotteau, V. Protection against experimental autoimmune encephalomyelitis by a proteasome modulator. *J. Neuroimmunol.* **2001**, *118*, 233–244. [CrossRef]
154. Gupta, R.; Debbaneh, M.G.; Liao, W. Genetic Epidemiology of Psoriasis. *Curr. Dermatol. Rep.* **2014**, *3*, 61–78. [CrossRef] [PubMed]
155. Yang, L.; Guo, W.; Zhang, S.; Wang, G. Ubiquitination-proteasome system: A new player in the pathogenesis of psoriasis and clinical implications. *J. Dermatol. Sci.* **2018**, *89*, 219–225. [CrossRef] [PubMed]
156. Boehncke, W.-H.; Schön, M.P. Psoriasis. *Lancet* **2015**, *386*, 983–994. [CrossRef]
157. Bakir-Gungor, B.; Remmers, E.F.; Meguro, A.; Mizuki, N.; Kastner, D.L.; Gül, A.; Sezerman, O.U. Identification of possible pathogenic pathways in Behçet's disease using genome-wide association study data from two different populations. *Eur. J. Hum. Genet.* **2014**, *23*, 678–687. [CrossRef]
158. Sánchez-Serrano, I. Success in translational research: Lessons from the development of bortezomib. *Nat. Rev. Drug Discov.* **2006**, *5*, 107–114. [CrossRef] [PubMed]

159. Stewart, A.K.; Rajkumar, S.V.; Dimopoulos, M.A.; Masszi, T.; Špička, I.; Oriol, A.; Hájek, R.; Rosiñol, L.; Siegel, D.S.; Mihaylov, G.G.; et al. Carfilzomib, Lenalidomide, and Dexamethasone for Relapsed Multiple Myeloma. *N. Engl. J. Med.* **2015**, *372*, 142–152. [CrossRef]
160. Richardson, P.; Sonneveld, P.; Schuster, M.; Irwin, D.; Stadtmauer, E.; Facon, T.; Harousseau, J.-L.; Ben-Yehuda, D.; Lonial, S.; Goldschmidt, H.; et al. Bortezomib or High-Dose Dexamethasone for Relapsed Multiple Myeloma. *N. Engl. J. Med.* **2005**, *352*, 2487–2498. [CrossRef]
161. Manasanch, E.E.; Orlowski, R.Z. Proteasome inhibitors in cancer therapy. *Nat. Rev. Clin. Oncol.* **2017**, *14*, 417–433. [CrossRef]
162. Ishii, T.; Tanaka, Y.; Kawakami, A.; Saito, K.; Ichinose, K.; Fujii, H.; Shirota, Y.; Shirai, T.; Fujita, Y.; Watanabe, R.; et al. Multicenter double-blind randomized controlled trial to evaluate the effectiveness and safety of bortezomib as a treatment for refractory systemic lupus erythematosus. *Mod. Rheumatol.* **2018**, *28*, 986–992. [CrossRef]
163. Van Dam, L.S.; Osmani, Z.; Kamerling, S.W.; Kraaij, T.; Bakker, J.; Scherer, H.U.; Rabelink, T.J.; Voll, R.; Alexander, T.; Isenberg, D.; et al. A reverse translational study on the effect of rituximab, rituximab plus belimumab, or bortezomib on the humoral autoimmune response in SLE. *Rheumatology* **2020**, *59*, 2734–2745. [CrossRef] [PubMed]
164. Hiepe, F.; Radbruch, F.H.A. Plasma cells as an innovative target in autoimmune disease with renal manifestations. *Nat. Rev. Nephrol.* **2016**, *12*, 232–240. [CrossRef] [PubMed]
165. Knops, N.; Emonds, M.; Herman, J.; Levtchenko, E.; Mekahli, D.; Pirenne, J.; Van Geet, C.; Dierickx, D. Bortezomib for autoimmune hemolytic anemia after intestinal transplantation. *Pediatr. Transplant.* **2020**, *24*, 13700. [CrossRef]
166. Beydoun, S.B.; Persaud, Y.; Lafferty, J.; Callaghan, M.U.; Savaşan, S. Bortezomib treatment of steroid-refractory Evans syndrome in children. *Pediatr. Blood Cancer* **2020**, *67*, 28725. [CrossRef]
167. Yates, S.; Matevosyan, K.; Rutherford, C.; Shen, Y.-M.; Sarode, R. Bortezomib for chronic relapsing thrombotic thrombocytopenic purpura: A case report. *Transfusion* **2014**, *54*, 2064–2067. [CrossRef] [PubMed]
168. Jakez-Ocampo, J.; Atisha-Fregoso, Y.; Llorente, L. Refractory Primary Sjögren Syndrome Successfully Treated with Bortezomib. *J. Clin. Rheumatol.* **2015**, *21*, 31–32. [CrossRef] [PubMed]
169. Berges, C.; Haberstock, H.; Fuchs, D.; Miltz, M.; Sadeghi, M.; Opelz, G.; Daniel, V.; Naujokat, C. Proteasome inhibition suppresses essential immune functions of human CD4+T cells. *Immunology* **2008**, *124*, 234–246. [CrossRef]
170. Pletinckx, K.; Vaßen, S.; Schlusche, I.; Nordhoff, S.; Bahrenberg, G.; Dunkern, T.R. Inhibiting the immunoproteasome's β5i catalytic activity affects human peripheral blood-derived immune cell viability. *Pharmacol. Res. Perspect.* **2019**, *7*, e00482. [CrossRef]
171. Scheibe, F.; Prüss, H.; Mengel, A.M.; Kohler, S.; Nümann, A.; Köhnlein, M.; Ruprecht, K.; Alexander, T.; Hiepe, F.; Meisel, A. Bortezomib for treatment of therapy-refractory anti-NMDA receptor encephalitis. *Neurology* **2016**, *88*, 366–370. [CrossRef]
172. Wickel, J.; Chung, H.-Y.; Platzer, S.; Lehmann, T.; Prüss, H.; Leypoldt, F.; Günther, A.; Scherag, A.; Geis, C.; on behalf of the GENERATE Study Group. Generate-Boost: Study protocol for a prospective, multicenter, randomized controlled, double-blinded phase II trial to evaluate efficacy and safety of bortezomib in patients with severe autoimmune encephalitis. *Trials* **2020**, *21*, 1–12. [CrossRef] [PubMed]
173. Meregalli, C. An Overview of Bortezomib-Induced Neurotoxicity. *Toxics* **2015**, *3*, 294–303. [CrossRef] [PubMed]
174. Johnson, H.W.B.; Lowe, E.; Anderl, J.L.; Fan, A.; Muchamuel, T.; Bowers, S.; Moebius, D.C.; Kirk, C.; McMINN, D.L. Required Immunoproteasome Subunit Inhibition Profile for Anti-Inflammatory Efficacy and Clinical Candidate KZR-616 ((2S,3R)-N-((S)-3-(Cyclopent-1-en-1-yl)-1-((R)-2-methyloxiran-2-yl)-1-oxopropan-2-yl)-3-hydroxy-3-(4-methoxyphenyl)-2-((S)-2-(2-morpholinoacetamido)propanamido)propenamide). *J. Med. Chem.* **2018**, *61*, 11127–11143. [CrossRef]
175. Von Brzezinski, L.; Säring, P.; Landgraf, P.; Cammann, C.; Seifert, U.; Dieterich, D.C. Low neurotoxicity of ONX-0914 supports the idea of specific immunoproteasome inhibition as a side-effect-limiting, therapeutic strategy. *Eur. J. Microbiol. Immunol.* **2017**, *7*, 234–245. [CrossRef]
176. Thibaudeau, T.A.; Smith, D.M. A Practical Review of Proteasome Pharmacology. *Pharmacol. Rev.* **2019**, *71*, 170–197. [CrossRef] [PubMed]
177. Zilberberg, J.; Matos, J.; Dziopa, E.; Dziopa, L.; Yang, Z.; Kirk, C.J.; Assefnia, S.; Korngold, R. Inhibition of the Immunoproteasome Subunit LMP7 with ONX 0914 Ameliorates Graft-versus-Host Disease in an MHC-Matched Minor Histocompatibility Antigen–Disparate Murine Model. *Biol. Blood Marrow Transplant.* **2015**, *21*, 1555–1564. [CrossRef]
178. Liu, H.; Wan, C.; Ding, Y.; Han, R.; He, Y.; Xiao, J.; Hao, J. PR-957, a selective inhibitor of immunoproteasome subunit low-MW polypeptide 7, attenuates experimental autoimmune neuritis by suppressing T h 17-cell differentiation and regulating cytokine production. *FASEB J.* **2016**, *31*, 1756–1766. [CrossRef]
179. Basler, M.; Groettrup, M. Recent insights how combined inhibition of immuno/proteasome subunits enables therapeutic efficacy. *Genes Immun.* **2020**, *21*, 273–287. [CrossRef]
180. Ladi, E.; Everett, C.; Stivala, C.E.; Daniels, B.E.; Durk, M.R.; Harris, S.F.; Huestis, M.P.; Purkey, H.E.; Staben, S.T.; Augustin, M.; et al. Design and Evaluation of Highly Selective Human Immunoproteasome Inhibitors Reveal a Compensatory Process That Preserves Immune Cell Viability. *J. Med. Chem.* **2019**, *62*, 7032–7041. [CrossRef]
181. Leestemaker, Y.; De Jong, A.; Witting, K.F.; Penning, R.; Schuurman, K.; Rodenko, B.; Zaal, E.A.; Van De Kooij, B.; Laufer, S.; Heck, A.J.; et al. Proteasome Activation by Small Molecules. *Cell Chem. Biol.* **2017**, *24*, 725–736.e7. [CrossRef] [PubMed]
182. Myeku, N.; Clelland, C.L.; Emrani, S.; Kukushkin, N.V.; Yu, W.H.; Goldberg, A.L.; Duff, K. Tau-driven 26S proteasome impairment and cognitive dysfunction can be prevented early in disease by activating cAMP-PKA signaling. *Nat. Med.* **2016**, *22*, 46–53. [CrossRef] [PubMed]

183. Liu, Y.; Hettinger, C.L.; Zhang, D.; Rezvani, K.; Wang, X.; Wang, H. Sulforaphane enhances proteasomal and autophagic activities in mice and is a potential therapeutic reagent for Huntington's disease. *J. Neurochem.* **2014**, *129*, 539–547. [CrossRef] [PubMed]
184. Lee, B.-H.; Lee, M.J.; Park, S.; Oh, D.-C.; Elsasser, S.; Chen, P.-C.; Gartner, C.; Dimova, N.; Hanna, J.V.; Gygi, S.P.; et al. Enhancement of proteasome activity by a small-molecule inhibitor of USP14. *Nat. Cell Biol.* **2010**, *467*, 179–184Bico. [CrossRef]

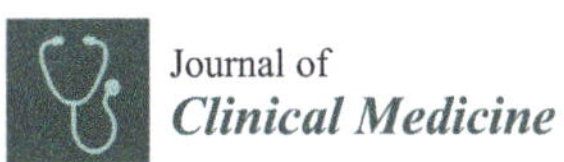
Journal of
Clinical Medicine

MDPI

Review

The Pathogenic Role of Interferons in the Hyperinflammatory Response on Adult-Onset Still's Disease and Macrophage Activation Syndrome: Paving the Way towards New Therapeutic Targets

Ilenia Di Cola [1,†], Piero Ruscitti [1,*,†], Roberto Giacomelli [2] and Paola Cipriani [1]

1 Department of Biotechnological and Applied Clinical Sciences, University of L'Aquila, 67100 L'Aquila, Italy; ilenia.dicola@graduate.univaq.it (I.D.C.); paola.cipriani@univaq.it (P.C.)
2 Rheumatology and Immunology Unit, Department of Medicine, University of Rome Campus Biomedico, 00128 Rome, Italy; r.giacomelli@unicampus.it
* Correspondence: piero.ruscitti@univaq.it; Tel.: +39-086-243-4742 or +39-086-243-3523
† Contributed equally.

Abstract: Adult-onset Still's disease (AOSD) is a systemic inflammatory disorder of unknown aetiology affecting young adults, which is burdened by life-threatening complications, mostly macrophage activation syndrome (MAS). Interferons (IFNs) are signalling molecules that mediate a variety of biological functions from defence against viral infections, to antitumor and immunomodulatory effects. These molecules have been classified into three major types: IFN I, IFN II, IFN III, presenting specific characteristics and functions. In this work, we reviewed the role of IFNs on AOSD and MAS, focusing on their pathogenic role in promoting the hyperinflammatory response and as new possible therapeutic targets. In fact, both preclinical and clinical observations suggested that these molecules could promote the hyperinflammatory response in MAS during AOSD. Furthermore, the positive results of inhibiting IFN-γ in primary hemophagocytic lymphohistiocytosis may provide a solid rationale to arrange further clinical studies, paving the way for reducing the high mortality rate in MAS during AOSD.

Keywords: adult-onset Still's disease; macrophage activation syndrome; IFN-γ

Citation: Di Cola, I.; Ruscitti, P.; Giacomelli, R.; Cipriani, P. The Pathogenic Role of Interferons in the Hyperinflammatory Response on Adult-Onset Still's Disease and Macrophage Activation Syndrome: Paving the Way towards New Therapeutic Targets. *J. Clin. Med.* **2021**, *10*, 1164. https://doi.org/10.3390/jcm10061164

Academic Editor: Eugen Feist

Received: 26 February 2021
Accepted: 8 March 2021
Published: 10 March 2021

1. Introduction

Adult-onset Still's disease (AOSD) is an inflammatory disease usually affecting young adults [1]. AOSD is associated with a very heterogeneous clinical picture, a triad of high fever, arthritis, and evanescent pink salmon skin rash are commonly observed [2]. Furthermore, a multiorgan involvement of the disease is recognised, including liver involvement, splenomegaly, and poly-serositis [2]. A typical hyperferritinemia is observed in these patients, associated with increases of C-reactive protein (CRP) and erythrocyte sedimentation rate (ESR) [1]. Additionally, patients with AOSD experience life-threatening complications, which may rapidly evolve into multiple-organ failure and death [3]. These patients would frequently develop macrophage activation syndrome (MAS), a secondary form of hemophagocytic lymphohistiocytosis (HLH) [4,5]. The latter is characterised by continuous high fever, extreme hyperferritinemia, pancytopenia, and histopathological evidence of hemophagocytosis by activated macrophages, typically in bone marrow [5,6].

Although it is typical, this histological finding is not mandatory for HLH diagnosis since it cannot be recognized at the beginning of the disease in bone marrow biopsies [4]. Another important characterisation of HLH is the organomegaly, splenomegaly, and hepatomegaly frequently recognized in these patients [4]. In addition, it was proposed that AOSD and MAS may be considered part of the same disease spectrum, sharing clinical and pathogenic features, and in which AOSD may represent a milder form [7]. Furthermore, these diseases have been recently included in the so-called hyperferritinemic syndrome, which, together with catastrophic anti-phospholipid syndrome and septic shock, share similar clinical and laboratory features, including very high levels of ferritin [8].

As far as the pathogenesis is concerned, AOSD is considered at the crossroads between auto-inflammatory and autoimmune diseases [9]. Both the innate and adaptative arms of the immune system are called upon in the pathogenic mechanisms underlying this disease [10]. The pathogenic mechanisms of MAS have not been fully clarified yet, but recently a multi-layer pathogenic model was proposed [6]. Both genetic predisposition and several triggers may contribute to the development of a cytolytic dysfunction, prolonging the survival of target cells and enhancing antigen presentation to overproduce proinflammatory cytokines, leading to full-blown MAS syndrome [5,6,11]. In this context, the role of interferons (IFNs) was pointed out mainly for inducing cytokine storm syndrome and MAS occurrence during AOSD [5,6,11]. On these bases, in this work we reviewed the role of IFNs on AOSD and MAS, focusing on their pathogenic role in promoting the hyperinflammatory response and as new possible therapeutic targets.

2. Interferons

In 1957, a molecule was first described with the ability to "interfere" with viral replication and protect cells from infection, which was called an IFN [12]. Since then, a growing body of evidence has shown that multiple IFNs exist which mediate a variety of biological functions from defence against viral infections to antitumor and immunomodulatory effects [13]. IFNs are classified into three main groups according to chromosomal location, their aminoacidic sequence, and specific receptors: i. type I IFNs (-α, -β, -δ, -ε, -ζ, -κ, -τ, and -ω); ii. type II IFN (-γ); iii. type III IFNs (-λ1, -λ2, -λ3). Type I IFNs and IFN-γ are physiologically expressed and are increased by stress and infections [13]. IFNs are critical effectors of both innate and adaptive immune responses, associated with the development of immune cell populations and their activation in response to pathogens, cancers, and other conditions [14]. In addition, the elevated production of IFNs is recognised during both autoimmune and autoinflammatory diseases [15]. This increases the expression of target genes and the canonical interferon-stimulated genes (ISGs) in affected tissues and in circulating blood cells, thus defining the "IFN signature" [14]. The latter is reported to be a typical characteristic of some diseases [16].

3. IFN I

3.1. Generalities

IFN-α and IFN-β are the most studied and characterised members of this class of IFNs [16]. IFN-α is encoded by more than 20 different genes. Among these, 13 lead to a functional protein in humans and 14 in mice, whereas IFN-β is encoded by a single gene in both humans and mice [16,17]. Although IFN-α and -β may regulate an overlapping set of genes, these two cytokines differ slightly in their downstream effects and in their expression pattern [18]. Other type I subtypes (IFN- δ, -ε, -ζ, -κ, -τ, and -ω) are less-often studied [16]. Type I IFNs act on most cell types and induce an antiviral state by increasing the major histocompatibility complex expression and inducing the production of chemokines and cytokines [19,20]. Furthermore, type I IFNs boost the innate arm of the immune system by stimulating the maturation of dendritic cells and the function of natural killer cells [16]. These IFNs also enhance the adaptive response of the immune system by promoting the activation of T and B cells [14]. As a major component of the innate immune system protecting against viruses, the expression of IFN-α and IFN-β is induced by viral infection [19,20]. Type I IFNs bind to the ubiquitously expressed type I IFN receptor (IFNAR) in an autocrine and paracrine manner, modulating the expression of numerous IFN-stimulated genes (ISG) which are involved in the antiviral and anti-inflammatory responses and the pro-apoptotic and anti-proliferative activities [18].

3.2. Pathogenic Implications in AOSD and MAS

Multiple lines of evidence indicate that type I IFNs also exert anti-inflammatory functions [21–23]. These anti-inflammatory phenomena were proposed because IFN-α may reduce both interleukin (IL)-1α and IL-1β production by two main pathways [23,24]. By acting on the signal transducer and activator of transcription 1 (STAT1), type I IFNs may repress the activity of the Nucleotide Binding Domain (NBD), Leucine-Rich Repeat (LRR) containing (NLR) protein 1 (NLRP1) and NLRP3 inflammasomes, thereby suppressing caspase-1-dependent IL-1β maturation [23]. These molecules could also induce the expression of IL-10 in a STAT1-dependent manner, which in turn may reduce the abundance of the pro-IL-1α and pro-IL-1β signals via STAT3 [23]. Such inflammasome inhibition by type I IFNs may also suggest a mechanism for the observed IFN-dependent suppression of IL-18 maturation, since it would also depend on inflammasome activity [23]. Because of these anti-inflammatory functions, an impaired response of type I IFNs may be implicated in the generation of the hyperinflammatory processes [18]. Patients with more severe COVID-19, during the ongoing catastrophic pandemic by SARS-CoV-2, may provide a virally induced representative model of cytokine storm syndrome, thus suggesting similarities with the underlying pathogenic mechanisms of AOSD and MAS [25,26]. Interestingly, severe coronavirus disease 2019 (COVID-19) may display many common aspects with other disorders included in hyperferritinaemic syndrome, including continuous fever and high levels of ferritin [27]. In the context of COVID-19, Hadjadj et al. observed a distinct phenotype in severe and critical patients, associated with a highly impaired type I IFN response, associated with decreased production and reduced activity [28]. In addition, the presence of neutralizing autoantibodies against type I IFNs was supposed in the inhibition of the type I IFN response [29]. These autoantibodies against type I IFNs seemed to be clinically silent until the infection, suggesting that the small quantities of such molecules could be implicated in the onset of cytokine storm syndrome [29].

Taking these observations together, the impairment of the functions of type I IFNs or their delayed response may be implicated in the development of a cytokine storm syndrome. These pathogenic alterations could be also associated with the development of MAS during AOSD, thus providing food for thought for further mechanistic studies. In fact, limited data are available about the role of IFN I in the pathogenesis of AOSD and MAS, so far. In this setting, sera levels of both IFN-α and IFN-β were studied by enzyme-linked immunosorbent assay (ELISA) in 39 AOSD patients, both during a flare of the disease and when following therapies [30]. Levels of IFN-α were detected in only one of the AOSD patients. Instead, levels of IFN-β were found in both patients with an active flare of the disease and those following therapies, without any statistically significant difference [30]. Notably, the type I IFN response on the HLH experimental model was studied in a murine model with a specific deletion of IFNAR (IFNAR-KO) [31]. HLH was induced by stimulation with an IL-10 receptor-blocking antibody and a Toll-like receptor 9 (TLR9) agonist. When IL-10 signalling was maintained, the administration of the TLR9 agonist resulted in a milder HLH in wild-type (WT) mice, with less severe hepatitis and lack of hemophagocytosis. However, thrombocytopenia and IFN-γ were similar between the IFNAR-KO and the WT mice. Despite IFN-γ levels being comparable to those of the WT mice, the IFNAR-KO mice did not develop anaemia, suggesting that type I IFNs could be involved in leading to this feature during HLH [31]. In the same model, the simultaneous administration of both an IL-10 receptor-blocking antibody and a TLR9 agonist led to fulminant HLH. The IFNAR-KO mice had less weight loss than their WT counterparts but were comparable for thrombocytopenia, hepatitis, and splenic hemophagocytosis. Furthermore, the IFNAR-KO mice treated for fulminant HLH conditions experienced the same degree of anaemia when compared to WT mice. Taking together these findings, a complex interaction between type I and type II IFNs in the pathogenesis of TLR9-mediated HLH could be suggested [31].

4. IFN II

4.1. Generalities

The type II IFN subtype is made of a single gene product: IFN-γ [16,32,33]. Its structure is different from type I IFNs, but it is classified in this family of molecules due to its antiviral effects [16]. IFN-γ binds to the nearly ubiquitously expressed receptor (IFNGR), and signals through Janus kinase 1 (JAK1) and JAK2 to phosphorylate STAT1 [13]. IFN-γ is involved in the modulation of the immune and inflammatory responses and is predominantly produced by natural killer (NK), NKT, and activated T cells [18]. It has weaker antiviral effects than type I IFNs, but potent effects on increasing major histocompatibility complex expression, antigen presentation, and chemokine production, while suppressing cell proliferation [18]. IFN-γ would be the prototypic "macrophage-activating factor" increasing cytokine and chemokine production, phagocytosis, and the intracellular killing of microbial pathogens by macrophages [33]. Furthermore, IFN-γ boosts type 1 adaptive immunity by promoting the differentiation of type 1 helper T cells, the generation of follicular helper T cells, B cell class switching, autoantibody production, and the generation of autoimmunity-associated B cells [18]. This molecule may also have protective functions by suppressing responses mediated by type 2 helper- and IL-17-producing helper T cells, inducing specialized regulatory T cells and restraining tissue damage [18]. Moreover, IFN-γ may directly enhance antigen presentation by promoting antigen processing and by inducing the expression of major histocompatibility complex molecules [18].

In this context, the involvement of the IFN-γ pathway in the pathogenic mechanisms of HLH, either primary or secondary, was proposed [30]. Although the mechanisms leading to IFN-γ-mediated immunopathology remain to be fully clarified, many data would suggest this cytokine is a crucial mediator in HLH occurrence [30,34–36].

4.2. Pathogenic Implications, Ex Vivo Observations

The pathogenic implications of IFN-γ in HLH were studied through the evaluation of neopterin levels in HLH patients [37]. Neopterin is a marker of inflammation belonging to a group of pteridines, and it is biosynthetically derived from guanosine triphosphate. It is secreted by human monocyte-derived macrophage and dendritic cells upon stimulation with IFN-γ. On these bases, it may be considered as a surrogate marker of this cytokine. Sera neopterin levels obtained at the time of diagnosis of 21 HLH patients and 50 untreated children with active juvenile dermatomyositis were evaluated by competitive enzyme immunoassay. HLH patients had higher levels of neopterin than the control group. Furthermore, neopterin significantly correlated with ferritin, suggesting a possible pathogenic link. Moreover, a cut-off of 38.9 nmol/L was derived by a ROC curve with a 70% sensitivity, and 95% specificity in diagnosing HLH, thus suggesting that neopterin levels could be an accurate marker of the disease [37].

Considering that IFN-γ is rapidly catabolized, it may be difficult to use it as a biomarker, thus highlighting the assessment of IFN-γ-induced chemokines in studying this pathway. In an elegant study, sera levels of the IFN-γ-induced chemokines (C-X-C motif) ligand 9 (CXCL9), and CXCL10 were evaluated in 14 patients with active HLH. These chemokines were higher than those collected from patients with a non-active disease or following therapies. Furthermore, the correlations among IFN-γ, CXCL9, and CXCL10 and the laboratory features of HLH were evaluated, including neutrophil and platelet counts, ferritin, lactate dehydrogenase, and alanine transaminase levels. CXCL9 correlated with all studied laboratory parameters. IFN-γ and CXCL10 correlated with all the parameters except for platelet counts for IFN-γ, and ferritin levels for CXCL10 [38]. In a further study, IFN-γ and IFN-γ-induced chemokines, CXCL9, CXCL10, and CXCL11, were studied using ELISA. Sera samples of 39 active and untreated AOSD patients, 30 rheumatoid arthritis patients, and 28 healthy controls were collected. IFN-γ, CXCL9, CXCL10, and CXCL11 were higher in AOSD patients when compared with RA patients or healthy controls. Furthermore, CXCL9, CXCL10, and CXCL11 were significantly higher in AOSD patients with MAS than those without it. In addition, these chemokines correlated with inflammatory markers and systemic scores. Notably, a decrease of these chemokines except for IFN-γ was observed after the reduction of disease activity during the follow-up. Finally, on immunohistochemistry, more inflammatory cells expressing CXCL10 were observed in skin biopsy samples from AOSD patients than in healthy controls [30].

4.3. Pathogenic Implications and In Vivo Observations

The importance of IFN-γ in the pathogenesis of both primary and secondary HLH would be enhanced by the data obtained in experimental models. In fact, IFN-γ may be suggested as a pivotal mediator in murine models of HLH [39,40]. In this setting, the first experimental model of HLH was provided in perforin-deficient mice infected by lymphocytic choriomeningitis virus (LMCV). After this infection, the mice manifested the typical features of HLH, including fever, pancytopenia, and hypofibrinogenemia, associated with evidence of tissue hemophagocytosis. Furthermore, in this model, a marked increase of pro-inflammatory cytokines was shown with a remarkable quantity of IFN-γ. The latter was related due to a persistent antigen presentation and an increase in the antigen responsiveness of cytotoxic T cells [39]. Subsequently, in Rab 27a-deficient (Rab27a−/−) mice, it was also shown that infection with LCMV led to HLH [40]. Interestingly, in both these models, the administration of an IFN-γ blocking agent had a therapeutic effect [39,40]. In fact, the authors described how this treatment improved survival and led to an improvement of haematological and histopathological features in these mice. Indeed, the inhibition of IFN-γ increased blood cell counts. A significant reduction of triglyceride and ferritin levels was also observed over time in these experimental models. Furthermore, following IFN-γ inhibition, complete normalization of the histopathological features of the spleen was described in these models. The authors also noted a reduction of macrophage activation, as evidenced by the reduction of haemophagocytosis in the liver of both murine models [40].

In another study, it was shown that experimental HLH could be induced by repeated stimulation of TLR9 [34]. The authors also tested if IFN-γ could be required for the induction of HLH. Compared with WT mice, the IFN-γ−/−mice did not develop anaemia, thrombocytopenia, or hepatic inflammation, and these mice preserved the splenic structure. However, some features could not be dependent on IFN-γ, since leukopenia and hyperferritinemia were observed in both the WT and the IFN-γ −/− mice. Furthermore, the authors described the protective role of IL-10 in this setting, showing that the inhibition of its signal and/or the IL-10 receptor led to the development of hemophagocytosis. These data could reinforce the idea that IL-10 may also contribute by modulating both the variability and severity of this disease [34]. These findings were investigated in a later work in which IFN-γ-deficient mice underwent stimulation with a TLR9 agonist, IFN-γ, or a combination of both [35]. Following singular and repeated stimulation with a TLR9 agonist or IFN-γ, HLH features were not developed. However, mice treated with both a TLR9 agonist and IFN-γ reproduced the main features of HLH, developing cytopenias, hepatitis, and hepatosplenomegaly. On these bases, the authors suggested that TLR9- and IFN-γ-dependent signals could synergize in enhancing the myeloid progenitor function and inducing myelopoiesis. Thus, in this study, TLR9-driven signals would potentiate the effects of IFN-γ, leading to the development of HLH [35]. In a subsequent study, HLH in WT, transgenic, and cytokine-inhibited mice was assessed following stimulation with an IL-10 receptor-blocking antibody and a TLR9 agonist. Interestingly, fulminant HLH and hemophagocytosis developed independently of the presence of IFN-γ, whereas anaemia and dyserythropoiesis did not suggest an IFN-γ dependence [31]. IFN-γ dependent anaemia during HLH was also confirmed and detailed [41]. In fact, it was shown that IFN-γ could induce cytopenia and hemophagocytosis. The latter may have derived from the direct action of IFN-γ on macrophages in vivo, altering endocytosis and consequently leading to severe anaemia, the so-called consumptive anaemia of inflammation [41]. Other processes involved in HLH-associated anaemia could be blood loss, haemolysis, and decreased bone marrow output [41]. In addition, the IFN-γ-induced chemokines CXCL9 and

CXCL10 were identified as possible biomarkers to be correlated with disease parameters including thrombocytopenia, hyperferritinemia, and lymphopenia [38]. These results provided the rationale for studying these IFN-γ-induced chemokines as possible predictors of HLH occurrence in humans, as previously mentioned [38].

In addition, some authors used a murine model of HLH induced by the administration of a TLR9 ligand in IL-6 transgenic mice to study the pathogenic mechanisms of the disease [36]. These mice, when injected with TLR ligands, may develop this condition by mimicking an acute infection on a background of high levels of IL-6 [36]. This experimental approach would more closely resemble what occurs in AOSD and its juvenile counterpart, an infectious trigger on an inflammatory background leading to MAS occurrence [36]. In addition, these IL-6 transgenic mice, following the administration of a TLR9 agonist, were associated with reduced survival, low neutrophils and platelet counts, and high levels of ferritin, LDH, and pro-inflammatory cytokines. In this experimental model, it was observed that IFN-γ and the IFN-γ-induced chemokines CXCL9 and CXCL10, were significantly increased in the liver, spleen, and plasma of the IL-6 transgenic mice, as compared to the WT mice. Furthermore, IFN-γ inhibition significantly decreased circulating levels of CXCL9, CXCL10, IL-1β, IL-6, TNF, and ferritin. Thus, a complex interplay between IL-6 and IFN-γ could be suggested in generating HLH [36].

4.4. Therapeutic Strategies

As previously discussed, experimental mouse models and ex vivo observations provide the rationale behind the use of IFN-γ inhibiting strategies for the treatment of HLH on account of the importance of the underlying IFN-γ-associated pathogenetic mechanisms of the disease [31,34–36,38–41].

Emapalumab is a fully human monoclonal antibody that neutralises both free- and receptor-bound IFN-γ by inhibiting receptor dimerization and the transduction of the signalling pathway of this molecule [42]. The efficacy of emapalumab was recently assessed in a clinical trial enrolling thirty-four patients aged between 0–18 years with a diagnosis of primary HLH, some were previously treated, while others were untreated. As main endpoints, the overall response was codified into patients with a complete response (defined absence of fever, cytopenia, hyperferritinemia, coagulopathy, neurological manifestations, increase of soluble CD25, and a normal spleen size), a partial response (three or more abnormalities that met the criteria for a complete response), or an improvement larger than 50% from baseline in at least three abnormalities associated with HLH. Twenty-six patients completed the eight-week treatment study. The percentage of previously treated patients with a response as assessed by the pre-defined parameters was 63%, while for the whole population of patients it was 65%. Of the previously treated patients, 26% achieved a complete response, 30% a partial response, 7% had improvement of HLH features, and 37% had no response. In the untreated patients, 43% achieved a partial response, 28.5% an improvement, and 28.5% no response. In this study, the authors also assessed CXCL9, which significantly decreased following the administration of emapalumab. Interestingly, low CXCL9 levels were associated with the clinical response during this clinical trial, suggesting possible predictors of efficacy following the administration of this drug [43].

In addition, a case report of a patient with refractory Epstein–Barr virus-associated HLH treated with emapalumab was recently described, with the resolution of all clinical symptoms and an improvement of laboratory markers of the disease [44]. Although IFN-γ inhibition would commonly be employed as a bridge to allogeneic stem cell transplantation, the successful use of emapalumab was also reported after transplant rejection in three relapsed primary HLH patients [45,46]. Finally, despite emapalumab being licensed for the treatment of primary HLH, several ongoing studies are assessing its use in the additional clinical settings of secondary HLH to systemic juvenile idiopathic arthritis (SJIA), and occurrence in adult ages (NCT03985423, NCT03311854).

5. IFN III

The third class of IFNs is composed of IFN-λ1, -λ2, -λ3, and -λ4 [16,47]. These are produced by most cell types, mainly from plasmacytoid dendritic cells following either viral or bacterial infection. Type III IFNs bind to the type III IFN receptor (IFNLR), preferentially expressed on certain myeloid cell types and epithelial cells of the respiratory, gastrointestinal, and reproductive tracts. This expression pattern is associated with local viral control at the site of entry. Furthermore, type III IFNs activate similar signalling pathways and partly induce the same genes as type I IFNs, resulting in a potent antiviral response [48]. The pathogenic role of type III IFNs in AOSD and MAS has yet to be defined.

6. Discussion and Appraisal of Literature

During AOSD, the difficult clinical scenario of MAS makes it difficult to manage patients, since genetic background, pro-inflammatory milieu, and triggers are mixed with a high mortality rate [5,6]. Thus, a growing body of studies has focused on investigating new therapeutic targets to better manage these patients [11,49]. Although IL-1 and IL-6 inhibiting agents were shown to be efficacious in AOSD [50,51], findings from clinical trials of canakinumab and tocilizumab on SJIA suggested that these therapies could not fully abrogate the risk of MAS development, even if the disease could be well controlled [52,53]. Consequently, these data suggest that additional pathogenic mechanisms could be implicated in MAS occurrence and together with the preclinical data, provided the rationale for IFN-γ inhibition in this field [31,34–36,38–41]. Thus, IFNs could be implicated in the development of this life-threatening complication during AOSD, as shown in Figure 1. In fact, Locatelli F et al. demonstrated the efficacy of emapalumab in children with primary HLH [43], which could be considered a genetic model of cytokine storm syndrome [54]. These clinical results may further confirm the pathogenic role of IFN-γ. It could also be possible to postulate the efficacy of emapalumab on cytokine storm syndromes from other aetiologies, including inflammatory or iatrogenic, and in adult ages. However, the data mined from children to adults with HLH would be limited by the presence of comorbidities, which may contribute to a higher rate of mortality in adulthood (almost 40%) [55,56]. In fact, patients with cytokine storm syndrome and comorbidities may be at high risk of poor prognosis, less able to tolerate medical procedures, and less responsive to any treatment, as recently shown in severe COVID-19 cases [57,58].

In addition, considering the poor prognosis of MAS occurring in AOSD, one crucial point would be a more accurate estimation of the subsequent clinical response. In this context, IFN-γ-induced chemokines were correlated with markers of MAS disease severity and clinical response to emapalumab [43,44], thus suggesting possible predictors of clinical response to treatment. Furthermore, IFN-γ-induced chemokines could be considered as mechanistic biomarkers, better reproducing the ongoing pathogenic mechanisms in MAS during AOSD and possibly more accurately reflecting the manipulated signalling pathways. In this context, specific HLH features such as anaemia and thrombocytopenia would be more correlated to IFN-γ [31]. In the heterogenous scenario of these patients, some clinical features should be considered as possible predictors of clinical response to IFN-γ inhibition when more relevant than others. Looking at new therapeutic strategies targeting IFN-γ, the possible role of JAK inhibitors was proposed in animal models of HLH as a further therapeutic option in these patients [59,60]. By the modulation of IFN-γ and other cytokines, the JAK1/2 inhibitor ruxolitinib reduced immune cell proliferation and activation, and reversed organ pro-inflammatory damage on experimental models of HLH [59,60]. Since they were concomitantly affecting different proinflammatory pathways, these drugs could simultaneously target IFN-γ and other pathogenic mechanisms of MAS during AOSD, possibly allowing for better management of cytokine storm syndrome in these patients [61]. On these bases, recent evidence has shown ruxolitinib may be considered for patients with secondary HLH with contraindications to glucocorticoids, with a good clinical response [62–64].

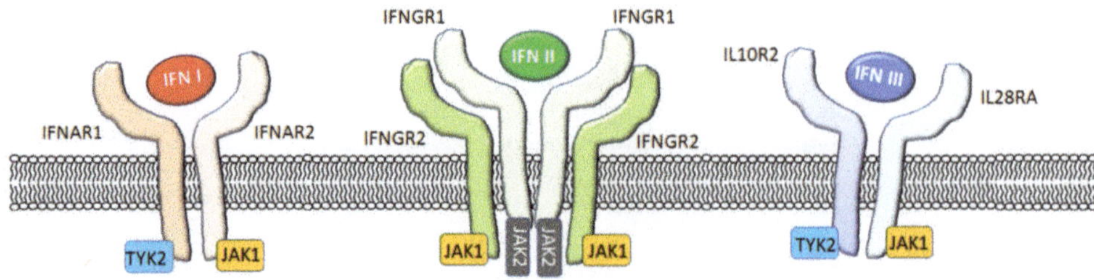

Pathogenic implications in cytokine storm syndrome occurrence

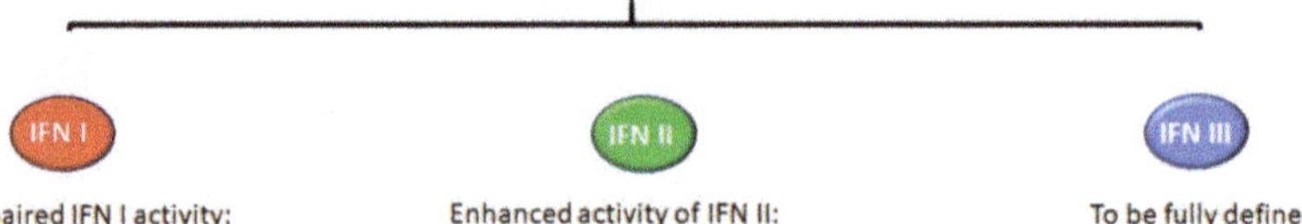

Delayed and impaired IFN I activity:
- Lack of negative control on production of pro-inflammatory cytokines;
- Lack of negative control on maturation of pro-inflammatory cytokines;
- Lack of positive control on the production of anti-inflammatory cytokines.

Enhanced activity of IFN II:
- Increased production of pro-inflammatory cytokines;
- Increased production of pro-inflammatory chemokines;
- Increased activation of macrophages;
- Increased activation of cytotoxic T cells;
- Increased expression of MCHs;
- Increased antigen presentation.

To be fully defined.

Figure 1. Pathogenic implications of IFNs in a cytokine storm syndrome occurrence. Type I IFNs bind to the IFNAR complex, consisting of two different chains, IFNAR1 and IFNAR2. Type II IFN activates the IFNGR, which is composed of two different chains, IFNGR1 and IFNGR2, and type III IFNs signal through a receptor complex made up of IL28RA and IL10R2. The impairment of the functions of type I IFNs or its delayed response may be implicated in the development of a cytokine storm syndrome lacking the negative control of production and maturation of pro-inflammatory cytokines as well as lacking the positive control on the production of anti-inflammatory cytokines. The enhanced activity of IFN II results in occurrences of cytokine storm syndrome via increased production of pro-inflammatory cytokines and chemokines and the increased activation of macrophages and cytotoxic T cells. The role of IFN III in this context has yet to be fully defined. Abbreviations: IFN: Interferon; IFNAR: interferon-alpha/beta receptor; IFNGR: interferon-gamma receptor; IL28RA: interleukin 28 receptor, alpha subunit; IL10R2: interleukin 10 receptor 2; TYK2: tyrosine kinase 2; JAK 1: Janus kinase 1; JAK 2: Janus kinase 2.

Finally, it must be pointed out that HLH could be also observed in patients with severe combined immunodeficiency lacking the main pathogenic effectors of the disease, T- and NK-cells. In these patients with severe combined immunodeficiency, the aberrant activation of macrophages and the subsequent cytokine storm syndrome may occur despite the complete absence of lymphocytes [65]. Furthermore, IFNGR1 deficiency is a rare immune deficiency characterized by selective susceptibility to mycobacterial disease due to IFNGR1 gene mutations [66]. Complete autosomal recessive IFNGR1 deficiency is characterized by the early onset of disseminated life-threatening infections from low-virulent mycobacteria, lack of response to IFN-γ cytokine replacement therapy, and high mortality [67]. A hematopoietic stem cell transplant is the only curative therapy available for these patients. Taking these observations together in the context of HLH, early identification of these patients would be needed to avoid unnecessary exposure to IFN-γ inhibition during cytokine storm syndrome.

7. Conclusions

In conclusion, IFNs are signalling molecules that mediate a variety of biological functions from defence against viral infections to antitumor and immunomodulatory effects. Preclinical and clinical observations suggest that these molecules could promote the hyperinflammatory response in MAS during AOSD, although additional evidence is needed to fully elucidate this topic. Finally, the positive results of inhibiting IFN-γ in primary HLH may provide a solid rationale to arrange further clinical studies, paving the way towards new therapeutic targets and reducing the high mortality rate in MAS during AOSD.

Author Contributions: Conceptualization, I.D.C., P.R., R.G. and P.C.; methodology, I.D.C., P.R., R.G., P.C.; validation, I.D.C., P.R., R.G., P.C.; formal analysis, I.D.C., P.R., R.G., P.C.; investigation, I.D.C., P.R., R.G., P.C.; resources, I.D.C., P.R., R.G., P.C.; data curation, I.D.C., P.R., R.G., P.C.; writing—original draft preparation, I.D.C., P.R., R.G., P.C.; writing—review and editing, I.D.C., P.R., R.G., P.C.; visualization, I.D.C., P.R., R.G., P.C.; supervision, I.D.C., P.R., R.G., P.C.; project administration, I.D.C., P.R., R.G., P.C. All authors have read and agreed to the published version of the manuscript.

Funding: This research received no external funding.

Institutional Review Board Statement: Not applicable.

Informed Consent Statement: Not applicable.

Data Availability Statement: Not applicable.

Acknowledgments: The authors thank Federica Sensini for her technical assistance.

Conflicts of Interest: The authors declare that they have no conflict of interest for this work.

References

1. Feist, E.; Mitrovic, S.; Fautrel, B. Mechanisms, biomarkers and targets for adult-onset Still's disease. *Nat. Rev. Rheumatol.* **2018**, *14*, 603–618. [CrossRef]
2. Giacomelli, R.; Ruscitti, P.; Shoenfeld, Y. A comprehensive review on adult onset Still's disease. *J. Autoimmun.* **2018**, *93*, 24–36. [CrossRef]
3. Ruscitti, P.; Iacono, D.; Ciccia, F.; Emmi, G.; Cipriani, P.; Grembiale, R.D.; Perosa, F.; Emmi, L.; Triolo, G.; Giacomelli, R.; et al. Macrophage Activation Syndrome in Patients Affected by Adult-onset Still Disease: Analysis of Survival Rates and Predictive Factors in the Gruppo Italiano di Ricerca in Reumatologia Clinica e Sperimentale Cohort. *J. Rheumatol.* **2018**, *45*, 864–872. [CrossRef]
4. La Rosée, P.; Horne, A.; Hines, M.; Greenwood, T.V.B.; Machowicz, R.; Berliner, N.; Birndt, S.; Gil-Herrera, J.; Girschikofsky, M.; Jordan, M.B.; et al. Recommendations for the management of hemophagocytic lymphohistiocytosis in adults. *Blood* **2019**, *133*, 2465–2477. [CrossRef] [PubMed]
5. Ramos-Casals, M.; Brito-Zerón, P.; López-Guillermo, A.; Khamashta, M.A.; Bosch, X. Adult haemophagocytic syndrome. *Lancet* **2014**, *383*, 1503–1516. [CrossRef]
6. Grom, A.A.; Horne, A.; De Benedetti, F. Macrophage activation syndrome in the era of biologic therapy. *Nat. Rev. Rheumatol.* **2016**, *12*, 259–268. [CrossRef]
7. Efthimiou, P.; Kadavath, S.; Mehta, B. Life-threatening complications of adult-onset Still's disease. *Clin. Rheumatol.* **2014**, *33*, 305–314. [CrossRef]
8. Rosário, C.; Zandman-Goddard, G.; Meyron-Holtz, E.G.; D'Cruz, D.P.; Shoenfeld, Y. The Hyperferritinemic Syndrome: Macrophage activation syndrome, Still's disease, septic shock and catastrophic antiphospholipid syndrome. *BMC Med.* **2013**, *11*, 185. [CrossRef] [PubMed]
9. Gerfaud-Valentin, M.; Jamilloux, Y.; Iwaz, J.; Sève, P. Adult-onset Still's disease. *Autoimmun. Rev.* **2014**, *13*, 708–722. [CrossRef] [PubMed]
10. Ruscitti, P.; Ursini, F.; Cipriani, P.; De Sarro, G.; Giacomelli, R. Biologic drugs in adult onset Still's disease: A systematic review and meta-analysis of observational studies. *Expert Rev. Clin. Immunol.* **2017**, *13*, 1089–1097. [CrossRef]
11. Ruscitti, P.; Cipriani, P.; Di Benedetto, P.; Liakouli, V.; Carubbi, F.; Berardicurti, O.; Ciccia, F.; Guggino, G.; Triolo, G.; Giacomelli, R. Advances in immunopathogenesis of macrophage activation syndrome during rheumatic inflammatory diseases: Toward new therapeutic targets? *Expert Rev. Clin. Immunol.* **2017**, *13*, 1041–1047. [CrossRef] [PubMed]
12. Isaacs, A.; Lindenmann, J. Pillars Article: Virus Interference. I. The Interferon. *Proc. R. Soc. Lond. B Biol. Sci.* **1957**, *147*, 258–267.
13. Pestka, S.; Krause, C.D.; Walter, M.R. Interferons, interferon-like cytokines, and their receptors. *Immunol. Rev.* **2004**, *202*, 8–32. [CrossRef] [PubMed]
14. Wang, B.X.; Fish, E.N. Global virus outbreaks: Interferons as 1st responders. *Semin. Immunol.* **2019**, *43*, 101300. [CrossRef] [PubMed]
15. Kretschmer, S.; Lee-Kirsch, M.A. Type I interferon-mediated autoinflammation and autoimmunity. *Curr. Opin. Immunol.* **2017**, *49*, 96–102. [CrossRef] [PubMed]

16. Ludigs, K.; Parfenov, V.; Du Pasquier, R.A.; Guarda, G. Type I IFN-mediated regulation of IL-1 production in inflammatory disorders. *Cell. Mol. Life Sci.* **2012**, *69*, 3395–3418. [CrossRef] [PubMed]
17. Goodbourn, S.; Didcock, L.; Randall, R.E. Interferons: Cell signalling, immune modulation, antiviral response and virus countermeasures. *J. Gen. Virol.* **2000**, *81*, 2341–2364. [CrossRef]
18. Barrat, F.J.; Crow, M.K.; Ivashkiv, L.B. Interferon target-gene expression and epigenomic signatures in health and disease. *Nat. Immunol.* **2019**, *20*, 1574–1583. [CrossRef]
19. Randall, R.E.; Goodbourn, S. Interferons and viruses: An interplay between induction, signalling, antiviral responses and virus countermeasures. *J. Gen. Virol.* **2008**, *89*, 1–47. [CrossRef]
20. Sadler, A.J.; Williams, B.R.G. Interferon-inducible antiviral effectors. *Nat. Rev. Immunol.* **2008**, *8*, 559–568. [CrossRef]
21. Billiau, A. Anti-inflammatory properties of Type I interferons. *Antivir. Res.* **2006**, *71*, 108–116. [CrossRef]
22. Theofilopoulos, A.N.; Baccala, R.; Beutler, B.; Kono, D.H. Type I Interferons (α/β) in Immunity and Autoimmunity. *Annu. Rev. Immunol.* **2005**, *23*, 307–335. [CrossRef]
23. Guarda, G.; Braun, M.; Staehli, F.; Tardivel, A.; Mattmann, C.; Förster, I.; Farlik, M.; Decker, T.; Du Pasquier, R.A.; Romero, P.; et al. Type I Interferon Inhibits Interleukin-1 Production and Inflammasome Activation. *Immunity* **2011**, *34*, 213–223. [CrossRef] [PubMed]
24. Schindler, R.; Ghezzi, P.; Dinarello, C.A. IL-1 induces IL-IV. IFN-gamma suppresses IL-1 but not lipopolysaccha-ride-induced transcription of IL-1. *J. Immunol.* **1990**, *144*, 2216–2222.
25. Ruscitti, P.; Berardicurti, O.; Di Benedetto, P.; Cipriani, P.; Iagnocco, A.; Shoenfeld, Y.; Giacomelli, R. Severe COVID-19, Another Piece in the Puzzle of the Hyperferritinemic Syndrome. An Immunomodulatory Perspective to Alleviate the Storm. *Front. Immunol.* **2020**, *11*, 1130. [CrossRef] [PubMed]
26. Ruscitti, P.; Bruno, F.; Berardicurti, O.; Acanfora, C.; Pavlych, V.; Palumbo, P.; Conforti, A.; Carubbi, F.; Di Cola, I.; Di Benedetto, P.; et al. Lung involvement in macrophage activation syndrome and severe COVID-19: Results from a cross-sectional study to assess clinical, laboratory and artificial intelligence–radiological differences. *Ann. Rheum. Dis.* **2020**, *79*, 1152–1155. [CrossRef]
27. Ruscitti, P.; Berardicurti, O.; Barile, A.; Cipriani, P.; Shoenfeld, Y.; Iagnocco, A.; Giacomelli, R. Severe COVID-19 and related hyperferritinaemia: More than an innocent bystander? *Ann. Rheum. Dis.* **2020**, *79*, 1515–1516. [CrossRef] [PubMed]
28. Hadjadj, J.; Yatim, N.; Barnabei, L.; Corneau, A.; Boussier, J.; Smith, N.; Péré, H.; Charbit, B.; Bondet, V.; Chenevier-Gobeaux, C.; et al. Impaired type I interferon activity and inflammatory responses in severe COVID-19 patients. *Science* **2020**, *369*, 718–724. [CrossRef]
29. Bastard, P.; Rosen, L.B.; Zhang, Q.; Michailidis, E.; Hoffmann, H.-H.; Zhang, Y.; Dorgham, K.; Philippot, Q.; Rosain, J.; Béziat, V.; et al. Auto-antibodies against type I IFNs in patients with life-threatening COVID-19. *Science* **2020**, *370*, eabd4585. [CrossRef] [PubMed]
30. Han, J.H.; Suh, C.-H.; Jung, J.-Y.; Ahn, M.-H.; Han, M.H.; Kwon, J.E.; Yim, H.; Kim, H.-A. Elevated circulating levels of the interferon-γ–induced chemokines are associated with disease activity and cutaneous manifestations in adult-onset Still's disease. *Sci. Rep.* **2017**, *7*, srep46652. [CrossRef] [PubMed]
31. Canna, S.W.; Wrobel, J.; Chu, N.; Kreiger, P.A.; Paessler, M.; Behrens, E.M. Interferon-γ Mediates Anemia but Is Dispensable for Fulminant Toll-like Receptor 9-Induced Macrophage Activation Syndrome and Hemophagocytosis in Mice. *Arthritis Rheum.* **2013**, *65*, 1764–1775. [CrossRef]
32. Young, H.A.; Bream, J.H. IFN-γ: Recent Advances in Understanding Regulation of Expression, Biological Functions, and Clinical Applications. *Curr. Top. Microbiol. Immunol.* **2007**, *316*, 97–117. [CrossRef] [PubMed]
33. Platanias, L.C. Mechanisms of type-I- and type-II-interferon-mediated signalling. *Nat. Rev. Immunol.* **2005**, *5*, 375–386. [CrossRef]
34. Behrens, E.M.; Canna, S.W.; Slade, K.; Rao, S.; Kreiger, P.A.; Paessler, M.; Kambayashi, T.; Koretzky, G.A. Repeated TLR9 stimulation results in macrophage activation syndrome–like disease in mice. *J. Clin. Investig.* **2011**, *121*, 2264–2277. [CrossRef] [PubMed]
35. Weaver, L.K.; Chu, N.; Behrens, E.M. Interferon-γ–Mediated Immunopathology Potentiated by Toll-Like Receptor 9 Activation in a Murine Model of Macrophage Activation Syndrome. *Arthritis Rheumatol.* **2019**, *71*, 161–168. [CrossRef]
36. Prencipe, G.; Caiello, I.; Pascarella, A.; Grom, A.A.; Bracaglia, C.; Chatel, L.; Ferlin, W.G.; Marasco, E.; Strippoli, R.; de Min, C.; et al. Neutralization of IFN-γ reverts clinical and laboratory features in a mouse model of macrophage activation syndrome. *J. Allergy Clin. Immunol.* **2018**, *141*, 1439–1449. [CrossRef] [PubMed]
37. Ibarra, M.F.; Klein-Gitelman, M.; Morgan, E.; Proytcheva, M.; Sullivan, C.; Morgan, G.; Pachman, L.M.; O'Gorman, M.R.G. Serum Neopterin Levels as a Diagnostic Marker of Hemophagocytic Lymphohistiocytosis Syndrome. *Clin. Vaccine Immunol.* **2011**, *18*, 609–614. [CrossRef]
38. Buatois, V.; Chatel, L.; Cons, L.; Lory, S.; Richard, F.; Guilhot, F.; Johnson, Z.; Bracaglia, C.; De Benedetti, F.; De Min, C.; et al. Use of a mouse model to identify a blood biomarker for IFNγ activity in pediatric secondary hemophagocytic lymphohistiocytosis. *Transl. Res.* **2017**, *180*, 37–52. [CrossRef]
39. Jordan, M.B.; Hildeman, D.; Kappler, J.; Marrack, P. An animal model of hemophagocytic lymphohistiocytosis (HLH): CD8+ T cells and interferon gamma are essential for the disorder. *Blood* **2004**, *104*, 735–743. [CrossRef]
40. Schmid, J.P.; Ho, C.-H.; Chrétien, F.; Lefebvre, J.M.; Pivert, G.; Kosco-Vilbois, M.; Ferlin, W.; Geissmann, F.; Fischer, A.; Basile, G.D.S. Neutralization of IFNγ defeats haemophagocytosis in LCMV-infected perforin- and Rab27a-deficient mice. *EMBO Mol. Med.* **2009**, *1*, 112–124. [CrossRef] [PubMed]

41. Zoller, E.E.; Lykens, J.E.; Terrell, C.E.; Aliberti, J.; Filipovich, A.H.; Henson, P.M.; Jordan, M.B. Hemophagocytosis causes a consumptive anemia of inflammation. *J. Exp. Med.* **2011**, *208*, 1203–1214. [CrossRef]
42. Hatterer, E.; Richard, F.; Malinge, P.; Serge, A.; Startchick, S.; Kosco-Vilbois, M.; Deehan, M.; Ferlin, W.; Guilhot, F. P156 Investigating the novel mechanism of action for NI-0501, a human interferon gamma monoclonal antibody. *Cytokine* **2012**, *59*, 570. [CrossRef]
43. Henter, J.-I.; von Bahr Greenwood, T.; Bergsten, E. Emapalumab in Primary Hemophagocytic Lymphohistiocytosis. *N. Engl. J. Med.* **2020**, *383*, 596–599. [CrossRef]
44. Lounder, D.T.; Bin, Q.; De Min, C.; Jordan, M.B. Treatment of refractory hemophagocytic lymphohistiocytosis with emapalumab despite severe concurrent infections. *Blood Adv.* **2019**, *3*, 47–50. [CrossRef] [PubMed]
45. Merli, P.; Algeri, M.; Gaspari, S.; Locatelli, F. Novel Therapeutic Approaches to Familial HLH (Emapalumab in FHL). *Front. Immunol.* **2020**, *11*, 608492. [CrossRef] [PubMed]
46. Locatelli, F.; Lucarelli, B.; Merli, P. Current and future approaches to treat graft failure after allogeneic hematopoietic stem cell transplantation. *Expert Opin. Pharmacother.* **2013**, *15*, 23–36. [CrossRef] [PubMed]
47. Coccia, E.M.; Severa, M.; Giacomini, E.; Monneron, D.; Remoli, M.E.; Julkunen, I.; Cella, M.; Lande, R.; Uzé, G. Viral infection and Toll-like receptor agonists induce a differential expression of type I and λ interferons in human plasmacytoid and monocyte-derived dendritic cells. *Eur. J. Immunol.* **2004**, *34*, 796–805. [CrossRef]
48. Kotenko, S.V.; Gallagher, G.; Baurin, V.V.; Lewis-Antes, A.; Shen, M.; Shah, N.K.; Langer, J.A.; Sheikh, F.; Dickensheets, H.; Donnelly, R.P. IFN-λs mediate antiviral protection through a distinct class II cytokine receptor complex. *Nat. Immunol.* **2002**, *4*, 69–77. [CrossRef] [PubMed]
49. Bracaglia, C.; Prencipe, G.; De Benedetti, F. Macrophage Activation Syndrome: Different mechanisms leading to a one clinical syndrome. *Pediatr. Rheumatol.* **2017**, *15*, 1–7. [CrossRef] [PubMed]
50. Giacomelli, R.; Sota, J.; Ruscitti, P.; Campochiaro, C.; Colafrancesco, S.; Dagna, L.; Iacono, D.; Iannone, F.; Lopalco, G.; Sfriso, P.; et al. The treatment of adult-onset Still's disease with anakinra, a recombinant human IL-1 receptor antagonist: A systematic review of literature. *Clin. Exp. Rheumatol.* **2020**, *39*, 187–195.
51. Castañeda, S.; Martínez-Quintanilla, D.; Martín-Varillas, J.L.; García-Castañeda, N.; Atienza-Mateo, B.; González-Gay, M.A. Tocilizumab for the treatment of adult-onset Still's disease. *Expert Opin. Biol. Ther.* **2019**, *19*, 273–286. [CrossRef]
52. Grom, A.A.; Ilowite, N.T.; Pascual, V.; Brunner, H.I.; Martini, A.; Lovell, D.J.; Ruperto, N.; Leon, K.; Lheritier, K.; Abrams, K.; et al. Rate and Clinical Presentation of Macrophage Activation Syndrome in Patients With Systemic Juvenile Idiopathic Arthritis Treated With Canakinumab. *Arthritis Rheumatol.* **2016**, *68*, 218–228. [CrossRef] [PubMed]
53. Yokota, S.; Itoh, Y.; Morio, T.; Sumitomo, N.; Daimaru, K.; Minota, S. Macrophage Activation Syndrome in Patients with Systemic Juvenile Idiopathic Arthritis under Treatment with Tocilizumab. *J. Rheumatol.* **2015**, *42*, 712–722. [CrossRef] [PubMed]
54. Behrens, E.M.; Koretzky, G.A. Review: Cytokine Storm Syndrome: Looking Toward the Precision Medicine Era. *Arthritis Rheumatol.* **2017**, *69*, 1135–1143. [CrossRef]
55. Ruscitti, P.; Cipriani, P.; Ciccia, F.; Masedu, F.; Liakouli, V.; Carubbi, F.; Berardicurti, O.; Guggino, G.; Di Benedetto, P.; Di Bartolomeo, S.; et al. Prognostic factors of macrophage activation syndrome, at the time of diagnosis, in adult patients affected by autoimmune disease: Analysis of 41 cases collected in 2 rheumatologic centers. *Autoimmun. Rev.* **2017**, *16*, 16–21. [CrossRef]
56. Ruscitti, P.; Cipriani, P.; Masedu, F.; Iacono, D.; Ciccia, F.; Liakouli, V.; Guggino, G.; Carubbi, F.; Berardicurti, O.; Di Benedetto, P.; et al. Adult-onset Still's disease: Evaluation of prognostic tools and validation of the systemic score by analysis of 100 cases from three centers. *BMC Med.* **2016**, *14*, 1–11. [CrossRef] [PubMed]
57. Berardicurti, O.; Ruscitti, P.; Ursini, F.; D'Andrea, S.; Ciaffi, J.; Meliconi, R.; Iagnocco, A.; Cipriani, P.; Giacomelli, R. Mortal-ity in tocilizumab-treated patients with COVID-19: A systematic review and meta-analysis. *Clin. Exp. Rheumatol.* **2020**, *38*, 1247–1254.
58. Klopfenstein, T.; Zayet, S.; Lohse, A.; Selles, P.; Zahra, H.; Kadiane-Oussou, N.J.; Toko, L.; Royer, P.-Y.; Balblanc, J.-C.; Gendrin, V.; et al. Impact of tocilizumab on mortality and/or invasive mechanical ventilation requirement in a cohort of 206 COVID-19 patients. *Int. J. Infect. Dis.* **2020**, *99*, 491–495. [CrossRef] [PubMed]
59. Maschalidi, S.; Sepulveda, F.E.; Garrigue, A.; Fischer, A.; Basile, G.D.S. Therapeutic effect of JAK1/2 blockade on the manifestations of hemophagocytic lymphohistiocytosis in mice. *Blood* **2016**, *128*, 60–71. [CrossRef]
60. Das, R.; Guan, P.; Sprague, L.; Verbist, K.; Tedrick, P.; An, Q.A.; Cheng, C.; Kurachi, M.; Levine, R.; Wherry, E.J.; et al. Janus kinase inhibition lessens inflammation and ameliorates disease in murine models of hemophagocytic lymphohistiocytosis. *Blood* **2016**, *127*, 1666–1675. [CrossRef]
61. Favoino, E.; Prete, M.; Catacchio, G.; Ruscitti, P.; Navarini, L.; Giacomelli, R.; Perosa, F. Working and safety profiles of JAK/STAT signaling inhibitors. Are these small molecules also smart? *Autoimmun. Rev.* **2021**, *20*, 102750. [CrossRef] [PubMed]
62. Wang, J.; Zhang, R.; Wu, X.; Li, F.; Yang, H.; Liu, L.; Guo, H.; Zhang, X.; Mai, H.; Li, H.; et al. Ruxolitinib-combined doxorubicin-etoposide-methylprednisolone regimen as a salvage therapy for refractory/relapsed haemophagocytic lymphohistiocytosis: A single-arm, multicentre, phase 2 trial. *Br. J. Haematol.* **2021**. [CrossRef]
63. Zhang, Q.; Wei, A.; Ma, H.H.; Zhang, L.; Lian, H.Y.; Wang, D.; Zhao, Y.Z.; Cui, L.; Li, W.J.; Yang, Y.; et al. A pilot study of ruxolitinib as a front-line therapy for 12 children with secondary hemophagocytic lymphohistiocytosis. *Haematologica* **2020**. [CrossRef]
64. Hansen, S.; Alduaij, W.; Biggs, C.M.; Belga, S.; Luecke, K.; Merkeley, H.; Chen, L.Y.C. Ruxolitinib as adjunctive therapy for secondary hemophagocytic lymphohistiocytosis: A case series. *Eur. J. Haematol.* **2021**. [CrossRef] [PubMed]

65. Bode, S.F.; Ammann, S.; Al-Herz, W.; Bataneant, M.; Dvorak, C.C.; Gehring, S.; Gennery, A.; Gilmour, K.C.; Gonzalez-Granado, L.I.; Gross-Wieltsch, U.; et al. The syndrome of hemophagocytic lymphohistiocytosis in primary immunodeficiencies: Implications for differential diagnosis and pathogenesis. *Haematologica* **2015**, *100*, 978–988. [CrossRef] [PubMed]
66. Dorman, S.E.; Picard, C.; Lammas, D.; Heyne, K.; Van Dissel, J.T.; Baretto, R.; Rosenzweig, S.D.; Newport, M.; Levin, M.; Roesler, J.; et al. Clinical features of dominant and recessive interferon γ receptor 1 deficiencies. *Lancet* **2004**, *364*, 2113–2121. [CrossRef]
67. Olbrich, P.; Martínez-Saavedra, M.T.; Pérez-Hurtado, J.M.; Sanchez, C.; Sánchez, B.; Deswarte, C.; Obando, I.; Casanova, J.-L.; Speckmann, C.; Bustamante, J.; et al. Diagnostic and therapeutic challenges in a child with complete Interferon-γ Receptor 1 deficiency. *Pediatr. Blood Cancer* **2015**, *62*, 2036–2039. [CrossRef]

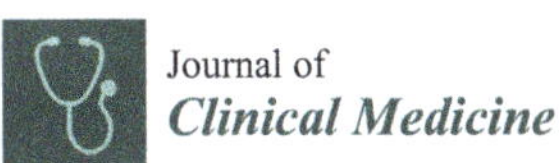
Journal of
Clinical Medicine

MDPI

Review

Adult-Onset Still's Disease: Clinical Aspects and Therapeutic Approach

Stylianos Tomaras [1,*], Carl Christoph Goetzke [2,3,4], Tilmann Kallinich [2,3,4] and Eugen Feist [1]

1 Department of Rheumatology, Helios Clinic Vogelsang-Gommern, 39245 Gommern, Germany; Eugen.Feist@helios-gesundheit.de
2 Department of Pediatrics, Division of Pulmonology, Immunology and Critical Care Medicine, Charité–Universitätsmedizin Berlin, Corporate Member of Freie Universität Berlin, Humboldt-Universität zu Berlin, and Berlin Institute of Health (BIH), 10117 Berlin, Germany; carl-christoph.goetzke@charite.de (C.C.G.); tilmann.kallinich@charite.de (T.K.)
3 German Rheumatism Research Center (DRFZ), Leibniz Association, 10117 Berlin, Germany
4 Berlin Institute of Health, 10178 Berlin, Germany
* Correspondence: Stylianos.Tomaras@helios-gesundheit.de

Abstract: Adult-onset Still's disease (AoSD) is a rare systemic autoinflammatory disease characterized by arthritis, spiking fever, skin rash and elevated ferritin levels. The reason behind the nomenclature of this condition is that AoSD shares certain symptoms with Still's disease in children, currently named systemic-onset juvenile idiopathic arthritis. Immune dysregulation plays a central role in AoSD and is characterized by pathogenic involvement of both arms of the immune system. Furthermore, the past two decades have seen a large body of immunological research on cytokines, which has attributed to both a better understanding of AoSD and revolutionary advances in treatment. Additionally, recent studies have introduced a new approach by grouping patients with AoSD into only two phenotypes: one with predominantly systemic features and one with a chronic articular disease course. Diagnosis presupposes an extensive diagnostic workup to rule out infections and malignancies. The severe end of the spectrum of this disease is secondary haemophagocytic lymphohistiocytosis, better known as macrophage activation syndrome. In this review, we discuss current research conducted on the pathogenesis, diagnosis, classification, biomarkers and complications of AoSD, as well as the treatment strategy at each stage of the disease course. We also highlight the similarities and differences between AoSD and systemic-onset juvenile idiopathic arthritis. There is a considerable need for large multicentric prospective trials.

Keywords: adult-onset Still's disease; autoinflammatory disorder; systemic-onset juvenile idiopathic arthritis; haemophagocytic lymphohistiocytosis; macrophage activation syndrome

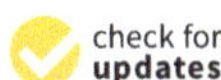

Citation: Tomaras, S.; Goetzke, C.C.; Kallinich, T.; Feist, E. Adult-Onset Still's Disease: Clinical Aspects and Therapeutic Approach. *J. Clin. Med.* **2021**, *10*, 733. https://doi.org/10.3390/jcm10040733

Academic Editor: Ferdinando Nicoletti

Received: 18 December 2020
Accepted: 7 February 2021
Published: 12 February 2021

1. Introduction

Adult-onset Still's disease (AoSD) is a rare systemic autoinflammatory disease characterized by arthritis, spiking fever, skin rash and elevated ferritin levels. The cause of this complex disorder, which usually affects young adults, remains unknown [1]. A London doctor named Bywaters first introduced the term AoSD in the medical literature in 1971 by describing this condition in a small group of 14 patients with an age range of 17 to 35 years [2]. The reason behind the nomenclature of this disease is that AoSD shares certain symptoms with Still's disease in children, which is currently named systemic-onset juvenile idiopathic arthritis (SoJIA). Based on gene expression analysis, some regard SoJIA and AoSD as a single nosological entity [3]. Most recent estimates place AoSD incidence at 0.16 to 0.4 per 100,000 persons [4].

One of the most interesting current discussions in immunology is the newly introduced concept of a "crossroads between autoinflammation and autoimmunity due to the pathogenic involvement of both arms of the immune system" [5]. AoSD, like PFAPA (periodic fever with aphthous stomatitis, pharyngitis and adenitis) and Behçet's disease, is a complex disorder with malfunctioning dysregulated immune system. On the one hand, it lacks the classical characteristics of autoimmune diseases, such as autoantibodies, but on the other hand, it has negative genetic testing in family histories, which is opposite to other autoinflammatory conditions [6].

The past two decades have seen a large body of immunological research on cytokines, which has attributed to both a better understanding of AoSD and significant advances in treatment. One major problem is that although biological drugs have made revolutionary changes in the management of a range of rheumatic conditions, many patients with AoSD are not benefiting from most of them [7]. In addition, every rheumatologist with a patient who had a life-threatening cytokine storm during macrophage activation syndrome (MAS) has deep respect for AoSD.

The goal of our paper is to summarize the current (2020) state of knowledge on the pathogenesis, diagnosis, classification, biomarkers and complications of AoSD, as well as the treatment strategy at each stage of the disease course.

2. Autoinflammation and Autoimmunity

Autoimmunity was, historically, defined as a dysregulation of the adaptive immune system, exclusively involving B and T lymphocytes and leading to the production of autoantibodies directed against self. Autoinflammation, on the other hand, was strictly separated from autoimmunity and was previously considered to have a solely innate autoimmune aetiology. Recent studies on pattern recognition receptors (PRRs) were the breakthrough discovery that changed the way we approach these two phenomena and elucidated the pathology of a group of disorders where both arms interfere and contribute to the inflammatory response [8].

Autoinflammation in periodic fever syndromes is caused by an inborn error of the innate immune system that results in the perturbation of pattern recognition receptors (PRRs), such as the leucine-rich repeat containing family (NLR), leading to an inappropriate chain reaction towards both pathogen-associated molecular patterns (PAMPs) and damage-associated molecular patterns molecules released from injured tissues (DAMPs) [9].

In concert with this theory, genetic errors in the NLR pathway can trigger the onset of Crohn's disease, a very well-known disorder that was classified as an autoimmune disease until recently. Currently, Crohn's disease is considered an autoimmune disease with a prevalent autoinflammatory pathogenesis [10]. Moreover, a small subgroup of patients with rheumatoid arthritis show systemic inflammatory symptoms, such as fever and serositis, although this disease is not supposed to have a coexistent autoinflammatory background [11].

AoSD belongs to this group of disorders and is thought to be "the archetype of non-familial, or sporadic, systemic autoinflammatory disorders" [12].

2.1. *Pathogenesis Part I: Who Started the Fire*

The exact underlying cause of AoSD is not fully understood. We still do not know what exactly triggers DAMPs and PAMPs.

The causal inferences between genetics and AoSD are controversial. Human genetic factors apparently contribute to SoJIA in children, whereas the underlying genomic susceptibility in the adult form is unclear [13].

On the other hand, there is a high degree of similarity between infections and the onset of AoSD for fever, leucocytosis and elevated C-reactive protein (CRP). Logically, many investigators focused on identifying infectious triggers and described the occurrence of AoSD after infection with cytomegalovirus, Epstein-Barr, influenza, *Mycoplasma*, hepatitis, etc. [4]. We now know that cytomegalovirus may also trigger a relapse of AoSD [14]. Blood cultures and polymerase chain reaction (PCR) tests may, therefore, be useful for a differential diagnosis, although no specific diagnostic algorithms exist to date. It is currently still not clear which pathogenic viruses and bacteria should be included in the diagnostic workup. Remarkably, procalcitonin is not a reliable marker, since patients suffering from AoSD can show elevated procalcitonin levels without confirmed infection [15].

Other studies have examined the relationship between cancer and AoSD [16] and reported malignancy-mediated autoinflammation in breast cancer [17], thyroid cancer [18], melanoma, lung cancer and haematological malignancies, mostly lymphomas [19]. Despite increasing sophistication in the diagnostic workup for possible malignancies, there are no universally accepted guidelines for patients with AoSD, which makes daily clinical work more difficult. Positron emission tomography and computed tomography (PET/CT) scanning could be useful in difficult case scenarios to rule out solid tumours or large vessel vasculitis mimicking AoSD, but it is not routine practice because of the relatively high costs [20]. Bone marrow examination can rule out a haematologic malignancy or support the diagnosis of MAS.

In short, AoSD is a diagnosis of exclusion. The process of eliminating similar medical conditions is most likely to take a considerable amount of time. Table 1 summarizes the broad spectrum of differential diagnoses.

Table 1. Differential diagnosis of AoSD [12].

Infections	Tuberculosis, toxoplasmosis, brucellosis, yersiniosis HIV, Epstein-Barr, cytomegalovirus, hepatitis, herpes, influenza, parvovirus B19, measles, rubella
Malignancies	Lymphoma, Castleman disease, myeloproliferative disorders, melanoma and colon, breast, lung, kidney and thyroid cancer In pediatrics also: leukemia
Systemic diseases	Systemic lupus erythematosus, idiopathic inflammatory myopathies, vasculitis, hereditary autoinflammatory syndromes, neutrophilic dermatosis, Sweet syndrome, reactive arthritis, sarcoidosis, Schnitzler syndrome, Kikuchi-Fujimoto disease In pediatrics also: other types of inflammatory arthritis

2.2. Pathogenesis Part II: What Keeps the Fire Burning

PAMPs and DAMPs stimulate macrophages and neutrophils, leading to activation of specific inflammasomes via Toll-like receptors. Inflammasomes are multiprotein units that act as catalysts by activating the caspase pathway immediately after they come into contact with damage or illness. Caspase enzymes lead to overproduction of IL-1β, the hallmark of AoSD, and IL-18. IL-1β and IL-18 then promote further abnormal inflammation by several cytokine bursts, including IL-6, IL-8, IL-17, IL-18 and TNF-α. At this point, the patient is experiencing heavy systemic symptoms [21–24].

Furthermore, activated macrophages stimulate the release of excessive levels of ferritin. In addition to functioning as an iron storage molecule, ferritin also plays a central role in many conditions with an amplified inflammatory response, currently called "hyperferritinemic syndromes", such as AoSD, MAS, catastrophic antiphospholipid syndrome and septic shock [25]. Ferritin has a key role in inflammation by promoting cytokine production, and at the same time, cytokines can regulate ferritin synthesis.

Moreover, analysis of accumulating data over the past years showed an enhancement of neutrophil extracellular traps (NET) in AoSD, which promotes the acute phase response by activating the NLRP3 inflammasome [26].

Additionally, dysfunctional natural killer (NK) cells, elevated T-helper Th1 and Th17 cells, enhanced IFN-γ and IL-17 levels, different alarmins, such as the S100 proteins, significantly higher IFN-γ-producing Th1 cells and Th1/Th2 cells ratios and advanced glycation end products complete the proinflammatory environment in many ways, which favours the abnormal response of the human immune system [27–29].

2.3. Pathogenesis Part III: Why Is Firefighting so Hard

The massive release of cytokines in patients with AoSD over a prolonged period of time can be fatal. Deficient resolution of inflammation may be mostly due to failures in immune system self-regulation. Deficient regulatory T cells, decreased or defective NK cells, insufficient production of anti-inflammatory cytokines or problematic circulation of advanced glycation end products (AGEs) have been hypothesized to cause these complex problems [30–33]. Surprisingly, the anti-inflammatory cytokine IL-10 levels are elevated during the higher state of inflammation and correlate with disease activity in AoSD [34].

3. Clinical Symptoms

Nonspecific symptoms such as fever, sore throat or arthralgia that usually bring patients with AoSD to medical attention are rather misleading. The similarities with an infection often obscure the diagnosis and lead to empirical antibiotic therapies. Italian and French studies have shown a diagnostic delay ranging from 1.5 to 4 years between the onset of symptoms and the final diagnosis of AoSD [4,35]. When all conservative treatments fail, practitioners realize they are facing a prolonged febrile illness without an obvious aetiology. The diagnostic journey then begins.

In a large retrospective study, which set out to analyse 1641 patients with fever of unknown origin (FUO), AoSD was responsible for 5.4% of cases [36]. Overall, rheumatic diseases comprise approximately 30% of cases with FUO, with AoSD being the most frequent group [37].

Fever is a cardinal symptom in AoSD and occurs in 60 to 100% of cases. Patients typically report two fever spikes daily, one in the morning and one in the evening, usually >39 °C. In 60 to 80% of patients, a macular or maculopapular evanescent salmon-pink skin rash on the proximal limbs and trunk accompanies high fever. Interestingly, this rash can disappear completely during afebrile intervals. Permanent skin rashes, on the other hand, presenting with urticaria, are warning signs for haematological complications. Both fever and skin rash are correlated with disease activity. Along with other nonspecific constitutional symptoms, such as weight loss and malaise, patients with active AoSD feel sick and miserable [1,4,38].

Arthralgia is also a cardinal symptom that is observed in 70 to 100% of patients, often accompanied by polyarthritis involving small joints, imitating rheumatoid arthritis. Some patients with chronic articular AoSD show severe osteodestructive features, which cause ankyloses and functional disability [39].

Other concomitant symptoms, such as pharyngitis, odynophagia, lymphadenopathy, splenomegaly, myalgia, pleuritis or abdominal pain vary from person to person. National registries and patient cohorts are a major determinant for successful characterization of clinical phenotypes in the field of rare diseases, such as AoSD. Table 2 shows the summary statistics of some observational studies and illustrates the heterogeneity of AoSD and SoJIA.

Table 2. Comparison of clinical features (%) of patients with AoSD and SoJIA.

	Di Benedetto P, Cipriani P, Iacono D, et al. (2020) [40]	**Hu QY, Zeng T, Sun CY et al. (2019) [41]**	**Sfriso P, Priori R, Valesini G, et al. (2016) [35]**	**Gerfaud-Valentin M, Maucort-Boulch D, Hot A, et al. (2014) [42]**	**Fautrel B. et al. (2002) [43]**	**Tsai H. et al. (2012) [44]**	**Behrens E. D. et al. (2008) [45]**
Case number	147	517	245	57	72	28	136
Nationality	Italy	China	Italy	France	France	Taiwan	United States
Female	39.5	72	47.3	53	nk	53.6	54
Average age at onset	45.2	37.7	38.8	36	35.2	8.7	5.7 Median 2
Fever $\geq$ 39 °C	100	91.3	92.6	95	84.7	100	98
Rash	74.8	79.9	67.7	77	70.8	67.9	81

Table 2. *Cont.*

	Di Benedetto P, Cipriani P, Iacono D, et al. (2020) [40]	Hu QY, Zeng T, Sun CY et al. (2019) [41]	Sfriso P, Priori R, Valesini G, et al. (2016) [35]	Gerfaud-Valentin M, Maucort-Boulch D, Hot A, et al. (2014) [42]	Fautrel B. et al. (2002) [43]	Tsai H. et al. (2012) [44]	Behrens E. D. et al. (2008) [45]
Arthralgia/arthritis	88.4	73.1	93	95	88.8	89.3	88
Sore throat	56.5	60.5	62	53	52.7	nk	nk
Lymphadenopathy	54.4	51.1	60.4 *	60	44.4 *	46.4	31
Hepatomegaly	nk	6.6	41.7	21	nk	nk	~7
Splenomegaly	66.7	34.4	60.4 *	30	44.4 *	21.4 *	~5
Pericarditis	21.1	14.1	17.3	19	20.8	nk	10
Pleuritis	19.7	nk	nk	18	nk	7.1 *	nk
Myalgia	64.6	32.5	nk	44	nk	nk	nk
AoSD pneumonia	12.2	nk	nk	nk	nk	nk	nk
Abdominal pain	13.6	nk	nk	18	nk	nk	nk

nk = not known. * reported together as single variable.

4. Laboratory Findings and Biomarkers

There are no pathognomonic laboratory findings in AoSD. Negative acute phase proteins allow exclusion of an active AoSD. Laboratory tests will almost always detect high levels of both CRP and leukocytes (>10,000/mm^3), yet highly elevated leukocyte counts of >50,000/mm^3 are usually associated with haematological malignancies. In contrast, leukopenia is related to an unfortunate course of disease with complications such as reactive haemophagocytic lymphohistiocytosis or thrombotic angiopathy.

Diagnostic workup should also include liver function tests, as nearly 50% of the patients show elevated transaminases, mostly due to non-steroidal anti-inflammatory drugs (NSAIDs) or antibiotics and rarely due to fulminant hepatitis [35].

Moreover, ferritin is a very helpful serologic marker for diagnosis and follow-up, especially when it increases >5-fold. Current propositions for hyperferritinaemia in AoSD include increased production by macrophages, liver and erythrocytes due to parallel erythrophagocytosis [46–49]. Furthermore, high circulating ferritin has a positive feedback mechanism that can further exacerbate its own inflammatory properties [24]. Ferritin contains two types of subunits: heavy (H) and light (L). In the bone marrow of patients with MAS, high levels of H-ferritin are found, and they correlate with disease severity. Correspondingly, lymph nodes and skin are infiltrated with CD68/H-ferritin cells.

Several studies have pointed out the diagnostic utility of glycosylated ferritin (GF). A low percentage of GF is significantly related to amplifying inflammation in AoSD. A combined laboratory approach of GF <20% with ferritin levels >5-fold can optimize the diagnosis and yield a sensitivity of 43.2% and specificity of 92.9% [47]. Low GF can also be used as a biomarker for haemophagocytosis [50]. Remarkably, GF does not perform well in the assessment of disease activity in AoSD, since it remains low for several weeks or months after flare up [51]. Unfortunately, measurement of GF is not a common marker in routine laboratory diagnostics so far and few studies have been published supporting its relevance.

Serum cytokine levels, such as IL-1, IL-6 or IL-18, could be helpful to diagnose AoSD, but they are not yet recommended for routine practice [52–54].

Furthermore, studies investigating the members of the S100 protein family and how they interact with proinflammatory signalling pathways show that they could be a potential biomarker. However, more studies are needed to consider them a routine test [55,56].

High levels of serum amyloid A can predict the development of systemic amyloidosis [53].

5. Diagnostic Criteria

During the diagnostic process, most physicians use the Yamaguchi and Fautrel classification criteria for AoSD in actual practice, although they are primarily designed to select patients for clinical trials (Table 3).

Table 3. Classification criteria for AoSD and the revised definition of the International League of Associations for Rheumatology (ILAR) diagnostic criteria for SoJIA.

Criteria	1992 Yamaguchi [57]	2002 Fautrel [47]	2004 ILAR [58]
Major	• Fever ≥39 °C lasting ≥1 week • Arthralgia or arthritis ≥ 2 weeks • Typical rash • Leucocytosis ≥ 10,000/µL with ≥80% neutrophils	• Spiking fever ≥39 °C • Arthralgia • Transient erythema • ≥80% granulocytes • Pharyngitis • Glycosylated ferritin ≤20%	• Arthritis in at least one joint • Fever >2 weeks, daily for at least 3 days
Minor	• Sore throat • Lymphadenopathy • Hepatomegaly or splenomegaly • Abnormal liver function tests • Negative rheumatoid factor and anti-nuclear antibodies	• Maculopapular rash • Leucocytes ≥10,000/µL	• Evanescent erythematous rash • Generalized lymph node enlargement • Hepatomegaly • Splenomegaly • Serositis
Exclusion criteria	Infection, malignancy or other rheumatic disorders than mimic AoSD	None	Other forms of JIA must be excluded
Algorithm	Five criteria, at least two major ones AND no exclusion criteria	Four major criteria OR three majors with two minor ones	All major criteria AND at least one minor criteria
Sensitivity	96.2%	80.6%	Not applicable
Specificity	92.1%	98.5%	Not applicable

One major limitation of the Yamaguchi criteria set is its exclusion criteria. This approach is not beneficial in clinical practice, as it presupposes an extensive diagnostic workup, whereas the needed laboratory and imaging tests are not specified. Another problem is that helpful biomarkers such as ferritin are not included. In contrast, Fautrel's criteria provide a core set without exclusion criteria and refer to the usability of glycosylated ferritin as a diagnostic marker.

To validate the performance of the Fautrel criteria in 2018 in a different cohort than the original in 2002, a French working group included 54 patients with AoSD and 278 controls. The sensitivity was 87.0%, the specificity was 97.8%, and the positive and negative predictive values were 88.7% and 97.5%, respectively. In the same study, the Yamaguchi criteria (without exclusion restrictions) performed better and showed a sensitivity of 96.3% and a specificity 98.9%, with positive and negative predictive values of 94.5% and 99.3%, respectively [59].

6. The Course of the Disease Splits in Two

Several disease patterns have been observed in patient cohort studies. For approximately 19–44% of affected patients, AoSD has a monocyclic course without relapses. A polycyclic course is identified in 10–41% of affected patients and is characterized by unpredictable periods of exacerbation after a few months or years. Approximately 35–57% of affected patients show a chronic progressive course, which is the most frequent one, which is characterized by steady progression, continuous inflammation and often erosive joint involvement [60].

However, recent studies have introduced a new approach by grouping patients with AoSD into only two phenotypes: one with predominantly systemic features and one with a chronic articular disease course. Treatment of the systemic form is different from the treatment used for adults with progressive joint involvement, due to a higher inflammatory status and possible multi-organ damage with haematological complications. The non-systemic subgroup, on the other hand, may begin with systemic symptoms and evolve to a disease resembling rheumatoid arthritis at the end stage. This phenotypic dichotomy may also simplify the design of future clinical trials [4,61–64].

Predictive factors for the systemic subset of AoSD include high fever (>39 °C) and high levels of liver enzymes or CRP, while female sex, polyarthritis at disease onset and steroid dependence are associated with the chronic articular subgroup [65,66]. To close, this simplified theory of dichotomous disease courses is supported, at least partially, by studies on cytokine profiles and responses to biologic treatments [65,67,68].

7. Complications

7.1. Cytokine Storm

The most severe complication of the spectrum of Still's disease and AoSD is secondary haemophagocytic lymphohistiocytosis (HLH), better known as MAS. The term cytokine storm best describes excessive cytokinaemia during MAS. The prevalence varies from 10 to 15% and is associated with high mortality [64]. Possible triggers such as infections or medications in combination with uncontrolled and prolonged inflammation in patients with genetic predisposition may lead to this life-threatening condition [69–71].

Researchers from France developed diagnostic criteria for MAS to shorten the critical process of reaching an accurate diagnosis. In this multicentre retrospective cohort study of 312 patients, the diagnosis relied on a set of nine variables: known underlying immunosuppression, high temperature, organomegaly, triglyceride, ferritin, serum aspartate transaminase, fibrinogen levels, cytopenia and haemophagocytosis features on bone marrow aspirate (Table 4). Based on a scoring system, physicians can then calculate the "HScore" and assess the probability of the patient having MAS. MAS can be ruled out with an HScore of ≤90 MAS, whereas an HScore ≥ 250 has a diagnostic accuracy of >99% [72].

Table 4. HScore † ‡ for diagnosis of haemophagocytic lymphohistiocytosis [72].

Variable	Number of Points
Temperature	
<38.4 °C	0
38.4–39.4 °C	33
>39.4 °C	49
Organomegaly	
None	0
Hepatomegaly or splenomegaly	23
Hepatomegaly and splenomegaly	38
Cytopenia	
One lineage	0
Two lineages	24
Three lineages	34
Triglycerides (mmol/L)	
<1.5	0
1.5–4.0	44
>4.0	64
Fibrinogen (g/L)	
>2.5	0
≤2.5	30

Table 4. *Cont.*

Variable	Number of Points
Ferritin (ng/mL)	
<2000	0
2000–6000	35
>6000	50
Serum aspartate aminotransferase (IU/L)	
<30	0
≥30	19
Haemophagocytosis on bone marrow aspirate	
No	0
Yes	35
Known immunosuppression	
No	0
Yes	18

† The probability of having haemophagocytic syndrome ranges from <1% with an HScore of ≤90 to >99% with an HScore of ≥250. ‡ The HScore is freely available online (http://saintantoine.aphp.fr/score/ (accessed on 19 September 2020)).

Knowing how to diagnose MAS could be life-saving because of its short therapeutic window of opportunity. Even if the full diagnostic criteria are not met, treatment should be started as soon as possible to silence the cytokine storm and prevent hyperinflammatory complications, critical illness and death. Cross-specialty collaboration is the key to success.

Once a diagnosis of MAS has been made, serum ferritin concentrations are useful for monitoring disease activity and response to treatment. Very high peak levels as well as a limited decrease (less than 50% from first measurement near diagnosis) after initiation of treatment are associated with high mortality in paediatric patients [73].

7.2. Parenchymal Lung Disease and PAH

The latest research in paediatrics reported lung involvement in children with SoJIA, a rare but potentially fatal complication [74,75]. Correspondingly, 12% of the 147 adult patients with AoSD included in Gruppo Italiano di Ricerca in Reumatologia Clinica e Sperimentale (GIRRCS) cohort have been diagnosed with parenchymal lung disease. Older age and higher inflammation status were independent predictors. Overall, the survival rate was significantly decreased in this subgroup [76]. The reason behind the high mortality rate is the association with MAS. Lung involvement seems to trigger accelerating mechanisms of inflammation. This observation reflects the data about the occurrence of MAS in children with lung damage [77,78]. Bronchiolitis and nonspecific interstitial pneumonia are the most common histological patterns [79]. Pulmonary hypertension in AoSD is a rare complication but it represents a life-threatening condition with a mortality of about 40%. This disorder mostly affects women and leads to rapidly progressive respiratory distress [80,81].

7.3. Coagulation Disorders

Disseminated intravascular coagulation (DIC) is a rare complication in patients, mainly in those with the systemic phenotype of AoSD and it occurs in 1–5% of cases. Cutaneous or mucosal bleeding and/or signs of thromboembolism are suggestive of DIC [82]. The DIC-Score by the International Society on Thrombosis and Haemostasis (ISTH) criteria is shown in Table 5.

Table 5. DIC-Score by ISTH [83].

Variables	Points
Platelet count (/μL)	
50,000–100,000	1
<50,000	2
Prolongation of PT (seconds)	
3–6	1
>6	2
Fibrinogen (mg/dL)	
<100	1
D-dimer (μg/mL)	
0.5–1	1
1–2	2
>2	3
If score ≥ 5: compatible with DIC. Repeat daily. If score < 5: suggestive of DIC. Repeat after 1–2 days.	

DIC = Disseminated intravascular coagulation, ISTH = International Society on Thrombosis and Haemostasis.

Moreover, thrombotic microangiopathy (TMA) in the context of hyperinflammatory conditions, such as AoSD, is another feared coagulation disorder. TMA causes small vessel thrombosis and could lead to strokes or multi-organ failure. Acute blurred vision may be an early symptom of ocular involvement in TMA [84].

8. Treatment Management

The establishment of a default management strategy for rare diseases such as AoSD is not easy (Figure 1). Steroids and NSAIDs are almost always the first-line treatment regimen in both clinical phenotypes; unfortunately, they have a poor overall response. To achieve satisfactory control of the disease, many physicians offer their patients disease modifying antirheumatic drugs (DMARDs) such as methotrexate, ciclosporin or azathioprine, although there is no robust evidence to support this practice [85]. However, the anticipated response rate in patients with the chronic articular phenotype of AoSD should be higher when the therapy protocol for rheumatoid arthritis is adopted [67].

Moreover, systematic reviews on AoSD are problematic because of the heterogeneity of clinical disease courses, the different organ manifestations and used treatment approaches. There is a great need for large multicentric prospective trials.

8.1. Anti-TNF Therapy

In contrast to numerous trials in the field of rheumatoid arthritis and spondyloarthritis, the efficacy of TNFα blockers in AoSD is controversial. They should probably only be prescribed for patients in the end stage of the articular type to inhibit erosion progression [86–88].

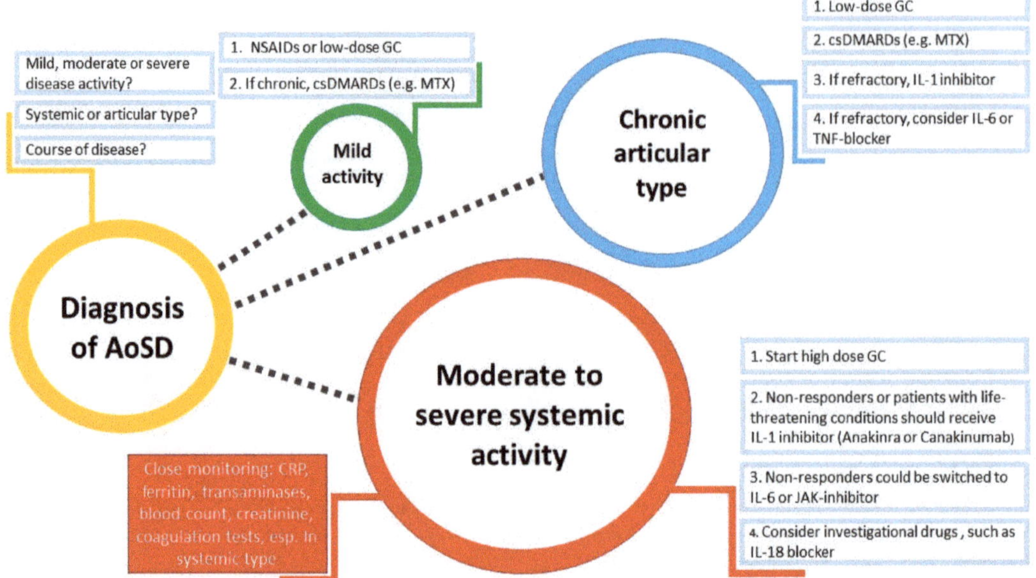

Figure 1. Suggested strategy for management of AoSD. Diameter of the circles represents the challenge in clinical practice. AoSD = Adult-onset Still's disease, NSAIDs = Non-steroidal anti-inflammatory drugs, MTX = Methotrexate, csDMARDs = Conventional synthetic disease-modifying antirheumatic drugs, IL = Interleukin, TNF = Tumor necrosis factor, JAK = Janus kinase, GC = Glucocorticoids, CRP = C-reactive protein.

8.2. Anti-IL-1 Therapy

Evidence over the last twenty years has explained the central functional role of IL-1 in the pathogenesis of autoinflammatory conditions. Anakinra, a recombinant humanized IL-1 receptor antagonist, is the first choice for AoSD, yet patients with mainly articular phenotypes do not always benefit. Anakinra is licensed for subcutaneous use for systemic juvenile idiopathic arthritis, periodic fever syndromes, rheumatoid arthritis and AoSD (only by the European Medicines Agency) [12,89–91]. Rapid improvement in the systemic features of AoSD following anakinra administration was well demonstrated in a recent large observational retrospective multicentre study in 140 Italian patients [92].

However, the slower absorption of the subcutaneous route is a major disadvantage when facing a cytokine storm in patients with critical illness. This issue was addressed in a study with 46 patients with MAS, where 18 of them were treated with intravenous anakinra. Its pharmacokinetic and safety profile looks promising, yet the dosing scheme remains unclear. The authors concluded that intravenous anakinra could be used as a first-line treatment in MAS [69].

The other strategy for inhibiting IL-1 that has been intensively studied to date consists of a fully human antibody against IL-1β, canakinumab [93–95]. Canakinumab is currently licensed for AoSD, SoJIA, periodic fever syndromes and gout [96]. The CONSIDER study (Canakinumab for Treatment of Adult-Onset Still's Disease to Achieve Reduction of Arthritic Manifestation), a phase II, randomized, double-blind, placebo-controlled, multicentre, investigator-initiated trial was terminated prematurely and did not reach the primary outcome (ΔDAS28 > 1.2). However, this trial demonstrated that in AoSD, treatment with canakinumab yielded improvement in several clinical aspects of the disease, while showing a favourable safety profile [97–99].

The efficacy and safety of another IL-inhibitor, rilonacept, was analyzed in a randomized, double-blind, placebo-controlled trial with seventy-one children with SoJIA. Rilonacept showed some benefit with an acceptable safety profile, although the primary end point was not met [100].

8.3. Anti-IL-6 Therapy

Tocilizumab, a humanized monoclonal antibody against the IL-6 receptor, showed promising results in the treatment of AoSD in a pilot study. Both the systemic features and the arthritic manifestations improved [101–103]. A 2018 meta-analysis investigated the benefits of tocilizumab in patients with AoSD and definitely showed signals of efficacy compared to conventional therapy regimes and was well acceptable in terms of safety [104]. The other IL-6 receptor antagonist, sarilumab, was reported to be effective as a steroid-sparing agent [105].

8.4. JAK Inhibitors

Contrary to anti-IL-1 and anti-IL-6 therapies, Janus kinase (JAK) inhibitors block a wide variety of proinflammatory cells and can therefore become a very promising treatment approach in heterogeneous disorders, such as AoSD. In a study with 14 patients with refractory AoSD, seven of them achieved complete remission under tofacitinib, while six responded partially. This trial also showed the steroid sparing effect of tofacitinib, especially in the articular phenotype [106]. Furthermore, a reported case of AoSD complicated by MAS describes remission with tofacitinib after failure of response to tocilizumab [107]. Another case report describes successful treatment of AoSD with tofacitinib in a HIV-positive female patient [108]. Baricitinib could also be an option, although current data are debatable [109].

8.5. Anti-IL-18 Therapy

Given the new insights into the pathogenic role of IL-18 in AoSD, this cytokine quickly became a drug target. Tadekinig alpha, a recombinant human IL-18 binding protein, demonstrated its potential effectiveness and acceptable safety profile in a phase 2 multicentred European study in 2018. The low number of participants (21) and the short period of treatment duration (12 weeks) could be considered limiting factors [110].

9. Still's Disease in Children and Adults—Is There a Difference?

SoJIA was first described by Georg F. Still in 1897 as a novel disease entity differing from other forms of juvenile onset arthritis [111]. As AoSD and SoJIA share certain symptoms, it is worth investigating whether AoSD is a continuum of SoJIA in adult patients.

A closer look at the age-dependent disease prevalence gives first indications that the two entities may be a continuum of one and the same entity. Unpublished data from German registries for pediatric and adult patients with rheumatic diseases yields a continuous decline of SoJIA prevalence by age with highest prevalence in age group 0–4 years. The prevalence in the 15–20 years old patients closely corresponds to the prevalence of young adults with AoSD, which also further declines by age.

Even on closer inspection, SoJIA and AoSD show multiple other similarities. The differences described below may be based primarily on different research strategies as well as the inclusion of various patient cohorts and therefore do not contradict the thesis of a common disease continuum. Understanding the pathology and clinical manifestation of both entities should therefore be considered synergistically to identify age-dependent differences and define age-independent similarities.

Investigating drivers of paediatric diseases frequently focus on underlying genetic conditions. Therefore, multiple genome association studies have been performed to answer whether the fire ignites particularly easily in the presence of a certain genotype. First genetic studies on SoJIA were already published in 1976 and showed that SoJIA differs from other forms of JIA [112]. More recently a locus on chromosome 1 and loci within the HLA class II and III region on chromosome 6 have been associated with SoJIA [113]. Furthermore, HLA-DRB1*11 was found to be a major risk factor for SoJIA indicating the involvement of antigen-specific T cells [114]. In combination, these studies suggest a complex pathogenesis with multiple levels of genetic diversity. Furthermore, there is also emerging evidence for a rare familial monogenic form of SoJIA, which is associated with mutations in *LACC1* leading to a reduced autophagy flux in primary macrophages [115–117].

In SoJIA, a model assumes a biphasic disease course with an initial systemic phase dominated by fever, followed by an intermediate phase and finally a phase in which arthritis is in the foreground [118]. Especially during the early phase of SoJIA PAMPs and DAMPs, prominently S100A8/9 and SA10012 initiate a fever-syndrome with signs of autoinflammation [119,120]. In this respect, it was shown that leukocytes from SoJIA patients overreact to TLR4 and TLR 8 stimuli leading to a strongly increased IL-1 production by monocytes [121]. In a landmark paper, Pascual et al. described that sera derived from patients with SoJIA can induce–amongst others–the transcription of IL-1 in cells derived from healthy controls [122]. Additionally, unstimulated cells from patients with active SoJIA and AOSD express genes related to innate immunity including members of the IL-1 pathway [3,122]. This perspective is broadened by recent work, which demonstrate an association of high expression of certain transcription factors with early active SoJIA, indicating a role of B-cell activation and autoimmunity during that phase of disease [123].

Similar to AoSD it is suggested, that this first autoinflammatory phase is furthermore sustained by IL-18 and IL-6 [124]. IL-18 is part of the IL-1-family and induces the expression of Interferon-γ mainly by cytotoxic lymphocytes, which robustly express the IL-18 receptor. The naturally occurring antagonist IL-18 binding protein (IL-18BP) which is again induced by Interferon-γ controls the action of IL-18 [125].

Due to their central role in the differentiation of Th17 cells, the two cytokines IL-1β and IL-6 may be a key to understand the disease evolution of SoJIA [126,127]. Two recent studies analysing cells from patients with SoJIA give evidence that an IL-1-blockade prevents and/or reverses the differentiation of ɣ/δ T cells and regulatory T cells into a Th17 phenotype [128,129].

A central role of an impaired NK cell function in the perpetuation of SoJIA pathogenesis has been studied by analysing patient's cells as well as applying a corresponding murine model [130–132].

Differently from adult patients, MAS is well known in paediatric patients. The transition from SoJIA to MAS (for classification criteria see Table 6) is sought to be initiated by the constant inflammatory trigger and often corresponds to a massive increase in IFNγ. Furthermore, as effective treatment of SoJIA using IL-1 and IL-6 blockade does not completely protect from MAS in these patients further mechanism must be involved in the development of MAS [78]. There is evidence, that a major driver for MAS is free IL-18 overcoming the inhibitory levels of IL-18-binding protein [125]. The close link of SoJIA to MAS is further demonstrated by whole-exome-sequencing showing overlaps between both diseases [133].

Table 6. Classification criteria for MAS in SoJIA (EULAR/ACR-approved [134]).

Major criteria	• Febrile patient with (suspected) SoJIA • Serum ferritin > 684 ng/mL
Minor criteria	• Platelet count $\leq$ 181 $\times$ 109/L • Aspartate aminotransferase > 48 U/L • Triglycerides > 156 mg/dL • Fibrinogen $\leq$ 360 mg/gL
Algorithm	Both major criteria with at least two minor criteria

Clinical presentation can vary but most patients initially present very ill. The most common initial clinical features are fever, (most commonly a polyarticular) arthritis, and rash. Especially a fever pattern with one or two peaks on a daily basis, with rapid return to baseline is highly suggestive. The fever is classically accompanied by a discrete, salmon pink, erythematous macular rash. Furthermore, inflammatory affections of all organs can occur [135]. Emerging evidence for a lung disease, a rare but life-threatening complication in SoJIA patients comes from a multicentre retrospective study. The found pathology was mostly an alveolar proteinosis and lung disease was associated with macrophage dysfunction. Contrary to AoSD very young age was a predictor and despite a suggested macrophage dysfunction it is not associated with MAS in paediatric patients [74].

Similar to the AoSD classification criteria from Yamaguchi [57] and from Fautrel [43] the International League of Associations for Rheumatology (ILAR) defined criteria for the diagnosis of SoJIA (see Table 3) [58]. As the paediatric criteria require the presence of an arthritis a subset of SoJIA patients can have a severe delay in diagnosis as the systemic symptoms can proceed the arthritis by up to 10 years [135]. Retrospective testing of the Yamaguchi criteria in paediatric patients with suspected SoJIA with and without arthritis has yielded promising results especially for SoJIA patients with a delay in onset of arthritis [136]. Combining both sets of criteria might improve the time until diagnosis, especially in patients with a long time between systemic onset and beginning of arthritis [137]. A treatment window targeting the cytokine driven first phase of the disease might otherwise close [138].

Consensus-based treatment strategies exist from the German Society for Pediatric Rheumatology (GKJR) (Figure 2) [139] and the North American Childhood Arthritis and Rheumatology Research Alliance (CARRA) [140]. These are summarized as "treatment-to-target". The main goal is achieving a clinical remission with the secondary goal of avoiding long-term glucocorticoids [139]. According to the CARRA and GKJR consensus statements methotrexate therapy is an option in articular diseases courses, either as sole long-term or adjunctive therapy. Besides glucocorticoids, IL-1 [141] and IL-6-receptor-targeting drugs are established cornerstones of modern therapeutical approaches [142]. The later ones have been proven successful in randomized trials [141–143]. Use of biologics is already suggested for initial treatment as monotherapy [139], whilst only results for initial treatment with anakinra have been published [144]. Furthermore, current data from the German National Pediatric Rheumatologic Database shows an increased usage of these biologicals as well as an improved initial response to treatment [145]. Other explanations for this effect could be an improved access to specialized care and a more rapid start of treatment. Furthermore, patient recruitment for a trial with the Janus-kinase bariticinib is active (ClinicalTrials.gov Identifier: NCT04088396). There is also an ongoing trial of tofacitinib in children with SoJIA (ClinicalTrials.gov Identifier: NCT03000439).

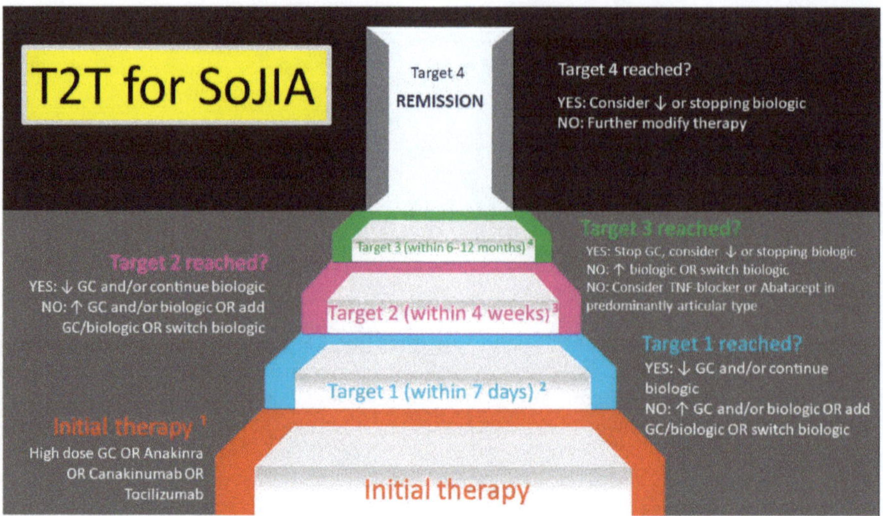

Figure 2. Treat-to-target consensus treatment strategy from the German Society for Pediatric Rheumatology for definitive SoJIA. In addition, non-steroidal anti-inflammatory drugs, intraarticular GC or Methotrexate may be used throughout.[1] Maximal doses for glucocorticoids: intravenous methylprednisolone pulse therapy (20–30 mg/kg/day (max. 1000 mg/day) for 5 days or prednisolone equivalent 1–2 mg/kg/day (max. 80 mg/day). Maximal doses for biologics: Anakinra 8 mg/kg/day (max. 300 mg/day), Canakinumab max. 300 mg every 4 weeks, Tocilizumab (for body weight > 30 kg) 8 mg/kg (max. 800 mg) i.v. every 2 weeks and (for body weight < 30 kg) 12 mg/kg every 2 weeks.[2] Treatment target 1-definition: resolution of fever or improvement of CRP by at least 50%. [3] Treatment target 2-definition: improvement of the physician global assessment by at least 50% AND reduction of the active joint count by at least 50% OR JADAS-10 score of maximally 5.4. [4] Treatment target 3-definition: clinically inactive disease without GC. T2T = Treat to target, SoJIA = Systemic-onset juvenile idiopathic arthritis, GC = Glucocorticoids, TNF = Tumor necrosis factor, JADAS = juvenile arthritis disease activity score (JADAS), "Biologic" refers to Anakinra, Canakinumab or Tocilizumab. ↓ = reduce drug dose. ↑ = increase drug dose.

Although individual studies show certain differences between AOSD and SoJIA, a comparative analysis indicates that both findings most likely describe different ends of a common disease continuum.

10. Conclusions

AoSD is characterized by pathogenic involvement of both arms of the immune system. Despite extensive progress in understanding the pathophysiology and targeting the right cytokines, there are few large prospective cohort studies and randomized trials compared to other rare diseases, such as vasculitis. The new dichotomous classification of patients with AoSD into systemic and articular phenotypes may be a simple but very important step in designing and conducting future clinical trials. Furthermore, the development of activity score and treatment to target is required. These tasks should be addressed in cooperation between paediatric and adult rheumatologists.

Author Contributions: S.T. and C.C.G. drafted the manuscript. S.T. is responsible for the figure drawing. All authors edited and finalized the manuscript for submission. E.F. and T.K. reviewed and approved the submitted manuscript. All authors have read and agreed to the published version of the manuscript.

Funding: This research received no external funding.

Acknowledgments: C.C.G. is a fellow in the BIH Charité Clinician Scientist Program funded by the Charité–Universitätsmedizin Berlin and the Berlin Institute of Health. T.K. is a fellow of the BIH.

Conflicts of Interest: The authors report no declarations of interest.

Abbreviations

AoSD	Adult-onset Still's disease
SoJIA	Systemic-onset juvenile idiopathic arthritis
MAS	Macrophage activation syndrome
HLH	Haemophagocytic lymphohistiocytosis
PRRs	Pattern recognition receptors
NLR	Leucine-rich repeat containing family
PAMPs	Pathogen-associated molecular patterns
DAMPs	Damage-associated molecular patterns
IL	Interleukin
TNF	Tumor necrosis factor
GF	Glycosylated ferritin
DIC	Disseminated intravascular coagulation
TMA	Thrombotic microangiopathy
PET/CT	Positron Emission Tomography/Computer Tomography
ILAR	International League of Associations for Rheumatology

References

1. Fautrel, B. Adult-onset Still disease. *Best Pract. Res. Clin. Rheumatol.* **2008**, *22*, 773–792. [CrossRef]
2. Bywaters, E.G. Still's disease in the adult. *Ann. Rheum. Dis.* **1971**, *30*, 121–133. [CrossRef] [PubMed]
3. Nirmala, N.; Brachat, A.; Feist, E.; Blank, N.; Specker, C.; Witt, M.; Zernicke, J.; Martini, A.; Junge, G. Gene-expression analysis of adult-onset Still's disease and systemic juvenile idiopathic arthritis is consistent with a continuum of a single disease entity. *Pediatr Rheumatol. Online J.* **2015**, *13*, 50. [CrossRef] [PubMed]
4. Gerfaud-Valentin, M.; Jamilloux, Y.; Iwaz, J.; Sève, P. Adult-onset Still's disease. *Autoimmun. Rev.* **2014**, *13*, 708–722. [CrossRef] [PubMed]
5. McGonagle, D.; McDermott, M.F. A proposed classification of the immunological diseases. *PLoS Med.* **2006**, *3*, e297. [CrossRef]
6. McGonagle, D.; Aziz, A.; Dickie, L.J.; McDermott, M.F. An integrated classification of pediatric inflammatory diseases, based on the concepts of autoinflammation and the immunological disease continuum. *Pediatr Res.* **2009**, *65*, 38r–45r. [CrossRef]
7. Ruscitti, P.; Cipriani, P.; Masedu, F.; Iacono, D.; Ciccia, F.; Liakouli, V.; Guggino, G.; Carubbi, F.; Berardicurti, O.; Di Benedetto, P.; et al. Adult-onset Still's disease: Evaluation of prognostic tools and validation of the systemic score by analysis of 100 cases from three centers. *BMC Med.* **2016**, *14*, 194. [CrossRef]
8. Gordon, S. Pattern recognition receptors: Doubling up for the innate immune response. *Cell* **2002**, *111*, 927–930. [CrossRef]
9. McGonagle, D.; Savic, S.; McDermott, M.F. The NLR network and the immunological disease continuum of adaptive and innate immune-mediated inflammation against self. *Semin. Immunopathol.* **2007**, *29*, 303–313. [CrossRef]
10. Caso, F.; Costa, L.; Nucera, V.; Barilaro, G.; Masala, I.F.; Talotta, R.; Caso, P.; Scarpa, R.; Sarzi-Puttini, P.; Atzeni, F. From autoinflammation to autoimmunity: Old and recent findings. *Clin. Rheumatol.* **2018**, *37*, 2305–2321. [CrossRef]
11. Savic, S.; Mistry, A.; Wilson, A.G.; Barcenas-Morales, G.; Doffinger, R.; Emery, P.; McGonagle, D. Autoimmune-autoinflammatory rheumatoid arthritis overlaps: A rare but potentially important subgroup of diseases. *RMD Open* **2017**, *3*, e000550. [CrossRef]
12. Feist, E.; Mitrovic, S.; Fautrel, B. Mechanisms, biomarkers and targets for adult-onset Still's disease. *Nat. Rev. Rheumatol.* **2018**, *14*, 603–618. [CrossRef]
13. Li, Z.; Liu, H.L.; Chen, J.; Zeng, T.; He, L.; Li, M.; Luo, C.; Liu, S.; Ding, T.T.; Yimaiti, K.; et al. Both HLA class I and II regions identified as genome-wide significant susceptibility loci for adult-onset Still's disease in Chinese individuals. *Ann. Rheum. Dis.* **2020**, *79*, 161–163. [CrossRef]
14. Jia, J.; Shi, H.; Liu, M.; Liu, T.; Gu, J.; Wan, L.; Teng, J.; Liu, H.; Cheng, X.; Ye, J.; et al. Cytomegalovirus Infection May Trigger Adult-Onset Still's Disease Onset or Relapses. *Front. Immunol* **2019**, *10*, 898. [CrossRef]
15. Scirè, C.A.; Cavagna, L.; Perotti, C.; Bruschi, E.; Caporali, R.; Montecucco, C. Diagnostic value of procalcitonin measurement in febrile patients with systemic autoimmune diseases. *Clin. Exp. Rheumatol.* **2006**, *24*, 123–128.
16. Fukuoka, K.; Miyamoto, A.; Ozawa, Y.; Ikegaya, N.; Maesono, T.; Komagata, Y.; Kaname, S.; Arimura, Y. Adult-onset Still's disease-like manifestation accompanied by the cancer recurrence after long-term resting state. *Mod. Rheumatol.* **2019**, *29*, 704–707. [CrossRef]
17. Neishi, J.; Tsukada, Y.; Maehara, T.; Ueki, K.; Maezawa, A.; Nojima, Y. Adult Still's disease as a paraneoplastic manifestation of breast cancer. *Scand. J. Rheumatol.* **2000**, *29*, 328–330. [CrossRef]
18. Ahn, J.K.; Oh, J.M.; Lee, J.; Kim, S.W.; Cha, H.S.; Koh, E.M. Adult onset Still's disease diagnosed concomitantly with occult papillary thyroid cancer: Paraneoplastic manifestation or coincidence? *Clin. Rheumatol.* **2010**, *29*, 221–224. [CrossRef]
19. Liozon, E.; Ly, K.H.; Vidal-Cathala, E.; Fauchais, A.L. Adult-onset Still's disease as a manifestation of malignancy: Report of a patient with melanoma and literature review. *La Rev. De Med. Interne* **2014**, *35*, 60–64. [CrossRef]
20. Kim, Y.J.; Kim, S.I.; Hong, K.W.; Kang, M.W. Diagnostic value of 18F-FDG PET/CT in patients with fever of unknown origin. *Intern. Med. J.* **2012**, *42*, 834–837. [CrossRef]

21. Church, L.D.; Cook, G.P.; McDermott, M.F. Primer: Inflammasomes and interleukin 1beta in inflammatory disorders. *Nat. Clin. Pract. Rheumatol.* **2008**, *4*, 34–42. [CrossRef]
22. Wang, M.Y.; Jia, J.C.; Yang, C.D.; Hu, Q.Y. Pathogenesis, disease course, and prognosis of adult-onset Still's disease: An update and review. *Chin. Med. J.* **2019**, *132*, 2856–2864. [CrossRef] [PubMed]
23. Hsieh, C.W.; Chen, Y.M.; Lin, C.C.; Tang, K.T.; Chen, H.H.; Hung, W.T.; Lai, K.L.; Chen, D.Y. Elevated Expression of the NLRP3 Inflammasome and Its Correlation with Disease Activity in Adult-onset Still Disease. *J. Rheumatol.* **2017**, *44*, 1142–1150. [CrossRef] [PubMed]
24. Jamilloux, Y.; Gerfaud-Valentin, M.; Martinon, F.; Belot, A.; Henry, T.; Sève, P. Pathogenesis of adult-onset Still's disease: New insights from the juvenile counterpart. *Immunol. Res.* **2015**, *61*, 53–62. [CrossRef] [PubMed]
25. Ruddell, R.G.; Hoang-Le, D.; Barwood, J.M.; Rutherford, P.S.; Piva, T.J.; Watters, D.J.; Santambrogio, P.; Arosio, P.; Ramm, G.A. Ferritin functions as a proinflammatory cytokine via iron-independent protein kinase C zeta/nuclear factor kappaB-regulated signaling in rat hepatic stellate cells. *Hepatology* **2009**, *49*, 887–900. [CrossRef]
26. Hu, Q.; Shi, H.; Zeng, T.; Liu, H.; Su, Y.; Cheng, X.; Ye, J.; Yin, Y.; Liu, M.; Zheng, H.; et al. Increased neutrophil extracellular traps activate NLRP3 and inflammatory macrophages in adult-onset Still's disease. *Arthritis Res. Ther.* **2019**, *21*, 9. [CrossRef]
27. Foell, D.; Roth, J. Proinflammatory S100 proteins in arthritis and autoimmune disease. *Arthritis Rheum.* **2004**, *50*, 3762–3771. [CrossRef]
28. Chen, D.Y.; Lan, J.L.; Lin, F.J.; Hsieh, T.Y.; Wen, M.C. Predominance of Th1 cytokine in peripheral blood and pathological tissues of patients with active untreated adult onset Still's disease. *Ann. Rheum. Dis.* **2004**, *63*, 1300–1306. [CrossRef] [PubMed]
29. Chen, D.Y.; Chen, Y.M.; Lan, J.L.; Lin, C.C.; Chen, H.H.; Hsieh, C.W. Potential role of Th17 cells in the pathogenesis of adult-onset Still's disease. *Rheumatology* **2010**, *49*, 2305–2312. [CrossRef] [PubMed]
30. Hofmann, S.R.; Kubasch, A.S.; Ioannidis, C.; Rösen-Wolff, A.; Girschick, H.J.; Morbach, H.; Hedrich, C.M. Altered expression of IL-10 family cytokines in monocytes from CRMO patients result in enhanced IL-1β expression and release. *Clin. Immunol.* **2015**, *161*, 300–307. [CrossRef]
31. Chen, D.Y.; Chen, Y.M.; Lin, C.C.; Hsieh, C.W.; Wu, Y.C.; Hung, W.T.; Chen, H.H.; Lan, J.L. The potential role of advanced glycation end products (AGEs) and soluble receptors for AGEs (sRAGE) in the pathogenesis of adult-onset still's disease. *BMC Musculoskelet. Disord.* **2015**, *16*, 111. [CrossRef] [PubMed]
32. Shimojima, Y.; Kishida, D.; Ueno, K.I.; Ushiyama, S.; Ichikawa, T.; Sekijima, Y. Characteristics of Circulating Natural Killer Cells and Their Interferon-γ Production in Active Adult-onset Still Disease. *J. Rheumatol.* **2019**, *46*, 1268–1276. [CrossRef]
33. Park, J.H.; Kim, H.S.; Lee, J.S.; Kim, J.J.; Jung, K.H.; Park, Y.W.; Yoo, D.H. Natural killer cell cytolytic function in Korean patients with adult-onset Still's disease. *J. Rheumatol.* **2012**, *39*, 2000–2007. [CrossRef]
34. Sun, Y.; Wang, Z.; Chi, H.; Hu, Q.; Ye, J.; Liu, H.; Cheng, X.; Shi, H.; Zhou, Z.; Teng, J.; et al. Elevated serum levels of interleukin-10 in adult-onset Still's disease are associated with disease activity. *Clin. Rheumatol.* **2019**, *38*, 3205–3210. [CrossRef]
35. Sfriso, P.; Priori, R.; Valesini, G.; Rossi, S.; Montecucco, C.M.; D'Ascanio, A.; Carli, L.; Bombardieri, S.; LaSelva, G.; Iannone, F.; et al. Adult-onset Still's disease: An Italian multicentre retrospective observational study of manifestations and treatments in 245 patients. *Clin. Rheumatol.* **2016**, *35*, 1683–1689. [CrossRef]
36. Zhou, G.; Zhou, Y.; Zhong, C.; Ye, H.; Liu, Z.; Liu, Y.; Tang, G.; Qu, J.; Lv, X. Retrospective analysis of 1,641 cases of classic fever of unknown origin. *Ann. Transl Med.* **2020**, *8*, 690. [CrossRef] [PubMed]
37. Wright, W.F.; Auwaerter, P.G. Fever and Fever of Unknown Origin: Review, Recent Advances, and Lingering Dogma. *Open Forum Infect. Dis.* **2020**, *7*, ofaa132. [CrossRef]
38. Bagnari, V.; Colina, M.; Ciancio, G.; Govoni, M.; Trotta, F. Adult-onset Still's disease. *Rheumatol. Int.* **2010**, *30*, 855–862. [CrossRef]
39. Elkon, K.B.; Hughes, G.R.; Bywaters, E.G.; Ryan, P.F.; Inman, R.D.; Bowley, N.B.; James, M.P.; Eady, R.A. Adult-onset Still's disease. Twenty-year followup and further studies of patients with active disease. *Arthritis Rheum.* **1982**, *25*, 647–654. [CrossRef]
40. Di Benedetto, P.; Cipriani, P.; Iacono, D.; Pantano, I.; Caso, F.; Emmi, G.; Grembiale, R.D.; Cantatore, F.P.; Atzeni, F.; Perosa, F.; et al. Ferritin and C-reactive protein are predictive biomarkers of mortality and macrophage activation syndrome in adult onset Still's disease. Analysis of the multicentre Gruppo Italiano di Ricerca in Reumatologia Clinica e Sperimentale (GIRRCS) cohort. *PLoS ONE* **2020**, *15*, e0235326. [CrossRef] [PubMed]
41. Hu, Q.Y.; Zeng, T.; Sun, C.Y.; Luo, C.N.; Liu, S.; Ding, T.T.; Ji, Z.F.; Lu, A.; Yimaiti, K.; Teng, J.L.; et al. Clinical features and current treatments of adult-onset Still's disease: A multicentre survey of 517 patients in China. *Clin. Exp. Rheumatol.* **2019**, *37* (Suppl. 121), 52–57.
42. Gerfaud-Valentin, M.; Maucort-Boulch, D.; Hot, A.; Iwaz, J.; Ninet, J.; Durieu, I.; Broussolle, C.; Sève, P. Adult-onset still disease: Manifestations, treatment, outcome, and prognostic factors in 57 patients. *Medicine* **2014**, *93*, 91–99. [CrossRef]
43. Fautrel, B.; Zing, E.; Golmard, J.L.; Le Moel, G.; Bissery, A.; Rioux, C.; Rozenberg, S.; Piette, J.C.; Bourgeois, P. Proposal for a new set of classification criteria for adult-onset still disease. *Medicine* **2002**, *81*, 194–200. [CrossRef] [PubMed]
44. Tsai, H.Y.; Lee, J.H.; Yu, H.H.; Wang, L.C.; Yang, Y.H.; Chiang, B.L. Initial manifestations and clinical course of systemic onset juvenile idiopathic arthritis: A ten-year retrospective study. *J. Formos. Med. Assoc.* **2012**, *111*, 542–549. [CrossRef] [PubMed]
45. Behrens, E.M.; Beukelman, T.; Gallo, L.; Spangler, J.; Rosenkranz, M.; Arkachaisri, T.; Ayala, R.; Groh, B.; Finkel, T.H.; Cron, R.Q. Evaluation of the presentation of systemic onset juvenile rheumatoid arthritis: Data from the Pennsylvania Systemic Onset Juvenile Arthritis Registry (PASOJAR). *J. Rheumatol.* **2008**, *35*, 343–348.

46. Giacomelli, R.; Ruscitti, P.; Shoenfeld, Y. A comprehensive review on adult onset Still's disease. *J. Autoimmun* **2018**, *93*, 24–36. [CrossRef]
47. Fautrel, B.; Le Moël, G.; Saint-Marcoux, B.; Taupin, P.; Vignes, S.; Rozenberg, S.; Koeger, A.C.; Meyer, O.; Guillevin, L.; Piette, J.C.; et al. Diagnostic value of ferritin and glycosylated ferritin in adult onset Still's disease. *J. Rheumatol.* **2001**, *28*, 322–329.
48. Schiller, D.; Mittermayer, H. Hyperferritinemia as a marker of Still's disease. *Clin. Infect. Dis. Off. Publ. Infect. Dis. Soc. Am.* **1998**, *26*, 534–535. [CrossRef] [PubMed]
49. Rosário, C.; Zandman-Goddard, G.; Meyron-Holtz, E.G.; D'Cruz, D.P.; Shoenfeld, Y. The hyperferritinemic syndrome: Macrophage activation syndrome, Still's disease, septic shock and catastrophic antiphospholipid syndrome. *BMC Med.* **2013**, *11*, 185. [CrossRef] [PubMed]
50. Fardet, L.; Coppo, P.; Kettaneh, A.; Dehoux, M.; Cabane, J.; Lambotte, O. Low glycosylated ferritin, a good marker for the diagnosis of hemophagocytic syndrome. *Arthritis Rheum.* **2008**, *58*, 1521–1527. [CrossRef]
51. Vignes, S.; Le Moël, G.; Fautrel, B.; Wechsler, B.; Godeau, P.; Piette, J.C. Percentage of glycosylated serum ferritin remains low throughout the course of adult onset Still's disease. *Ann. Rheum. Dis.* **2000**, *59*, 347–350. [CrossRef]
52. Kudela, H.; Drynda, S.; Lux, A.; Horneff, G.; Kekow, J. Comparative study of Interleukin-18 (IL-18) serum levels in adult onset Still's disease (AOSD) and systemic onset juvenile idiopathic arthritis (sJIA) and its use as a biomarker for diagnosis and evaluation of disease activity. *BMC Rheumatol.* **2019**, *3*, 4. [CrossRef]
53. Mitrovic, S.; Fautrel, B. New Markers for Adult-Onset Still's Disease. *Jt. Bone Spine* **2018**, *85*, 285–293. [CrossRef] [PubMed]
54. Rau, M.; Schiller, M.; Krienke, S.; Heyder, P.; Lorenz, H.; Blank, N. Clinical manifestations but not cytokine profiles differentiate adult-onset Still's disease and sepsis. *J. Rheumatol.* **2010**, *37*, 2369–2376. [CrossRef]
55. Kim, H.A.; An, J.M.; Nam, J.Y.; Jeon, J.Y.; Suh, C.H. Serum S100A8/A9, but not follistatin-like protein 1 and interleukin 18, may be a useful biomarker of disease activity in adult-onset Still's disease. *J. Rheumatol.* **2012**, *39*, 1399–1406. [CrossRef] [PubMed]
56. Bae, C.B.; Suh, C.H.; An, J.M.; Jung, J.Y.; Jeon, J.Y.; Nam, J.Y.; Kim, H.A. Serum S100A12 may be a useful biomarker of disease activity in adult-onset Still's disease. *J. Rheumatol.* **2014**, *41*, 2403–2408. [CrossRef] [PubMed]
57. Yamaguchi, M.; Ohta, A.; Tsunematsu, T.; Kasukawa, R.; Mizushima, Y.; Kashiwagi, H.; Kashiwazaki, S.; Tanimoto, K.; Matsumoto, Y.; Ota, T.; et al. Preliminary criteria for classification of adult Still's disease. *J. Rheumatol.* **1992**, *19*, 424–430.
58. Petty, R.E.; Southwood, T.R.; Manners, P.; Baum, J.; Glass, D.N.; Goldenberg, J.; He, X.; Maldonado-Cocco, J.; Orozco-Alcala, J.; Prieur, A.M.; et al. International League of Associations for Rheumatology classification of juvenile idiopathic arthritis: Second revision, Edmonton, 2001. *J. Rheumatol.* **2004**, *31*, 390–392.
59. Lebrun, D.; Mestrallet, S.; Dehoux, M.; Golmard, J.L.; Granger, B.; Georgin-Lavialle, S.; Arnaud, L.; Grateau, G.; Pouchot, J.; Fautrel, B. Validation of the Fautrel classification criteria for adult-onset Still's disease. *Semin. Arthritis Rheum.* **2018**, *47*, 578–585. [CrossRef] [PubMed]
60. Pouchot, J.; Sampalis, J.S.; Beaudet, F.; Carette, S.; Décary, F.; Salusinsky-Sternbach, M.; Hill, R.O.; Gutkowski, A.; Harth, M.; Myhal, D.; et al. Adult Still's disease: Manifestations, disease course, and outcome in 62 patients. *Medicine* **1991**, *70*, 118–136. [CrossRef]
61. Maria, A.T.; Le Quellec, A.; Jorgensen, C.; Touitou, I.; Rivière, S.; Guilpain, P. Adult onset Still's disease (AOSD) in the era of biologic therapies: Dichotomous view for cytokine and clinical expressions. *Autoimmun. Rev.* **2014**, *13*, 1149–1159. [CrossRef] [PubMed]
62. Franchini, S.; Dagna, L.; Salvo, F.; Aiello, P.; Baldissera, E.; Sabbadini, M.G. Adult onset Still's disease: Clinical presentation in a large cohort of Italian patients. *Clin. Exp. Rheumatol.* **2010**, *28*, 41–48.
63. Ichida, H.; Kawaguchi, Y.; Sugiura, T.; Takagi, K.; Katsumata, Y.; Gono, T.; Ota, Y.; Kataoka, S.; Kawasumi, H.; Yamanaka, H. Clinical manifestations of Adult-onset Still's disease presenting with erosive arthritis: Association with low levels of ferritin and Interleukin-18. *Arthritis Care Res.* **2014**, *66*, 642–646. [CrossRef]
64. Hot, A.; Toh, M.L.; Coppéré, B.; Perard, L.; Madoux, M.H.; Mausservey, C.; Desmurs-Clavel, H.; Ffrench, M.; Ninet, J. Reactive hemophagocytic syndrome in adult-onset Still disease: Clinical features and long-term outcome: A case-control study of 8 patients. *Medicine* **2010**, *89*, 37–46. [CrossRef]
65. Chen, D.Y.; Lan, J.L.; Lin, F.J.; Hsieh, T.Y. Proinflammatory cytokine profiles in sera and pathological tissues of patients with active untreated adult onset Still's disease. *J. Rheumatol.* **2004**, *31*, 2189–2198. [PubMed]
66. Fujii, T.; Nojima, T.; Yasuoka, H.; Satoh, S.; Nakamura, K.; Kuwana, M.; Suwa, A.; Hirakata, M.; Mimori, T. Cytokine and immunogenetic profiles in Japanese patients with adult Still's disease. Association with chronic articular disease. *Rheumatology* **2001**, *40*, 1398–1404. [CrossRef]
67. Franchini, S.; Dagna, L.; Salvo, F.; Aiello, P.; Baldissera, E.; Sabbadini, M.G. Efficacy of traditional and biologic agents in different clinical phenotypes of adult-onset Still's disease. *Arthritis Rheum.* **2010**, *62*, 2530–2535. [CrossRef]
68. Pouchot, J.; Arlet, J.B. Biological treatment in adult-onset Still's disease. *Best Pract. Res. Clin. Rheumatol.* **2012**, *26*, 477–487. [CrossRef] [PubMed]
69. Mehta, P.; Cron, R.Q.; Hartwell, J.; Manson, J.J.; Tattersall, R.S. Silencing the cytokine storm: The use of intravenous anakinra in haemophagocytic lymphohistiocytosis or macrophage activation syndrome. *Lancet Rheumatol.* **2020**, *2*, e358–e367. [CrossRef]
70. Carter, S.J.; Tattersall, R.S.; Ramanan, A.V. Macrophage activation syndrome in adults: Recent advances in pathophysiology, diagnosis and treatment. *Rheumatology* **2019**, *58*, 5–17. [CrossRef]

71. Crayne, C.B.; Albeituni, S.; Nichols, K.E.; Cron, R.Q. The Immunology of Macrophage Activation Syndrome. *Front. Immunol.* **2019**, *10*, 119. [CrossRef] [PubMed]
72. Fardet, L.; Galicier, L.; Lambotte, O.; Marzac, C.; Aumont, C.; Chahwan, D.; Coppo, P.; Hejblum, G. Development and validation of the HScore, a score for the diagnosis of reactive hemophagocytic syndrome. *Arthritis Rheumatol.* **2014**, *66*, 2613–2620. [CrossRef] [PubMed]
73. Lin, T.F.; Ferlic-Stark, L.L.; Allen, C.E.; Kozinetz, C.A.; McClain, K.L. Rate of decline of ferritin in patients with hemophagocytic lymphohistiocytosis as a prognostic variable for mortality. *Pediatric Blood Cancer* **2011**, *56*, 154–155. [CrossRef] [PubMed]
74. Saper, V.E.; Chen, G.; Deutsch, G.H.; Guillerman, R.P.; Birgmeier, J.; Jagadeesh, K.; Canna, S.; Schulert, G.; Deterding, R.; Xu, J.; et al. Emergent high fatality lung disease in systemic juvenile arthritis. *Ann. Rheum. Dis.* **2019**, *78*, 1722–1731. [CrossRef]
75. Schulert, G.S.; Yasin, S.; Carey, B.; Chalk, C.; Do, T.; Schapiro, A.H.; Husami, A.; Watts, A.; Brunner, H.I.; Huggins, J.; et al. Systemic Juvenile Idiopathic Arthritis-Associated Lung Disease: Characterization and Risk Factors. *Arthritis Rheumatol.* **2019**, *71*, 1943–1954. [CrossRef]
76. Ruscitti, P.; Berardicurti, O.; Iacono, D.; Pantano, I.; Liakouli, V.; Caso, F.; Emmi, G.; Grembiale, R.D.; Cantatore, F.P.; Atzeni, F.; et al. Parenchymal lung disease in adult onset Still's disease: An emergent marker of disease severity-characterisation and predictive factors from Gruppo Italiano di Ricerca in Reumatologia Clinica e Sperimentale (GIRRCS) cohort of patients. *Arthritis Res. Ther.* **2020**, *22*, 151. [CrossRef]
77. Ruscitti, P.; Cipriani, P.; Di Benedetto, P.; Liakouli, V.; Carubbi, F.; Berardicurti, O.; Ciccia, F.; Guggino, G.; Triolo, G.; Giacomelli, R. Advances in immunopathogenesis of macrophage activation syndrome during rheumatic inflammatory diseases: Toward new therapeutic targets? *Expert Rev. Clin. Immunol.* **2017**, *13*, 1041–1047. [CrossRef]
78. Grom, A.A.; Horne, A.; De Benedetti, F. Macrophage activation syndrome in the era of biologic therapy. *Nat. Rev. Rheumatol.* **2016**, *12*, 259–268. [CrossRef]
79. Gerfaud-Valentin, M.; Cottin, V.; Jamilloux, Y.; Hot, A.; Gaillard-Coadon, A.; Durieu, I.; Broussolle, C.; Iwaz, J.; Sève, P. Parenchymal lung involvement in adult-onset Still disease: A STROBE-compliant case series and literature review. *Medicine* **2016**, *95*, e4258. [CrossRef]
80. Mehta, M.V.; Manson, D.K.; Horn, E.M.; Haythe, J. An atypical presentation of adult-onset Still's disease complicated by pulmonary hypertension and macrophage activation syndrome treated with immunosuppression: A case-based review of the literature. *Pulm. Circ.* **2016**, *6*, 136–142. [CrossRef]
81. Efthimiou, P.; Kadavath, S.; Mehta, B. Life-threatening complications of adult-onset Still's disease. *Clin. Rheumatol.* **2014**, *33*, 305–314. [CrossRef]
82. Mitrovic, S.; Fautrel, B. Complications of adult-onset Still's disease and their management. *Expert Rev. Clin. Immunol.* **2018**, *14*, 351–365. [CrossRef]
83. Gando, S.; Levi, M.; Toh, C.H. Disseminated intravascular coagulation. *Nat. Rev. Dis Primers* **2016**, *2*, 16037. [CrossRef]
84. El Karoui, K.; Karras, A.; Lebrun, G.; Charles, P.; Arlet, J.B.; Jacquot, C.; Orssaud, C.; Nochy, D.; Pouchot, J. Thrombotic microangiopathy and purtscher-like retinopathy associated with adult-onset Still's disease: A role for glomerular vascular endothelial growth factor? *Arthritis Rheum.* **2009**, *61*, 1609–1613. [CrossRef] [PubMed]
85. Kontzias, A.; Efthimiou, P. Adult-onset Still's disease: Pathogenesis, clinical manifestations and therapeutic advances. *Drugs* **2008**, *68*, 319–337. [CrossRef] [PubMed]
86. Fautrel, B.; Sibilia, J.; Mariette, X.; Combe, B. Tumour necrosis factor alpha blocking agents in refractory adult Still's disease: An observational study of 20 cases. *Ann. Rheum. Dis.* **2005**, *64*, 262–266. [CrossRef] [PubMed]
87. Kraetsch, H.G.; Antoni, C.; Kalden, J.R.; Manger, B. Successful treatment of a small cohort of patients with adult onset of Still's disease with infliximab: First experiences. *Ann. Rheum. Dis.* **2001**, *60* (Suppl. 3), iii55–iii57. [CrossRef]
88. Cavagna, L.; Caporali, R.; Epis, O.; Bobbio-Pallavicini, F.; Montecucco, C. Infliximab in the treatment of adult Still's disease refractory to conventional therapy. *Clin. Exp. Rheumatol.* **2001**, *19*, 329–332.
89. Kötter, I.; Wacker, A.; Koch, S.; Henes, J.; Richter, C.; Engel, A.; Günaydin, I.; Kanz, L. Anakinra in patients with treatment-resistant adult-onset Still's disease: Four case reports with serial cytokine measurements and a review of the literature. *Semin. Arthritis Rheum.* **2007**, *37*, 189–197. [CrossRef]
90. Giampietro, C.; Ridene, M.; Lequerre, T.; Costedoat Chalumeau, N.; Amoura, Z.; Sellam, J.; Sibilia, J.; Bourgeois, P.; Fautrel, B. Anakinra in adult-onset Still's disease: Long-term treatment in patients resistant to conventional therapy. *Arthritis Care Res.* **2013**, *65*, 822–826. [CrossRef]
91. Ortiz-Sanjuán, F.; Blanco, R.; Riancho-Zarrabeitia, L.; Castañeda, S.; Olivé, A.; Riveros, A.; Velloso-Feijoo, M.L.; Narváez, J.; Jiménez-Moleón, I.; Maiz-Alonso, O.; et al. Efficacy of Anakinra in Refractory Adult-Onset Still's Disease: Multicenter Study of 41 Patients and Literature Review. *Medicine* **2015**, *94*, e1554. [CrossRef] [PubMed]
92. Colafrancesco, S.; Priori, R.; Valesini, G.; Argolini, L.; Baldissera, E.; Bartoloni, E.; Cammelli, D.; Canestrari, G.; Cantarini, L.; Cavallaro, E.; et al. Response to Interleukin-1 Inhibitors in 140 Italian Patients with Adult-Onset Still's Disease: A Multicentre Retrospective Observational Study. *Front. Pharm.* **2017**, *8*, 369. [CrossRef] [PubMed]
93. Feist, E.; Burmester, G.R. Canakinumab for treatment of cryopyrin-associated periodic syndrome. *Expert Opin. Biol. Ther.* **2010**, *10*, 1631–1636. [CrossRef] [PubMed]
94. Sfriso, P.; Bindoli, S.; Doria, A.; Feist, E.; Galozzi, P. Canakinumab for the treatment of adult-onset Still's disease. *Expert Rev. Clin. Immunol.* **2020**, *16*, 129–138. [CrossRef]

95. Feist, E.; Quartier, P.; Fautrel, B.; Schneider, R.; Sfriso, P.; Efthimiou, P.; Cantarini, L.; Lheritier, K.; Leon, K.; Karyekar, C.S.; et al. Efficacy and safety of canakinumab in patients with Still's disease: Exposure-response analysis of pooled systemic juvenile idiopathic arthritis data by age groups. *Clin. Exp. Rheumatol.* **2018**, *36*, 668–675. [PubMed]
96. Kontzias, A.; Efthimiou, P. The use of Canakinumab, a novel IL-1β long-acting inhibitor, in refractory adult-onset Still's disease. *Semin. Arthritis Rheum.* **2012**, *42*, 201–205. [CrossRef]
97. Kedor, C.; Listing, J.; Zernicke, J.; Weiß, A.; Behrens, F.; Blank, N.; Henes, J.C.; Kekow, J.; Rubbert-Roth, A.; Schulze-Koops, H.; et al. Canakinumab for Treatment of Adult-Onset Still's Disease to Achieve Reduction of Arthritic Manifestation (CONSIDER): Phase II, randomised, double-blind, placebo-controlled, multicentre, investigator-initiated trial. *Ann. Rheum. Dis.* **2020**, *79*, 1090–1097. [CrossRef]
98. Kedor, C.; Listing, J.; Zernicke, J.; Feist, E. Response to: 'Changing the outcome measures, changing the results? The urgent need of a specific Disease Activity Score to adult-onset Still's disease' by Ruscitti et al. *Ann. Rheum. Dis.* **2020**. [CrossRef]
99. Kedor, C.; Zernicke, J.; Feist, E. Response to: 'Correspondence on 'Changing the outcome measures, changing the results? The urgent need of a specific disease activity score to adult-onset Still's disease" by Muraviov and Muraviova. *Ann. Rheum. Dis.* **2020**. [CrossRef] [PubMed]
100. Ilowite, N.T.; Prather, K.; Lokhnygina, Y.; Schanberg, L.E.; Elder, M.; Milojevic, D.; Verbsky, J.W.; Spalding, S.J.; Kimura, Y.; Imundo, L.F.; et al. Randomized, double-blind, placebo-controlled trial of the efficacy and safety of rilonacept in the treatment of systemic juvenile idiopathic arthritis. *Arthritis Rheumatol.* **2014**, *66*, 2570–2579. [CrossRef]
101. Song, S.T.; Kim, J.J.; Lee, S.; Kim, H.A.; Lee, E.Y.; Shin, K.C.; Lee, J.H.; Lee, K.H.; Choi, S.T.; Cha, H.S.; et al. Efficacy of tocilizumab therapy in Korean patients with adult-onset Still's disease: A multicentre retrospective study of 22 cases. *Clin. Exp. Rheumatol.* **2016**, *34*, S64–S71.
102. Li, T.; Gu, L.; Wang, X.; Guo, L.; Shi, H.; Yang, C.; Chen, S. A Pilot Study on Tocilizumab for Treating Refractory Adult-Onset Still's Disease. *Sci Rep.* **2017**, *7*, 13477. [CrossRef] [PubMed]
103. Kaneko, Y.; Kameda, H.; Ikeda, K.; Ishii, T.; Murakami, K.; Takamatsu, H.; Tanaka, Y.; Abe, T.; Takeuchi, T. Tocilizumab in patients with adult-onset still's disease refractory to glucocorticoid treatment: A randomised, double-blind, placebo-controlled phase III trial. *Ann. Rheum. Dis.* **2018**, *77*, 1720–1729. [CrossRef]
104. Ma, Y.; Wu, M.; Zhang, X.; Xia, Q.; Yang, J.; Xu, S.; Pan, F. Efficacy and safety of tocilizumab with inhibition of interleukin-6 in adult-onset Still's disease: A meta-analysis. *Mod. Rheumatol.* **2018**, *28*, 849–857. [CrossRef] [PubMed]
105. Simeni Njonnou, S.R.; Soyfoo, M.S.; Vandergheynst, F.A. Efficacy of sarilumab in adult-onset Still's disease as a corticosteroid-sparing agent. *Rheumatology* **2019**, *58*, 1878–1879. [CrossRef]
106. Hu, Q.; Wang, M.; Jia, J.; Teng, J.; Chi, H.; Liu, T.; Liu, H.L.; Cheng, X.; Ye, J.; Su, Y.; et al. Tofacitinib in refractory adult-onset Still's disease: 14 cases from a single centre in China. *Ann. Rheum. Dis.* **2020**, *79*, 842–844. [CrossRef] [PubMed]
107. Honda, M.; Moriyama, M.; Kondo, M.; Kumakura, S.; Murakawa, Y. Tofacitinib-induced remission in refractory adult-onset Still's disease complicated by macrophage activation syndrome. *Scand. J. Rheumatol.* **2020**, *49*, 336–338. [CrossRef]
108. Hoff, P.; Walther, M.; Wesselmann, H.; Weinerth, J.; Feist, E.; Ohrndorf, S. Successful treatment of adult Still's disease with tofacitinib in a HIV-2 positive female patient. *Z. Fur Rheumatol.* **2020**. [CrossRef]
109. Kacar, M.; Fitton, J.; Gough, A.K.; Buch, M.H.; McGonagle, D.G.; Savic, S. Mixed results with baricitinib in biological-resistant adult-onset Still's disease and undifferentiated systemic autoinflammatory disease. *RMD Open* **2020**, 6. [CrossRef]
110. Gabay, C.; Fautrel, B.; Rech, J.; Spertini, F.; Feist, E.; Kötter, I.; Hachulla, E.; Morel, J.; Schaeverbeke, T.; Hamidou, M.A.; et al. Open-label, multicentre, dose-escalating phase II clinical trial on the safety and efficacy of tadekinig alfa (IL-18BP) in adult-onset Still's disease. *Ann. Rheum. Dis.* **2018**, *77*, 840–847. [CrossRef]
111. Still, G.F. On a Form of Chronic Joint Disease in Children. *Med. Chir. Trans.* **1897**, *80*, 47-60.9. [CrossRef]
112. Schaller, J.G.; Ochs, H.D.; Thomas, E.D.; Nisperos, B.; Feigl, P.; Wedgwood, R.J. Histocompatibility antigens in childhood-onset arthritis. *J. Pediatr.* **1976**, *88*, 926–930. [CrossRef]
113. Ombrello, M.J.; Arthur, V.L.; Remmers, E.F.; Hinks, A.; Tachmazidou, I.; Grom, A.A.; Foell, D.; Martini, A.; Gattorno, M.; Özen, S.; et al. Genetic architecture distinguishes systemic juvenile idiopathic arthritis from other forms of juvenile idiopathic arthritis: Clinical and therapeutic implications. *Ann. Rheum. Dis.* **2017**, *76*, 906–913. [CrossRef] [PubMed]
114. Ombrello, M.J.; Remmers, E.F.; Tachmazidou, I.; Grom, A.; Foell, D.; Haas, J.P.; Martini, A.; Gattorno, M.; Özen, S.; Prahalad, S.; et al. HLA-DRB1*11 and variants of the MHC class II locus are strong risk factors for systemic juvenile idiopathic arthritis. *Proc. Natl. Acad. Sci. USA* **2015**, *112*, 15970–15975. [CrossRef] [PubMed]
115. Wakil, S.M.; Monies, D.M.; Abouelhoda, M.; Al-Tassan, N.; Al-Dusery, H.; Naim, E.A.; Al-Younes, B.; Shinwari, J.; Al-Mohanna, F.A.; Meyer, B.F.; et al. Association of a mutation in LACC1 with a monogenic form of systemic juvenile idiopathic arthritis. *Arthritis Rheumatol.* **2015**, *67*, 288–295. [CrossRef]
116. Singh, A.; Suri, D.; Vignesh, P.; Anjani, G.; Jacob, P.; Girisha, K.M. LACC1 gene mutation in three sisters with polyarthritis without systemic features. *Ann. Rheum. Dis.* **2020**, *79*, 425–426. [CrossRef]
117. Sulliman Ommar Omarjee, A.-L.M.; Quiniou, G.; Moreews, M.; Ainouze, M.; Frachette, C.; Melki, I.; Dumaine, C.; Gerfaud-Valentin, M.; Duquesne, A.; Tilmann, K.; et al. LACC1 deficiency defines a novel form of juvenile arthritis associated with reduced autophagy and metabolism in macrophages. *J. Exp. Med.* **2020**, accepted.
118. Reiff, A. Treatment of Systemic Juvenile Idiopathic Arthritis with Tocilizumab—the Role of Anti-Interleukin-6 Therapy after a Decade of Treatment. *Biol. Ther.* **2012**, *2*, 1. [CrossRef]

119. Holzinger, D.; Foell, D.; Kessel, C. The role of S100 proteins in the pathogenesis and monitoring of autoinflammatory diseases. *Mol. Cell Pediatr.* **2018**, *5*, 7. [CrossRef]
120. Kessel, C.; Holzinger, D.; Foell, D. Phagocyte-derived S100 proteins in autoinflammation: Putative role in pathogenesis and usefulness as biomarkers. *Clin. Immunol.* **2013**, *147*, 229–241. [CrossRef]
121. Cepika, A.M.; Banchereau, R.; Segura, E.; Ohouo, M.; Cantarel, B.; Goller, K.; Cantrell, V.; Ruchaud, E.; Gatewood, E.; Nguyen, P.; et al. A multidimensional blood stimulation assay reveals immune alterations underlying systemic juvenile idiopathic arthritis. *J. Exp. Med.* **2017**, *214*, 3449–3466. [CrossRef]
122. Pascual, V.; Allantaz, F.; Arce, E.; Punaro, M.; Banchereau, J. Role of interleukin-1 (IL-1) in the pathogenesis of systemic onset juvenile idiopathic arthritis and clinical response to IL-1 blockade. *J. Exp. Med.* **2005**, *201*, 1479–1486. [CrossRef] [PubMed]
123. Hügle, B.; Schippers, A.; Fischer, N.; Ohl, K.; Denecke, B.; Ticconi, F.; Vastert, B.; Costa, I.G.; Haas, J.P.; Tenbrock, K. Transcription factor motif enrichment in whole transcriptome analysis identifies STAT4 and BCL6 as the most prominent binding motif in systemic juvenile idiopathic arthritis. *Arthritis Res. Ther.* **2018**, *20*, 98. [CrossRef]
124. Gohar, F.; McArdle, A.; Jones, M.; Callan, N.; Hernandez, B.; Kessel, C.; Miranda-Garcia, M.; Lavric, M.; Holzinger, D.; Pretzer, C.; et al. Molecular signature characterisation of different inflammatory phenotypes of systemic juvenile idiopathic arthritis. *Ann. Rheum. Dis.* **2019**, *78*, 1107–1113. [CrossRef]
125. Weiss, E.S.; Girard-Guyonvarc'h, C.; Holzinger, D.; de Jesus, A.A.; Tariq, Z.; Picarsic, J.; Schiffrin, E.J.; Foell, D.; Grom, A.A.; Ammann, S.; et al. Interleukin-18 diagnostically distinguishes and pathogenically promotes human and murine macrophage activation syndrome. *Blood* **2018**, *131*, 1442–1455. [CrossRef]
126. Yang, L.; Anderson, D.E.; Baecher-Allan, C.; Hastings, W.D.; Bettelli, E.; Oukka, M.; Kuchroo, V.K.; Hafler, D.A. IL-21 and TGF-beta are required for differentiation of human T(H)17 cells. *Nature* **2008**, *454*, 350–352. [CrossRef] [PubMed]
127. Zhou, L.; I Ivanov, I.; Spolski, R.; Min, R.; Shenderov, K.; Egawa, T.; Levy, D.E.; Leonard, W.J.; Littman, D.R. IL-6 programs T(H)-17 cell differentiation by promoting sequential engagement of the IL-21 and IL-23 pathways. *Nat. Immunol.* **2007**, *8*, 967–974. [CrossRef]
128. Henderson, L.A.; Hoyt, K.J.; Lee, P.Y.; Rao, D.A.; Jonsson, A.H.; Nguyen, J.P.; Rutherford, K.; Julé, A.M.; Charbonnier, L.M.; Case, S.; et al. Th17 reprogramming of T cells in systemic juvenile idiopathic arthritis. *JCI Insight* **2020**, 5. [CrossRef] [PubMed]
129. Kessel, C.; Lippitz, K.; Weinhage, T.; Hinze, C.; Wittkowski, H.; Holzinger, D.; Fall, N.; Grom, A.A.; Gruen, N.; Foell, D. Proinflammatory Cytokine Environments Can Drive Interleukin-17 Overexpression by γ/δ T Cells in Systemic Juvenile Idiopathic Arthritis. *Arthritis Rheumatol.* **2017**, *69*, 1480–1494. [CrossRef]
130. Vandenhaute, J.; Avau, A.; Filtjens, J.; Malengier-Devlies, B.; Imbrechts, M.; Van den Berghe, N.; Ahmadzadeh, K.; Mitera, T.; Boon, L.; Leclercq, G.; et al. Regulatory Role for NK Cells in a Mouse Model of Systemic Juvenile Idiopathic Arthritis. *J. Immunol.* **2019**, *203*, 3339–3348. [CrossRef]
131. Wulffraat, N.M.; Rijkers, G.T.; Elst, E.; Brooimans, R.; Kuis, W. Reduced perforin expression in systemic juvenile idiopathic arthritis is restored by autologous stem-cell transplantation. *Rheumatology* **2003**, *42*, 375–379. [CrossRef] [PubMed]
132. Put, K.; Vandenhaute, J.; Avau, A.; van Nieuwenhuijze, A.; Brisse, E.; Dierckx, T.; Rutgeerts, O.; Garcia-Perez, J.E.; Toelen, J.; Waer, M.; et al. Inflammatory Gene Expression Profile and Defective Interferon-γ and Granzyme K in Natural Killer Cells from Systemic Juvenile Idiopathic Arthritis Patients. *Arthritis Rheumatol.* **2017**, *69*, 213–224. [CrossRef] [PubMed]
133. Kaufman, K.M.; Linghu, B.; Szustakowski, J.D.; Husami, A.; Yang, F.; Zhang, K.; Filipovich, A.H.; Fall, N.; Harley, J.B.; Nirmala, N.R.; et al. Whole-Exome Sequencing Reveals Overlap Between Macrophage Activation Syndrome in Systemic Juvenile Idiopathic Arthritis and Familial Hemophagocytic Lymphohistiocytosis. *Arthritis Rheumatol.* **2014**, *66*, 3486–3495. [CrossRef]
134. Ravelli, A.; Minoia, F.; Davì, S.; Horne, A.; Bovis, F.; Pistorio, A.; Aricò, M.; Avcin, T.; Behrens, E.M.; De Benedetti, F.; et al. 2016 Classification Criteria for Macrophage Activation Syndrome Complicating Systemic Juvenile Idiopathic Arthritis: A European League Against Rheumatism/American College of Rheumatology/Paediatric Rheumatology International Trials Organisation Collaborative Initiative. *Arthritis Rheumatol.* **2016**, *68*, 566–576. [CrossRef] [PubMed]
135. De Benedetti, F.; Schneider, R. Chapter 16—Systemic Juvenile Idiopathic Arthritis. In *Textbook of Pediatric Rheumatology*, 7th ed.; Petty, R.E., Laxer, R.M., Lindsley, C.B., Wedderburn, L.R., Eds.; W.B. Saunders: Philadelphia, PA, USA, 2016; pp. 205–216.e206.
136. Kumar, S.; Kunhiraman, D.S.; Rajam, L. Application of the Yamaguchi criteria for classification of "suspected" systemic juvenile idiopathic arthritis (sJIA). *Pediatr. Rheumatol. Online J.* **2012**, *10*, 40. [CrossRef]
137. Silva, J.R.; Brito, I. Systemic juvenile idiopathic arthritis versus adult-onset Still´s disease: The pertinence of changing the current classification criteria. *Acta Reum. Port.* **2020**, *45*, 150–151.
138. Föll, D.; Wittkowski, H.; Hinze, C. Still's disease as biphasic disorder: Current knowledge on pathogenesis and novel treatment approaches. *Z. Rheumatol.* **2020**, *79*, 639–648. [CrossRef] [PubMed]
139. Hinze, C.H.; Holzinger, D.; Lainka, E.; Haas, J.P.; Speth, F.; Kallinich, T.; Rieber, N.; Hufnagel, M.; Jansson, A.F.; Hedrich, C.; et al. Practice and consensus-based strategies in diagnosing and managing systemic juvenile idiopathic arthritis in Germany. *Pediatr. Rheumatol. Online J.* **2018**, *16*, 7. [CrossRef]
140. DeWitt, E.M.; Kimura, Y.; Beukelman, T.; Nigrovic, P.A.; Onel, K.; Prahalad, S.; Schneider, R.; Stoll, M.L.; Angeles-Han, S.; Milojevic, D.; et al. Consensus treatment plans for new-onset systemic juvenile idiopathic arthritis. *Arthritis Care Res.* **2012**, *64*, 1001–1010. [CrossRef] [PubMed]

141. Ruperto, N.; Brunner, H.I.; Quartier, P.; Constantin, T.; Wulffraat, N.; Horneff, G.; Brik, R.; McCann, L.; Kasapcopur, O.; Rutkowska-Sak, L.; et al. Two randomized trials of canakinumab in systemic juvenile idiopathic arthritis. *N. Engl. J. Med.* **2012**, *367*, 2396–2406. [CrossRef]
142. De Benedetti, F.; Brunner, H.I.; Ruperto, N.; Kenwright, A.; Wright, S.; Calvo, I.; Cuttica, R.; Ravelli, A.; Schneider, R.; Woo, P.; et al. Randomized trial of tocilizumab in systemic juvenile idiopathic arthritis. *N. Engl. J. Med.* **2012**, *367*, 2385–2395. [CrossRef] [PubMed]
143. Quartier, P.; Allantaz, F.; Cimaz, R.; Pillet, P.; Messiaen, C.; Bardin, C.; Bossuyt, X.; Boutten, A.; Bienvenu, J.; Duquesne, A.; et al. A multicentre, randomised, double-blind, placebo-controlled trial with the interleukin-1 receptor antagonist anakinra in patients with systemic-onset juvenile idiopathic arthritis (ANAJIS trial). *Ann. Rheum. Dis.* **2011**, *70*, 747–754. [CrossRef] [PubMed]
144. Ter Haar, N.M.; van Dijkhuizen, E.H.P.; Swart, J.F.; van Royen-Kerkhof, A.; El Idrissi, A.; Leek, A.P.; de Jager, W.; de Groot, M.C.H.; Haitjema, S.; Holzinger, D.; et al. Treatment to Target Using Recombinant Interleukin-1 Receptor Antagonist as First-Line Monotherapy in New-Onset Systemic Juvenile Idiopathic Arthritis: Results From a Five-Year Follow-Up Study. *Arthritis Rheumatol.* **2019**, *71*, 1163–1173. [CrossRef] [PubMed]
145. Klotsche, J.; Raab, A.; Niewerth, M.; Sengler, C.; Ganser, G.; Kallinich, T.; Niehues, T.; Hufnagel, M.; Thon, A.; Hospach, T.; et al. Outcome and Trends in Treatment of Systemic Juvenile Idiopathic Arthritis in the German National Pediatric Rheumatologic Database, 2000–2013. *Arthritis Rheumatol* **2016**, *68*, 3023–3034. [CrossRef] [PubMed]

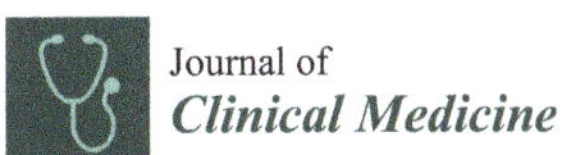
Journal of
Clinical Medicine

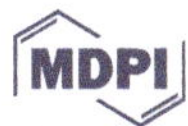

Review

Diagnosis and Management of the Cryopyrin-Associated Periodic Syndromes (CAPS): What Do We Know Today?

Tatjana Welzel [1,2] and Jasmin B. Kuemmerle-Deschner [1,*]

[1] Pediatric Rheumatology and Autoinflammation Reference Center Tuebingen (arcT), University Children's Hospital Tuebingen, D-72076 Tuebingen, Germany; tatjana.welzel@ukbb.ch
[2] Pediatric Pharmacology and Pharmacometrics, University Children's Hospital Basel (UKBB), University of Basel, CH-4031 Basel, Switzerland
* Correspondence: jasmin.kuemmerle-deschner@med.uni-tuebingen.de

Abstract: The cryopyrin-associated periodic syndromes (CAPS) are usually caused by heterozygous *NLRP3* gene variants, resulting in excessive inflammasome activation with subsequent overproduction of interleukin (IL)-1β. The CAPS spectrum includes mild, moderate, and severe phenotypes. The mild phenotype is called familial cold autoinflammatory syndrome (FCAS), the moderate phenotype is also known as Muckle–Wells syndrome (MWS), and the neonatal-onset multisystem inflammatory disease (NOMID)/chronic infantile neurologic cutaneous articular syndrome (CINCA) describes the severe phenotype. The CAPS phenotypes display unspecific and unique clinical signs. Dermatologic, musculoskeletal, ocular, otologic, and neurologic disease symptoms combined with chronic systemic inflammation are characteristic. Nevertheless, making the CAPS diagnosis is challenging as several patients show a heterogeneous multi-system clinical presentation and the spectrum of genetic variants is growing. Somatic mosaicisms and low-penetrance variants lead to atypical clinical symptoms and disease courses. To avoid morbidity and to reduce mortality, early diagnosis is crucial, and a targeted anti-IL-1 therapy should be started as soon as possible. Furthermore, continuous and precise monitoring of disease activity, organ damage, and health-related quality of life is important. This review summarizes the current evidence in diagnosis and management of patients with CAPS.

Keywords: CAPS; FCAS; MWS; CINCA; NOMID; hearing loss; urticarial-like rash; autoinflammatory disease; anti-IL-1 treatment

Citation: Welzel, T.; Kuemmerle-Deschner, J.B. Diagnosis and Management of the Cryopyrin-Associated Periodic Syndromes (CAPS): What Do We Know Today?. *J. Clin. Med.* **2021**, *10*, 128. https://doi.org/10.3390/jcm10010128

Received: 12 December 2020
Accepted: 30 December 2020
Published: 1 January 2021

1. Introduction

Autoinflammatory diseases (AID) are rare, often severe illnesses caused by genetic variants in innate immunity genes resulting in a constitutive overproduction of proinflammatory cytokines [1,2]. The genetic origin of monogenic interleukin-1 (IL-1) mediated AID was first determined for the familial Mediterranean fever (FMF) in 1997 [3,4]. In 1999, mutations in the *TNFRSF1A* gene were shown to be associated with Hibernian fever subsequently relabeled as tumor necrosis factor (TNF) receptor-associated periodic syndrome (TRAPS) [5,6]. Furthermore, for the hyperimmunoglobulinemia D syndrome (HIDS)/mevalonate kinase deficiency (MKD) the *MVK* gene was described in 1999 [7,8]. In 2001/2002, the *NLRP3* gene (also known as *CIAS1* or *NALP3* gene) was discovered, coding for the protein cryopyrin or synonymously called NLRP3/NALP3 protein [9–11]. Variants of this gene usually cause the cryopyrin-associated periodic syndromes (CAPS), a clinical spectrum of different autoinflammatory phenotypes with varying disease activity and phenotype-related risk for morbidity and mortality [12]. The CAPS spectrum includes mild, moderate, and severe phenotypes. The mild phenotype is also called familial cold autoinflammatory syndrome (FCAS, OMIM 120100), the moderate phenotype is known as Muckle–Wells syndrome (MWS, OMIM 191900), and the neonatal-onset multisystem inflammatory disease (NOMID)/chronic infantile neurologic cutaneous articular syndrome

(CINCA) (OMIM 607115) describes the severe phenotype. In a recent consensus proposal of a new taxonomy for monogenetic AID, it was proposed to use the name *NLRP3*-associated autoinflammatory diseases (*NLRP3*-AID) for the CAPS spectrum [13]. The different levels of phenotypic severity of the same disease should be reflected by using the adjectives: mild, moderate, and severe [13]. However, it seems that this new taxonomy has yet failed to receive broad recognition, therefore, the, up until now, more prevalent term CAPS is used in this paper.

The CAPS phenotypes display unspecific and unique clinical signs. Dermatologic, musculoskeletal, ocular, otologic, and neurologic disease symptoms combined with chronic systemic inflammation are characteristic. Nevertheless, making the CAPS diagnosis is challenging as several patients show a heterogeneous multi-system clinical presentation and the spectrum of genetic variants is growing. Somatic mosaicisms and frequent variants of uncertain significance also known as low-penetrance variants lead to atypical clinical symptoms and disease courses.

The CAPS phenotypes are an important differential diagnosis in patients with systemic inflammation and suspected AID. Prompt diagnosis and early start of targeted anti-IL-1 treatment is crucial to avoid disease burden and organ damage. Furthermore, effective multidisciplinary management of patients with CAPS including, treat-to-target (T2T) strategies, as well as standardized monitoring of disease activity, organ damage, and disease-related psychosocial burden is important. In this review, we summarize what we know today, nearly 20 years after *NLRP3* gene discovery, give an overview of the current evidence in making the diagnosis, and give an update regarding the current management recommendations for patients with CAPS.

2. Epidemiology

CAPS belong to the orphan diseases or so-called rare diseases. Their true incidence is unknown due to underdiagnosis, underreporting, and selection bias, similar to other rare disease [14]. However, the prevalence is estimated to be 2.7 to 5.5 per 1 million and might be higher, as CAPS is still not widely known, and therefore often not diagnosed correctly [15,16]. The different CAPS phenotypes seem to vary in incidence and prevalence over the globe. Caucasians are more often affected, whereas no gender differences could be observed so far [15,17]. CAPS has been reported on nearly every continent, and the geographical distribution of CAPS might be influenced by external factors such as weather [14]. For example, patients with FCAS can avoid flares if not exposed to cold, and therefore they might prefer to live in areas with a mild climate. In North America, a founder mutation (L353P) associated with the mild CAPS phenotype FCAS is observed in up to 75% of CAPS patients, whereas in Europe the moderate MWS seems to be the most common CAPS phenotype [14,18,19]. The more severe phenotypes, such as CINCA or NOMID, are rare and mostly caused by de novo variants [20].

3. Genetics

In 2001, heterozygous gain-of-function variants in the *NLRP3* gene were identified in patients with FCAS and MWS and later in NOMID/CINCA [9–11]. This discovery led to the conclusion that FCAS, MWS, and NOMID/CINCA represent different phenotypes that belong to the same disease spectrum, called CAPS [12]. Today, genetic variants can be classified as "pathogenic", "likely pathogenic", "uncertain significance", "likely benign", and "benign" [21]. The Infevers database (https://infevers.umai-montpellier.fr/web/), an exhaustive registry for sequence variants identified in different AID related genes, listed more than 240 sequence variants of the *NLRP3* gene in November 2020 [22]. Of these, more than 100 are known to be pathogenic/likely pathogenic and the majority is located in exon 3.

3.1. Frequent Variants of Uncertain Significance

Frequent variants of uncertain significance (VUS), also known as low-penetrance variants, can be present in asymptomatic healthy individuals. Nevertheless, some of these frequent VUS, also described as risk alleles, may contribute to an AID phenotype in affected carriers [23–25]. The systemic inflammation might be mediated by different pathways parallel to the caspase 1 activation, including IL-1β and non-IL-1β mediated inflammatory pathways [23,26]. Schuh et al. analyzed peripheral blood mononuclear cells of several symptomatic patients with *NLRP3* VUS and found increased NLRP3-specific IL-1β release upon stimulation and elevated NLRP3-independent IL-6 and TNF-α levels [27]. Furthermore, frequent VUS seem to act as susceptibility alleles to inflammation [28,29]. Well known frequent VUS in the *NLRP3* gene are the following variants: V198M, R488K, and Q703K. Symptomatic carriers display a distinct clinical phenotype, which includes typical CAPS symptoms of headache, urticarial-like rashes, and arthralgia, as well as atypical CAPS symptoms, such as severe gastrointestinal symptoms [23]. In addition, symptomatic patients with *NLRP3* VUS seem to have significantly more fever (76%) [23] and can present with cranial nerve inflammation [27]. Moreover, it seems that Q703K variants can be also associated with pharyngitis and oral aphthosis [24]. Whereas Kuemmerle-Deschner et al. stated that patients with frequent VUS in the *NLRP3* gene were at lower risk for eye disease, hearing loss, and renal involvement [23], Theodoropoulou et al. concluded that patients with clinical CAPS phenotype and Q703K variants had a comparable complication risk to patients with pathogenic *NLRP3* gene variants [24]. However, patients with low-penetrance *NLRP3* gene variants seem to display an intermediate biologic phenotype, with traditional markers of inflammation being elevated less frequently [23]. It is important to notice that the detection of a frequent VUS in the *NLRP3* gene does not genetically confirm the diagnosis of CAPS.

3.2. Somatic Mutation/Somatic Mosaicism

Somatic mutation/somatic mosaicism is a term which describes the occurrence of a new mutation post-zygotically in an embryo after the single cell stage with inheritance by all subsequent cells of that lineage, resulting in genetically different cell populations within an individual [30]. Whereas germline mutations are present in the first fertilized egg and, consequently, expressed in all cells of the body, the body distribution of somatic mutations depends on the time when the post-zygotic mutation occurs. If the somatic mutation occurs early in embryonic development, it results in a high frequency of altered cells across many different tissues and cell types; while those occurring later affect a lower frequency of mutant cells in a more limited distribution, potentially leading to a delayed onset of disease [30]. In 2005, Saito et al. identified a somatic mutation in a CINCA/NOMID patient [31]. Subsequently, somatic mosaicism was reported in 70% of former genetically negative NOMID/CINCA patients [32]. Labrousse et al. estimated that the proportion of CAPS-like patients carrying mosaicism ranged between 0.5% and 19% [33]. One of the most common somatic mutations is the E567K [33]. Up to now, there are 35 different somatic mutations that have been identified in the *NLRP3* gene [33]. Somatic mutations can result in an atypical AID phenotype, milder disease course, or late onset [32,34–36]. Furthermore, vertical transmission of somatic mosaicism has been reported [37]. Additionally, the phenotypic spectrum of CAPS appears to be related to the germinal/mosaic status and localization of the underlying variant [38]. Louvrier et al. reported that somatic mutations for *NLRP3* were mainly situated in the core of the NLRP3-inflammasome activating domain, while germline mutations were scattered throughout this domain [38]. Furthermore, it seems that there are two hotspots for somatic mutations. One is located in the HD2 domain of *NLRP3* and the second mosaic mutational hotspot involves Phe304 to Gly309 amino acids that overlap the Walker B motif of the nucleotide binding domain [38]. Due to the low or extremely low frequency of the mutant allele, somatic mutations can be missed using conventional methods of genetic analysis, such as Sanger sequencing. To detect somatic mutations, usually novel technologies are needed, such as next generation sequencing (NGS)-based methods with greater depth.

4. Pathogenesis

The *NLRP3* gene encodes for the protein NLRP3, which is part of the cytoplasmatic nucleotid-binding domain, a family member of the intracellular "NOD like" receptor (NLR) [39]. NLRP3 nucleates an intracellular multi-molecular complex, called the NLRP3 inflammasome [40]. The NLRP3 inflammasome consists of specific adaptor proteins such as ASC (apoptosis-associated speck-like protein containing a caspase recruitment domain) and several chaperone proteins [41,42] and the formation of this complex enables the activation of proinflammatory protease caspase-1. Caspase-1 can cleave pro-interleukin (IL)-1β and pro-IL-18 in their biological active forms (IL-1β, IL-18) [42–44]. IL-1β, and to a less extent IL-18, can elicit neutrophilic inflammation [14]. Once released, IL-1β causes a cascade of downstream signals, which finally result in the activation of nuclear factor κB (NFκB) and the production and release of other inflammatory cytokines. The NLRP3 inflammasome can be activated by a large variety of pathogen-associated molecular patterns (PAMPs) and danger-associated molecular patterns (DAMPs). Additionally, it seems that cells of CAPS patients have increased levels of reactive oxygen species due to increased redox stress, resulting in overactivation or ineffective anti-inflammatory mechanisms [45]. A unique feature of monocytes isolated from patients with FCAS is inflammasome activation when cultured at a slightly cooler temperature of 32 °C instead of the traditional 37 °C, resulting in increased IL-1β, IL-6, und TNF-α secretion [46].

5. Three Distinct Phenotypes Versus One Cryopyrin-Associated Periodic Syndromes (CAPS) Spectrum

Historically, FCAS, MWS, and NOMID/CINCA have been described as three distinct diseases. The first clinical reports of FCAS date back to 1940, when Kile and Rusk described FCAS as an inherited disorder with cold-induced skin and musculoskeletal symptoms [47]. MWS was first described in 1962 by Muckle and Wells as a syndrome of urticarial rash, neurosensory hearing loss, and amyloidosis [48]. CINCA/NOMID was first described by Prieur, in 1980, as a chronic inflammatory disease with rash, articular involvement, and chronic aseptic meningitis [49,50]. However, in all three phenotypes, the disease-causing variant was identified in the *NLRP3* gene [12]. Furthermore, patients can present with overlapping symptoms between the historically distinct phenotypes. Therefore, today CAPS is conceived as a continuous spectrum of disease. Although anti-IL-1 treatment is recommended for all phenotypes and is known to be effective throughout the complete CAPS severity spectrum [51], it is still important to distinguish among the subphenotypes, particularly in the moderate to severe CAPS phenotypes, because more intensive treatment is necessary to achieve remission and to prevent organ damage [52–54].

6. Clinical Manifestations

Similar to several other AID, CAPS is a multi-system inflammatory disease, affecting eyes, skin, muscles, joints, bones, kidneys, and the central nervous system. Some signs of inflammation are commonly associated with distinct subtypes of the CAPS spectrum (Table 1), whereas others are present in all subgroups. Characteristic CAPS symptoms can result from acute inflammation (flares) but they can also be caused by organ damage due to chronic inflammation. A chronic disease course was reported by 57% of 136 patients with CAPS, whereas 43% experienced only symptoms during acute inflammatory flares [55]. The age of CAPS onset ranges between perinatal/early infancy and adulthood. The median disease onset is 0.8 years (0.1–5), but a late-onset, with a median age of 50 years in patients with somatic mutations, has been described [36,55]. The duration of acute inflammatory flares can vary between <24 h up to more than 3 days [55]. CAPS flares can be triggered typically by cold, stress, infections, or trauma and lack of sleep [55]. In particular, cold is a commonly reported and potent trigger for the mild CAPS phenotypes, such as FCAS.

In FCAS, inflammatory flares might be more frequent in the winter, on damp and windy days, and following exposure to air conditioning [14,56].

Table 1. Clinical manifestations and characteristics of cryopyrin-associated periodic syndromes (CAPS) (adapted from [14,18]).

	Clinical Manifestations and Characteristics of CAPS		
	Mild Phenotype (FCAS)	**Moderate Phenotype (MWS)**	**Sever Phenotype (CINCA/NOMID)**
Disease onset	<6 months–adulthood	Early childhood–adulthood	Perinatal
Family history	Often positive	Often positive	Often negative (sporadic de novo mutations)
Inflammatory flares	Yes	Yes + continuous disease symptoms	Yes + continuous disease symptoms
Duration of inflammatory flares	30 min–72 h	1–3 Days ± subclinical	Persistent inflammation
Cold trigger	Yes	Possible	Rare
Dermatological manifestations	Cold-induced neutrophilic urticaria	Neutrophilic urticaria	Neutrophilic urticaria
Fever	6–24 h after cold exposure possible	Particularly in childhood	Yes
Fatigue	Rare	Yes	Yes
Hearing loss	No	Yes	Yes
Ocular manifestation	Conjunctivitis	Conjunctivitis, episcleritis, optic disc edema/papilledema	Conjunctivitis, episcleritis, optic disc edema/papilledema
Muskulosceletal manifestations	Myalgia, arthralgia	Myalgia, arthralgia, oligoarthritis	Myalgia, arthralgia, (poly-) arthritis. epiphyseal bony overgrowth, limb-length discrepancies, contractures
Central nervous system manifestations	Headache	Headache, intermittent aseptic meningitis	Headache, chronic aseptic meningitis increased intracranial pressure, brain atrophy

Abbreviations: FCAS, familial cold autoinflammatory syndrome; MWS, Muckle–Wells syndrome; NOMID, neonatal-onset multisystem inflammatory disease; CINCA, chronic infantile neurologic cutaneous articular syndrome.

6.1. *Unspecific General Symptoms*

Common unspecific signs associated with CAPS are fever/subfebrile temperature, fatigue, and influenza-like muscle pains. While CAPS is classified as a hereditary fever disorder, it is important to know that fever is not always a complaint and, often, objective measurement of body temperature in patients with CAPS does not meet standard criteria for fever [14]. In particular, fatigue is a major component of CAPS and, together with emotional irritability, both can affect a patient's quality of life [57,58].

6.2. *Skin Manifestation*

The characteristic dermatological manifestation of CAPS is a neutrophilic dermatitis that presents clinically with "urticaria-like" lesions, but it can appear also as erythematous and edematous papules or plaques. The rashes are rarely itchy, but often painful and sensitive to touch [14]. Typically, the rashes are located at the trunk and limbs, but can be seen also on the face, upper arms, thighs, and abdomen [14]. In the mild CAPS phenotypes, such as FCAS, the rashes are usually not induced by direct contact with cold objects or water, but often appear 1–4 h after cold exposure in areas not necessarily subjected directly to cold. Additionally, painful extremity swelling is reported [59]. Histologically perivascular neutrophilic infiltrations with leucozytoclasia without vasculitis and eosinophilic infiltrations can be detected in a skin biopsy [60,61].

6.3. Musculoskeletal Involvement

The involvement of muscles, bones, and joints depends on the clinical phenotype. Whereas patients with a mild CAPS phenotype may complain about limb pain, painful periarticular swelling and myalgia limited to inflammatory flares, patients with moderate CAPS often also experience arthralgia and arthritis [58,59]. Joints such as wrists, knees, and ankles are often affected [58]. Patients with severe CAPS may have skeletal abnormalities with bone deformation and may suffer from chronic polyarthritis. Several patients with NOMID/CINCA show characteristic arthropathy with bone and joint deformation caused by overgrowth and asymmetry of the cartilage, excessive uncontrolled growth of the patella and of the long bones, and abnormal epiphyseal and metaphyseal calcification [56,62]. Osseous lesions often affect growth plates asymmetrically with unilaterally reduced longitudinal growth of affected bones causing severe asymmetric limb length discrepancies [14]. In one third of patients, the arthropathy and bone changes are disabling [56]. Other features in patients with severe CAPS are chronic hydrocephalus, atypical facies with frontal bossing, macrocrania, and flattening of the nasal dorsum ("saddle nose") [56,63,64].

6.4. Eye Involvement

Interstitial keratitis, conjunctivitis, episcleritis, iridocyclitis and anterior and posterior uveitis, band keratopathy, and corneal abnormalities can be present in patients with CAPS [65,66]. Less common are posterior stromal corneal opacification with edema, anterior iris snychecia, and cataract [65]. The most common eye manifestation is the conjunctivitis occurring during flares in many CAPS patients [65]. Patients with moderate to severe CAPS often report dry eyes with chronic conjunctivitis or perilimbal redness. In up to 40% of patients, the cornea is involved [58]. Chronic anterior uveitis and anterior segment manifestation varying from mild to severe are seen in up to 55% of patients with NOMID/CINCA [67]. Inflammation of the posterior eye segments is less frequent and can be present as vitritis, retinal vasculitis, and focal chorioretinitis. Elevated intracranial pressure in patients with severe CAPS (NOMID/CINCA) may cause papillary edema and subsequent optic disc atrophy [67]. Typically, ocular manifestations present bilaterally [68]. In more than 80% of NOMID/CINCA patients, the optic nerve head is affected, the most frequent ocular manifestation in this group of patients [58]. Ocular manifestations can progress to blindness and ocular disability.

6.5. Hearing Loss

Neurosensory hearing loss is a major symptom in moderate and severe CAPS. Usually, in untreated CAPS patients, hearing loss starts in childhood and early adulthood [56]. At onset, initially high frequencies are affected, which are often not detected in the routine otologic assessment [69,70]. Therefore, regular monitoring to provide early detection of hearing loss with high frequency pure tone averages (HF-PTA) is important [71]. In some patients, it is possible to detect a cochlear enhancement in the FLAIR magnet resonance imaging, representing inflammation of the inner ear [69]. The mechanism of hearing loss in CAPS is still under research. Nakanashi et al. raised the hypothesis that macrophages/monocyte-like cells in the cochlea might mediate local autoinflammation via activation the NLRP3 inflammasome [72]. They demonstrated that the inflammasome could be activated in macrophage/monocyte-like cells in a mouse cochlea with secretion of IL-1β and concluded that local cochlear activation of the NLRP3 inflammasome could induce cochlear autoinflammation and sensorineural hearing loss [72]. Depending on the type of variant, the hearing loss increases in extent and intensity throughout the course of the disease and with age [73]. Particularly, the variants T348M and E311K are associated with progressive linear deafness if patients are untreated [73], whereas the variant R918Q seems to cause a late onset of hearing loss and moderate progression [74]. A reversal or halt in progress of hearing loss may be achieved by timely induction of treatment but it can be irreversible if the start of treatment is delayed [75,76].

6.6. Central Nervous Impairment

Abnormalities of the central nervous system (CNS) can be caused by aseptic meningitis, in which polymorphonuclear cells infiltrate the cerebrospinal fluid (CSF) [56]. The CNS involvement varies with CAPS phenotype. In moderate CAPS, aseptic meningitis may occur only during inflammatory flares with headache and vomiting, whereas chronic aseptic meningitis and increased intracranial pressure including its consequences, such as chronic headache, papilledema, and CNS degeneration, is frequently observed in severe CAPS [56]. Brain atrophy and cognitive impairment may occur, depending on the severity of the disease. Mild cognitive deficits with need for specialized educational support are reported for the mild to moderate CAPS phenotypes [77]. Further CNS symptoms are seizures, strokes, and stroke-like episodes with hemiparesis, and vascular occlusions [64,78] have been reported. Early onset of CAPS is predictive of more severe CNS involvement and neurological complications [55].

7. Diagnostic Approach

A median delay between symptom onset and CAPS diagnosis has been reported to be 1.4 years (0.2–8.9) [79]. Particularly, in the mild phenotypes, a diagnosis is often delayed (median age 23.3 years) as compared with the more severe CAPS phenotypes [80]. Although early age of onset is a very strong indicator for CAPS, diagnosis of CAPS also has to be considered in adults due to the rarity of the disease, mild phenotypes, and somatic mutation. If CAPS is suggested, a systematic stepwise diagnostic approach (Figure 1) similar to other AID is recommended including patient's history, family history, physical examinations, and inflammatory markers during inflammatory flares and symptom-free intervals [81,82]. Red flags in patient history are specific triggers, such as cold exposure, characteristic disease symptoms, or a family history of early hearing loss or renal transplants. The autoinflammatory disease activity index (AIDAI), a standardized symptom diary [83], captures AID characteristic symptoms and can help to identify CAPS phenotypic patterns. Furthermore, a complete and thorough physical examination is important. The patients should be examined for typical clinical CAPS manifestations, such as urticarial-like rashes. In addition, laboratory inflammatory markers, such as the c-reactive protein (CRP), serum amyloid A (SAA), and the whole blood count, are considered to be first line laboratory examinations during inflammatory flares and in symptom-free intervals [82]. Characteristics of systemic inflammation are blood leukocytosis, neutrophilia, thrombocytosis, anemia, increased erythrocyte sedimentation rate (ESR), elevated CRP and SAA, and myeloid-related protein 8 and 14 (MRP8/MRP14, also known as S100A8/S100A9) [84–86]. Particularly, SAA is one crucial parameter to detect subclinical inflammation and risk evaluation for the development of AA-amyloidosis [87]. Additionally, S100A12 and MRP8/MRP14 can be used for the monitoring of inflammation with a good correlation to inflammation and treatment response [86,88]. Other disorders associated with recurrent systemic inflammation, such as immunodeficiencies, infections, autoimmune diseases, and malignancies, need to be excluded. If these first steps support the suspicion of CAPS, musculoskeletal, neurological, and ophthalmologic examination is suggested [51]. Moreover, HF-PTA, including 0.5 to 10 kHz, formal cognitive testing, brain MRI studies, lumbar punctures with opening pressure, cell counts, protein concentration, and lesional skin biopsy should be considered [51]. During inflammatory flares, elevated neopterin and elevated protein can be detected in the CSF [89]. In patients with severe musculoskeletal involvement, X-ray and bone MRI should be performed [51]. Molecular diagnosis should be attempted when the clinical phenotype, laboratory, and functional tests are suggestive for CAPS.

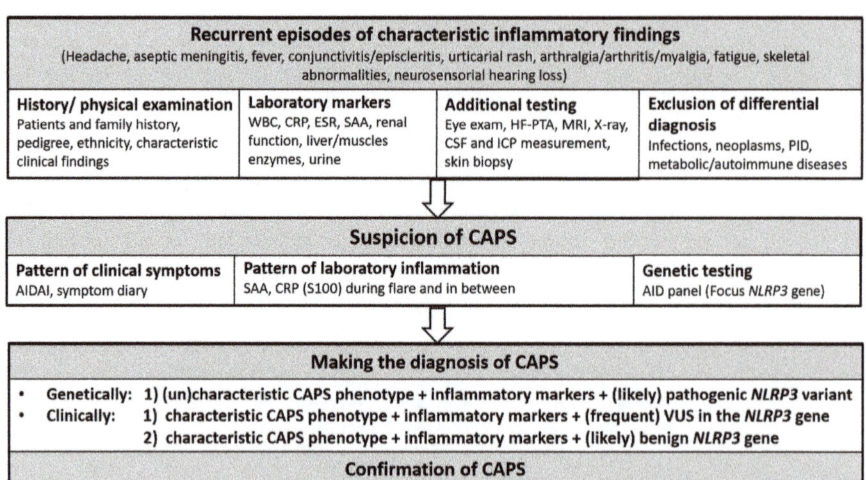

Figure 1. Diagnostic approach to CAPS. WBC, whole blood count; CRP, c reactive protein; ESR, erythrocyte sedimentation rate; SAA, serum amyloid A; HF-PTA, high frequency pure tone audiogram; MRI, magnet resonance imaging; CSF, cerebrospinal fluid; ICP, intracranial pressure; PID, primary immune deficiency; AIDAI, autoinflammatory disease activity index; S100, S 100 proteins (S100A12, S100A8/A9); VUS, variant of uncertain significance. Bold format and grey background indicate headings.

7.1. Diagnostic and Classification Criteria

7.1.1. Diagnostic Criteria

CAPS is diagnosed clinically and genetically. Diagnostic criteria are used to guide the care of individual patients, and therefore must have a very high sensitivity and specificity in order that patients receive the correct diagnosis and treatment [90]. The diagnostic criteria of CAPS recognize that all but a few patients with CAPS have detectable systemic inflammation and use unique CAPS-specific clinical features along the whole disease spectrum to achieve reasonable specificity and sensitivity to aid clinicians in making the CAPS diagnosis [91]. These diagnostic criteria do not include genetic confirmation, and therefore can be applied in places where genetic testing is not available. If genetic testing is not available or it is negative, making a CAPS diagnosis is possible if raised inflammatory markers (CRP/SAA) can be detected plus at least two of the following symptoms: urticarial-like rash (neutrophilic dermatitis), cold-triggered episodes, sensorineural hearing loss, musculoskeletal symptoms, chronic aseptic meningitis, and skeletal abnormalities (Table 2) [91].

Table 2. Diagnostic criteria for CAPS (data from [91]).

Diagnostic Criteria for CAPS	
mandatory	+ ≥2 of 6 clinical characteristic symptoms/signs
Raised inflammatory markers (C-reactive protein, serum amyloid A)	• Urticarial rash • Cold/stress-triggered flares • Chronic aseptic meningitis • Neurosensorial hearing loss • Muskoloskeletal symptoms (arthralgia, arthritis, myalgia) • Skeletal abnormalities (epipysial overgrowth/frontal bossing)

7.1.2. Classification Criteria

Classification criteria are primarily used to define cohorts of patients that can be included in clinical research. Using classification criteria may result in some patients with the disease not being captured (false negative); however, the chance of patients not having the indicated diagnosis (false positive) is very low [90]. In 2019, Gattorno et al. developed validated evidence-based classification criteria for hereditary AID with high sensitivity and specificity [92]. The classification criteria for CAPS are summarized in Table 3.

Table 3. Classification criteria for CAPS (data from [92]).

Eurofever/Printo Classification Criteria for CAPS	
Genetic Criteria	**Clinical Criteria**
Presence of a pathogenic/likely pathogenic *NLRP3* gene variant	At least one among the following: • Urticarial rash • Red eye (conjunctivitis, episclereitis, uveietis) • Neurosensorial hearing loss
Presence of a frequent *NLRP3* gene variant of uncertain significance	At least two among the following: • Urticarial rash • Red eye (conjunctivitis, episclereitis, uveitis) • Neurosensorial hearing loss
No presence of one of the above mentioned *NLRP3* gene variants	At least two among the following: • Urticarial rash • Cold/stress-triggered flares • Chronic aseptic meningitis • Neurosensorial hearing loss • Skeletal abnormalities (epipysial overgrowth/frontal bossing)

7.2. Diagnostic Challenges

As mentioned above, patients with low-penetrance variants or somatic mosaicism might present with atypical clinical CAPS phenotypes. AID panels and targeted NGS may be negative or inconclusive and the correlation of clinical phenotype and genetic result is critical [93]. Furthermore, patients might present with a heterogeneous multi-systemic clinical presentation. Advanced genetic testing can enable a diagnosis in some AID patients [94,95].

8. Treatment

CAPS treatment is a multidisciplinary effort including medication, psychosocial support, physiotherapy and supportive care. Treatment aims are to suppress systemic inflammation, to improve functionality, to prevent organ damage, and to increase patients' quality of life. To achieve these aims, cytokine targeting drugs are important and evidence-based treatment plans including treat-to-target (T2T) strategies play a pivotal role in CAPS management [51,96]. The key component of T2T is the definition of a clinical target, such as disease remission or the lowest possible disease activity. Standardized and repeated examinations are required to determine if a previously defined target is achieved [97]. Different levels of disease activity may require different treatment selections and dosing approaches [51,96]. Since IL-1 plays a central role in CAPS pathogenesis, the anti-IL-1 treatment is recommended for the whole CAPS spectrum [51]. Currently, three anti-IL-1 treatments (anakinra, canakinumab, and rilonacept) are available, and several studies have addressed their safety and efficacy. However, symptomatic patients with low-penetrance variants are at risk to achieve only a partial response to anti-IL-1 treatment, as inflammation seems to be mediated due to NLRP3 specific IL-1β release and NLRP3-independent IL-6 or TNF-α production [23,27].

8.1. Anti-IL-1 Treatment

Anakinra is a short-acting recombinant IL-1 receptor antagonist, which has been proven to have long-term efficacy and safety in several studies [54,98–101]. Anakinra is administered daily subcutaneously and blocks the binding of IL-1α and IL-1β to the IL-1 receptor. In a study of 43 CAPS patients treated with anakinra, for up to 5 years, the most reported serious adverse events were pneumonia and gastroenteritis [101]. Anakinra has been approved by the European Medicines Agency (EMA) and the Food and Drug Administration (FDA) for CAPS. For anakinra, the typical dosing regimen varies from 1 to 2 mg/kg/day for patients with FCAS, up to 10 mg/kg/day for critically ill patients with NOMID/CINCA [14]. The CNS penetrance of anakinra seems to be superior, and therefore this might be the treatment of choice in cases with aseptic meningitis [102]. The recombinant soluble IL-1 receptor rilonacept binds to IL-1α and IL-1β. Weekly subcutaneous administration has shown a good safety and efficacy profile against CAPS [103,104]. So far, rilonacept has only been approved by the FDA. The dose of rilonacept for adults is 160 mg/week and varies from 2.2 to 4.4 mg/kg/week in children [14]. Canakinumab is a fully humanized anti-IL-1β monoclonal antibody that selectively binds to soluble IL-1β and has to be administered subcutaneously every four to eight weeks. Several studies have confirmed long-term efficacy and safety against CAPS [52,105–109]. In patients with mild to moderate CAPS, 150 mg of canakinumab can be administered if the body weight is >40 kg or it can be dosed with 2 mg/kg for patients from $\geq$15 to $\leq$ 40 kg, every four to eight weeks [14]. For children (15–40 kg) with an inadequate response, a dose increase, up to 3–4 mg/kg, might be necessary and dosing up to 8 mg/kg every four weeks has been described for NOMID/CINCA patients [110]. Canakinumab has been approved by the EMA and FDA.

8.2. Supportive Therapy

In patients with CAPS, supportive care plays an important role and can consist, for example, of hearing aids, physiotherapy, and orthopedic devices. Furthermore, adjunctive therapies, such as non-steroidal anti-inflammatory drugs for pain and fever or corticosteroid eye drops and tear substitutes, might help to overcome the disease symptoms. Particularly for patients with the mild CAPS phenotype, warming therapies and local protection for cold (gloves, wristlets) can be beneficial for flair prophylaxis.

8.3. Psychosocial Needs

In addition to anti-IL-1 treatment, CAPS patients can profit from psychosocial support. AID have been shown to be associated with depression, lower health-related quality of life, anxiety, and risk of isolation due to frequent canceling of social events [111–113]. Since AID can affect all areas of life and well-being is linked to psychological factors such as illness beliefs, coping strategies, and the distribution of dependency, these aspects have to be taken into account in the long-term management of CAPS [111,114]. Furthermore, patient support networks can provide emotional support.

8.4. Outlook Drug Development

Currently, there are new treatment approaches under development, which might be used to treat CAPS in the future. For example, small molecule inhibitors targeting NLRP3 directly are one promising drug development [115]. The diarylsulfonylurea compound MCC950 seems to be a potent selective small inhibitor of NLRP3, blocking canonical and non-canonical NLRP3 activation by closing the "open" confirmation of active NLRP3 [116,117]. MCC950-based therapies may effectively treat inflammation driven by wild-type NLRP3, and an evaluation of its ability to inhibit CAPS mutant variants has provided a mechanistic framework for advancing therapeutic development and for understanding its therapeutic potential in patients [118]. Furthermore, Youm et al. showed that β-hydroxybutyrate (BHB) suppressed the activation of the NLRP3 inflammasome by preventing K+ efflux and reducing ASC oligomerization and speck formation [119]. In addition, several other ways to inhibit the NLRP3 inflammasome, such as autophagy or microRNAs, are under research [115].

9. Monitoring

Regular monitoring of disease activity is crucial to determine disease activity and organ damage [51]. Monitoring includes serial physical examinations, measurements of weight and height, audiology and ophthalmologic exams, radiographs and MRIs, as well as musculoskeletal, neurological, and laboratory examinations, such as blood count, liver and muscle enzymes, renal function, urine analysis, CSF measurements, and determination of SAA and CRP levels to detect ongoing inflammation. For monitoring of disease activity in CAPS, longitudinal patient diaries, such as the MWS disease activity score (MWS-DAS) or the AIDAI, can be used for systematic assessment of daily diseases symptoms. Both were initially developed for clinical trials but can be used by clinicians as well. The MWS-DAS captures disease symptoms in 10 domains; nine domains reflect the organ involvement in MWS (fever, headache, eye involvement, hearing impairment, oral ulcers, abdominal pain, renal disease, musculoskeletal disease, and rash), and the tenth is the patient's global assessment score [100,120]. The validated AIDAI is a simple tool for outpatients to assess CAPS disease activity at home [83], allowing treating physicians to better differentiate between inactive or active disease and the need for treatment adjustments. The autoinflammatory disease damage index (ADDI) is a reliable instrument for assessing disease-related organ damage [121]. The ADDI consists of 18 items grouped into the following eight categories: reproductive, renal/amyloidosis, developmental, serosal, neurological, auditory, ocular, and musculoskeletal damage [121,122]. The ADDI can be used to monitor structural damage in individual patients and allows outcome analysis and comparison of results in clinical trials [121].

10. Prognosis

The prognosis in CAPS patients depends, on the one hand, on the CAPS phenotype and, on the other hand, on an early diagnosis allowing the start of effective treatment. The prevalence for AA-amyloidosis in CAPS patients without treatment varies between 10% for mild phenotypes and 25% for moderate phenotype [123]. With the availability of anti-IL-1 treatment, the prognosis of patients with CAPS has improved considerably. However, early and aggressive treatment is crucial to improve quality of life and to avoid organ damage. Only an early start of treatment will prevent organ damage and avoid progress. Furthermore, starting treatment early can result in reversibility, for example, of hearing loss.

Author Contributions: Conceptualization, T.W. and J.B.K.-D.; writing—original draft preparation, T.W.; writing—review and editing, J.B.K.-D.; visualization, T.W.; supervision, J.B.K.-D. Both authors have read and agreed to the published version of the manuscript.

Funding: This research received no external funding.

Conflicts of Interest: T.W. declares no conflict of interest. J.B.K.-D. received grant support and speaker's fees from Novartis and SOBI. No funder had a role in the design of this article; in the collection, analyses, or interpretation of data; in the writing of the manuscript, or in the decision to publish this article.

References

1. Broderick, L. Hereditary Autoinflammatory Disorders: Recognition and Treatment. *Immunol. Allergy Clin. N. Am.* **2019**, *39*, 13–29. [CrossRef] [PubMed]
2. Broderick, L.; De Nardo, D.; Franklin, B.S.; Hoffman, H.M.; Latz, E. The Inflammasomes and Autoinflammatory Syndromes. *Annu. Rev. Pathol. Mech. Dis.* **2015**, *10*, 395–424. [CrossRef] [PubMed]
3. French FMF Consortium. A candidate gene for familial Mediterranean fever. *Nat. Genet.* **1997**, *17*, 25–31. [CrossRef] [PubMed]
4. International FMF Consortium. Ancient missense mutations in a new member of the RoRet gene family are likely to cause familial Mediterranean fever. *Cell* **1997**, *90*, 797–807. [CrossRef]
5. McDermott, M.F.; Aksentijevich, I.; Galon, J.; McDermott, E.M.; Ogunkolade, B.; Centola, M.; Mansfield, E.; Gadina, M.; Karenko, L.; Pettersson, T.; et al. Germline Mutations in the Extracellular Domains of the 55 kDa TNF Receptor, TNFR1, Define a Family of Dominantly Inherited Autoinflammatory Syndromes. *Cell* **1999**, *97*, 133–144. [CrossRef]
6. Kastner, D.L. Autoinflammation: Past, Present, and Future. In *Textbook of Autoinflammation*; Hashkes, P.J., Laxer, R.M., Simon, A., Eds.; Springer: Berlin/Heidelberg, Germany, 2019; Chapter 1; pp. 3–15.
7. Drenth, J.P.; Cuisset, L.; Grateau, G.; Vasseur, C.; van de Velde-Visser, S.D.; de Jong, J.G.; Beckmann, J.S.; van der Meer, J.W.; Delpech, M. Mutations in the gene encoding mevalonate kinase cause hyper-IgD and periodic fever syndrome. *International Hyper-IgD Study Group. Nat. Genet.* **1999**, *22*, 178–181. [CrossRef]
8. Houten, S.M.; Kuis, W.; Duran, M.; De Koning, T.J.; Van Royen-Kerkhof, A.; Romeijn, G.J.; Frenkel, J.; Dorland, L.; De Barse, M.M.; Huijbers, W.A.; et al. Mutations in MVK, encoding mevalonate kinase, cause hyperimmunoglobulinaemia D and periodic fever syndrome. *Nat. Genet.* **1999**, *22*, 175–177. [CrossRef]
9. Hoffman, H.M.; Mueller, J.L.; Broide, D.H.; Wanderer, A.A.; Kolodner, R.D. Mutation of a new gene encoding a putative pyrin-like protein causes familial cold autoinflammatory syndrome and Muckle–Wells syndrome. *Nat. Genet.* **2001**, *29*, 301–305. [CrossRef]
10. Feldmann, J.; Prieur, A.-M.; Quartier, P.; Berquin, P.; Certain, S.; Cortis, E.; Teillac-Hamel, D.; Fischer, A.; Basile, G.D.S. Chronic Infantile Neurological Cutaneous and Articular Syndrome Is Caused by Mutations in CIAS1, a Gene Highly Expressed in Polymorphonuclear Cells and Chondrocytes. *Am. J. Hum. Genet.* **2002**, *71*, 198–203. [CrossRef]
11. Aksentijevich, I.; Nowak, M.; Mallah, M.; Chae, J.J.; Watford, W.T.; Hofmann, S.R.; Stein, L.; Russo, R.; Goldsmith, D.; Dent, P.; et al. De novoCIAS1 mutations, cytokine activation, and evidence for genetic heterogeneity in patients with neonatal-onset multisystem inflammatory disease (NOMID): A new member of the expanding family of pyrin-associated autoinflammatory diseases. *Arthritis Rheum.* **2002**, *46*, 3340–3348. [CrossRef]
12. Aksentijevich, I.; Putnam, C.D.; Remmers, E.F.; Mueller, J.L.; Le, J.; Kolodner, R.D.; Moak, Z.; Chuang, M.; Austin, F.; Goldbach-Mansky, R.; et al. The clinical continuum of cryopyrinopathies: Novel CIAS1 mutations in North American patients and a new cryopyrin model. *Arthritis Rheum.* **2007**, *56*, 1273–1285. [CrossRef] [PubMed]
13. Ben-Chetrit, E.; Gattorno, M.; Gul, A.; Kastner, D.L.; Lachmann, H.J.; Touitou, I.; Ruperto, N. Consensus proposal for taxonomy and definition of the autoinflammatory diseases (AIDs): A Delphi study. *Ann. Rheum. Dis.* **2018**, *77*, 1558–1565. [CrossRef] [PubMed]
14. Hoffman, H.M.; Kuemmerle-Deschner, J.B.; Goldbach-Mansky, R. Cryopyrine-Associated Periodic Syndromes (CAPS). In *Textbook of Autoinflammation*; Hashkes, P.J., Laxer, R.M., Simon, A., Eds.; Springer: Berlin/Heidelberg, Germany, 2019; Chapter 19; pp. 347–365.
15. Cuisset, L.; Jeru, I.; Dumont, B.; Fabre, A.; Cochet, E.; Le Bozec, J.; Delpech, M.; Amselem, S.; Touitou, I.; French CAPS study group. Mutations in the autoinflammatory cryopyrin-associated periodic syndrome gene: Epidemiological study and lessons from eight years of genetic analysis in France. *Ann. Rheum. Dis.* **2010**, *70*, 495–499. [CrossRef] [PubMed]
16. Lainka, E.; Neudorf, U.; Lohse, P.; Timmann, C.; Bielak, M.; Stojanov, S.; Huss, K.; Von Kries, R.; Niehues, T. Analysis of Cryopyrin-Associated Periodic Syndromes (CAPS) in German Children: Epidemiological, Clinical and Genetic Characteristics. *Klin. Pädiatr.* **2010**, *222*, 356–361. [CrossRef]
17. Giat, E.; Lidar, M. Cryopyrin-associated periodic syndrome. *Isr. Med. Assoc. J.* **2014**, *16*, 659–661.
18. Kummerle-Deschner, J.B. Cryopyrin-associated periodic syndrome. *Z. Rheumatol.* **2012**, *71*, 199–208. [CrossRef]
19. Hoffman, H.M.; Gregory, S.G.; Mueller, J.L.; Tresierras, M.; Broide, D.H.; Wanderer, A.A.; Kolodner, R.D. Fine structure mapping of CIAS1: Identification of an ancestral haplotype and a common FCAS mutation, L353P. *Qual. Life Res.* **2003**, *112*, 209–216. [CrossRef]
20. Booshehri, L.M.; Hoffman, H.M. CAPS and NLRP3. *J. Clin. Immunol.* **2019**, *39*, 277–286. [CrossRef]
21. Richards, S.; Aziz, N.; Bale, S.; Bick, D.; Das, S.; Gastier-Foster, J.; Grody, W.W.; Hegde, M.; Lyon, E.; Spector, E.; et al. Standards and guidelines for the interpretation of sequence variants: A joint consensus recommendation of the American College of Medical Genetics and Genomics and the Association for Molecular Pathology. *Genet. Med.* **2015**, *17*, 405–423. [CrossRef]
22. Sarrauste de Menthière, C.; Terriere, S.; Pugnere, D.; Ruiz, M.; Demaille, J.; Touitou, I. INFEVERS: The Registry for FMF and hereditary inflammatory disorders mutations. *Nucleic Acids Res.* **2003**, *31*, 282–285. [CrossRef]
23. Kuemmerle-Deschner, J.B.; Verma, D.; Endres, T.; Broderick, L.; De Jesus, A.A.; Hofer, F.; Blank, N.; Krause, K.; Rietschel, C.; Horneff, G.; et al. Brief Report: Clinical and Molecular Phenotypes of Low-Penetrance Variants of NLRP3: Diagnostic and Therapeutic Challenges. *Arthritis Rheumatol.* **2017**, *69*, 2233–2240. [CrossRef] [PubMed]

24. Theodoropoulou, K.; Wittkowski, H.; Busso, N.; Von Scheven-Gête, A.; Moix, I.; Vanoni, F.; Hengten, V.; Horneff, G.; Haas, J.-P.; Fischer, N.; et al. Increased Prevalence of NLRP3 Q703K Variant Among Patients with Autoinflammatory Diseases: An International Multicentric Study. *Front. Immunol.* **2020**, *11*, 877. [CrossRef] [PubMed]
25. Shinar, Y.; Ceccherini, I.; Rowczenio, D.; Aksentijevich, I.; Arostegui, J.; Ben-Chétrit, E.; Boursier, G.; Gattorno, M.; Hayrapetyan, H.; Ida, H.; et al. ISSAID/EMQN Best Practice Guidelines for the Genetic Diagnosis of Monogenic Autoinflammatory Diseases in the Next-Generation Sequencing Era. *Clin. Chem.* **2020**, *66*, 525–536. [CrossRef] [PubMed]
26. Rieber, N.; Gavrilov, A.; Hofer, L.; Singh, A.; Öz, H.; Endres, T.; Schäfer, I.; Handgretinger, R.; Hartl, D.; Kuemmerle-Deschner, J. A functional inflammasome activation assay differentiates patients with pathogenic NLRP3 mutations and symptomatic patients with low penetrance variants. *Clin. Immunol.* **2015**, *157*, 56–64. [CrossRef]
27. Schuh, E.; Groß, C.J.; Wagner, D.; Schlüter, M.; Groß, O.; Kümpfel, T. MCC950 blocks enhanced interleukin-1beta production in patients with NLRP3 low penetrance variants. *Clin. Immunol.* **2019**, *203*, 45–52. [CrossRef]
28. D'Osualdo, A.; Ferlito, F.; Prigione, I.; Obici, L.; Meini, A.; Zulian, F.; Pontillo, A.; Corona, F.; Barcellona, R.; Di Duca, M.; et al. Neutrophils from patients withTNFRSF1A mutations display resistance to tumor necrosis factor—Induced apoptosis: Pathogenetic and clinical implications. *Arthritis Rheum.* **2006**, *54*, 998–1008. [CrossRef]
29. Touitou, I.; Askentijevich, I. Genetic Approach to the Diagnosis of Autoinflammatory Diseases. In *Textbook of Autoinflammation*; Hashkes, P.J., Laxer, R.M., Simon, A., Eds.; Springer: Berlin/Heidelberg, Germany, 2019; Chapter 12; pp. 225–237.
30. Hoffman, H.M.; Broderick, L. Editorial: It Just Takes One: Somatic Mosaicism in Autoinflammatory Disease. *Arthritis Rheumatol.* **2017**, *69*, 253–256. [CrossRef]
31. Saito, M.; Fujisawa, A.; Nishikomori, R.; Kambe, N.; Nakata-Hizume, M.; Yoshimoto, M.; Ohmori, K.; Okafuji, I.; Yoshioka, T.; Kusunoki, T.; et al. Somatic mosaicism of CIAS1 in a patient with chronic infantile neurologic, cutaneous, articular syndrome. *Arthritis Rheum.* **2005**, *52*, 3579–3585. [CrossRef]
32. Tanaka, N.; Izawa, K.; Saito, M.K.; Sakuma, M.; Oshima, K.; Ohara, O.; Nishikomori, R.; Morimoto, T.; Kambe, N.; Goldbach-Mansky, R.; et al. High incidence of NLRP3 somatic mosaicism in patients with chronic infantile neurologic, cutaneous, articular syndrome: Results of an international multicenter collaborative study. *Arthritis Rheum.* **2011**, *63*, 3625–3632. [CrossRef]
33. Labrousse, M.; Kevorkian-Verguet, C.; Boursier, G.; Rowczenio, D.; Maurier, F.; Lazaro, E.; Aggarwal, M.; Lemelle, I.; Mura, T.; Belot, A.; et al. Mosaicism in autoinflammatory diseases: Cryopyrin-associated periodic syndromes (CAPS) and beyond. A systematic review. *Crit. Rev. Clin. Lab. Sci.* **2018**, *55*, 432–442. [CrossRef]
34. Nakagawa, K.; Gonzalez-Roca, E.; Souto, A.; Kawai, T.; Umebayashi, H.; Campistol, J.M.; Cañellas, J.; Takei, S.; Kobayashi, N.; Callejas-Rubio, J.L.; et al. SomaticNLRP3mosaicism in Muckle-Wells syndrome. A genetic mechanism shared by different phenotypes of cryopyrin-associated periodic syndromes. *Ann. Rheum. Dis.* **2013**, *74*, 603–610. [CrossRef] [PubMed]
35. Mensa-Vilaro, A.; Bosque, M.T.; Magri, G.; Honda, Y.; Martínez-Banaclocha, H.; Casorran-Berges, M.; Sintes, J.; González-Roca, E.; Ruiz-Ortiz, E.; Heike, T.; et al. Brief Report: Late-Onset Cryopyrin-Associated Periodic Syndrome Due to Myeloid-Restricted Somatic NLRP3 Mosaicism. *Arthritis Rheumatol.* **2016**, *68*, 3035–3041. [CrossRef] [PubMed]
36. Rowczenio, D.; Gomes, S.M.; Aróstegui, J.I.; Mensa-Vilaro, A.; Omoyinmi, E.; Trojer, H.; Baginska, A.; Baroja-Mazo, A.; Pelegrin, P.; Savic, S.; et al. Late-Onset Cryopyrin-Associated Periodic Syndromes Caused by Somatic NLRP3 Mosaicism—UK Single Center Experience. *Front. Immunol.* **2017**, *8*, 1410. [CrossRef] [PubMed]
37. Jiménez-Treviño, S.; González-Roca, E.; Ruiz-Ortiz, E.; Yagüe, J.; Ramos, E.; Aróstegui, J.I. First report of vertical transmission of a somatic NLRP3 mutation in cryopyrin-associated periodic syndromes: Table 1. *Ann. Rheum. Dis.* **2013**, *72*, 1109–1110. [CrossRef]
38. Louvrier, C.; Assrawi, E.; El Khouri, E.; Melki, I.; Copin, B.; Bourrat, E.; Lachaume, N.; Cador-Rousseau, B.; Duquesnoy, P.; Piterboth, W.; et al. NLRP3-associated autoinflammatory diseases: Phenotypic and molecular characteristics of germline versus somatic mutations. *J. Allergy Clin. Immunol.* **2020**, *145*, 1254–1261. [CrossRef]
39. Ye, Z.; Ting, J. NLR, the nucleotide-binding domain leucine-rich repeat containing gene family. *Curr. Opin. Immunol.* **2008**, *20*, 3–9. [CrossRef]
40. Pétrilli, V.; Dostert, C.; Muruve, D.A.; Tschopp, J. The inflammasome: A danger sensing complex triggering innate immunity. *Curr. Opin. Immunol.* **2007**, *19*, 615–622. [CrossRef]
41. Agostini, L.; Martinon, F.; Burns, K.; McDermott, M.F.; Hawkins, P.N.; Tschopp, J. NALP3 forms an IL-1beta-processing inflammasome with increased activity in Muckle-Wells autoinflammatory disorder. *Immunity* **2004**, *20*, 319–325. [CrossRef]
42. Martinon, F.; Burns, K.; Tschopp, J. The inflammasome: A molecular platform triggering activation of inflammatory caspases and processing of proIL-beta. *Mol. Cell* **2002**, *10*, 417–426. [CrossRef]
43. Tran, T.A.T.; Grievink, H.W.; Lipinska, K.; Kluft, C.; Burggraaf, J.; Moerland, M.; Tasev, D.; Malone, K.E. Whole blood assay as a model for in vitro evaluation of inflammasome activation and subsequent caspase-mediated interleukin-1 beta release. *PLoS ONE* **2019**, *14*, e0214999. [CrossRef]
44. Afonina, I.S.; Müller, C.; Martin, S.J.; Beyaert, R. Proteolytic Processing of Interleukin-1 Family Cytokines: Variations on a Common Theme. *Immunity* **2015**, *42*, 991–1004. [CrossRef] [PubMed]
45. Tassi, S.; Carta, S.; Delfino, L.; Caorsi, R.; Martini, A.; Gattorno, M.; Rubartelli, A. Altered redox state of monocytes from cryopyrin-associated periodic syndromes causes accelerated IL-1beta secretion. *Proc. Natl. Acad. Sci. USA* **2010**, *107*, 9789–9794. [CrossRef] [PubMed]

46. Rosengren, S.; Mueller, J.L.; Anderson, J.P.; Niehaus, B.L.; Misaghi, A.; Anderson, S.; Boyle, D.L.; Hoffman, H.M. Monocytes from familial cold autoinflammatory syndrome patients are activated by mild hypothermia. *J. Allergy Clin. Immunol.* **2007**, *119*, 991–996. [CrossRef]
47. Kile, R.L.; Rusk, H.A. A Case of Cold Urticaria with an Unusual Family History. *J. Am. Med. Assoc.* **1940**, *114*, 1067–1068. [CrossRef]
48. Muckle, T.J.; Wells, M. Urticaria, deafness, and amyloidosis: A new heredo-familial syndrome. *Q. J. Med.* **1962**, *31*, 235–248. [CrossRef] [PubMed]
49. Prieur, A.M.; Griscelli, C. Chronic meningo-cutaneo-articular syndrome in children. *Rev. Rhum. Mal. Osteo-articul.* **1980**, *47*, 645–649.
50. Prieur, A.-M.; Griscelli, C. Arthropathy with rash, chronic meningitis, eye lesions, and mental retardation. *J. Pediatr.* **1981**, *99*, 79–83. [CrossRef]
51. Ter Haar, N.; Oswald, M.; Jeyaratnam, J.; Anton, J.; Barron, K.; Brogan, P.; Cantarini, L.; Galeotti, C.; Grateau, G.; Hentgen, V.; et al. Recommendations for the management of autoinflammatory diseases. *Pediatr. Rheumatol.* **2015**, *13*, P133. [CrossRef]
52. Caorsi, R.; Lepore, L.; Zulian, F.; Alessio, M.; Stabile, A.; Insalaco, A.; Finetti, M.; Battagliese, A.; Martini, G.; Bibalo, C.; et al. The schedule of administration of canakinumab in cryopyrin associated periodic syndrome is driven by the phenotype severity rather than the age. *Arthritis Res. Ther.* **2013**, *15*, R33. [CrossRef]
53. Kuemmerle-Deschner, J.B.; Hofer, F.; Endres, T.; Kortus-Goetze, B.; Blank, N.; Weißbarth-Riedel, E.; Schuetz, C.; Kallinich, T.; Krause, K.; Rietschel, C.; et al. Real-life effectiveness of canakinumab in cryopyrin-associated periodic syndrome. *Rheumatology (Oxford)* **2016**, *55*, 689–696. [CrossRef]
54. Neven, B.; Marvillet, I.; Terrada, C.; Ferster, A.; Boddaert, N.; Couloignier, V.; Pinto, G.; Pagnier, A.; Bodemer, C.; Bodaghi, B.; et al. Long-term efficacy of the interleukin-1 receptor antagonist anakinra in ten patients with neonatal-onset multisystem inflammatory disease/chronic infantile neurologic, cutaneous, articular syndrome. *Arthritis Rheum.* **2010**, *62*, 258–267. [CrossRef]
55. Levy, R.; Gérard, L.; Kuemmerle-Deschner, J.; Lachmann, H.J.; Koné-Paut, I.; Cantarini, L.; Woo, P.; Naselli, A.; Bader-Meunier, B.; Insalaco, A.; et al. Phenotypic and genotypic characteristics of cryopyrin-associated periodic syndrome: A series of 136 patients from the Eurofever Registry. *Ann. Rheum. Dis.* **2015**, *74*, 2043–2049. [CrossRef] [PubMed]
56. Neven, B.; Prieur, A.-M.; Maire, P.Q.D. Cryopyrinopathies: Update on pathogenesis and treatment. *Nat. Clin. Pr. Rheumatol.* **2008**, *4*, 481–489. [CrossRef] [PubMed]
57. Yadlapati, S.; Efthimiou, P. Impact of IL-1 inhibition on fatigue associated with autoinflammatory syndromes. *Mod. Rheumatol.* **2015**, *26*, 3–8. [CrossRef]
58. Kuemmerle-Deschner, J.B. CAPS—Pathogenesis, presentation and treatment of an autoinflammatory disease. *Semin. Immunopathol.* **2015**, *37*, 377–385. [CrossRef]
59. Hoffman, D.H.M.; Wanderer, A.A.; Broide, D.H. Familial cold autoinflammatory syndrome: Phenotype and genotype of an autosomal dominant periodic fever. *J. Allergy Clin. Immunol.* **2001**, *108*, 615–620. [CrossRef] [PubMed]
60. Sathishkumar, D.; Al-Abadi, E.; Nicklaus-Wollenteit, I.; Moss, C.; Hawkins, P.N.; Gach, J.E. Early-onset urticaria: A marker of cryopyrin-associated periodic syndrome. *Clin. Exp. Dermatol.* **2017**, *42*, 579–581. [CrossRef]
61. Herbert, V.; Ahmadi-Simab, K.; Reich, K.; Böer-Auer, A. Neutrophilic urticarial dermatosis (NUD) indicating Cryopyrin-associated periodic syndrome associated with a novel mutation of the NLRP3 gene. *J. Eur. Acad. Dermatol. Venereol.* **2016**, *30*, 852–853. [CrossRef]
62. Hill, S.C.; Namde, M.; Dwyer, A.; Poznanski, A.; Canna, S.; Goldbach-Mansky, R. Arthropathy of neonatal onset multisystem inflammatory disease (NOMID/CINCA). *Pediatr. Radiol.* **2007**, *37*, 145–152. [CrossRef]
63. Finetti, M.; Omenetti, A.; Efederici, S.; Caorsi, R.; Gattorno, M. Chronic Infantile Neurological Cutaneous and Articular (CINCA) syndrome: A review. *Orphanet J. Rare Dis.* **2016**, *11*, 167. [CrossRef]
64. Goldbach-Mansky, R.; Dailey, N.J.; Canna, S.W.; Gelabert, A.; Jones, J.; Rubin, B.I.; Kim, H.J.; Brewer, C.; Zalewski, C.; Wiggs, E.; et al. Neonatal-onset multisystem inflammatory disease responsive to interleukin-1beta inhibition. *N. Engl. J. Med.* **2006**, *355*, 581–592. [CrossRef] [PubMed]
65. Cekic, S.; Yalcinbayir, O.; Kilic, S.S. Ocular Involvement in Muckle-Wells Syndrome. *Ocul. Immunol. Inflamm.* **2018**, *28*, 70–78. [CrossRef]
66. Alejandre, N.; Ruiz-Palacios, A.; García-Aparicio, A.M.; Blanco-Kelly, F.; Bermúdez, S.; Fernández-Sanz, G.; Romero, F.I.; Aróstegui, J.I.; Ayuso, C.; Jiménez-Alfaro, I.; et al. Description of a new family with cryopyrin-associated periodic syndrome: Risk of visual loss in patients bearing the R260W mutation. *Rheumatolog* **2014**, *53*, 1095–1099. [CrossRef] [PubMed]
67. Dollfus, H.; Häfner, R.; Hofmann, H.M.; Russo, R.A.G.; Denda, L.; Gonzales, L.D.; Decunto, C.; Premoli, J.; Melo-Gomez, J.; Jorge, J.P.; et al. Chronic Infantile Neurological Cutaneous and Articular/Neonatal Onset Multisystem Inflammatory Disease Syndrome Ocular Manifestations in a Recently Recognized Chronic Inflammatory Disease of Childhood. *Arch. Ophthalmol.* **2000**, *118*, 1386–1392. [CrossRef]
68. Yoshikawa, T.; Kawai, M.M.; Nishikomori, R.; Heike, T.; Takahashi, K. Obvious optic disc swelling in a patient with cryopyrin-associated periodic syndrome. *Clin. Ophthalmol.* **2013**, *7*, 1581–1585. [CrossRef]
69. Ahmadi, N.; Brewer, C.C.; Zalewski, C.; King, K.A.; Butman, J.A.; Plass, N.; Henderson, C.; Goldbach-Mansky, R.; Kim, H.J. Cryopyrin-associated periodic syndromes: Otolaryngologic and audiologic manifestations. *Otolaryngol. Head Neck Surg.* **2011**, *145*, 295–302. [CrossRef]

70. Koitschev, A.; Gramlich, K.; Hansmann, S.; Benseler, S.; Plontke, S.K.; Koitschev, C.; Koetter, I.; Kuemmerle-Deschner, J.B. Progressive familial hearing loss in Muckle-Wells syndrome. *Acta Oto-Laryngol.* **2012**, *132*, 756–762. [CrossRef] [PubMed]
71. Kuemmerle-Deschner, J.B.; Koitschev, A.; Tyrrell, P.N.; Plontke, S.K.; Deschner, N.; Hansmann, S.; Ummenhofer, K.; Lohse, P.; Koitschev, C.; Benseler, S.M. Early detection of sensorineural hearing loss in Muckle-Wells-syndrome. *Pediatr. Rheumatol.* **2015**, *13*, 43. [CrossRef]
72. Nakanishi, H.; Prakash, P.; Ito, T.; Kim, H.J.; Brewer, C.C.; Harrow, D.; Roux, I.; Hosokawa, S.; Griffith, A.J. Genetic Hearing Loss Associated with Autoinflammation. *Front. Neurol.* **2020**, *11*, 141. [CrossRef]
73. Kuemmerle-Deschner, J.B.; Koitschev, A.; Ummenhofer, K.; Hansmann, S.; Plontke, S.K.; Koitschev, C.; Koetter, I.; Angermair, E.; Benseler, S.M. Hearing loss in Muckle-Wells syndrome. *Arthritis Rheum.* **2013**, *65*, 824–831. [CrossRef]
74. Nakanishi, H.; Kawashima, Y.; Kurima, K.; Chae, J.J.; Ross, A.M.; Pinto-Patarroyo, G.; Patel, S.K.; Muskett, J.A.; Ratay, J.S.; Chattaraj, P.; et al. NLRP3 mutation and cochlear autoinflammation cause syndromic and nonsyndromic hearing loss DFNA34 responsive to anakinra therapy. *Proc. Natl. Acad. Sci. USA* **2017**, *114*, E7766–E7775. [CrossRef] [PubMed]
75. Iida, Y.; Wakiguchi, H.; Okazaki, F.; Nakamura, T.; Yasudo, H.; Kubo, M.; Sugahara, K.; Yamashita, H.; Suehiro, Y.; Okayama, N.; et al. Early canakinumab therapy for the sensorineural deafness in a family with Muckle-Wells syndrome due to a novel mutation of NLRP3 gene. *Clin. Rheumatol.* **2018**, *38*, 943–948. [CrossRef] [PubMed]
76. Klein, A.K.; Horneff, G. Improvement of sensoneurinal hearing loss in a patient with Muckle-Wells syndrome treated with anakinra. *Klin. Padiatr.* **2010**, *222*, 266–268. [CrossRef] [PubMed]
77. Mamoudjy, N.; Maurey, H.; Marie, I.; Koné-Paut, I.; Deiva, K. Neurological outcome of patients with cryopyrin-associated periodic syndrome (CAPS). *Orphanet J. Rare Dis.* **2017**, *12*, 1–7. [CrossRef]
78. Parker, T.D.; Keddie, S.; Kidd, D.; Lane, T.; Maviki, M.; Hawkins, P.N.; Lachmann, H.J.; Ginsberg, L. Neurology of the cryopyrin-associated periodic fever syndrome. *Eur. J. Neurol.* **2016**, *23*, 1145–1151. [CrossRef]
79. Toplak, N.; Frenkel, J.; Ozen, S.; Lachmann, H.J.; Woo, P.; Koné-Paut, I.; De Benedetti, F.; Neven, B.; Hofer, M.; Dolezalova, P.; et al. An International registry on Autoinflammatory diseases: The Eurofever experience. *Ann. Rheum. Dis.* **2012**, *71*, 1177–1182. [CrossRef]
80. Mehr, S.; Allen, R.; Boros, C.; Adib, N.; Kakakios, A.; Turner, P.J.; Rogers, M.; Zurynski, Y.; Singh-Grewal, D. Cryopyrin-associated periodic syndrome in Australian children and adults: Epidemiological, clinical and treatment characteristics. *J. Paediatr. Child. Health* **2016**, *52*, 889–895. [CrossRef]
81. Soon, G.S.; Laxer, R.M. Approach to recurrent fever in childhood. *Can. Fam. Physician* **2017**, *63*, 756–762.
82. Georgin-Lavialle, S.; Fayand, A.; Rodrigues, F.; Bachmeyer, C.; Savey, L.; Grateau, G. Autoinflammatory diseases: State of the art. *Presse Médicale* **2019**, *48*, e25–e48. [CrossRef]
83. Piram, M.; Koné-Paut, I.; Lachmann, H.J.; Frenkel, J.; Ozen, S.; Kuemmerle-Deschner, J.; Stojanov, S.; Simon, A.; Finetti, M.; Sormani, M.P.; et al. Validation of the Auto-Inflammatory Diseases Activity Index (AIDAI) for hereditary recurrent fever syndromes. *Ann. Rheum. Dis.* **2013**, *73*, 2168–2173. [CrossRef]
84. Hawkins, P.; Lachmann, H.J.; Aganna, E.; McDermott, M.F. Spectrum of clinical features in Muckle-Wells syndrome and response to anakinra. *Arthritis Rheum.* **2004**, *50*, 607–612. [CrossRef] [PubMed]
85. Li, C.; Tan, X.; Zhang, J.; Li, S.; Mo, W.; Han, T.; Kuang, W.; Zhou, Y.; Deng, J. Gene mutations and clinical phenotypes in 15 Chinese children with cryopyrin-associated periodic syndrome (CAPS). *Sci. China Life Sci.* **2017**, *60*, 1436–1444. [CrossRef] [PubMed]
86. Wittkowski, H.; Kuemmerle-Deschner, J.B.; Austermann, J.; Holzinger, D.; Goldbach-Mansky, R.; Gramlich, K.; Lohse, P.; Jung, T.; Roth, J.; Benseler, S.M.; et al. MRP8 and MRP14, phagocyte-specific danger signals, are sensitive biomarkers of disease activity in cryopyrin-associated periodic syndromes. *Ann. Rheum. Dis.* **2011**, *70*, 2075–2081. [CrossRef] [PubMed]
87. Lachmann, H.J.; Goodman, H.J.B.; Gilbertson, J.A.; Gallimore, J.R.; Sabin, C.A.; Gillmore, J.D.; Hawkins, P.N. Natural History and Outcome in Systemic AA Amyloidosis. *N. Engl. J. Med.* **2007**, *356*, 2361–2371. [CrossRef] [PubMed]
88. Nirmala, N.; Grom, A.; Gram, H. Biomarkers in systemic juvenile idiopathic arthritis: A comparison with biomarkers in cryopyrin-associated periodic syndromes. *Curr. Opin. Rheumatol.* **2014**, *26*, 543–552. [CrossRef]
89. Serrano, M.; Ormazábal, A.; Anton, J.; Arostegui, J.I.; García-Cazorla, À. Cerebrospinal Fluid Neopterin and Cryopyrin-Associated Periodic Syndrome. *Pediatr. Neurol.* **2009**, *41*, 448–450. [CrossRef]
90. Hashkes, P.J.; Barron, K.S.; Laxer, R.M. Clinical Approach to the Diagnosis of Autoinflammatory Diseases. In *Textbook of Autoinflammation*; Springer: Berlin/Heidelberg, Germany, 2019; pp. 203–223.
91. Kuemmerle-Deschner, J.B.; Özen, S.; Tyrrell, P.N.; Kone-Paut, I.; Goldbach-Mansky, R.; Lachmann, H.; Blank, N.; Hoffman, H.M.; Weissbarth-Riedel, E.; Hügle, B.; et al. Diagnostic criteria for cryopyrin-associated periodic syndrome (CAPS). *Ann. Rheum. Dis.* **2017**, *76*, 942–947. [CrossRef]
92. Gattorno, M.; Hofer, M.; Federici, S.; Vanoni, F.; Bovis, F.; Aksentijevich, I.; Anton, J.; Arostegui, J.I.; Barron, K.; Ben-Cherit, E.; et al. Classification criteria for autoinflammatory recurrent fevers. *Ann. Rheum. Dis.* **2019**, *78*, 1025–1032. [CrossRef]
93. Boursier, G.; Rittore, C.; Georgin-Lavialle, S.; Belot, A.; Galeotti, C.; Hachulla, E.; Hentgen, V.; Rossi-Semerano, L.; Sarrabay, G.; Touitou, A.I.; et al. Positive Impact of Expert Reference Center Validation on Performance of Next-Generation Sequencing for Genetic Diagnosis of Autoinflammatory Diseases. *J. Clin. Med.* **2019**, *8*, 1729. [CrossRef]
94. Papa, R.; Rusmini, M.; Volpi, S.; Caorsi, R.; Picco, P.; Grossi, A.; Caroli, F.; Bovis, F.; Musso, V.; Obici, L.; et al. Next generation sequencing panel in undifferentiated autoinflammatory diseases identifies patients with colchicine-responder recurrent fevers. *Rheumatology (Oxford)* **2019**, *59*, 344–360. [CrossRef]

95. Kuemmerle-Deschner, J.B.; Welzel, T.; Hoertnagel, K.; Tsiflikas, I.; Hospach, A.; Liu, X.; Schlipf, S.; Hansmann, S.; Samba, S.D.; Griesinger, A.; et al. New variant in the IL1RN-gene (DIRA) associated with late-onset, CRMO-like presentation. *Rheumatology* **2020**, *59*, 3259–3263. [CrossRef] [PubMed]
96. Hansmann, S.; Lainka, E.; Horneff, G.; Holzinger, D.; Rieber, N.; Jansson, A.F.; Rösen-Wolff, A.; Erbis, G.; Prelog, M.; Brunner, J.; et al. Consensus protocols for the diagnosis and management of the hereditary autoinflammatory syndromes CAPS, TRAPS and MKD/HIDS: A German PRO-KIND initiative. *Pediatr. Rheumatol.* **2020**, *18*, 1–11. [CrossRef]
97. Smolen, J.S. Treat-to-target: Rationale and strategies. *Clin. Exp. Rheumatol.* **2012**, *30* (Suppl. 73), S2–S6. [PubMed]
98. Lepore, L.; Paloni, G.; Caorsi, R.; Alessio, M.; Rigante, D.; Ruperto, N.; Cattalini, M.; Tommasini, A.; Zulian, F.; Ventura, A.; et al. Follow-Up and Quality of Life of Patients with Cryopyrin-Associated Periodic Syndromes Treated with Anakinra. *J. Pediatr.* **2010**, *157*, 310–315.e1. [CrossRef] [PubMed]
99. Sibley, C.H.; Plass, N.; Snow, J.; Wiggs, E.A.; Brewer, C.C.; King, K.A.; Zalewski, C.; Kim, H.J.; Bishop, R.; Hill, S.; et al. Sustained response and prevention of damage progression in patients with neonatal-onset multisystem inflammatory disease treated with anakinra: A cohort study to determine three- and five-year outcomes. *Arthritis Rheum.* **2012**, *64*, 2375–2386. [CrossRef] [PubMed]
100. Kuemmerle-Deschner, J.B.; Tyrrell, P.N.; Koetter, I.; Wittkowski, H.; Bialkowski, A.; Tzaribachev, N.; Lohse, P.; Koitchev, A.; Deuter, C.; Foell, D.; et al. Efficacy and safety of anakinra therapy in pediatric and adult patients with the autoinflammatory Muckle-Wells syndrome. *Arthritis Rheum.* **2011**, *63*, 840–849. [CrossRef] [PubMed]
101. Kullenberg, T.; Löfqvist, M.; Leinonen, M.; Goldbach-Mansky, R.; Olivecrona, H. Long-term safety profile of anakinra in patients with severe cryopyrin-associated periodic syndromes. *Rheumatology* **2016**, *55*, 1499–1506. [CrossRef]
102. Rodriguez-Smith, J.; Lin, Y.; Tsai, W.L.; Kim, H.; Montealegre-Sanchez, G.; Chapelle, D.; Huang, Y.; Sibley, C.H.; Gadina, M.; Wesley, R.; et al. Cerebrospinal Fluid Cytokines Correlate with Aseptic Meningitis and Blood–Brain Barrier Function in Neonatal-Onset Multisystem Inflammatory Disease: Central Nervous System Biomarkers in Neonatal-Onset Multisystem Inflammatory Disease Correlate with Central Nervous System Inflammation. *Arthritis Rheumatol.* **2017**, *69*, 1325–1336. [CrossRef]
103. Hoffman, H.M.; Throne, M.L.; Amar, N.J.; Sebai, M.; Kivitz, A.J.; Kavanaugh, A.; Weinstein, S.P.; Belomestnov, P.; Yancopoulos, G.D.; Stahl, N.; et al. Efficacy and safety of rilonacept (interleukin-1 Trap) in patients with cryopyrin-associated periodic syndromes: Results from two sequential placebo-controlled studies. *Arthritis Rheum.* **2008**, *58*, 2443–2452. [CrossRef]
104. Hoffman, H.M.; Throne, M.L.; Amar, N.J.; Cartwright, R.C.; Kivitz, A.J.; Soo, Y.; Weinstein, S.P. Long-Term Efficacy and Safety Profile of Rilonacept in the Treatment of Cryopryin-Associated Periodic Syndromes: Results of a 72-Week Open-Label Extension Study. *Clin. Ther.* **2012**, *34*, 2091–2103. [CrossRef]
105. Lachmann, H.J.; Kone-Paut, I.; Kuemmerle-Deschner, J.B.; Leslie, K.S.; Hachulla, E.; Quartier, P.; Gitton, X.; Widmer, A.; Patel, N.; Hawkins, P.N. Use of Canakinumab in the Cryopyrin-Associated Periodic Syndrome. *N. Engl. J. Med.* **2009**, *360*, 2416–2425. [CrossRef] [PubMed]
106. Kuemmerle-Deschner, J.B.; Hachulla, E.; Cartwright, R.; Hawkins, P.N.; Tran, T.A.; Bader-Meunier, B.; Hoyer, J.; Gattorno, M.; Gul, A.; Smith, J.; et al. Two-year results from an open-label, multicentre, phase III study evaluating the safety and efficacy of canakinumab in patients with cryopyrin-associated periodic syndrome across different severity phenotypes. *Ann. Rheum. Dis.* **2011**, *70*, 2095–2102. [CrossRef]
107. Brogan, P.A.; Hofer, M.; Kuemmerle-Deschner, J.B.; Koné-Paut, I.; Roesler, J.; Kallinich, T.; Horneff, G.; Penadés, I.C.; Sevilla-Perez, B.; Goffin, L.; et al. Rapid and Sustained Long-Term Efficacy and Safety of Canakinumab in Patients with Cryopyrin-Associated Periodic Syndrome Ages Five Years and Younger. *Arthritis Rheumatol.* **2019**, *71*, 1955–1963. [CrossRef] [PubMed]
108. Russo, R.A.G.; Melo-Gomes, S.; Lachmann, H.J.; Wynne, K.; Rajput, K.; Eleftheriou, D.; Edelsten, C.; Hawkins, P.N.; Brogan, P.A. Efficacy and safety of canakinumab therapy in paediatric patients with cryopyrin-associated periodic syndrome: A single-centre, real-world experience. *Rheumatology* **2014**, *53*, 665–670. [CrossRef] [PubMed]
109. Kuemmerle-Deschner, J.B.; Ramos, E.; Blank, N.; Roesler, J.; Felix, S.D.; Jung, T.; Stricker, K.; Chakraborty, A.; Tannenbaum, S.; Wright, A.M.; et al. Canakinumab (ACZ885, a fully human IgG1 anti-IL-1beta mAb) induces sustained remission in pediatric patients with cryopyrin-associated periodic syndrome (CAPS). *Arthritis Res. Ther.* **2011**, *13*, R34. [CrossRef]
110. Sibley, C.H.; Chioato, A.; Felix, S.; Colin, L.; Chakraborty, A.; Plass, N.; Rodriguez-Smith, J.; Brewer, C.; King, K.; Zalewski, C.; et al. A 24-month open-label study of canakinumab in neonatal-onset multisystem inflammatory disease. *Ann. Rheum. Dis.* **2015**, *74*, 1714–1719. [CrossRef]
111. Cipolletta, S.; Giudici, L.; Punzi, L.; Galozzi, P.; Sfriso, P. Health-related quality of life, illness perception, coping strategies and the distribution of dependency in autoinflammatory diseases. *Clin. Exp. Rheumatol.* **2019**, *37*, 156–157.
112. Makay, B.; Emiroğlu, N.; Ünsal, E. Depression and anxiety in children and adolescents with familial Mediterranean fever. *Clin. Rheumatol.* **2009**, *29*, 375–379. [CrossRef]
113. Giese, A.; Örnek, A.; Kılıç, L.; Kurucay, M.; Şendur, S.N.; Lainka, E.; Henning, B.F. Anxiety and depression in adult patients with familial Mediterranean fever: A study comparing patients living in Germany and Turkey. *Int. J. Rheum. Dis.* **2014**, *20*, 2093–2100. [CrossRef]
114. Erbis, G.; Schmidt, K.; Hansmann, S.; Sergiichuk, T.; Michler, C.; Kuemmerle-Deschner, J.B.; Benseler, S. Living with autoinflammatory diseases: Identifying unmet needs of children, adolescents and adults. *Pediatr. Rheumatol.* **2018**, *16*, 1–10. [CrossRef]
115. Shao, B.Z.; Xu, Z.Q.; Han, B.Z.; Su, D.F.; Liu, C. NLRP3 inflammasome and its inhibitors: A review. *Front Pharmacol.* **2015**, *6*, 262. [CrossRef] [PubMed]

116. Coll, R.C.; Robertson, A.A.B.; Chae, J.J.; Higgins, S.C.; Muñoz-Planillo, R.; Inserra, M.C.; Vetter, I.; Dungan, L.S.; Monks, B.G.; Stutz, A.; et al. A small-molecule inhibitor of the NLRP3 inflammasome for the treatment of inflammatory diseases. *Nat. Med.* **2015**, *21*, 248–255. [CrossRef] [PubMed]
117. Tapia-Abellán, A.; Angosto-Bazarra, D.; Martínez-Banaclocha, H.; De Torre-Minguela, C.; Cerón-Carrasco, J.P.; Pérez-Sánchez, H.; Arostegui, J.I.; Pelegrín, P. MCC950 closes the active conformation of NLRP3 to an inactive state. *Nat. Chem. Biol.* **2019**, *15*, 560–564. [CrossRef] [PubMed]
118. Walle, L.V.; Stowe, I.B.; Šácha, P.; Lee, B.L.; Demon, D.; Fossoul, A.; Van Hauwermeiren, F.; Saavedra, P.H.; Šimon, P.; Šubrt, V.; et al. MCC950/CRID3 potently targets the NACHT domain of wild-type NLRP3 but not disease-associated mutants for inflammasome inhibition. *PLoS Biol.* **2019**, *17*, e3000354. [CrossRef]
119. Youm, Y.H.; Nguyen, K.Y.; Grant, R.W.; Goldberg, E.L.; Bodogai, M.; Kim, D.; D'agostino, D.; Planavsky, N.; Lupfer, C.; Kanneganti, T.D.; et al. The ketone metabolite beta-hydroxybutyrate blocks NLRP3 inflammasome-mediated inflammatory disease. *Nat. Med.* **2015**, *21*, 263–269. [CrossRef]
120. Kümmerle-Deschner, J.B.; Tyrrell, P.N.; Reess, F.; Kotter, I.; Lohse, P.; Girschick, H.; Huemer, C.; Horneff, G.; Haas, J.-P.; Koitschev, A.; et al. Risk factors for severe Muckle-Wells syndrome. *Arthritis Rheum.* **2010**, *62*, 3783–3791. [CrossRef]
121. Ter Haar, N.M.; Annink, K.V.; Al-Mayouf, S.M.; Amaryan, G.; Anton, J.; Barron, K.S.; Benseler, S.M.; Brogan, P.A.; Cantarini, L.; Cattalini, M.; et al. Development of the autoinflammatory disease damage index (ADDI). *Ann. Rheum. Dis.* **2016**, *76*, 821–830. [CrossRef]
122. Ter Haar, N.M.; Van Delft, A.L.J.; Annink, K.V.; Van Stel, H.; Al-Mayouf, S.M.; Amaryan, G.; Anton, J.; Barron, K.; Benseler, S.; Brogan, P.A.; et al. In silico validation of the Autoinflammatory Disease Damage Index. *Ann. Rheum. Dis.* **2018**, *77*, 1599–1605. [CrossRef]
123. Obici, L.; Merlini, G. Amyloidosis in autoinflammatory syndromes. *Autoimmun. Rev.* **2012**, *12*, 14–17. [CrossRef]

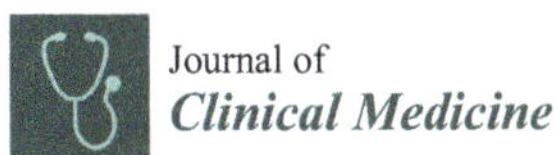

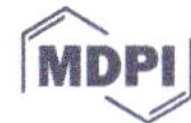

Review

Imaging of Joints and Bones in Autoinflammation

Katharina Ziegeler [1,*], Iris Eshed [2], Torsten Diekhoff [1] and Kay Geert Hermann [1]

1 Department of Radiology, Charité—Universitätsmedizin Berlin, 10117 Berlin, Germany; torsten.diekhoff@charite.de (T.D.); kgh@charite.de (K.G.H.)

2 Department of Diagnostic Imaging, Sheba Medical Center, Tel Giborim Affiliated with the Sackler School of Medicine, Tel Aviv University, 52621 Tel Aviv, Israel; iris.eshed@sheba.health.gov.il

* Correspondence: katharina.ziegeler@charite.de

Received: 21 November 2020; Accepted: 14 December 2020; Published: 17 December 2020

Abstract: Autoinflammatory disorders are commonly characterized by seemingly unprovoked systemic inflammation mainly driven by cells and cytokines of the innate immune system. In many disorders on this spectrum, joint and bone involvement may be observed and imaging of these manifestations can provide essential diagnostic information. This review aimed to provide a comprehensive overview of the imaging characteristics for major diseases and disease groups on the autoinflammatory spectrum, including familial Mediterranean fever (FMF), Behçet disease (BD), crystal deposition diseases (including gout), adult-onset Still's disease (AoSD), and syndromatic synovitis, acne, pustulosis, hyperostosis, and osteitis (SAPHO)/chronic recurrent multifocal osteomyelitis (CRMO). Herein, we discuss common and distinguishing imaging characteristics, phenotypical overlaps with related diseases, and promising fields of future research.

Keywords: imaging; autoinflammation; arthritis

1. Introduction

Autoinflammatory disorders, in contrast to classical autoimmune disorders, are commonly characterized by seemingly unprovoked systemic inflammation without auto-reactive T-lymphocytes or auto-antibodies [1]. The inflammatory process is mainly driven by cells and cytokines of the innate immune system. During the past decade, the understanding of auto-inflammation and auto-immunity has shifted away from a concept of two distinct groups of disorders towards a spectrum of disorders [1,2]. Although joint involvement in varying degrees may be observed in many autoinflammatory diseases, there are a number of diseases within this spectrum where imaging has special significance in the diagnostic process, i.e., familial Mediterranean fever (FMF), Behçet disease (BD), crystal deposition diseases, adult-onset Still's disease (AOSD), and syndromic synovitis, acne, pustulosis, hyperostosis, and osteitis (SAPHO)/chronic recurrent multifocal osteomyelitis (CRMO). The aim of this article was to provide an overview of the state of the art joint imaging techniques in these disease groups, and to point out promising fields of future research.

2. Familial Mediterranean Fever

Familial Mediterranean fever (FMF) is an autoinflammatory autosomal recessive disorder that usually begins before the age of 20 and causes recurrent fever and serosal inflammation of the abdomen, lungs, and joints, leading to severe pain [3]. FMF is commonly seen in people of Mediterranean and Middle Eastern descent, including Jews, Armenians, Arabs, Kurds, Greeks, Turks, Iranians, and Italians. It is caused by mutations in the Mediterranean fever (MEFV) gene, the product of which, the pyrin protein, is involved in the control of inflammation [4].

Arthralgia of the large joints of lower extremities including hip, knee, or ankle joints is common. The patient often presents with severe pain in one joint. Very rarely, multiple joints are affected simultaneously. The pattern of involvement of a large, lower extremity joint conjures a clinical resemblance to spondyloarthropathy (SpA). Indeed, the incidence of SpA in FMF patients was reported to be up to 7% of the total patient population. Moreover, up to 27% of patients with sacroiliitis had joint involvement [5] and a significantly higher frequency of M694V. Nonetheless, these patients maintained low HLA-B27 positivity [6].

Enthesitis, which is the hallmark of SpA, was also reported in FMF, mainly in the calcaneal insertion of the Achilles tendon, the plantar fascia, and/or the long plantar ligament [7]. The characteristic MRI features of this ankle enthesitis reported in SpA are insertional bone marrow edema (BME), thickening and high signal intensity of the affected tendon, and increased synovial fluid in the adjacent bursa [8]. A unique MRI feature in FMF is significant calcaneal BME along the insertion site of the long plantar tendon—an imaging example is given in Figure 1 [9]. This ankle enthesopathy of FMF patients is related to exertional leg pain that is a common debilitating symptom of FMF.

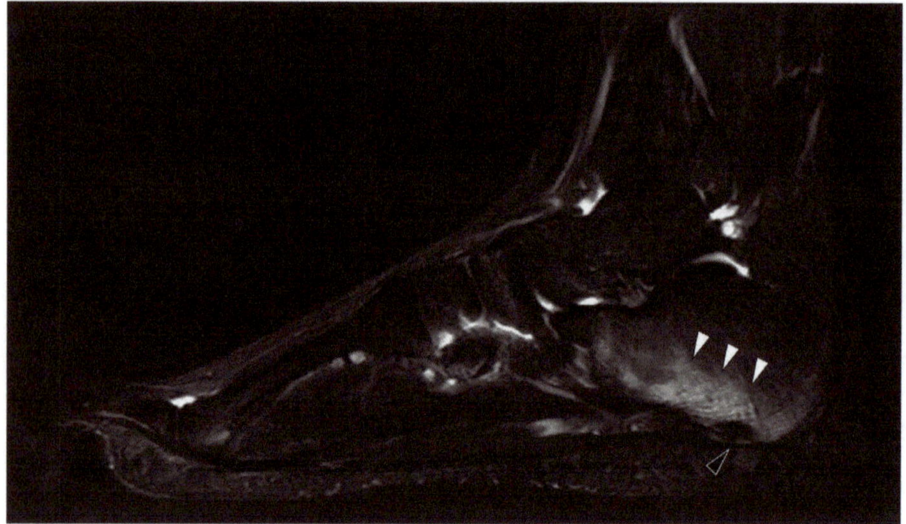

Figure 1. MRI in Familial Mediterranean fever (FMF). Sagittal T2 weighted with fat saturation image of an ankle of an 18 years old male with known FMF and exertional leg pain. There is characteristic enthesitis (black arrowhead) with extensive calcaneal bone marrow edema (white arrow heads) at the insertion of the long plantar tendon.

3. Behçet Disease

Behçet disease (BD) is an auto-inflammatory systemic vasculitis of unknown etiology. BD is characterized by mucocutaneous manifestations (i.e., recurrent oral and genital ulcerations), ocular manifestations (especially chronic relapsing uveitis and systemic vasculitis involving arteries and veins of all sizes), and peripheral arthritis [10]. Although BD does not follow a Mendelian inheritance, it is associated with HLA-B51/B5, and carriers are at high risk of developing BD compared to non-carriers [11].

Arthritic manifestation is one of the minor manifestations and it is usually overlooked. Joint involvement is typically non-erosive and non-deforming arthritis, seen in 50% of BD patients [12,13]. The most commonly involved joints include the knees, ankles, elbows, wrists, fingers, and toes [13,14]. Erosive forms of arthritis in BD are uncommon, and the most affected locations are the axial joint (sacroiliac), enthesis (calcaneal), and peripheral joints, such as metatarsophalangeal and interphalangeal joints of the feet [15]. Repeated attacks of synovitis in the same joint leads to a destructive arthritis resembling the radiological changes of rheumatoid arthritis. There are various variable reports on the prevalence of sacroiliitis and enthesitis in BD. While some report high prevalence, others claim that there is only rare involvement [15–17].

The coexistence of BD and SpA, as well as the presence of clinical overlap between BD and some SpA subgroups (i.e., inflammatory bowel disease and reactive disease) suggest a potential common pathogenesis. However, this has not yet been proven.

4. Crystal Deposition

In terms of prevalence, crystal-induced arthritides are the most common diseases on the autoinflammatory spectrum [18]. The establishment of their inflammatory nature dates back less than 20 years [19,20]. Since then, the capacity of both mono-sodium urate (MSU) and calcium species to activate the NLRP3 inflammasome [21], as well as the production and secretion of pro-inflammatory cytokines, has been widely accepted [22,23]. To date, the gold standard for diagnosis remains the demonstration of crystals in synovial fluid [24,25]. As joint aspiration is an invasive procedure, the need for improved diagnostic imaging is well established. Over the last few years, a number of imaging studies have greatly advanced the detection of MSU, calcium pyrophosphate (CPP), and basic calcium species (BCP). A common denominator of all crystal deposition diseases, however, is the fact that deposition on imaging should not be equated with disease. For CPP, community-based cross-sectional studies estimate the prevalence of deposition between 7.0% [26] and 8.1% [27], while estimates of symptomatic disease are well below 1% of the general population [28]. Asymptomatic hyperuricemia is estimated to affect approximately 2.6% of the general population [29], while the prevalence of symptomatic gout lies much lower, between 0.46% [28] and 1.1% [29]. Therefore, imaging of crystal deposition disease poses unique challenges, which are addressed in the following paragraphs.

5. Gout

Historically, radiography has been the main imaging modality for investigating gout [30]. However, as a radiograph is only able to reliably capture advanced stages of the disease, recent years have seen a shift towards cross-sectional imaging techniques. One of the most available, inexpensive, and non-invasive imaging techniques in point-of-care rheumatology is the ultrasound. Using ultrasounds, MSU depositions may be demonstrated in tendons, periarticular soft tissue, and articular cartilage (i.e., the double-contour sign) [31] with high sensitivity and specificity [32,33]. Longitudinal studies have also demonstrated the capacity of ultrasound to monitor diseases [34]. Additionally, ultrasounds can visualize erosions, joint effusion, and synovitis as surrogates of inflammation [35]. Dual-energy computed tomography (DECT) has become a well-established tool in gout imaging and was included in the 2018 update of the American College of Rheumatology (ACR) and European League Against Rheumatism (EULAR) classification criteria [24]. Its specificity and sensitivity have estimated to be 93.6% and 84.7% in a recent meta-analysis [36], yet its diagnostic accuracy may be lower in cases of recent onset gout [37,38]. Apart from establishing the diagnosis, DECT can be used as a tool for quantification of urate burden [39]. As such, it may be applied as a surveillance tool in urate lowering therapy [40]. Additionally, there is evidence that DECT may be useful to depict bone marrow edema, allowing for a more direct visualization of acute inflammation [41]. Clinical imaging examples of gout are supplied in Figure 2.

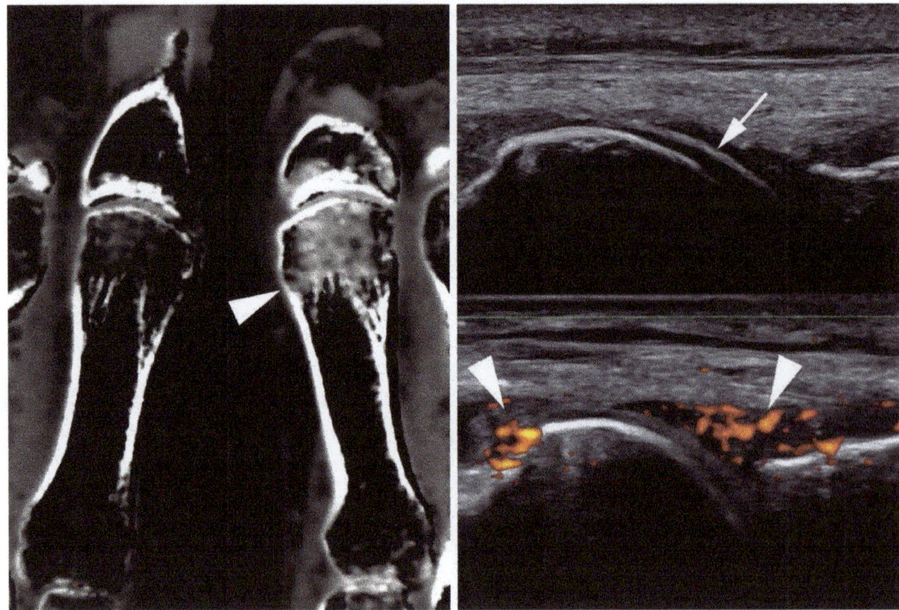

Figure 2. Multimodality imaging for gout. (**Left**): Virtual calcium subtraction imaging from dual-energy computed tomography. The arrowhead indicates bone marrow edema in the first metacarpal head. (**Right**): Ultrasound image of the same patient. The arrow indicates double-contour sign and arrowheads indicate synovitis on the power Doppler.

6. Calcium Pyrophosphate Dihydrate Deposition (CPPD)

The most widely applied and accepted imaging modality for the diagnosis of CPPD remains radiography [25], where linear or flake-like calcifications in typical localizations (e.g., the hyaline cartilage of the knee, or the triangular fibrocartilage of the wrist) may be demonstrated. Nevertheless, CPPD imaging has seen a steady advance in cross-sectional imaging techniques in recent years. Already embedded in the 2015 EULAR recommendations for the diagnosis of CPPD [25], ultrasonography has gained increased attention in recent years. This has been facilitated by the establishment and preliminary validation of ultrasonographic criteria for CPPD by the dedicated Outcome Measures in Rheumatology (OMERACT) taskforce [42,43]. A major strength of ultrasonography in CPPD imaging is its capacity to visualize inflammation by demonstration of synovitis using a power Doppler [35]. Computed tomography (CT) has long been established as an imaging tool in CPPD manifestations at the axial skeleton, especially the atlanto-axial joint (crowned dens syndrome) [44], but recent studies have applied it to the wrist [45] and knee [46], thus putting a new focus on crystal depositions, not only in cartilage but also in ligaments. The use of DECT in the diagnosis of CPPD remains controversial. Although in vitro and in vivo studies show an encouragingly high capacity for differentiation between different calcium species [47–49], evidence of added diagnostic value of DECT vs. conventional CT remains sparse [50,51]. However, DECT may be a valuable tool for strengthening the understanding of the development of specific patterns of arthropathy in CPPD as it can be used to non-invasively detect tissue remodeling [52]. To date, evidence of the usefulness of MRI in CPPD imaging is sparse. In spinal imaging, MRI may be useful for assessing acute inflammation when CPP deposition is established using alternative imaging, such as CT [53]. Imaging examples from different modalities are given in Figure 3.

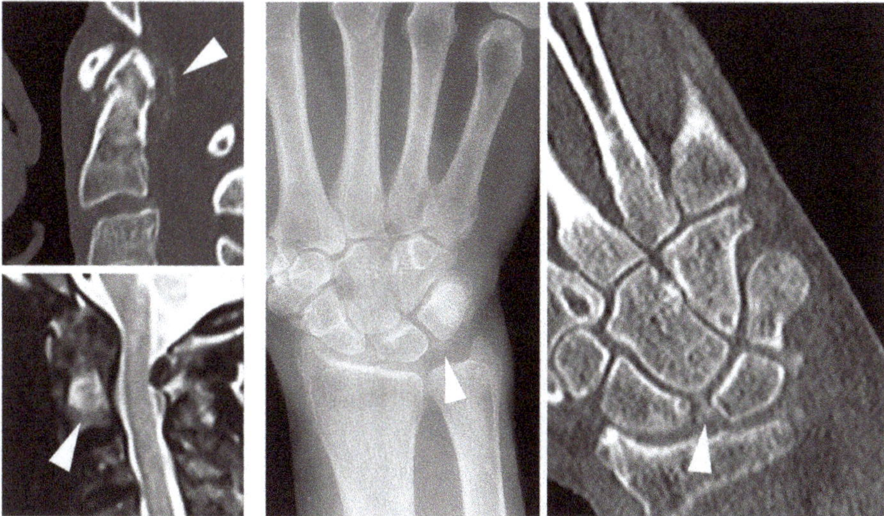

Figure 3. Multimodality imaging in Calcium Pyrophosphate Dihydrate Deposition (CPPD). (**Left**): Crowned dens syndrome with flake-like calcifications in the CT image (arrowhead) and concurring bone marrow edema on MRI (arrowhead). (**Right**): CPPD of the wrist, showing calcifications of the luno-triquetral ligament on radiography and additional calcifications of the scapho-lunate ligament on CT (arrowhead).

7. BCP and Mixed Crystal Disease

Basic calcium deposition (BCP) comprises a heterogeneous spectrum of conditions associated with a number of different calcium containing crystal species, the most common of which is hydroxy-apatite deposition disease (HADD) [54]. In terms of imaging characteristics, BCP may be distinguished from CPP crystal deposition, both by localization and calcification morphology. While HADD typically manifests as circumscribed calcific deposits inside of tendons, especially at the tendons of the rotator cuff [55], CPP crystals are typically found in ligaments and hyaline or fibrocartilage as ill defined, flake-like depositions [56]. An example of a symptomatic BCP deposit is provided in Figure 4. The most commonly applied imaging modality is radiography, which is usually sufficient for visualizing these depositions. Identification of calcium deposition on MRI imaging can be challenging, but three-dimensional imaging allows for the direct visualization of invasion of the deposit into the bursa or bone. The size of the calcific deposit does not correspond with the intensity of symptoms [57]. Symptom onset is typically observed when resorption of the calcification commences [58]. In this phase, macrophages invade [59] and, as a result, local edema, redness, swelling, and tenderness may be observed. This can be accompanied by intense pain and decreased range of motion. During this phase, calcium crystals may enter the subacromial-subdeltoid bursa [55].

A special subtype of BCP is the Milwaukee (shoulder/knee) syndrome [60]. This rare arthropathy exhibits a rapidly progressive joint destruction, often affects older women, and is connected with rotator cuff tears [61]. Synovial fluid aspiration yields a mixture of calcium crystals (predominantly hydroxy-apatite) and sero-hematic synovial fluid with low leucocyte counts [62].

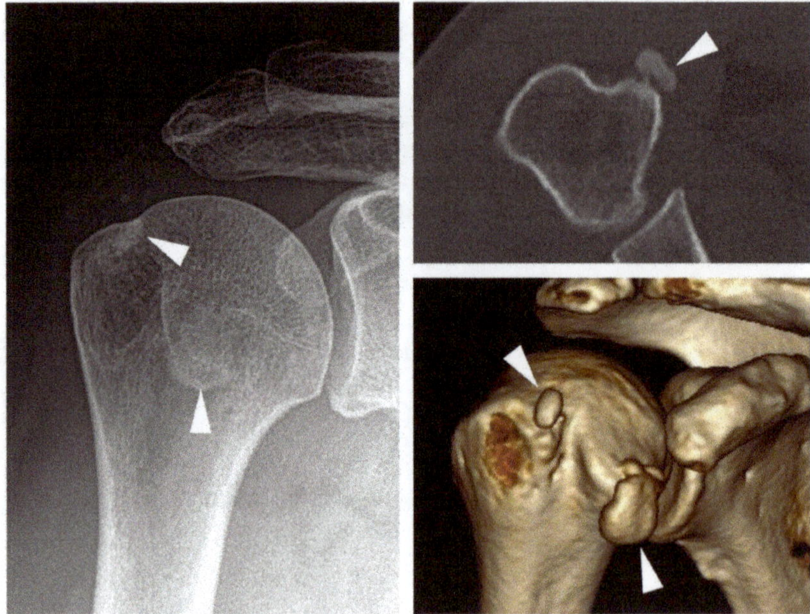

Figure 4. BCP deposition. (**Left**): White arrowheads indicate calcific deposition on radiography. (**Right**): Axial and 3D reconstructions of the same shoulder with better visualization of the depositions.

8. Adult-Onset Still's Disease (AOSD)

Still's disease is a rare systemic auto-inflammatory disease that often poses a diagnostic challenge to clinicians. Among the clinical features of the disease are arthralgia and arthritis, which typically concur with classical fever spikes. Joint involvement is considered a common manifestation and may be observed in at least two-thirds of affected patients. It may present at any joint, including the axial skeleton [63]. Biopsy of the synovium typically reveals non-specific synovitis [64] and synovial fluid analysis shows high cellularity with neutrophil predominance [65]. Although the arthritis is non-destructive in the majority of patients, approximately 30% of patients may develop erosions. In these patients, bilateral destruction of the carpus, with subsequent carpal ankylosis in the absence of erosive changes at the metacarpophalangeal and proximal interphalangeal joints, may be a valuable imaging feature for the distinction from rheumatoid arthritis [64]. Additionally, destructive arthritis of the distal interphalangeal joints in younger patients may be observed [66].

9. SAPHO and CRMO

The syndromes synovitis, acne, pustulosis, hyperostosis, and osteitis (SAPHO)/chronic recurrent multifocal osteomyelitis (CRMO) are considered related diseases, characterized mainly by neutrophilic inflammation, skin eruptions, and osteitis with bone hypertrophy [67]. Alternatively, the diseases are sometimes termed chronic non-bacterial osteomyelitis (CNO) [68]. The distribution of disease involvement differs in children and adults [69]. While the former typically presents with lesions in the long tubular bones and less frequently the spine and clavicles [70,71], the latter usually presents with involvement of the anterior chest wall, spine, and pelvis [72]. As many affected patients are children or adolescents, MRI is widely applied in the imaging of this disease family and may reliably depict osteitis in commonly affected sites [73]. An imaging example is supplied in Figure 5. However, radiography, and especially CT, are superior in the detection of hyperostosis and osteosclerosis, which are both well-established imaging characteristics of SAPHO/CRMO [74]. In adults with primary manifestations at the axial skeleton, differentiation from axial spondyloarthritis (axSpA) can be challenging; however, a valuable diagnostic clue is that generally sclerosis is more pronounced in patients with SAPHO/CRMO [69]. This imaging feature represents an interesting pathophysiological bridge towards the related axSpA spectrum. The predominantly auto-immune (e.g., B- and T-cell mediated) inflammation of the entheses in axSpA and psoriatic arthritis [75] shares many characteristics with the predominantly neutrophilic osteitis of SAPHO/CRMO [76].

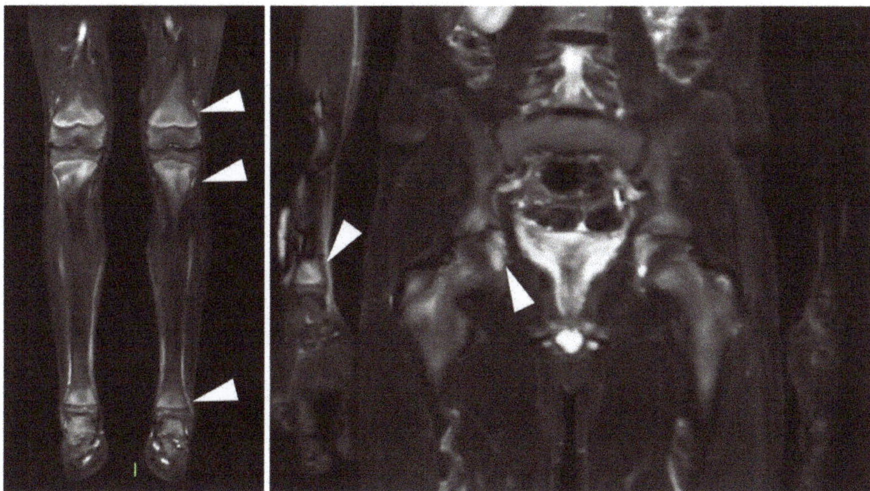

Figure 5. MRI in CRMO. Coronal T2 weighted with fat saturation images of a whole-body MRI in a 12 year old boy with chronic recurrent multifocal osteomyelitis (CRMO). There is evidence of bilateral bone marrow edema in the distal femur, distal/proximal tibia and talus, triradiate cartilage, and unilateral BME on the right distal radius (indicated by arrowheads. In the case of bilateral lesions, only one side was annotated).

10. Conclusions

Imaging is a vital tool to diagnose and follow-up on auto-inflammatory spectrum diseases. Although our knowledge of imaging features of specific auto-inflammatory diseases are steadily increasing, they remain particularly challenging to distinguish from auto-immune diseases in many cases, as cellular and cytokine profiles do not translate directly to imaging features. A better understanding of both common and distinguishing imaging features of auto-immune and auto-inflammatory diseases may increase our understanding of disease pathways in the future.

Author Contributions: Conceptualization, K.Z. and K.G.H.; investigation, K.Z., I.E., T.D.; writing—original draft preparation, K.Z., I.E.; writing—review and editing, K.Z., I.E., T.D., K.G.H.; visualization, I.E., T.D., K.Z.; supervision, K.G.H.; project administration, K.G.H.; funding acquisition, K.Z. All authors have read and agreed to the published version of the manuscript.

Funding: We acknowledge support from the German Research Foundation (DFG) and the Open Access Publication Fund of Charité–Universitätsmedizin Berlin.

Conflicts of Interest: The authors declare no conflict of interest.

References

1. McGonagle, D.; McDermott, M.F. A Proposed Classification of the Immunological Diseases. *PLoS Med.* **2006**, *3*, e297. [CrossRef] [PubMed]
2. Hedrich, C.M. Shaping the spectrum—From autoinflammation to autoimmunity. *Clin. Immunol.* **2016**, *165*, 21–28. [CrossRef] [PubMed]

3. Ozdogan, H.; Ugurlu, S. Familial Mediterranean Fever. *Press. Méd.* **2019**, *48*, e61–e76. [CrossRef] [PubMed]
4. Touitou, I. The spectrum of Familial Mediterranean Fever (FMF) mutations. *Eur. J. Hum. Genet.* **2001**, *9*, 473–483. [CrossRef]
5. Kaşifoğlu, T.; Çalışır, C.; Cansu, D.Ü.; Korkmaz, E.H.C. The frequency of sacroiliitis in familial Mediterranean fever and the role of HLA-B27 and MEFV mutations in the development of sacroiliitis. *Clin. Rheumatol.* **2008**, *28*, 41–46. [CrossRef]
6. Cosan, F.; Üstek, D.; Oku, B.; Duymaz-Tozkir, J.; Cakiris, A.; Abaci, N.; Ocal, L.; Aral, O.; Gul, A. Association of familial Mediterranean fever-related MEFV variations with ankylosing spondylitis. *Arthritis Rheum.* **2010**, *62*, 3232–3236. [CrossRef]
7. Eshed, I.; Rosman, Y.; Livneh, A.; Kedem, R.; Langevitz, P.; Lidar, M.; Ben-Zvi, I. Exertional Leg Pain in Familial Mediterranean Fever: A Manifestation of an Underlying Enthesopathy and a Marker of More Severe Disease. *Arthritis Rheumatol.* **2014**, *66*, 3221–3226. [CrossRef]
8. Eshed, I.; Bollow, M.; McGonagle, D.G.; Tan, A.L.; Althoff, C.; Asbach, P.; Hermann, K.-G. MRI of enthesitis of the appendicular skeleton in spondyloarthritis. *Ann. Rheum. Dis.* **2007**, *66*, 1553–1559. [CrossRef]
9. Eshed, I.; Kushnir, T.; Livneh, A.; Langevitz, P.; Ben-Zvi, I.; Konen, E.; Lidar, M. Exertional leg pain as a manifestation of occult spondyloarthropathy in familial Mediterranean fever: An MRI evaluation. *Scand. J. Rheumatol.* **2012**, *41*, 482–486. [CrossRef]
10. Feigenbaum, A. Description of Behcet's Syndrome in the Hippocratic Third Book of Endemic Diseases. *Br. J. Ophthalmol.* **1956**, *40*, 355–357. [CrossRef]
11. De Menthon, M.; LaValley, M.P.; Maldini, C.; Guillevin, L.; Mahr, A. HLA-B51/B5and the risk of Behçet's disease: A systematic review and meta-analysis of case-control genetic association studies. *Arthritis Rheum.* **2009**, *61*, 1287–1296. [CrossRef] [PubMed]
12. Kaklamani, V.G.; Vaiopoulos, G.; Kaklamanis, P.G. Behçet's Disease. *Semin. Arthritis Rheum.* **1998**, *27*, 197–217. [CrossRef]
13. Adil, A.; Goyal, A.; Bansal, P.; Quint, J.M. Behcet Disease. In *StatPearls*; StatPearls Publishing: Treasure Island, FL, USA, 2020.
14. Park, J.H. Clinical Analysis of Behcet Disease; Arthritic Manifestations in Behcet Disease may present as Seronegative Rheumatoid Arthritis or Palindromic Rheumatism. *Korean J. Intern. Med.* **1999**, *14*, 66–72. [CrossRef] [PubMed]
15. Bicer, A. Musculoskeletal Findings in Behcet's Disease. *Pathol. Res. Int.* **2011**, *2012*, 1–5. [CrossRef] [PubMed]
16. Yazici, H.; Tuzlaci, M.; Yurdakul, S. A controlled survey of sacroiliitis in Behcet's disease. *Ann. Rheum. Dis.* **1981**, *40*, 558–559. [CrossRef] [PubMed]
17. Hatemi, G.; Fresko, I.; Tascilar, K.; Yazici, H. Increased enthesopathy among Behçet's syndrome patients with acne and arthritis: An ultrasonography study. *Arthritis Rheum.* **2008**, *58*, 1539–1545. [CrossRef]
18. Dehlin, M.; Jacobsson, L.; Roddy, E. Global epidemiology of gout: Prevalence, incidence, treatment patterns and risk factors. *Nat. Rev. Rheumatol.* **2020**, *16*, 380–390. [CrossRef]
19. Punzi, L.; Scanu, A.; Ramonda, R.; Oliviero, F. Gout as autoinflammatory disease: New mechanisms for more appropriated treatment targets. *Autoimmun. Rev.* **2012**, *12*, 66–71. [CrossRef]
20. Shi, Y.; Evans, J.E.; Rock, K.L. Molecular identification of a danger signal that alerts the immune system to dying cells. *Nat. Cell Biol.* **2003**, *425*, 516–521. [CrossRef]
21. Bjarnason, I.; O'Morain, C.; Levi, A.; Peters, T.J. Absorption of 151chromium-labeled ethylenediaminetetraacetate in inflammatory bowel disease. *Gastroenterology* **1983**, *85*, 318–322. [CrossRef]
22. McCarthy, G.M.; Dunne, A. Calcium crystals and auto-inflammation. *Rheumatology* **2019**, *59*, 247–248. [CrossRef] [PubMed]
23. Oliviero, F.; Bindoli, S.; Scanu, A.; Feist, E.; Doria, A.; Galozzi, P.; Sfriso, P. Autoinflammatory Mechanisms in Crystal-Induced Arthritis. *Front. Med.* **2020**, *7*, 166. [CrossRef] [PubMed]
24. Richette, P.; Doherty, M.; Pascual, E.; Barskova, V.; Becce, F.; Castaneda, J.; Coyfish, M.; Guillo, S.; Jansen, T.; Janssens, H.; et al. 2018 updated European League Against Rheumatism evidence-based recommendations for the diagnosis of gout. *Ann. Rheum. Dis.* **2020**, *79*, 31–38. [CrossRef] [PubMed]
25. Zhang, W.; Doherty, M.; Bardini, T.; Barskova, V.; Guerne, P.-A.; Jansen, T.L.; Leeb, B.F.; Perez-Ruiz, F.; Pimentao, J.; Punzi, L.; et al. European League Against Rheumatism recommendations for calcium pyrophosphate deposition. Part I: Terminology and diagnosis. *Ann. Rheum. Dis.* **2011**, *70*, 563–570. [CrossRef]

26. Neame, R.L.; Carr, A.J.; Muir, K.; Doherty, M. UK community prevalence of knee chondrocalcinosis: Evidence that correlation with osteoarthritis is through a shared association with osteophyte. *Ann. Rheum. Dis.* **2003**, *62*, 513–518. [CrossRef]
27. Felson, D.T.; Anderson, J.J.; Naimark, A.; Kannel, W.; Meenan, R.F. The prevalence of chondrocalcinosis in the elderly and its association with knee osteoarthritis: The Framingham Study. *J. Rheumatol.* **1989**, *16*, 1241–1245.
28. Salaffi, F.; De Angelis, R.; Grassi, W.; Prevalence, M.P.; INvestigation Group (MAPPING) study. Prevalence of musculoskeletal conditions in an Italian population sample: Results of a regional community-based study. I. The MAPPING study. *Clin. Exp. Rheumatol.* **2005**, *23*, 819–828.
29. Koto, R.; Nakajima, A.; Horiuchi, H.; Yamanaka, H. Real-world treatment of gout and asymptomatic hyperuricemia: A cross-sectional study of Japanese health insurance claims data. *Mod. Rheumatol.* **2020**, *10*, 1–9. [CrossRef]
30. Abdellatif, W.; Ding, J.; Khorshed, D.; Shojania, K.; Nicolaou, S. Unravelling the mysteries of gout by multimodality imaging. *Semin. Arthritis Rheum.* **2020**, *50*, S17–S23. [CrossRef]
31. Checa, A. Consistency of the sonographic image (double contour sign) in patients with gout after ambulation. *J. Med. Ultrasound* **2019**, *27*, 40–42. [CrossRef]
32. Ogdie, A.; Taylor, W.; Neogi, T.; Fransen, J.; Jansen, T.L.; Schumacher, H.R.; Louthrenoo, W.; Vazquez-Mellado, J.; Eliseev, M.; McCarthy, G.; et al. Performance of Ultrasound in the Diagnosis of Gout in a Multicenter Study: Comparison with Monosodium Urate Monohydrate Crystal Analysis as the Gold Standard. *Arthritis Rheumatol.* **2017**, *69*, 429–438. [CrossRef] [PubMed]
33. Ogdie, A.; Taylor, W.J.; Weatherall, M.; Fransen, J.; Jansen, T.L.; Neogi, T.; Schumacher, H.R.; Dalbeth, N. Imaging modalities for the classification of gout: Systematic literature review and meta-analysis. *Ann. Rheum. Dis.* **2015**, *74*, 1868–1874. [CrossRef] [PubMed]
34. Peiteado, D.; Villalba, A.; Martín-Mola, E.; Balsa, A.; De Miguel, E. Ultrasound sensitivity to changes in gout: A longitudinal study after two years of treatment. *Clin. Exp. Rheumatol.* **2017**, *35*, 746–751. [PubMed]
35. Löffler, C.; Sattler, H.; Peters, L.; Tuleweit, A.; Löffler, U.; Wadsack, D.; Uppenkamp, M.; Bergner, R. In arthritis the Doppler based degree of hypervascularisation shows a positive correlation with synovial leukocyte count and distinguishes joints with leukocytes greater and less than 5/nL. *Jt. Bone Spine* **2016**, *83*, 517–523. [CrossRef]
36. Lee, Y.H.; Song, G.G. Diagnostic accuracy of dual-energy computed tomography in patients with gout: A meta-analysis. *Semin. Arthritis Rheum.* **2017**, *47*, 95–101. [CrossRef]
37. Gamala, M.; Jacobs, J.W.G.; Van Laar, J.M. The diagnostic performance of dual energy CT for diagnosing gout: A systematic literature review and meta-analysis. *Rheumatology* **2019**, *58*, 2117–2121. [CrossRef]
38. Bongartz, T.; Glazebrook, K.N.; Kavros, S.J.; Murthy, N.S.; Merry, S.P.; Franz, W.B.; Michet, C.J.; Veetil, B.M.A.; Davis, J.M.I.; Ii, T.G.M.; et al. Dual-energy CT for the diagnosis of gout: An accuracy and diagnostic yield study. *Ann. Rheum. Dis.* **2015**, *74*, 1072–1077. [CrossRef]
39. Kotlyarov, M.; Hermann, K.G.A.; Mews, J.; Hamm, B.; Diekhoff, T. Development and validation of a quantitative method for estimation of the urate burden in patients with gouty arthritis using dual-energy computed tomography. *Eur. Radiol.* **2020**, *30*, 404–412. [CrossRef]
40. Dalbeth, N.; Choi, H.K. Dual-Energy Computed Tomography for Gout Diagnosis and Management. *Curr. Rheumatol. Rep.* **2013**, *15*, 301. [CrossRef]
41. Diekhoff, T.; Scheel, M.; Hermann, S.; Mews, J.; Hamm, B.; Hermann, K.-G.A. Osteitis: A retrospective feasibility study comparing single-source dual-energy CT to MRI in selected patients with suspected acute gout. *Skelet. Radiol.* **2017**, *46*, 185–190. [CrossRef]
42. Filippou, G.; Scirè, C.A.; Adinolfi, A.; Damjanov, N.S.; Carrara, G.; Bruyn, G.A.W.; Cazenave, T.; D'Agostino, M.A.; Sedie, A.D.; Di Sabatino, V.; et al. Identification of calcium pyrophosphate deposition disease (CPPD) by ultrasound: Reliability of the OMERACT definitions in an extended set of joints—An international multiobserver study by the OMERACT Calcium Pyrophosphate Deposition Disease Ultrasound Subtask Force. *Ann. Rheum. Dis.* **2018**, *77*, 1194–1199. [CrossRef] [PubMed]
43. Filippou, G.; Scirè, C.A.; Damjanov, N.; Adinolfi, A.; Carrara, G.; Picerno, V.; Toscano, C.; Bruyn, G.A.; D'Agostino, M.A.; Sedie, A.D.; et al. Definition and Reliability Assessment of Elementary Ultrasonographic Findings in Calcium Pyrophosphate Deposition Disease: A Study by the OMERACT Calcium Pyrophosphate Deposition Disease Ultrasound Subtask Force. *J. Rheumatol.* **2017**, *44*, 1744–1749. [CrossRef] [PubMed]

44. Chang, E.Y.; Lim, W.Y.; Wolfson, T.; Gamst, A.; Chung, C.B.; Bae, W.C.; Resnick, D.L. Frequency of Atlantoaxial Calcium Pyrophosphate Dihydrate Deposition at CT. *Radiology* **2013**, *269*, 519–524. [CrossRef] [PubMed]
45. Ziegeler, K.; Diekhoff, T.; Hermann, S.; Hamm, B.; Hermann, K.G. Low-dose computed tomography as diagnostic tool in calcium pyrophosphate deposition disease arthropathy: Focus on ligamentous calcifications of the wrist. *Clin. Exp. Rheumatol.* **2019**, *37*, 826–833.
46. Misra, D.; Guermazi, A.; Sieren, J.P.; Lynch, J.A.; Torner, J.C.; Neogi, T.; Felson, D. CT imaging for evaluation of calcium crystal deposition in the knee: Initial experience from the Multicenter Osteoarthritis (MOST) study. *Osteoarthr. Cartil.* **2015**, *23*, 244–248. [CrossRef]
47. Diekhoff, T.; Kiefer, T.; Stroux, A.; Pilhofer, I.; Juran, R.; Mews, J.; Blobel, J.; Tsuyuki, M.; Ackermann, B.; Hamm, B.; et al. Detection and Characterization of Crystal Suspensions Using Single-Source Dual-Energy Computed Tomography. *Investig. Radiol.* **2015**, *50*, 255–260. [CrossRef]
48. Pascart, T.; Falgayrac, G.; Norberciak, L.; Lalanne, C.; Legrand, J.; Houvenagel, E.; Ea, H.-K.; Becce, F.; Budzik, J.-F. Dual-energy computed-tomography-based discrimination between basic calcium phosphate and calcium pyrophosphate crystal deposition in vivo. *Ther. Adv. Musculoskelet. Dis.* **2020**, *12*, 1759720. [CrossRef]
49. Pascart, T.; Norberciak, L.; Legrand, J.; Becce, F.; Budzik, J. Dual-energy computed tomography in calcium pyrophosphate deposition: Initial clinical experience. *Osteoarthr. Cartil.* **2019**, *27*, 1309–1314. [CrossRef]
50. Filippou, G.; Pascart, T.; Iagnocco, A. Utility of Ultrasound and Dual Energy CT in Crystal Disease Diagnosis and Management. *Curr. Rheumatol. Rep.* **2020**, *22*, 1–8. [CrossRef]
51. Ziegeler, K.; Hermann, S.; Hermann, K.G.A.; Hamm, B.; Diekhoff, T. Dual-energy CT in the differentiation of crystal depositions of the wrist: Does it have added value? *Skelet. Radiol.* **2019**, *49*, 707–713. [CrossRef]
52. Ziegeler, K.; Richter, S.-T.; Hermann, S.; Hermann, K.G.A.; Hamm, B.; Diekhoff, T. Dual-energy CT collagen density mapping of wrist ligaments reveals tissue remodeling in CPPD patients: First results from a clinical cohort. *Skelet. Radiol.* **2020**, 1–7. [CrossRef] [PubMed]
53. Moshrif, A.; Laredo, J.D.; Bassiouni, H.; Abdelkareem, M.; Richette, P.; Rigon, M.R.; Bardin, T. Spinal involvement with calcium pyrophosphate deposition disease in an academic rheumatology center: A series of 37 patients. *Semin. Arthritis Rheum.* **2019**, *48*, 1113–1126. [CrossRef] [PubMed]
54. Hongsmatip, P.; Cheng, K.Y.; Kim, C.; Lawrence, D.A.; Rivera, R.; Smitaman, E. Calcium hydroxyapatite deposition disease: Imaging features and presentations mimicking other pathologies. *Eur. J. Radiol.* **2019**, *120*, 108653. [CrossRef] [PubMed]
55. Chianca, V.; Albano, D.; Messina, C.; Midiri, F.; Mauri, G.; Aliprandi, A.; Catapano, M.; Pescatori, L.C.; Monaco, C.G.; Gitto, S.; et al. Rotator cuff calcific tendinopathy: From diagnosis to treatment. *Acta Biomed.* **2018**, *89*, 186–196. [PubMed]
56. Jacques, T.; Michelin, P.; Badr, S.; Nasuto, M.; Lefebvre, G.; Larkman, N.; Cotten, A. Conventional Radiology in Crystal Arthritis. *Radiol. Clin. N. Am.* **2017**, *55*, 967–984. [CrossRef] [PubMed]
57. Cho, N.S.; Lee, B.G.; Rhee, Y.G. Radiologic course of the calcific deposits in calcific tendinitis of the shoulder: Does the initial radiologic aspect affect the final results? *J. Shoulder Elb. Surg.* **2010**, *19*, 267–272. [CrossRef]
58. Uhthoff, H.; Sarkar, K. Calcifying tendinitis. *Baillières Clin. Rheumatol.* **1989**, *3*, 567–581. [CrossRef]
59. Greis, A.C.; Derrington, S.M.; McAuliffe, M. Evaluation and Nonsurgical Management of Rotator Cuff Calcific Tendinopathy. *Orthop. Clin. N. Am.* **2015**, *46*, 293–302. [CrossRef]
60. Ea, H.; Lioté, F. Calcium pyrophosphate dihydrate and basic calcium phosphate crystalinduced arthropathies: Update on pathogenesis, clinical features, and Therapy. *Curr. Rheumatol. Rep.* **2004**, *6*, 221–227. [CrossRef]
61. McCarty, D.J. Milwaukee shoulder syndrome. *Trans. Am. Clin. Climatol. Assoc.* **1991**, *102*, 271–283, discussion 283–274.
62. Santiago, T.; Coutinho, M.; Malcata, A.; Da Silva, J.A.P. Milwaukee shoulder (and knee) syndrome. *BMJ Case Rep.* **2014**, *2014*, bcr2013202183. [CrossRef] [PubMed]
63. Feist, E.; Mitrovic, S.; Fautrel, B. Mechanisms, biomarkers and targets for adult-onset Still's disease. *Nat. Rev. Rheumatol.* **2018**, *14*, 603–618. [CrossRef] [PubMed]
64. Fautrel, B. Adult-onset Still disease. *Best Pract. Res. Clin. Rheumatol.* **2008**, *22*, 773–792. [CrossRef] [PubMed]
65. Pouchot, J.; Sampalis, J.S.; Beaudet, F.; Carette, S.; Decary, F.; Salusinsky-Sternbach, M.; Hill, R.O.; Gutkowski, A.; Harth, M.; Myhal, D.; et al. Adult Still's disease: Manifestations, disease course, and outcome in 62 patients. *Medicine* **1991**, *70*, 118–136. [CrossRef]

66. Belghali, S.; El Amri, N.; Baccouche, K.; Laataoui, S.; Bouzaoueche, M.; Zeglaoui, H.; Bouajina, E. Atypical form of Adult-onset Still's Disease with Distal Interphalangeal Joints Involvement. *Curr. Rheumatol. Rev.* **2018**, *14*, 284–288. [CrossRef]
67. Jelušić, M.; Čekada, N.; Frković, M.; Potočki, K.; Skerlev, M.; Murat-Sušić, S.; Husar, K.; Đapić, T.; Šmigovec, I.; Bajramović, D. Chronic Recurrent Multifocal Osteomyelitis (CRMO) and Synovitis Acne Pustulosis Hyperostosis Osteitis (SAPHO) Syndrome—Two Presentations of the Same Disease? *Acta Dermatovenerol. Croat.* **2018**, *26*, 212–219.
68. Jansson, M.A.; Renner, E.D.; Ramser, J.; Mayer, A.; Haban, M.; Meindl, A.; Grote, V.; Diebold, J.; Schneider, K.; Belohradsky, B.H. Classification of Non-Bacterial Osteitis: Retrospective study of clinical, immunological and genetic aspects in 89 patients. *Rheumatology* **2007**, *46*, 154–160. [CrossRef]
69. Klicman, R.F.; Simoni, P.; Robinson, P.; Teh, J.; Jurik, A.G. SAPHO and CRMO: The Value of Imaging. *Semin. Musculoskelet. Radiol.* **2018**, *22*, 207–224. [CrossRef]
70. Falip, C.; Alison, M.; Boutry, N.; Job-Deslandre, C.; Cotten, A.; Azoulay, R.; Adamsbaum, C. Chronic recurrent multifocal osteomyelitis (CRMO): A longitudinal case series review. *Pediatr. Radiol.* **2013**, *43*, 355–375. [CrossRef]
71. Jurik, A.G. Chronic Recurrent Multifocal Osteomyelitis. *Semin. Musculoskelet. Radiol.* **2004**, *8*, 243–253. [CrossRef]
72. DePasquale, R.; Kumar, N.; Lalam, R.; Tins, B.; Tyrrell, P.; Singh, J.; Cassar-Pullicino, V. SAPHO: What radiologists should know. *Clin. Radiol.* **2012**, *67*, 195–206. [CrossRef] [PubMed]
73. Andronikou, S.; Kraft, J.K.; Offiah, A.C.; Jones, J.; Douis, H.; Thyagarajan, M.; Barrera, C.A.; Zouvani, A.; Ramanan, A.V. Whole-body MRI in the diagnosis of paediatric CNO/CRMO. *Rheumatology* **2020**. [CrossRef] [PubMed]
74. Buch, K.; Thuesen, A.C.B.; Brøns, C.; Schwarz, P. Chronic Non-bacterial Osteomyelitis: A Review. *Calcif. Tissue Int.* **2019**, *104*, 544–553. [CrossRef] [PubMed]
75. Chimenti, M.S.; Caso, F.; Alivernini, S.; De Martino, E.; Costa, L.; Tolusso, B.; Triggianese, P.; Conigliaro, P.; Gremese, E.; Scarpa, R.; et al. Amplifying the concept of psoriatic arthritis: The role of autoimmunity in systemic psoriatic disease. *Autoimmun. Rev.* **2019**, *18*, 565–575. [CrossRef]
76. Himuro, H.; Kurata, S.; Nagata, S.; Sumi, A.; Tsubaki, F.; Matsuda, A.; Fujimoto, K.; Abe, T. Imaging features in patients with SAPHO/CRMO: A pictorial review. *Jpn. J. Radiol.* **2020**, *38*, 622–629. [CrossRef]

Publisher's Note: MDPI stays neutral with regard to jurisdictional claims in published maps and institutional affiliations.

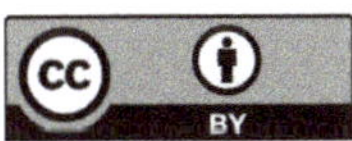

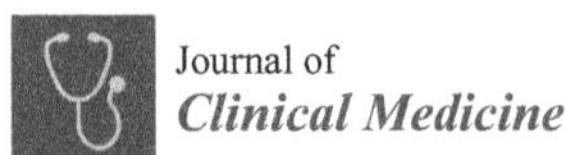
Journal of
Clinical Medicine

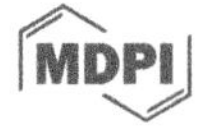

Review

The Impact of Dysphagia in Myositis: A Systematic Review and Meta-Analysis

Bendix Labeit [1,2,*], Marc Pawlitzki [1], Tobias Ruck [1], Paul Muhle [1,2], Inga Claus [1], Sonja Suntrup-Krueger [1,2], Tobias Warnecke [1], Sven G. Meuth [1], Heinz Wiendl [1] and Rainer Dziewas [1]

1 Department of Neurology with Institute of Translational Neurology, University Hospital Muenster, 48149 Muenster, Germany; Marc.Pawlitzki@ukmuenster.de (M.P.); Tobias.Ruck@ukmuenster.de (T.R.); Paul.Muhle@ukmuenster.de (P.M.); Inga.Claus@ukmuenster.de (I.C.); Sonja.Suntrup-Krueger@ukmuenster.de (S.S.-K.); Tobias.Warnecke@ukmuenster.de (T.W.); sven.meuth@ukmuenster.de (S.G.M.); heinz.wiendl@ukmuenster.de (H.W.); Rainer.Dziewas@ukmuenster.de (R.D.)

2 Institute for Biomagnetism and Biosignalanalysis, University of Muenster, 48149 Muenster, Germany

* Correspondence: Bendixruven.Labeit@ukmuenster.de; Tel.: +49-(0)251-835-6684

Received: 6 June 2020; Accepted: 6 July 2020; Published: 8 July 2020

Abstract: (1) Background: Dysphagia is a clinical hallmark and part of the current American College of Rheumatology/European League Against Rheumatism (ACR/EULAR) diagnostic criteria for idiopathic inflammatory myopathy (IIM). However, the data on dysphagia in IIM are heterogenous and partly conflicting. The aim of this study was to conduct a systematic review on epidemiology, pathophysiology, outcome and therapy and a meta-analysis on the prevalence of dysphagia in IIM. (2) Methods: Medline was systematically searched for all relevant articles. A random effect model was chosen to estimate the pooled prevalence of dysphagia in the overall cohort of patients with IIM and in different subgroups. (3) Results: 234 studies were included in the review and 116 (10,382 subjects) in the meta-analysis. Dysphagia can occur as initial or sole symptom. The overall pooled prevalence estimate in IIM was 36% and with 56% particularly high in inclusion body myositis. The prevalence estimate was significantly higher in patients with cancer-associated myositis and with NXP2 autoantibodies. Dysphagia is caused by inflammatory involvement of the swallowing muscles, which can lead to reduced pharyngeal contractility, cricopharyngeal dysfunction, reduced laryngeal elevation and hypomotility of the esophagus. Swallowing disorders not only impair the quality of life but can lead to serious complications such as aspiration pneumonia, thus increasing mortality. Beneficial treatment approaches reported include immunomodulatory therapy, the treatment of associated malignant diseases or interventional procedures targeting the cricopharyngeal muscle such as myotomy, dilatation or botulinum toxin injections. (4) Conclusion: Dysphagia should be included as a therapeutic target, especially in the outlined high-risk groups.

Keywords: myositis; inflammatory idiopathic myopathy; dysphagia; aspiration; pneumonia

1. Introduction

Idiopathic inflammatory myopathies (IIM) are a heterogeneous group of autoimmune diseases in which inflammation of the striated skeletal muscles leads to myalgia and weakness. As distinct subgroups, they include dermatomyositis (DM), inclusion body myositis (IBM) and polymyositis (PM), defined by clinical, serological and histological criteria. In DM, both muscles and skin tissues are affected. IBM owes its name to the histological findings of protein aggregates in muscle cells. In PM there is no skin involvement and an inflammation of the muscle tissue occurs without evidence of inclusion bodies in muscle biopsy. Besides these major groups, there are also overlap syndromes in which symptoms of other rheumatological diseases occur in combination with muscle impairment. In recent years, the role of autoantibodies has been increasingly recognized in both research and diagnostics. Specific autoantibodies are hypothesized to be involved in the pathophysiology of inflammation and thus are associated with distinct disease entities, e.g., the Jo-1 antibody is highly specific for the antisynthetase syndrome.

Swallowing is a complex neuromuscular process that requires the precise motor coordination of the oropharynx, larynx and esophagus [1,2]. While smooth muscles are located in the lower and middle part of the esophagus, the upper part and the oropharynx consist of striated skeletal muscle tissue [2], which is typically affected by inflammation in IIM. It is therefore not surprising that myositis can cause dysphagia via inflammatory involvement of the swallowing muscles. In fact, dysphagia is part of the current American College of Rheumatology/European League Against Rheumatism (ACR/EULAR) diagnostic criteria as an item indicating IIM in patients with symptoms of myalgia [3]. Instrumental assessments, e.g., flexible endoscopic evaluation of swallowing (FEES) or videofluoroscopy (VFSS) are considered the diagnostic gold standard [4,5].

The study data available on dysphagia in IIM are heterogeneous with partly conflicting results, e.g., the reported prevalence rates range from 0% [6] to 100% [7]. Similarly, heterogeneous study results can be found in the instrumental characterization of dysphagia, its consequences or therapeutic implications. The aim of this systematic review was therefore to summarize and analyze the existing evidence on epidemiology, pathophysiology, outcome and therapeutic effects and to estimate pooled prevalence rates in a meta-analysis.

2. Methods

2.1. Review

2.1.1. Inclusion and Exclusion Criteria in the Review

Studies had to meet the following inclusion criteria:

1. Cohort: the article had to report on dysphagia in at least one subject with IIM. If the cohort included less than five subjects, it had to be stated that diagnostic criteria of definitive or probable IIM according to either Bohan and Peter [8,9], Griggs [10], Needham and Mastaglia [11], the European Neuromuscular Center [12] or the ACR/EULAR criteria [3] were met. If this was not the case, articles were only included if based on the information provided the current ACR/EULAR criteria [3] for definitive or probable IIM were met or if the diagnosis was confirmed by muscle biopsy.
2. Topic: the articles had to report on at least one of the following topics:
    a. Epidemiology or prevalence of dysphagia in a population with a minimum of five subjects;
    b. Pathophysiology of dysphagia;
    c. Outcome of a patient cohort with dysphagia;
    d. Therapeutic effects on dysphagia or swallowing.

Articles were excluded if:

1. Patients had other diseases associated with dysphagia, e.g., myasthenia gravis. However, this exclusion criterion was not applied to diseases associated with IIM such as rheumatological diseases in case of overlap syndromes;
2. They exclusively reported on gastroesophageal reflux as manifestation of dysphagia;
3. Dysphagia was reported exclusively as manifestation of structures distal to the esophagus;
4. Conflicting results were reported within the article (e.g., differing prevalence rates).

2.1.2. Search Strategy

To identify studies, MEDLINE was searched for all relevant articles on dysphagia and myositis from inception to January 2020 (last update in January 2020). The following PubMed search algorithm was used:

("deglutition disorders"(MeSH Terms) OR ("deglutition"(All Fields) AND "disorders"(All Fields)) OR "deglutition disorders"(All Fields) OR "dysphagia"(All Fields)) AND (("myositis"(MeSH Terms) OR "myositis"(All Fields)) OR ("polymyositis"(MeSH Terms) OR "polymyositis"(All Fields)) OR ("dermatomyositis"(MeSH Terms) OR "dermatomyositis"(All Fields)) OR ("myositis, inclusion body"(MeSH Terms) OR ("myositis"(All Fields) AND "inclusion"(All Fields) AND "body"(All Fields)) OR "inclusion body myositis"(All Fields) OR ("inclusion"(All Fields) AND "body"(All Fields) AND "myositis"(All Fields))) OR ("Antisynthetase syndrome"(Supplementary Concept) OR "Antisynthetase syndrome"(All Fields] OR "antisynthetase syndrome"(All Fields)))".

Furthermore, reference lists of published articles were screened for additional studies.

2.2. *Meta-Analysis*

2.2.1. Inclusion and Exclusion Criteria in the Meta-Analysis

All studies that reported the prevalence of dysphagia in a cohort of a minimum of five subjects were included in the meta-analysis (Document S1). Only studies that reported directly on a cohort were included (no survey data with estimates of prevalence among physicians). If both instrumental and clinical results were available, the results of the instrumental diagnostics were used. If studies at the same institution had recruited subjects during overlapping periods, only the study with lowest bias risk (Section 2.2.2) was included, or, in case of equal bias risk, the study with the larger sample was included. An equivalent procedure was applied to overlapping cohorts of registry studies or precursor cohorts of a registry. If studies at the same institution did not report an overlapping recruitment period, studies were excluded only if one of the studies stated that all available patients at the institution were included. If studies reported on an identical patient cohort with the same bias risk and sample size, the study that allowed for more subgroup analyses was included.

In addition to the total cohort of IIM, pooled prevalence for dysphagia was estimated in the PM, DM and IBM subgroup and in the subgroup of studies with low bias risk regarding study cohort and dysphagia assessment (Section 2.2.2). Also, the pooled prevalence was estimated for cancer associated myositis, and non-cancer associated myositis in all studies that compared these two groups. All studies on myositis associated/specific antibodies were reviewed to determine whether dysphagia was reported to be associated with (or with the absence of) a specific antibody. If two or more studies compared the prevalence in a population with one of these reported antibodies to a population without the respective antibody, pooled prevalence was again estimated in both of these groups. Studies in the subgroup analysis were only included, if the sample size of the subgroup contained a minimum of five subjects.

2.2.2. Bias Risk in Individual Studies

In all studies included in the meta-analysis, the bias risk was assessed according to the two domains relevant for observational studies, "study participation" and "outcome measurement" of the "Quality in Prognosis Studies Tool" [13]. The domains were adapted to the topic of dysphagia, e.g., in the outcome measurement it was evaluated if studies relied on an instrumental gold-standard assessment including the pharyngeal phase of swallowing. The aim was to evaluate if the presence or absence of oropharyngoesophageal involvement had been assessed by an objective procedure and that dysphagia had not been determined by clinical examination or the presence of symptoms alone. The following criteria were evaluated:

Study participation criteria: (1) Study population represents the total population of IIM or one of its subgroups (DM, PM, IBM, JDM etc.) without additional clinical, demographic or diagnostic criteria, e.g., not only subjects with specific diagnostic procedure or additional clinical hallmark. Excluded from this were clinical criteria, which exclusively represented the contraindications of the instrumental diagnostics used. (2) Adequate description of recruitment: Either a defined period of time at a particular institution/region had to be specified, or it had to be evident that all available patients of an institution/region were included. (3) Adequate description of inclusion and exclusion criteria.

Outcome measures: (1) A clear definition of dysphagia or swallowing pathologies assessed is provided. (2) Dysphagia was assessed with an instrumental gold-standard procedure (flexible endoscopy of swallowing, VFSS, real-time MRI, scintigraphy) that includes the visualization of the pharyngeal phase of swallowing. (3) Identical method and setting of outcome measurement was applied for all study participants.

All points in this list had to have been fulfilled for a study to be classified as "low bias risk". If there was no indication of bias risk, the study was classified as "low bias risk", otherwise the study was classified as "significant bias risk".

2.2.3. Statistical Analysis

A random effect model (restricted maximum likelihood) was chosen to estimate the pooled prevalence rates. The effect size and standard deviation was calculated with Microsoft Excel 16 using the following approach [14]: If no patient had dysphagia in a study population (0 events), a "continuity correction" of 0.5 was added to the event column as well as to the sample size column to enable inverse variance weighting [15]. The further analysis was calculated with the software JASP 0.11.1. The pooled prevalence, the 95% confidence interval (CI), I^2 as a measure for heterogeneity and a funnel plot with the Egger's test as a measure for publication bias were calculated for each analyzed group. In the comparison of subjects with a parameter to subjects without the respective parameter (Section 2.2.1), prevalence rates were considered to be significantly different when the 95% CI did not overlap.

3. Results

Figure 1 illustrates the Preferred Reporting Items for Systematic Reviews and Meta-Analyses (PRISMA) flow diagram of the reviewed literature [16].

3.1. Review

A total of 139 articles reported on epidemiology and prevalence (Table S1), 101 articles on pathophysiology (Table S2), 34 articles on the outcome (Table S3) and 93 articles on therapeutic effects (Table S4).

3.1.1. Epidemiology

3.1.1.1. Dysphagia and Disease Course

In principle, IIM is a chronically progressive disease, but sometimes there are also relapsing–remitting episodes. The situation is similar with dysphagia in IIM. Besides relapsing–remitting episodes of dysphagia, several authors report that the prevalence of dysphagia increases as the disease progresses [17–26]. Nevertheless, dysphagia can also be the initial [17–21,23–32] or even the only symptom [18,29,31,33]. Therefore, dysphagia should not be considered a late symptom in IIM. Indeed, IIM might be the underlying disease in patients with unclear dysphagia, even if other investigations, such as laboratory results and electrophysiology, do not refer to IIM [32].

3.1.1.2. Factors Associated with Dysphagia

Several factors are reported to be associated with dysphagia. Among the subgroups, differences in prevalence are found: Higher prevalence is reported in DM compared to PM [34–37] but also vice versa [38], in IBM compared to other forms of IIM [39] and in overlap syndromes compared to other forms of IIM [39]. In addition, an increased risk of dysphagia is reported in patients with associated malignancy [37,40–45]. A number of antibodies are also linked to an increased risk of dysphagia: NXP2 [46–49], FHL-1 [50], SAE [47,51], HMGCR [47,52], NT5c1A [53], SRP [47,54,55], TIF1y [44,47], OJ [56] and myositis-specific or -associated autoantibodies in general [47]. ANA and MDA5 antibodies are reported to be associated with a reduced risk of dysphagia [47,57].

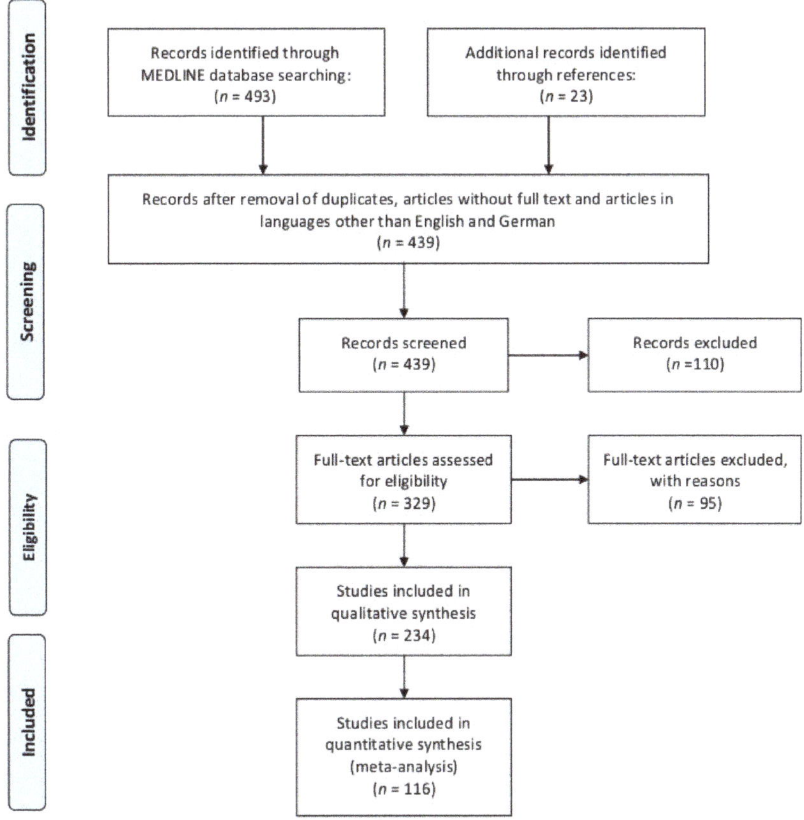

Figure 1. Preferred Reporting Items for Systematic Reviews and Meta-Analyses (PRISMA) flow diagram of the reviewed literature.

3.1.2. Pathophysiology

Inflammation of Swallowing Muscles

IIM can result in impairment of the oral [29,58–64], pharyngeal [7,23,24,27,29,31–33,44,58–116] and esophageal [24,29,38,59,62,73,81,85,89,90,93,95,98,99,101,103–105,112,114–131] phases of swallowing and pharyngeal dysfunction is associated with aspiration [27,29,31–33,58,60,61,70,76–79,81,83,84,86–89,91,93, 94,96–98,102,105,106,108,111,113]. Results from studies and case-reports with biopsies suggest that inflammatory involvement occurs in the affected swallowing muscles [29,31,32,86,90,91,94–97,100, 101,103,104,108,126,132,133], similarly to the well-known inflammatory reactions in the peripheral skeletal muscles in IIM. Interestingly, such changes also seem to occur in smooth muscle tissue of the esophagus [104,119,126]. Besides muscle biopsy, signs for inflammation can be detected by characteristic MRI findings, e.g., edema in the oropharynx [74,134–136]. However, presumably due to the small volume of the respective muscles, MRI findings are inconclusive and, if normal, cannot rule out myositis as cause of dysphagia [33]. The study data is conflicting on whether dysphagia is related to the clinical impairment of the peripheral skeletal muscles. Some studies report a correlation of peripheral symptoms with dysphagia [17,39,127], while other studies report the opposite [137,138].

Dysphagia Pathology

In general, four patterns of swallowing impairment can be distinguished depending on the muscle groups affected (illustrated in Figure 2): Reduced pharyngeal contractility, cricopharyngeal dysfunction, reduced laryngeal elevation and esophageal hypomotility. In case of unclear dysphagia, knowledge of these mechanisms and the corresponding findings in instrumental dysphagia assessment can be helpful in the differential diagnosis [33].

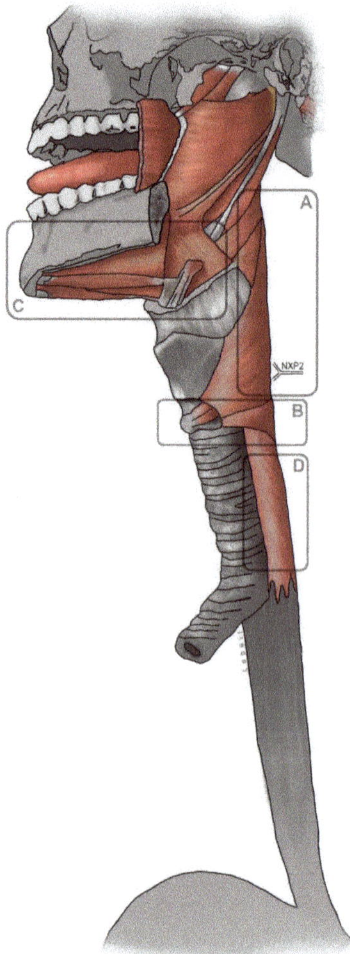

Figure 2. Skeletal swallowing muscles and the associated dysphagia mechanisms: A: Reduced pharyngeal contractility; B: Cricopharyngeal dysfunction; C: Reduced laryngeal elevation; D: Esophageal hypomotility.

Reduced pharyngeal contractility can result in insufficient pharyngeal bolus clearance [139]. Consequently, myositis patients often show pharyngeal residue after swallowing [7,27,29,31,33,44,58–61,65–67,69,71,73–80,83,84,86,87,91,93,96,100,101,103,104,106,111,112,115]. These can impact on swallowing safety and ultimately cause aspiration, which is a frequently reported finding [33,78,81,86]. Further findings indicating reduced pharyngeal contractility are absent or inadequate peristalsis or bolus propulsion [27,31,69,95,106,111], inadequate pharyngeal contraction [29,61,75,87,100,116,126], nasal regurgitation due to velopharyngeal insufficiency [31,44,62,74,79,80,97,98,104,109–111,116], piecemeal deglutition when swallowing larger boluses [82,140] or reduced pharyngeal pressure in manometry [7,29,32].

Numerous authors reported a dysfunction of the upper esophageal sphincter (UES) due to cricopharyngeal impairment [7,23,24,27,29,31,32,38,58,61,63,66,68,71,72,77,78,80,82,86,87,89–94,96,97,100–102,106,108]. Both, hypercontractility, e.g., a relaxation deficit of the UES [7,23,24,31,58,61,63,77,78,80,82,86,87,89,93,94,96,97,100,102,106,108], and hypocontractility [24,38,82,85,90,98,114] have been described. This may be explained by the fact that muscle physiology is affected in a different way during the acute inflammatory phase compared to the chronic phase when fibrosis occurs [82]. Cricopharyngeal hypercontractility often leads to an opening or relaxation disorder of the UES, resulting in pronounced residue or pooling of saliva in the piriform sinus [7,27,31,33,65–67,69,73,74,76–78,80,86,87,101,103,106,111,112,115], which is located directly above the UES. Typical findings in VFSS are a prominent cricopharyngeus muscle, also referred to as cricopharyngeal bar [23,32,61,68,86,91,93,97,99,106] and muscle propulsions or posterior indentations between C3 and C7 [7,71,96].

Another common finding in myositis is reduced laryngeal elevation [29,58,63,66,76,77,83,107,111]. This is probably caused by impaired contractility of the suprahyoid and longitudinal pharyngeal muscles [141]. Laryngeal elevation is a prerequisite for the UES to open [142] and reduced laryngeal elevation can lead to functional UES impairment. Therefore, the findings in dysphagia diagnostics can be similar to findings with primary UES disorder. Some studies suggest that the typical myositis-associated finding of residue in the piriform sinus may be primarily caused by reduced pharyngeal contractility of suprahyoid muscles rather than an actual dysfunction of the cricopharyngeus muscle itself [58,77]. In this context, one could speak of a pseudocricopharyngeal dysfunction due to reduced laryngeal elevation.

Various authors reported reduced or absent esophageal motility sometimes extending to the lower esophageal sphincter [29,38,114]. Most studies used manometry [24,29,38,59,85,90,98,105,114,117–119,122,129,130] some also VFSS, barium swallow or scintigraphy [62,73,81,89,99,104,120,121,124,125,127] to detect esophageal impairment.

3.1.3. Outcome

Dysphagia in patients with IIM not only affects quality of life [71], but is also associated with severe complications such as weight loss [30,138] or aspiration pneumonia [24,29,30,32,68,116,143–146]. Pneumonia after aspiration is particularly dangerous as this condition can be fatal [24,29,30,32,116,143–145,147]. The rates of pneumonia/aspiration pneumonia in cohorts with dysphagic patients are reported between 6% and 36% [24,30,32,68,99,116], are four times more prevalent and, thus, significantly higher in dysphagic than in non-dysphagic patients [24]. Some studies report that aspiration pneumonia is the leading cause of death [29,30,32,147]. In fact, a survey-based study among physicians on patient cases with IBM suggests that dysphagia-associated complications may even be the only cause of premature mortality [148]. It is therefore not surprising that dysphagia is associated with increased mortality [34,144,145,149]. Conversely, the survival rate is associated with dysphagia recovery [143]. Nevertheless, some studies also reported no association between dysphagia and mortality [25,35,150]. Besides mortality, dysphagia is associated with a worse functional status or general condition of the disease [24,39,110,151–153] and represents a negative predictive factor for further disease progression [151].

3.1.4. Therapy

Immunomodulatory Therapy

There are several articles reporting positive therapeutic effects of immunomodulatory medication on symptoms and/or on findings of objective swallowing evaluations. These include intravenous methylprednisolone pulse therapy [19,33,70,81,87,134,154–159], methotrexate [30,76,89,124,136,154,159–161], long-term prednisone/prednisolone [29,30,33,59,64,70,74,76,81,83,84,87,89,101,103,111,118,122,124,134,136,143,154,158,159,161–167], azathioprine [29,30,33,83,84,87,155,158,163], intravenous immunoglobulin (IVIG) [24,30,44,65,69,70,73,76,78,81,85,87,114,117,118,121,136,155,161,168–176], subcutaneous immunoglobulin [173,177,178], hydroxychloroquine [30,118,154], tacrolimus [162,172], cyclophosphamide [83,170,172], mycophenolate mofetil [118,179], cyclosporine [123] and rituximab [155]. If dysphagia does not respond to medical therapy, it may be helpful to switch to another group of medication, e.g., from steroids to IVIG [24]. The effects on swallowing function were reported in all forms of IIM including IBM [176].

Therapy of Malignancy

IIM is associated with malignant diseases and can occur as paraneoplastic syndrome. Therefore, treatment of malignancy can improve muscle symptoms. This effect is also described for dysphagia [44]. Both tumor resection [180–182] and chemotherapy [182–184] can improve or relieve impaired deglutition.

Non-Pharmacological Interventional Therapy

Non-pharmacological interventional therapies are symptomatic strategies without a modulatory effect on the disease course, aiming to improve swallowing physiology. Preliminary data suggest that the pneumonia rate can be reduced by interventional therapy if aspiration is reduced [68]. To date, all non-pharmacological interventional procedures attempt to relieve or eliminate the symptoms of cricopharyngeal dysfunction. Three different procedures have been reported:

Injection of botulinum toxin A in the cricopharyngeus muscle: This procedure can reduce the pressure in the UES [61,86] which may result in both symptom relief [61,68] and improvement in objective swallowing diagnostics [68,72]. The effect of this treatment usually lasts for a few months, hence repetitive treatments are necessary [72]. Some authors also reported no improvement [29].

Cricopharyngeal dilatation: This procedure is usually performed endoscopically via a balloon catheter. A clinical improvement of symptoms [29,30,32,80,102] as well as improvement in objective dysphagia diagnostics [78,80] have been described. Here, too, the effect may not be permanent, so that repetitive treatments may become necessary [32,80,102].

Cricopharyngeal myotomy: This is a non-reversible intervention with a surgical sectioning of the cricopharyngeus muscle. It can lead to an improvement of symptoms [24,29–32,86,91,96,97,100,102,108,110] and an improvement in objective swallowing diagnostics [91,96,97,100]. In some cases, improvement of symptoms without corresponding improvement in VFSS were reported [29]. Other articles reported improvement in swallowing diagnostics without benefits being perceived by the patients [91].

In the absence of interventional trials with clinically meaningful endpoints, the available studies do not allow for a direct comparison between these treatment options and related treatment-specific recommendations.

Behavioral Therapy

In myositis patients, various behavioral swallowing therapies such as diet modifications, compensatory techniques and exercises are used [29]. Unfortunately, there is little evidence for these techniques as there are few studies investigating behavioral therapy in IIM. In individual cases, it was reported that the Mendelson maneuver (pressing the back of the tongue against the palate when swallowing) has helped to maintain oral food intake without aspiration pneumonia or weight loss [29]. In addition, a case report suggests that isometric tongue strengthening has contributed to the maintenance of posterior tongue pressure [60].

3.2. Meta-Analysis

A total of 109 studies representing 10,382 subjects were included in the meta-analysis of the total patient cohort with IIM. The overall estimate of prevalence of dysphagia was 36%. In patients with IBM, a particularly high prevalence of 56% was estimated. No significant differences in prevalence were found between PM and DM (prevalence and CIs are visualized in Figure 3).

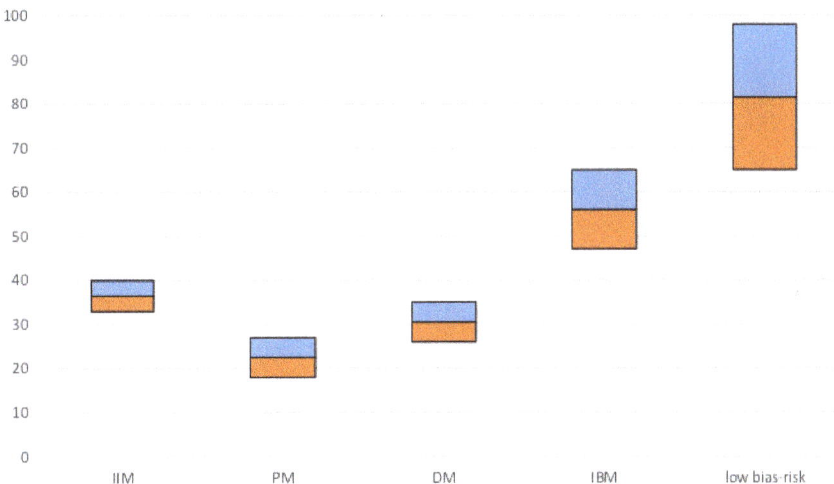

Figure 3. Pooled estimated prevalence of dysphagia: prevalence in % (y-axis): the blue and orange bars represent the 95% confidence interval; IIM: Idiopathic inflammatory myopathy, PM: Polymyositis, DM: Dermatomyositis, IBM: Inclusion body myositis, low bias risk studies: cohort of studies with low risk of bias.

Only six studies were classified as "low bias risk". In those studies, all with gold-standard instrumental assessments of dysphagia, the prevalence estimate was 82% and thus clearly higher compared to the total cohort. The estimate of dysphagia prevalence in non-cancer-associated IIM was 26% and 52% in cancer-associated IIM. In patients with NXP2-negative IIM, the estimated prevalence was 33% and 56% in patients with NXP2 antibodies. The CIs in these two comparative analyses did not overlap, so that a significant difference between patients with and without malignancy and NXP2-antibodies can be assumed. The forest plot for studies on malignancy is illustrated in Figure 4 and for studies on NXP2-antibodies in Figure 5. All other comparisons between patients with and without specific antibodies did not reveal significant differences in prevalence. Therefore, of the risk factors presented in Section 3.1.1.2, only malignancy and NXP2 antibodies could be confirmed in our meta-analysis. The estimate of the pooled prevalence, the 95% CI, the number of included studies, the number of included subjects, I^2 as measure for heterogeneity, the p-value of the Egger's test as measure for publication bias and the percentage of studies with low bias risk for all analyses are shown in Table 1. The included studies with prevalence and CI in forest and funnel plots for all analyses are shown in the Supplementary Materials S5.

Table 1. The estimate of the pooled prevalence, the 95% confidence interval (CI), the number of included studies and subjects, I^2 as measure for heterogeneity, *p*-value of the Egger's test and percentage of studies with low risk of bias for all meta-analyses.

Patient Group	*n*, Studies	*n*, Subjects	Prevalence	CI Lower	CI Upper	I-Squared	*p*-Value Egger's Test	Low Bias Risk
total cohort	109	10382	36%	33%	40%	87%	>0.01 *	6%
PM	21	882	23%	18%	27%	52%	0.03 *	5%
DM	49	3274	31%	26%	35%	80%	>0.01 *	2%
IBM	23	1352	56%	47%	65%	76%	>0.01 *	22%
low bias risk	6	115	82%	65%	98%	0%	0.70	100%
malignancy+	13	271	51%	43%	60%	0%	0.39	0%
malignancy−	13	1120	23%	17%	30%	85%	0.02 *	0%
NXP2+	5	196	56%	45%	66%	0%	0.42	0%
NXP2−	5	1188	33%	28%	37%	42%	0.22	0%
MDA5+	3	89	12%	0%	23%	61%	0.13	0%
MDA5−	3	538	21%	10%	32%	86%	0.22	0%
SEA+	2	17	76%	35%	100%	0%	n.a.	0%
SEA−	2	589	35%	20%	49%	81%	n.a.	0%
SRP+	3	51	62%	40%	84%	0%	0.69	0%
SRP−	3	943	36%	26%	45%	81%	0.15	0%
TIF1y+	3	103	45%	32%	58%	0%	0.67	0%
TIF1y−	3	519	23%	0%	48%	98%	0.12	0%

* Significant *p*-values.

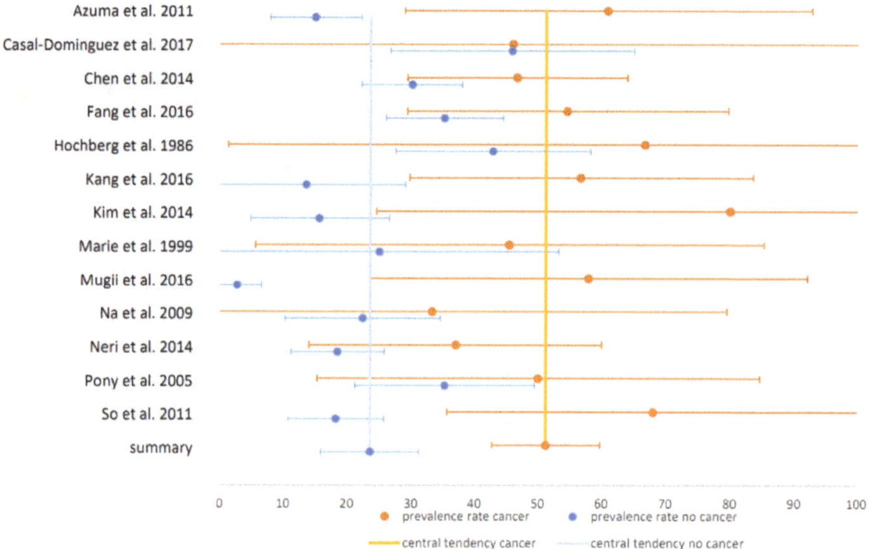

Figure 4. Forest plot for malignancy: Forest plot of the studies comparing prevalence in cancer and non-cancer-associated IIM: x-axis shows the prevalence in %.

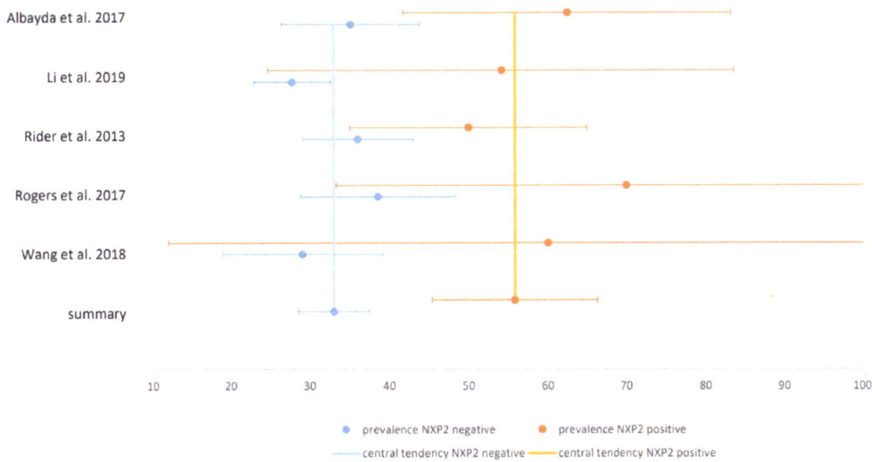

Figure 5. Forest plot for NXP2: Forest plot of the studies comparing prevalence in NXP2-positive and -negative IIM: x-axis shows the prevalence in %.

4. Discussion

Dysphagia is a frequent complication in IIM with an estimated pooled prevalence of 36% and a peak prevalence of 56% in IBM. Due to the worse outcome associated with dysphagia and the fact that standard immunomodulatory therapy as well as interventional treatment options can improve swallowing impairment, we propose to systematically evaluate swallowing function in patients with IIM and, if present, to include dysphagia as a therapeutic target. The association with malignancy and NXP2 antibodies may have diagnostic relevance in two ways: On the one hand, dysphagia should be considered early on in patients with these risk factors and therefore initiate instrumental swallowing assessment for detailed analysis. On the other hand, in patients with proven dysphagia it might be particularly relevant to carefully look for the presence of an associated malignancy, as dysphagia was shown to be associated with malignant comorbidities [40].

The fact that specific antibodies are associated with an increased risk of swallowing impairment could be an indication that specific pathophysiologic mechanisms might be prone to the oropharynx or the esophagus. The NXP2 antibody associated with dysphagia in this study is particularly common in patients with juvenile dermatomyositis [185]. In the studies on NXP2 antibodies included in our meta-analysis, there was one study in which only juvenile IIM was investigated [49], and another study in which juvenile IIM patients were included in addition to adult patients [47]. The remaining three studies were conducted in adult patients. In addition, the antibody is associated with calcinosis and in adult patients possibly also with malignancy [185]. Thus, an association with dysphagia may also seem possible by association with malignancy which, in turn, is associated with dysphagia. A connection between dysphagia and calcinosis also seems possible, although we did not find a supporting mechanistic explanation for this connection in the literature. However, other antibodies such as TIF-1y, for which in this study no increased prevalence of dysphagia could be proven, are also associated with malignancy [185] (although individual studies associate TIF-1y to dysphagia). Furthermore, in one of the studies on NXP2 antibodies from our meta-analysis, no association with malignancy and calcinosis in adult patients was found [186]. A higher prevalence of dysphagia is also observed in malignancy with compared to malignancy without active IIM [43]. This suggests that dysphagia is not due to an unspecific general deterioration caused by the malignant disease alone. Specific paraneoplastic immune-mediated mechanisms might therefore contribute to swallowing dysfunction. Further, the reported cases of isolated dysphagia (Section 3.1.1.1) might, similarly to orbital myositis [187], represent a distinct inflammatory entity.

A higher prevalence of dysphagia of 82% was estimated in the low bias risk studies with instrumental assessment. This finding corroborates previous studies showing that refined instrumental evaluation is more sensitive for detecting dysphagia than clinical testing [188,189]. Further, this suggests that oropharyngoesophageal dysfunction may also be present in patients who subjectively experience no swallowing complaints and, therefore, do not report symptoms of dysphagia [7,27,138]. Consistent with this, silent penetration and aspiration (clinically unapparent without symptoms, e.g., coughing or dyspnea) are reported in patients with IBM [71]. The reported prevalence rates vary widely which is also reflected by the strong heterogeneity of the overall cohort. There are four main explanations for these inconsistencies: (1) IIM is not a uniform disease but instead represents a heterogeneous group of diseases with different pathophysiologic mechanisms. Thus, there are presumably real differences in prevalence between different subgroups of the disease. If this is the case, heterogeneity in a meta-analysis should decrease when individual disease groups are analyzed separately; (2) Many different definitions of dysphagia were used, e.g., oropharyngeal vs. esophageal dysphagia. The prevalence rates of the different forms of dysphagia may differ; (3) Different forms of assessment of dysphagia were used, e.g., clinical (patient chart review, swallowing examination) vs. instrumental (FEES, VFSS, manometry, scintigraphy, real-time swallowing MRI). If this is a cause of different prevalence rates, heterogeneity in a meta-analysis should decrease when studies using a uniform assessment procedure are analyzed separately; (4) Dysphagia was determined at different points in the course of the disease (Section 3.1.1.1). Indeed, the heterogeneity partly decreased in the subgroup analysis of IBM, PM and DM and disappeared in the analysis of low bias risk studies with instrumental assessment. Therefore, the heterogeneity in the overall cohort seems to be due to both the different definitions and assessments of dysphagia and real differences in the investigated patient cohorts with differing pathophysiology. The low heterogeneity in most subgroup analysis with specific antibodies may indicate that in case of uniform pathophysiology prevalence rates converge.

Both the funnel plot and the Egger's test suggest that there was a publication bias in our overall cohort, i.e., studies with small sample sizes show higher prevalence rates than studies with large sample sizes. If the bias risk of individual studies is taken into account, an alternative conclusion emerges: Prospective studies with instrumental procedures generally had a smaller sample size, presumably due to the increased recruitment and data collection effort. However, they reported higher prevalence rates due to more sensitive and high-quality diagnostic procedures. In line with this explanatory approach, the funnel plot and the Egger's test no longer indicate a publication bias when studies with low bias risk are analyzed separately.

There are several limitations to this study that must be considered. First, in the overall cohort of the meta-analysis, only few studies had a low bias risk. Especially in the studies with a significant bias risk, different definitions of dysphagia were used and the classification as dysphagic and non-dysphagic was often based solely on clinical evaluation or symptoms. However, due to the lack of objective swallowing diagnostics, it is not possible to say with certainty whether oropharyngoesophageal dysfunction was actually present in these studies with significant bias risk. This has certainly contributed to the considerable heterogeneity and may have contributed to the publication bias. Second, in the meta-analysis of factors associated with increased risk of dysphagia, only studies comparing the prevalence in groups with and without the respective factors were included. However, several potential factors were reported where no such comparison was possible. Third, the majority of included studies were retrospective observational studies, some with small sample size or even only individual case reports. Thus, many conclusions are based on studies with low quality and evidence levels. This applies in particular to the therapy section, where not a single prospective randomized controlled trial could be included. Fourth, although studies at the same institutions with overlapping recruitment periods were excluded, it is possible that overlapping patient groups may also have occurred between registry studies and studies at individual institutions. Fifth, the review as well as the assessment of the bias risk were conducted by only one observer, which may reduce reliability. Sixth, for the systematic review of this meta-analysis, only Medline was searched with Pubmed, so studies that are only listed in other databases may not have been found. Seventh, due to different reporting standards and partially missing information, no demographic data were pooled and included in the meta-analysis. Especially when comparing groups (e.g., patients with malignant disease and without malignant disease), the groups may differ not only in the prevalence of dysphagia but also in demographic characteristics. For the available demographic data of the studies included in the meta-analysis, we refer to Table S1 (column "cohort") in the Supplementary Materials.

5. Conclusions

Dysphagia is common in patients with IIM, with an estimated overall prevalence rate of 36% and a particularly high prevalence in IBM. Factors with increased risk of dysphagia include malignancy and NXP2 autoantibodies. A refined instrumental assessment is more sensitive to detect dysphagia and should be included in the diagnostic work-up of swallowing impairment. Dysphagia in IIM is caused by inflammatory involvement of the swallowing muscles, which can lead to reduced pharyngeal contractility, cricopharyngeal dysfunction, reduced laryngeal elevation and esophageal hypomotility. In IIM, impaired deglutition can lead to life-threatening complications such as aspiration pneumonia and increasing mortality. Standard immunomodulatory therapy can improve swallowing function and dysphagia should, therefore, be included as a therapeutic target. Further positive therapeutic effects may result from the treatment of malignancy or from interventions targeting the cricopharyngeal muscle such as myotomy, dilatation or botulinum toxin injection.

Supplementary Materials: The following are available online at http://www.mdpi.com/2077-0383/9/7/2150/s1, Table S1: Articles reporting on epidemiology and prevalence, Table S2: Articles reporting on pathophysiology, Table S3: Articles reporting on outcome; Table S4: Articles reporting on therapeutic effects; Document S1: included studies with prevalence and CI in a forest plot and a funnel-plot for all meta-analysis;

Author Contributions: Conceptualization and study design, B.L.; formal analysis, B.L.; data curation, B.L.; writing—original draft preparation, B.L.; writing—review and editing, M.P. and T.R. and P.M. and I.C. and S.S.-K. and T.W. and S.G.M. and H.W. and R.D.; visualization, B.L.; supervision, R.D. and M.P.; All authors have read and agreed to the published version of the manuscript.

Funding: This research received no external funding.

Acknowledgments: We are especially grateful to Hanna Labeit, who helped to create the illustration. The authors acknowledge support from the Open Access Publication Fund of the University of Muenster.

Conflicts of Interest: Wiendl receives honoraria for acting as a member of Scientific Advisory Boards Biogen, Evgen, Genzyme, MedDay Pharmaceuticals, Merck Serono, Novartis, Roche Pharma AG, and Sanofi-Aventis as well as speaker honoraria and travel support from Alexion, Biogen, Cognomed, F. Hoffmann-La Roche Ltd., Gemeinnützige Hertie-Stiftung, Merck Serono, Novartis, Roche Pharma AG, Genzyme, TEVA, and Wiendl is acting as a paid consultant for Abbvie, Actelion, Biogen, IGES, Johnson & Johnson, Novartis, Roche, Sanofi-Aventis, and the Swiss Multiple Sclerosis Society. His research is funded by the German Ministry for Education and Research (BMBF), Deutsche Forschungsgesellschaft (DFG), Else Kröner Fresenius Foundation, Fresenius Foundation, the European Union, Hertie Foundation, NRW Ministry of Education and Research, Interdisciplinary Center for Clinical Studies (IZKF) Muenster and RE Children's Foundation, Biogen, GlaxoSmithKline GmbH, Roche Pharma AG, Sanofi-Genzyme. All other authors declare no conflict of interest.

References

1. Sasegbon, A.; Hamdy, S. The anatomy and physiology of normal and abnormal swallowing in oropharyngeal dysphagia. *Neurogastroenterol. Motil.* **2017**, *29*. [CrossRef] [PubMed]
2. Shaw, S.M.; Martino, R. The normal swallow: Muscular and neurophysiological control. *Otolaryngol. Clin. North Am.* **2013**, *46*, 937–956. [CrossRef] [PubMed]
3. Bottai, M.; Tjarnlund, A.; Santoni, G.; Werth, V.P.; Pilkington, C.; de Visser, M.; Alfredsson, L.; Amato, A.A.; Barohn, R.J.; Liang, M.H.; et al. EULAR/ACR classification criteria for adult and juvenile idiopathic inflammatory myopathies and their major subgroups: A methodology report. *RMD Open* **2017**, *3*, e000507. [CrossRef] [PubMed]

4. Dziewas, R.; auf dem Brinke, M.; Birkmann, U.; Bräuer, G.; Busch, K.; Cerra, F.; Damm-Lunau, R.; Dunkel, J.; Fellgiebel, A.; Garms, E.; et al. Safety and clinical impact of FEES – results of the FEES-registry. *Neurol. Res. Pract.* **2019**, *1*, 16. [CrossRef]
5. Wirth, R.; Dziewas, R.; Beck, A.M.; Clave, P.; Hamdy, S.; Heppner, H.J.; Langmore, S.; Leischker, A.H.; Martino, R.; Pluschinski, P.; et al. Oropharyngeal dysphagia in older persons-from pathophysiology to adequate intervention: A review and summary of an international expert meeting. *Clin. Interv. Aging* **2016**, *11*, 189–208. [CrossRef]
6. Weitoft, T. Occurrence of polymyositis in the county of Gavleborg, Sweden. *Scand. J. Rheumatol.* **1997**, *26*, 104–106. [CrossRef]
7. Murata, K.-Y.; Kouda, K.; Tajima, F.; Kondo, T. A dysphagia study in patients with sporadic inclusion body myositis (s-IBM). *Neurol. Sci.* **2012**, *33*, 765–770. [CrossRef]
8. Bohan, A.; Peter, J.B. Polymyositis and dermatomyositis (first of two parts). *N. Engl. J. Med.* **1975**, *292*, 344–347. [CrossRef]
9. Bohan, A.; Peter, J.B. Polymyositis and dermatomyositis (second of two parts). *N. Engl. J. Med.* **1975**, *292*, 403–407. [CrossRef]
10. Griggs, R.C.; Askanas, V.; DiMauro, S.; Engel, A.; Karpati, G.; Mendell, J.R.; Rowland, L.P. Inclusion body myositis and myopathies. *Ann. Neurol.* **1995**, *38*, 705–713. [CrossRef]
11. Needham, M.; Mastaglia, F.L. Inclusion body myositis: Current pathogenetic concepts and diagnostic and therapeutic approaches. *Lancet Neurol.* **2007**, *6*, 620–631. [CrossRef]
12. Rose, M.R. 188th ENMC International Workshop: Inclusion Body Myositis, 2–4 December 2011, Naarden, The Netherlands. *Neuromuscul. Disord.* **2013**, *23*, 1044–1055. [CrossRef]
13. Hayden, J.A.; van der Windt, D.A.; Cartwright, J.L.; Cote, P.; Bombardier, C. Assessing bias in studies of prognostic factors. *Ann. Intern. Med.* **2013**, *158*, 280–286. [CrossRef] [PubMed]
14. Neyeloff, J.L.; Fuchs, S.C.; Moreira, L.B. Meta-analyses and Forest plots using a microsoft excel spreadsheet: Step-by-step guide focusing on descriptive data analysis. *BMC Res. Notes* **2012**, *5*, 52. [CrossRef] [PubMed]
15. Higgins, J.P.T.; Green, S. *Cochrane Handbook of Systematic Reviews of Interventions*; Wiley: Chichester, New Hampshire, 2008; ISBN 9780470699515.
16. Moher, D.; Liberati, A.; Tetzlaff, J.; Altman, D.G. Preferred reporting items for systematic reviews and meta-analyses: The PRISMA statement. *PLoS Med.* **2009**, *6*, e1000097. [CrossRef]
17. Badrising, U.A.; Maat-Schieman, M.L.C.; van Houwelingen, J.C.; van Doorn, P.A.; van Duinen, S.G.; van Engelen, B.G.M.; Faber, C.G.; Hoogendijk, J.E.; de Jager, A.E.; Koehler, P.J.; et al. Inclusion body myositis. Clinical features and clinical course of the disease in 64 patients. *J. Neurol.* **2005**, *252*, 1448–1454. [CrossRef] [PubMed]
18. Benveniste, O.; Guiguet, M.; Freebody, J.; Dubourg, O.; Squier, W.; Maisonobe, T.; Stojkovic, T.; Leite, M.I.; Allenbach, Y.; Herson, S.; et al. Long-term observational study of sporadic inclusion body myositis. *Brain* **2011**, *134*, 3176–3184. [CrossRef] [PubMed]
19. 19. De Camargo, L.V.; de Carvalho, M.S.; Shinjo, S.K.; de Oliveira, A.S.B.; Zanoteli, E. Clinical, Histological, and Immunohistochemical Findings in Inclusion Body Myositis. *Biomed Res. Int.* **2018**, *2018*, 5069042. [CrossRef]
20. Chiu, S.K.; Yang, Y.H.; Wang, L.C.; Chiang, B.L. Ten-year experience of juvenile dermatomyositis: A retrospective study. *J. Microbiol. Immunol. Infect.* **2007**, *40*, 68–73.
21. Chwalinska-Sadowska, H.; Maldykowa, H. Polymyositis-dermatomyositis—A 25-year follow-up of 50 patients (analysis of clinical symptoms and signs and results of laboratory tests). *Mater. Med. Pol.* **1990**, *22*, 205–212.
22. Dobloug, C.; Garen, T.; Bitter, H.; Stjarne, J.; Stenseth, G.; Grovle, L.; Sem, M.; Gran, J.T.; Molberg, O. Prevalence and clinical characteristics of adult polymyositis and dermatomyositis; data from a large and unselected Norwegian cohort. *Ann. Rheum. Dis.* **2015**, *74*, 1551–1556. [CrossRef] [PubMed]
23. Lotz, B.P.; Engel, A.G.; Nishino, H.; Stevens, J.C.; Litchy, W.J. Inclusion body myositis. Observations in 40 patients. *Brain* **1989**, *112 Pt 3*, 727–747. [CrossRef]
24. Marie, I.; Menard, J.-F.; Hatron, P.Y.; Hachulla, E.; Mouthon, L.; Tiev, K.; Ducrotte, P.; Cherin, P. Intravenous immunoglobulins for steroid-refractory esophageal involvement related to polymyositis and dermatomyositis: A series of 73 patients. *Arthritis Care Res. (Hoboken)* **2010**, *62*, 1748–1755. [CrossRef]

25. Maugars, Y.M.; Berthelot, J.M.; Abbas, A.A.; Mussini, J.M.; Nguyen, J.M.; Prost, A.M. Long-term prognosis of 69 patients with dermatomyositis or polymyositis. *Clin. Exp. Rheumatol.* **1996**, *14*, 263–274. [PubMed]
26. Needham, M.; James, I.; Corbett, A.; Day, T.; Christiansen, F.; Phillips, B.; Mastaglia, F.L. Sporadic inclusion body myositis: Phenotypic variability and influence of HLA-DR3 in a cohort of 57 Australian cases. *J. Neurol. Neurosurg. Psychiatry* **2008**, *79*, 1056–1060. [CrossRef]
27. Cox, F.M.; Verschuuren, J.J.; Verbist, B.M.; Niks, E.H.; Wintzen, A.R.; Badrising, U.A. Detecting dysphagia in inclusion body myositis. *J. Neurol.* **2009**, *256*, 2009–2013. [CrossRef]
28. Lynn, S.J.; Sawyers, S.M.; Moller, P.W.; O'Donnell, J.L.; Chapman, P.T. Adult-onset inflammatory myopathy: North Canterbury experience 1989-2001. *Intern. Med. J.* **2005**, *35*, 170–173. [CrossRef] [PubMed]
29. Oh, T.H.; Brumfield, K.A.; Hoskin, T.L.; Kasperbauer, J.L.; Basford, J.R. Dysphagia in inclusion body myositis: Clinical features, management, and clinical outcome. *Am. J. Phys. Med. Rehabil.* **2008**, *87*, 883–889. [CrossRef]
30. Oh, T.H.; Brumfield, K.A.; Hoskin, T.L.; Stolp, K.A.; Murray, J.A.; Bassford, J.R. Dysphagia in inflammatory myopathy: Clinical characteristics, treatment strategies, and outcome in 62 patients. *Mayo Clin. Proc.* **2007**, *82*, 441–447. [CrossRef] [PubMed]
31. Riminton, D.S.; Chambers, S.T.; Parkin, P.J.; Pollock, M.; Donaldson, I.M. Inclusion body myositis presenting solely as dysphagia. *Neurology* **1993**, *43*, 1241–1243. [CrossRef]
32. Williams, R.B.; Grehan, M.J.; Hersch, M.; Andre, J.; Cook, I.J. Biomechanics, diagnosis, and treatment outcome in inflammatory myopathy presenting as oropharyngeal dysphagia. *Gut* **2003**, *52*, 471–478. [CrossRef] [PubMed]
33. Labeit, B.; Muhle, P.; Suntrup-Krueger, S.; Ahring, S.; Ruck, T.; Dziewas, R.; Warnecke, T. Dysphagia as Isolated Manifestation of Jo-1 Associated Myositis? *Front. Neurol.* **2019**, *10*, 739. [CrossRef] [PubMed]
34. Danko, K.; Ponyi, A.; Constantin, T.; Borgulya, G.; Szegedi, G. Long-term survival of patients with idiopathic inflammatory myopathies according to clinical features: A longitudinal study of 162 cases. *Medicine (Baltim.)* **2004**, *83*, 35–42. [CrossRef] [PubMed]
35. Galindo-Feria, A.S.; Rojas-Serrano, J.; Hinojosa-Azaola, A. Clinical and Prognostic Factors Associated With Survival in Mexican Patients with Idiopathic Inflammatory Myopathies. *J. Clin. Rheumatol.* **2016**, *22*, 51–56. [CrossRef]
36. Scola, R.H.; Werneck, L.C.; Prevedello, D.M.; Toderke, E.L.; Iwamoto, F.M. Diagnosis of dermatomyositis and polymyositis: A study of 102 cases. *Arq. Neuropsiquiatr.* **2000**, *58*, 789–799. [CrossRef]
37. So, M.W.; Koo, B.S.; Kim, Y.-G.; Lee, C.-K.; Yoo, B. Idiopathic inflammatory myopathy associated with malignancy: A retrospective cohort of 151 Korean patients with dermatomyositis and polymyositis. *J. Rheumatol.* **2011**, *38*, 2432–2435. [CrossRef]
38. Casal-Dominguez, M.; Pinal-Fernandez, I.; Mego, M.; Accarino, A.; Jubany, L.; Azpiroz, F.; Selva-O'callaghan, A. High-resolution manometry in patients with idiopathic inflammatory myopathy: Elevated prevalence of esophageal involvement and differences according to autoantibody status and clinical subset. *Muscle Nerve* **2017**, *56*, 386–392. [CrossRef]
39. Lilleker, J.B.; Vencovsky, J.; Wang, G.; Wedderburn, L.R.; Diederichsen, L.P.; Schmidt, J.; Oakley, P.; Benveniste, O.; Danieli, M.G.; Danko, K.; et al. The EuroMyositis registry: An international collaborative tool to facilitate myositis research. *Ann. Rheum. Dis.* **2018**, *77*, 30–39. [CrossRef] [PubMed]
40. Azuma, K.; Yamada, H.; Ohkubo, M.; Yamasaki, Y.; Yamasaki, M.; Mizushima, M.; Ozaki, S. Incidence and predictive factors for malignancies in 136 Japanese patients with dermatomyositis, polymyositis and clinically amyopathic dermatomyositis. *Mod. Rheumatol.* **2011**, *21*, 178–183. [CrossRef] [PubMed]
41. Chen, D.; Yuan, S.; Wu, X.; Li, H.; Qiu, Q.; Zhan, Z.; Ye, Y.; Lian, F.; Liang, L.; Xu, H.; et al. Incidence and predictive factors for malignancies with dermatomyositis: A cohort from southern China. *Clin. Exp. Rheumatol.* **2014**, *32*, 615–621.
42. Fang, Y.-F.; Wu, Y.-J.J.; Kuo, C.-F.; Luo, S.-F.; Yu, K.-H. Malignancy in dermatomyositis and polymyositis: Analysis of 192 patients. *Clin. Rheumatol.* **2016**, *35*, 1977–1984. [CrossRef]
43. Kang, E.H.; Lee, S.J.; Ascherman, D.P.; Lee, Y.J.; Lee, E.Y.; Lee, E.B.; Song, Y.W. Temporal relationship between cancer and myositis identifies two distinctive subgroups of cancers: Impact on cancer risk and survival in patients with myositis. *Rheumatology (Oxf.)* **2016**, *55*, 1631–1641. [CrossRef]
44. Mugii, N.; Hasegawa, M.; Matsushita, T.; Hamaguchi, Y.; Oohata, S.; Okita, H.; Yahata, T.; Someya, F.; Inoue, K.; Murono, S.; et al. Oropharyngeal Dysphagia in Dermatomyositis: Associations with Clinical and Laboratory Features Including Autoantibodies. *PLoS ONE* **2016**, *11*, e0154746. [CrossRef]

45. Neri, R.; Barsotti, S.; Iacopetti, V.; Iacopetti, G.; Pepe, P.; d'Ascanio, A.; Tavoni, A.G.; Mosca, M.; Bombardieri, S. Cancer-associated myositis: A 35-year retrospective study of a monocentric cohort. *Rheumatol. Int.* **2014**, *34*, 565–569. [CrossRef] [PubMed]
46. Albayda, J.; Pinal-Fernandez, I.; Huang, W.; Parks, C.; Paik, J.; Casciola-Rosen, L.; Danoff, S.K.; Johnson, C.; Christopher-Stine, L.; Mammen, A.L. Antinuclear Matrix Protein 2 Autoantibodies and Edema, Muscle Disease, and Malignancy Risk in Dermatomyositis Patients. *Arthritis Care Res. (Hoboken)* **2017**, *69*, 1771–1776. [CrossRef]
47. Li, S.; Ge, Y.; Yang, H.; Wang, T.; Zheng, X.; Peng, Q.; Lu, X.; Wang, G. The spectrum and clinical significance of myositis-specific autoantibodies in Chinese patients with idiopathic inflammatory myopathies. *Clin. Rheumatol.* **2019**, *38*, 2171–2179. [CrossRef] [PubMed]
48. Rogers, A.; Chung, L.; Li, S.; Casciola-Rosen, L.; Fiorentino, D.F. Cutaneous and Systemic Findings Associated With Nuclear Matrix Protein 2 Antibodies in Adult Dermatomyositis Patients. *Arthritis Care Res. (Hoboken)* **2017**, *69*, 1909–1914. [CrossRef] [PubMed]
49. Rider, L.G.; Shah, M.; Mamyrova, G.; Huber, A.M.; Rice, M.M.; Targoff, I.N.; Miller, F.W. The myositis autoantibody phenotypes of the juvenile idiopathic inflammatory myopathies. *Medicine (Baltim.)* **2013**, *92*, 223–243. [CrossRef] [PubMed]
50. Albrecht, I.; Wick, C.; Hallgren, A.; Tjarnlund, A.; Nagaraju, K.; Andrade, F.; Thompson, K.; Coley, W.; Phadke, A.; Diaz-Gallo, L.-M.; et al. Development of autoantibodies against muscle-specific FHL1 in severe inflammatory myopathies. *J. Clin. Invest.* **2015**, *125*, 4612–4624. [CrossRef]
51. Ge, Y.; Lu, X.; Shu, X.; Peng, Q.; Wang, G. Clinical characteristics of anti-SAE antibodies in Chinese patients with dermatomyositis in comparison with different patient cohorts. *Sci. Rep.* **2017**, *7*, 188. [CrossRef]
52. Ge, Y.; Lu, X.; Peng, Q.; Shu, X.; Wang, G. Clinical Characteristics of Anti-3-Hydroxy-3-Methylglutaryl Coenzyme A Reductase Antibodies in Chinese Patients with Idiopathic Inflammatory Myopathies. *PLoS ONE* **2015**, *10*, e0141616. [CrossRef] [PubMed]
53. Goyal, N.A.; Cash, T.M.; Alam, U.; Enam, S.; Tierney, P.; Araujo, N.; Mozaffar, F.H.; Pestronk, A.; Mozaffar, T. Seropositivity for NT5c1A antibody in sporadic inclusion body myositis predicts more severe motor, bulbar and respiratory involvement. *J. Neurol. Neurosurg. Psychiatry* **2016**, *87*, 373–378. [CrossRef]
54. Hengstman, G.J.D.; ter Laak, H.J.; Vree Egberts, W.T.M.; Lundberg, I.E.; Moutsopoulos, H.M.; Vencovsky, J.; Doria, A.; Mosca, M.; van Venrooij, W.J.; van Engelen, B.G.M. Anti-signal recognition particle autoantibodies: Marker of a necrotising myopathy. *Ann. Rheum. Dis.* **2006**, *65*, 1635–1638. [CrossRef] [PubMed]
55. Watanabe, Y.; Uruha, A.; Suzuki, S.; Nakahara, J.; Hamanaka, K.; Takayama, K.; Suzuki, N.; Nishino, I. Clinical features and prognosis in anti-SRP and anti-HMGCR necrotising myopathy. *J. Neurol. Neurosurg. Psychiatry* **2016**, *87*, 1038–1044. [CrossRef] [PubMed]
56. Noguchi, E.; Uruha, A.; Suzuki, S.; Hamanaka, K.; Ohnuki, Y.; Tsugawa, J.; Watanabe, Y.; Nakahara, J.; Shiina, T.; Suzuki, N.; et al. Skeletal Muscle Involvement in Antisynthetase Syndrome. *JAMA Neurol.* **2017**, *74*, 992–999. [CrossRef] [PubMed]
57. Hoesly, P.M.; Sluzevich, J.C.; Jambusaria-Pahlajani, A.; Lesser, E.R.; Heckman, M.G.; Abril, A. Association of antinuclear antibody status with clinical features and malignancy risk in adult-onset dermatomyositis. *J. Am. Acad. Dermatol.* **2019**, *80*, 1364–1370. [CrossRef]
58. Azola, A.; Mulheren, R.; Mckeon, G.; Lloyd, T.; Christopher-Stine, L.; Palmer, J.; Chung, T.H. Dysphagia in myositis: A study of the structural and physiologic changes resulting in disordered swallowing. *Am. J. Phys. Med. Rehabil.* 2019. [CrossRef]
59. Cochicho, J.; Madaleno, J.; Louro, E.; Simao, A.; Carvalho, A. Polymyositis and the Spectrum of Scleroderma Disorders. *Eur. J. Case Rep. Intern. Med.* **2016**, *3*, 346. [CrossRef]
60. Malandraki, G.A.; Kaufman, A.; Hind, J.; Ennis, S.; Gangnon, R.; Waclawik, A.; Robbins, J. The effects of lingual intervention in a patient with inclusion body myositis and Sjogren's syndrome: A longitudinal case study. *Arch. Phys. Med. Rehabil.* **2012**, *93*, 1469–1475. [CrossRef]
61. Liu, L.W.C.; Tarnopolsky, M.; Armstrong, D. Injection of botulinum toxin A to the upper esophageal sphincter for oropharyngeal dysphagia in two patients with inclusion body myositis. *Can. J. Gastroenterol.* **2004**, *18*, 397–399. [CrossRef]
62. Korn, J.H.; Mauiyyedi, S. Case 26-2001. *N. Engl. J. Med.* **2001**, *345*, 596–605. [CrossRef]
63. Darrow, D.H.; Hoffman, H.T.; Barnes, G.J.; Wiley, C.A. Management of dysphagia in inclusion body myositis. *Arch. Otolaryngol. Head Neck Surg.* **1992**, *118*, 313–317. [CrossRef]

64. Tierney, D.; Jirjis, J.N. A woman with difficulty swallowing. *Tenn. Med.* **1997**, *90*, 462–463. [PubMed]
65. Takamiya, M.; Takahashi, Y.; Morimoto, M.; Morimoto, N.; Yamashita, S.; Abe, K. Effect of intravenous immunoglobulin therapy on anti-NT5C1A antibody-positive inclusion body myositis after successful treatment of hepatitis C: A case report. *eNeurologicalSci* **2019**, *16*, 100204. [CrossRef] [PubMed]
66. Shibata, S.; Izumi, R.; Hara, T.; Ohshima, R.; Nakamura, N.; Suzuki, N.; Kato, K.; Katori, Y.; Tateyama, M.; Kuroda, H.; et al. Five-year history of dysphagia as a sole initial symptom in inclusion body myositis. *J. Neurol. Sci.* **2017**, *381*, 325–327. [CrossRef]
67. Ofori, E.; Ramai, D.; Ona, M.; Reddy, M. Paraneoplastic Dermatomyositis Syndrome Presenting as Dysphagia. *Gastroenterology Res.* **2017**, *10*, 251–254. [CrossRef] [PubMed]
68. Schrey, A.; Airas, L.; Jokela, M.; Pulkkinen, J. Botulinum toxin alleviates dysphagia of patients with inclusion body myositis. *J. Neurol. Sci.* **2017**, *380*, 142–147. [CrossRef]
69. Giannini, M.; Macchia, L.; Amati, A.; Lia, A.; Girolamo, F.; D'Abbicco, D.; Trojano, M.; Iannone, F. A rare association of anti-alanine-transfer RNA synthetase (anti-PL12) syndrome and sporadic inclusion body myositis. *Scand. J. Rheumatol.* **2018**, *47*, 336–337. [CrossRef] [PubMed]
70. Butt, Z.; Patel, L.; Das, M.K.; Mecoli, C.A.; Ramji, A. NXP-2 Positive Dermatomyositis: A Unique Clinical Presentation. *Case Rep. Rheumatol.* **2017**, *2017*, 4817275. [CrossRef] [PubMed]
71. Olthoff, A.; Carstens, P.-O.; Zhang, S.; von Fintel, E.; Friede, T.; Lotz, J.; Frahm, J.; Schmidt, J. Evaluation of dysphagia by novel real-time MRI. *Neurology* **2016**, *87*, 2132–2138. [CrossRef] [PubMed]
72. Di Pede, C.; Masiero, S.; Bonsangue, V.; Ragona, R.M.; Del Felice, A. Botulinum toxin and rehabilitation treatment in inclusion body myositis for severe oropharyngeal dysphagia. *Neurol. Sci.* **2016**, *37*, 1743–1745. [CrossRef] [PubMed]
73. Iannone, F.; Giannini, M.; Lapadula, G. Recovery of barium swallow radiographic abnormalities in a patient with dermatomyositis and severe dysphagia after high-dose intravenous immunoglobulins. *J. Clin. Rheumatol.* **2015**, *21*, 227. [CrossRef] [PubMed]
74. Eura, N.; Sugie, K.; Kiriyama, T.; Ueno, S. Characteristic dysphagia as a manifestation of dermatomyositis on oropharyngeal muscle imaging. *J. Clin. Rheumatol.* **2015**, *21*, 105–106. [CrossRef] [PubMed]
75. Ko, E.H.; Rubin, A.D. Dysphagia due to inclusion body myositis: Case presentation and review of the literature. *Ann. Otol. Rhinol. Laryngol.* **2014**, *123*, 605–608. [CrossRef] [PubMed]
76. Dagan, A.; Markovits, D.; Braun-Moscovici, Y.; Rozin, A.; Toledano, K.; Balbir-Gurman, A. Life-threatening oropharyngeal aphagia as the major manifestation of dermatomyositis. *Isr. Med. Assoc. J.* **2013**, *15*, 453–455.
77. Langdon, P.C.; Mulcahy, K.; Shepherd, K.L.; Low, V.H.; Mastaglia, F.L. Pharyngeal dysphagia in inflammatory muscle diseases resulting from impaired suprahyoid musculature. *Dysphagia* **2012**, *27*, 408–417. [CrossRef]
78. Murata, K.-Y.; Kouda, K.; Tajima, F.; Kondo, T. Balloon dilation in sporadic inclusion body myositis patients with Dysphagia. *Clin. Med. Insights Case Rep.* **2013**, *6*, 1–7. [CrossRef]
79. Dakovic, Z.; Vesic, S.; Tomovic, M.; Vukovic, J. Oropharyngeal dysphagia as dominant and life-threatening symptom in dermatomyositis. *Vojnosanit. Pregl.* **2009**, *66*, 671–674. [CrossRef]
80. Nagano, H.; Yoshifuku, K.; Kurono, Y. Polymyositis with dysphagia treated with endoscopic balloon dilatation. *Auris Nasus Larynx* **2009**, *36*, 705–708. [CrossRef]
81. Hafejee, A.; Coulson, I.H. Dysphagia in dermatomyositis secondary to bladder cancer: Rapid response to combined immunoglobulin and methylprednisolone. *Clin. Exp. Dermatol.* **2005**, *30*, 93–94. [CrossRef]
82. Ertekin, C.; Secil, Y.; Yuceyar, N.; Aydogdu, I. Oropharyngeal dysphagia in polymyositis/dermatomyositis. *Clin. Neurol. Neurosurg.* **2004**, *107*, 32–37. [CrossRef] [PubMed]
83. Ramachandran, R.B.; Swash, M. Pharyngeal Dysphagia in dermatomyositis: Responsive to cyclophosphamide. *J. Clin. Neuromuscul. Dis.* **2004**, *5*, 166–167. [CrossRef] [PubMed]
84. Ryan, A.; Nor, A.M.; Costigan, D.; Foley-Nolan, D.; El-Rafie, A.; Farrell, M.A.; Hardiman, O. Polymyositis masquerading as motor neuron disease. *Arch. Neurol.* **2003**, *60*, 1001–1003. [CrossRef]
85. Cherin, P.; Pelletier, S.; Teixeira, A.; Laforet, P.; Simon, A.; Herson, S.; Eymard, B. Intravenous immunoglobulin for dysphagia of inclusion body myositis. *Neurology* **2002**, *58*, 326. [CrossRef] [PubMed]
86. Bachmann, G.; Streppel, M.; Krug, B.; Neuen-Jacob, E. Cricopharyngeal muscle hypertrophy associated with florid myositis. *Dysphagia* **2001**, *16*, 244–248. [CrossRef] [PubMed]
87. Kwon, K.M.; Lee, J.S.; Kim, Y.H. A case report of life-threatening acute dysphagia in dermatomyositis: Challenges in diagnosis and treatment. *Medicine (Baltim.)* **2018**, *97*, e0508. [CrossRef]

88. Gorelik, O.; Almoznino-Sarafian, D.; Alon, I.; Rapoport, M.J.; Goltsman, G.; Herbert, M.; Modai, D.; Cohen, N. Acute inflammatory myopathy with severe subcutaneous edema, a new variant? Report of two cases and review of the literature. *Rheumatol. Int.* **2001**, *20*, 163–166. [CrossRef] [PubMed]
89. Barrera, P.; den Broeder, A.A.; van den Hoogen, F.H.; van Engelen, B.G.; van de Putte, L.B. Postural changes, dysphagia, and systemic sclerosis. *Ann. Rheum. Dis.* **1998**, *57*, 331–338. [CrossRef] [PubMed]
90. Caramaschi, P.; Blasi, D.; Carletto, A.; Randon, M.; Bambara, L.M. Megaoesophagus in a patient affected by dermatomyositis. *Clin. Rheumatol.* **1997**, *16*, 106–107. [CrossRef]
91. Shapiro, J.; Martin, S.; DeGirolami, U.; Goyal, R. Inflammatory myopathy causing pharyngeal dysphagia: A new entity. *Ann. Otol. Rhinol. Laryngol.* **1996**, *105*, 331–335. [CrossRef]
92. St Guily, J.L.; Perie, S.; Willig, T.N.; Chaussade, S.; Eymard, B.; Angelard, B. Swallowing disorders in muscular diseases: Functional assessment and indications of cricopharyngeal myotomy. *Ear Nose Throat J.* **1994**, *73*, 34–40. [CrossRef]
93. Johnson, E.R.; McKenzie, S.W. Kinematic pharyngeal transit times in myopathy: Evaluation for dysphagia. *Dysphagia* **1993**, *8*, 35–40. [CrossRef] [PubMed]
94. Verma, A.; Bradley, W.G.; Adesina, A.M.; Sofferman, R.; Pendlebury, W.W. Inclusion body myositis with cricopharyngeus muscle involvement and severe dysphagia. *Muscle Nerve* **1991**, *14*, 470–473. [CrossRef] [PubMed]
95. Danon, M.J.; Friedman, M. Inclusion body myositis associated with progressive dysphagia: Treatment with cricopharyngeal myotomy. Can. *J. Neurol. Sci.* **1989**, *16*, 436–438. [CrossRef] [PubMed]
96. Wintzen, A.R.; Bots, G.T.; de Bakker, H.M.; Hulshof, J.H.; Padberg, G.W. Dysphagia in inclusion body myositis. *J. Neurol. Neurosurg. Psychiatry* **1988**, *51*, 1542–1545. [CrossRef]
97. Kagen, L.J.; Hochman, R.B.; Strong, E.W. Cricopharyngeal obstruction in inflammatory myopathy (polymyositis/dermatomyositis). Report of three cases and review of the literature. *Arthritis Rheum.* **1985**, *28*, 630–636. [CrossRef]
98. Jacob, H.; Berkowitz, D.; McDonald, E.; Bernstein, L.H.; Beneventano, T. The esophageal motility disorder of polymyositis. A prospective study. *Arch. Intern. Med.* **1983**, *143*, 2262–2264. [CrossRef]
99. De Merieux, P.; Verity, M.A.; Clements, P.J.; Paulus, H.E. Esophageal abnormalities and dysphagia in polymyositis and dermatomyositis. *Arthritis Rheum.* **1983**, *26*, 961–968. [CrossRef]
100. Dietz, F.; Logeman, J.A.; Sahgal, V.; Schmid, F.R. Cricopharyngeal muscle dysfunction in the differential diagnosis of dysphagia in polymyositis. *Arthritis Rheum.* **1980**, *23*, 491–495. [CrossRef]
101. Metheny, J.A. Dermatomyositis: A vocal and swallowing disease entity. *Laryngoscope* **1978**, *88*, 147–161. [CrossRef]
102. Porubsky, E.S.; Murray, J.P.; Pratt, L.L. Cricopharyngeal achalasia in dermatomyositis. *Arch. Otolaryngol.* **1973**, *98*, 428–429. [CrossRef] [PubMed]
103. Thomas, F.B.; LeBauer, S.; Greenberger, N.J. Polymyositis masquerading as carcinoma of the cervical esophagus. *Arch. Intern. Med.* **1972**, *129*, 984–986. [CrossRef] [PubMed]
104. O'Hara, J.M.; Szemes, G.; Lowman, R.M. The esophageal lesions in dermatomyositis. A correlation of radiologic and pathologic findings. *Radiology* **1967**, *89*, 27–31. [CrossRef]
105. Donoghue, F.E.; Winkelmann, R.K.; Moersch, H.J. Esophageal defects in dermatomyositis. *Ann. Otol. Rhinol. Laryngol.* **1960**, *69*, 1139–1145. [CrossRef] [PubMed]
106. Felice, K.J.; North, W.A. Inclusion body myositis in Connecticut: Observations in 35 patients during an 8-year period. *Medicine (Baltim.)* **2001**, *80*, 320–327. [CrossRef] [PubMed]
107. Paik, N.-J.; Kim, S.J.; Lee, H.J.; Jeon, J.Y.; Lim, J.-Y.; Han, T.R. Movement of the hyoid bone and the epiglottis during swallowing in patients with dysphagia from different etiologies. *J. Electromyogr. Kinesiol.* **2008**, *18*, 329–335. [CrossRef]
108. Vencovsky, J.; Rehak, F.; Pafko, P.; Jirasek, A.; Valesova, M.; Alusik, S.; Trnavsky, K. Acute cricopharyngeal obstruction in dermatomyositis. *J. Rheumatol.* **1988**, *15*, 1016–1018.
109. Porkodi, R.; Shanmuganandan, K.; Parthiban, M.; Madhavan, R.; Rajendran, P. Clinical spectrum of inflammatory myositis in South India—A ten year study. *J. Assoc. Physicians India* **2002**, *50*, 1255–1258.
110. Houser, S.M.; Calabrese, L.H.; Strome, M. Dysphagia in patients with inclusion body myositis. *Laryngoscope* **1998**, *108*, 1001–1005. [CrossRef]
111. Palace, J.; Losseff, N.; Clough, C. Isolated dysphagia due to polymyositis. *Muscle Nerve* **1993**, *16*, 680–681.

112. Margulis, A.R.; Koehler, R.E. Radiologic diagnosis of disordered esophageal motility: A unified physiologic approach. *Radiol. Clin. North Am.* **1976**, *14*, 429–439.
113. Cunningham, J.D., Jr.; Lowry, L.D. Head and neck manifestations of dermatomyositis-polymyositis. *Otolaryngol. Head Neck Surg.* **1985**, *93*, 673–677. [PubMed]
114. Marie, I.; Hachulla, E.; Levesque, H.; Reumont, G.; Ducrotte, P.; Cailleux, N.; Hatron, P.Y.; Devulder, B.; Courtois, H. Intravenous immunoglobulins as treatment of life threatening esophageal involvement in polymyositis and dermatomyositis. *J. Rheumatol.* **1999**, *26*, 2706–2709. [PubMed]
115. Kleine-Natrop, H.E.; Engel, S. Participation of smooth muscles in dermatomyositis. *I. Arch. Klin. Exp. Dermatol.* **1967**, *228*, 353–363. [CrossRef]
116. Degos, R.; Civatte, J.; Belaich, S.; Delarue, A. The prognosis of adult dermatomyositis. *Trans. St Johns. Hosp. Dermatol. Soc.* **1971**, *57*, 98–104. [PubMed]
117. De Sousa Gameiro, R.; Reis, A.I.A.; Grilo, A.C.; Noronha, C. Following leads: Connecting dysphagia to mixed connective tissue disease. *BMJ Case Rep.* **2018**, *2018*. [CrossRef]
118. Gyorffy, J.B.; Marowske, J.; Gancayco, J. A Rare Cause of Dysphagia and Weight Loss. *Case Rep. Gastroenterol.* **2018**, *12*, 640–645. [CrossRef]
119. Tang, Y.; Xiong, W.; Yu, T.; Wang, M.; Zhang, G.; Lin, L. Eosinophilic Esophageal Myositis a Plausible Cause of Histological Changes of Primary Jackhammer Esophagus: A Case Report. *Am. J. Gastroenterol.* **2018**, *113*, 150–152. [CrossRef]
120. Dobloug, G.C.; Antal, E.A.; Sveberg, L.; Garen, T.; Bitter, H.; Stjarne, J.; Grovle, L.; Gran, J.T.; Molberg, O. High prevalence of inclusion body myositis in Norway; a population-based clinical epidemiology study. *Eur. J. Neurol.* **2015**, *22*, 672-e41. [CrossRef]
121. Dobloug, C.; Walle-Hansen, R.; Gran, J.T.; Molberg, O. Long-term follow-up of sporadic inclusion body myositis treated with intravenous immunoglobulin: A retrospective study of 16 patients. *Clin. Exp. Rheumatol.* **2012**, *30*, 838–842.
122. Almodovar, R.; Lindo, D.P.; Martin, H.; Mazzuchelli, R.; Pardo, J.; Quiros, F.J.; Zarco, P. Dermatomyositis and meningioma in the same patient. *Reumatol. Clin.* **2012**, *8*, 87–89. [CrossRef]
123. Mii, S.; Niiyama, S.; Kusunoki, M.; Arai, S.; Katsuoka, K. Cyclosporine A as treatment of esophageal involvement in dermatomyositis. *Rheumatol. Int.* **2006**, *27*, 183–185. [CrossRef] [PubMed]
124. Wenzel, J.; Uerlich, M.; Gerdsen, R.; Bieber, T.; Boehm, I. Association of inclusion body myositis with subacute cutaneous lupus erythematosus. *Rheumatol. Int.* **2001**, *21*, 75–77. [CrossRef] [PubMed]
125. Uthman, I.; Vazquez-Abad, D.; Senecal, J.L. Distinctive features of idiopathic inflammatory myopathies in French Canadians. *Semin. Arthritis Rheum.* **1996**, *26*, 447–458. [CrossRef]
126. Horowitz, H.W.; Sanghera, K.; Goldberg, N.; Pechman, D.; Kamer, R.; Duray, P.; Weinstein, A. Dermatomyositis associated with Lyme disease: Case report and review of Lyme myositis. *Clin. Infect. Dis.* **1994**, *18*, 166–171. [CrossRef] [PubMed]
127. Horowitz, M.; McNeil, J.D.; Maddern, G.J.; Collins, P.J.; Shearman, D.J. Abnormalities of gastric and esophageal emptying in polymyositis and dermatomyositis. *Gastroenterology* **1986**, *90*, 434–439. [CrossRef]
128. Stevens, M.B.; Hookman, P.; Siegel, C.I.; Esterly, J.R.; Shulman, L.E.; Hendrix, T.R. Aperistalsis of the esophagus in patients with connective-tissue disorders and raynaud's phenomenon. *N. Engl. J. Med.* **1964**, *270*, 1218–1222. [CrossRef] [PubMed]
129. Marie, I.; Hatron, P.Y.; Levesque, H.; Hachulla, E.; Hellot, M.F.; Michon-Pasturel, U.; Courtois, H.; Devulder, B. Influence of age on characteristics of polymyositis and dermatomyositis in adults. *Medicine (Baltim.)* **1999**, *78*, 139–147. [CrossRef]
130. Marie, I.; Hachulla, E.; Hatron, P.Y.; Hellot, M.F.; Levesque, H.; Devulder, B.; Courtois, H. Polymyositis and dermatomyositis: Short term and longterm outcome, and predictive factors of prognosis. *J. Rheumatol.* **2001**, *28*, 2230–2237. [CrossRef]
131. Chiang, I.P.; Wang, J.; Tsang, Y.M.; Hsiao, C.H. Focal myositis of esophagus: A distinct inflammatory pseudotumor mimicking esophageal malignancy. *Am. J. Gastroenterol.* **1997**, *92*, 174–175.
132. Laurikainen, E.; Aitasalo, K.; Halonen, P.; Falck, B.; Kalimo, H. Muscle pathology in idiopathic cricopharyngeal dysphagia. Enzyme histochemical and electron microscopic findings. *Eur. Arch. Otorhinolaryngol.* **1992**, *249*, 216–223. [CrossRef]
133. Wolman, L.; Darke, C.S.; Young, A. The larynx in rheumatoid arthritis. *J. Laryngol. Otol.* **1965**, *79*, 403–434. [CrossRef]

134. Otao, G.; Yamashita, S.-I.; Kyoraku, I.; Shiomi, K.; Nakazato, M. Dysphagia due to inflammation of oral muscles as the first symptom of dermatomyositis. *Intern. Med.* **2007**, *46*, 923–924. [CrossRef] [PubMed]
135. Curiel, R.V.; Brindle, K.A.; Kressel, B.R.; Katz, J.D. Dysphagia after testicular cancer. *Arthritis Rheum.* **2005**, *52*, 3712. [CrossRef] [PubMed]
136. Zuber, M.A.; Kouba, M.; Rudolph, S.E.; Weller, M.; Hrdlicka, P. Severe dysphagia and erythrodermia in a 59-year-old man. *Internist (Berl.)* **2013**, *54*, 359–365. [CrossRef] [PubMed]
137. Kim, S.J.; Han, T.R.; Jeong, S.J.; Beom, J.W. Comparison between swallowing-related and limb muscle involvement in dermatomyositis patients. *Scand. J. Rheumatol.* **2010**, *39*, 336–340. [CrossRef]
138. McCann, L.J.; Garay, S.M.; Ryan, M.M.; Harris, R.; Riley, P.; Pilkington, C.A. Oropharyngeal dysphagia in juvenile dermatomyositis (JDM): An evaluation of videofluoroscopy swallow study (VFSS) changes in relation to clinical symptoms and objective muscle scores. *Rheumatology (Oxf.)* **2007**, *46*, 1363–1366. [CrossRef]
139. Lee, T.; Park, J.H.; Sohn, C.; Yoon, K.J.; Lee, Y.-T.; Park, J.H.; Jung, I.S. Failed Deglutitive Upper Esophageal Sphincter Relaxation Is a Risk Factor for Aspiration in Stroke Patients with Oropharyngeal Dysphagia. *J. Neurogastroenterol. Motil.* **2017**, *23*, 34–40. [CrossRef]
140. Ertekin, C.; Aydogdu, I.; Yuceyar, N. Piecemeal deglutition and dysphagia limit in normal subjects and in patients with swallowing disorders. *J. Neurol. Neurosurg. Psychiatry* **1996**, *61*, 491–496. [CrossRef]
141. Pearson, W.G.J.R.; Hindson, D.F.; Langmore, S.E.; Zumwalt, A.C. Evaluating swallowing muscles essential for hyolaryngeal elevation by using muscle functional magnetic resonance imaging. *Int. J. Radiat. Oncol. Biol. Phys.* **2013**, *85*, 735–740. [CrossRef]
142. Kelly, J.H. Management of upper esophageal sphincter disorders: Indications and complications of myotomy. *Am. J. Med.* **2000**, *108* (Suppl. 4a), 43S–46S. [CrossRef]
143. Ogawa-Momohara, M.; Muro, Y.; Kono, M.; Akiyama, M. Prognosis of dysphagia in dermatomyositis. *Clin. Exp. Rheumatol.* **2019**, *37*, 165.
144. Medsger, T.A.J.R.; Robinson, H.; Masi, A.T. Factors affecting survivorship in polymyositis. A life-table study of 124 patients. *Arthritis Rheum.* **1971**, *14*, 249–258. [CrossRef] [PubMed]
145. Carpenter, J.R.; Bunch, T.W.; Engel, A.G.; O'Brien, P.C. Survival in polymyositis: Corticosteroids and risk factors. *J. Rheumatol.* **1977**, *4*, 207–214. [PubMed]
146. Capkun, G.; Callan, A.; Tian, H.; Wei, Z.; Zhao, C.; Agashivala, N.; Barghout, V. Burden of illness and healthcare resource use in United States patients with sporadic inclusion body myositis. *Muscle Nerve* **2017**, *56*, 861–867. [CrossRef]
147. Peng, A.; Koffman, B.M.; Malley, J.D.; Dalakas, M.C. Disease progression in sporadic inclusion body myositis: Observations in 78 patients. *Neurology* **2000**, *55*, 296–298. [CrossRef]
148. Price, M.A.; Barghout, V.; Benveniste, O.; Christopher-Stine, L.; Corbett, A.; de Visser, M.; Hilton-Jones, D.; Kissel, J.T.; Lloyd, T.E.; Lundberg, I.E.; et al. Mortality and Causes of Death in Patients with Sporadic Inclusion Body Myositis: Survey Study Based on the Clinical Experience of Specialists in Australia, Europe and the USA. *J. Neuromuscul. Dis.* **2016**, *3*, 67–75. [CrossRef]
149. Benbassat, J.; Gefel, D.; Larholt, K.; Sukenik, S.; Morgenstern, V.; Zlotnick, A. Prognostic factors in polymyositis/dermatomyositis. A computer-assisted analysis of ninety-two cases. *Arthritis Rheum.* **1985**, *28*, 249–255. [CrossRef]
150. Hochberg, M.C.; Feldman, D.; Stevens, M.B. Adult onset polymyositis/dermatomyositis: An analysis of clinical and laboratory features and survival in 76 patients with a review of the literature. *Semin. Arthritis Rheum.* **1986**, *15*, 168–178. [CrossRef]
151. Challa, D.; Crowson, C.S.; Niewold, T.B.; Reed, A.M. Predictors of changes in disease activity among children with juvenile dermatomyositis enrolled in the Childhood Arthritis and Rheumatology Research Alliance (CARRA) Legacy Registry. *Clin. Rheumatol.* **2018**, *37*, 1011–1015. [CrossRef]
152. Suzuki, S.; Nishikawa, A.; Kuwana, M.; Nishimura, H.; Watanabe, Y.; Nakahara, J.; Hayashi, Y.K.; Suzuki, N.; Nishino, I. Inflammatory myopathy with anti-signal recognition particle antibodies: Case series of 100 patients. *Orphanet J. Rare Dis.* **2015**, *10*, 61. [CrossRef] [PubMed]
153. Kobayashi, S.; Higuchi, K.; Tamaki, H.; Wada, Y.; Wada, N.; Kubo, M.; Koike, Y.; Nagata, M.; Tatsuzawa, O.; Fujikawa, S. Characteristics of juvenile dermatomyositis in Japan. *Acta Paediatr. Jpn.* **1997**, *39*, 257–262. [CrossRef]

154. Cnop, K.; Martinez, B.; Austad, K.E. Resistant dermatomyositis in a rural indigenous Maya woman. *BMJ Case Rep.* **2019**, *12*. [CrossRef] [PubMed]
155. Chinniah, K.J.; Mody, G.M. Recovery from severe dysphagia in systemic sclerosis-myositis overlap: A case report. *Afr. Health Sci.* **2017**, *17*, 593–596. [CrossRef] [PubMed]
156. Raghu, P.; Manadan, A.M.; Schmukler, J.; Mathur, T.; Block, J.A. Pulse Dose Methylprednisolone Therapy for Adult Idiopathic Inflammatory Myopathy. *Am. J. Ther.* **2015**, *22*, 244–247. [CrossRef]
157. Bonin, C.C.; Santos Pires da Silva, B.; Mota, L.M.; de Carvalho, J.F. Severe and refractory myositis in mixed connective tissue disease: A description of a rare case. *Lupus* **2010**, *19*, 1659–1661. [CrossRef]
158. Tateyama, M.; Saito, N.; Fujihara, K.; Shiga, Y.; Takeda, A.; Narikawa, K.; Hasegawa, T.; Taguchi, Y.; Sakuma, R.; Onodera, Y.; et al. Familial inclusion body myositis: A report on two Japanese sisters. *Intern. Med.* **2003**, *42*, 1035–1038. [CrossRef]
159. Al-Mayouf, S.; Al-Mazyed, A.; Bahabri, S. Efficacy of early treatment of severe juvenile dermatomyositis with intravenous methylprednisolone and methotrexate. *Clin. Rheumatol.* **2000**, *19*, 138–141. [CrossRef]
160. MacFarlane, L.; Osman, N.; Ritter, S.; Miller, A.L.; Loscalzo, J. Clinical Problem-Solving. Eye of the Beholder. *N. Engl. J. Med.* **2016**, *374*, 1774–1779. [CrossRef]
161. Basnayake, S.K.; Blumbergs, P.; Tan, J.A.; Roberts-Thompson, P.J.; Limaye, V. Inflammatory myopathy with anti-SRP antibodies: Case series of a South Australian cohort. *Clin. Rheumatol.* **2015**, *34*, 603–608. [CrossRef]
162. Watanabe, M.; Natsuga, K.; Arita, K.; Abe, R.; Shimizu, H. Generalized acute subcutaneous edema as a rare cutaneous manifestation of severe dermatomyositis. *J. Eur. Acad. Dermatol. Venereol.* **2016**, *30*, e151–e152. [CrossRef] [PubMed]
163. Zedan, M.; El-Ayouty, M.; Abdel-Hady, H.; Shouman, B.; El-Assmy, M.; Fouda, A. Anasarca: Not a nephrotic syndrome but dermatomyositis. *Eur. J. Pediatr.* **2008**, *167*, 831–834. [CrossRef] [PubMed]
164. Chen, T.; Pu, C.; Shi, Q.; Wang, Q.; Cong, L.; Liu, J.; Luo, H.; Fei, L.; Tang, W.; Yu, S. Chronic progressive external ophthalmoplegia with inflammatory myopathy. *Int. J. Clin. Exp. Pathol.* **2014**, *7*, 8887–8892. [PubMed]
165. Black, M.; Marshman, G. Dermatomyositis and pemphigus vulgaris: Association or coincidence? *Australas. J. Dermatol.* **2011**, *52*, e11–e14. [CrossRef] [PubMed]
166. Wang, H.; Li, H.; Kai, C.; Deng, J. Polymyositis associated with hypothyroidism or hyperthyroidism: Two cases and review of the literature. *Clin. Rheumatol.* **2011**, *30*, 449–458. [CrossRef] [PubMed]
167. Noda, S.; Umezaki, H.; Itoh, H.; Hiromatsu, K.; Yamamoto, T. Chronic focal polymyositis. *J. Neurol. Neurosurg. Psychiatry* **1988**, *51*, 728. [CrossRef]
168. Milisenda, J.C.; Doti, P.I.; Prieto-Gonzalez, S.; Grau, J.M. Dermatomyositis presenting with severe subcutaneous edema: Five additional cases and review of the literature. *Semin. Arthritis Rheum.* **2014**, *44*, 228–233. [CrossRef]
169. Sitzia, C.; Sansone, V.A.; Corsi Romanelli, M.M. Creatine kinase elevation: A neglected clue to the diagnosis of polymyositis. A case report. *Clin. Chem. Lab. Med.* **2019**, *57*, e149–e151. [CrossRef]
170. Alqatari, S.; Riddell, P.; Harney, S.; Henry, M.; Murphy, G. MDA-5 associated rapidly progressive interstitial lung disease with recurrent Pneumothoraces: A case report. *BMC Pulm. Med.* **2018**, *18*, 59. [CrossRef]
171. Prossliner, V.; Philipp, M.; Moosbrugger, V.; Poewe, W.; Zangerle, R.; Wanschitz, J.; Schmuth, M. Severe dysphagia, myalgia, and rash in a 55-year-old man. *J. Dtsch. Dermatol. Ges.* **2016**, *14*, 438–441. [CrossRef]
172. Matsuoka, N.; Asano, T.; Sato, S.; Sasajima, T.; Fujita, Y.; Temmoku, J.; Yashiro Furuya, M.; Matsumoto, H.; Suzuki, E.; Kobayashi, H.; et al. A case of dermatomyositis complicated with pleural effusion and massive ascites. *Fukushima J. Med. Sci.* **2019**. [CrossRef] [PubMed]
173. Pars, K.; Garde, N.; Skripuletz, T.; Pul, R.; Dengler, R.; Stangel, M. Subcutaneous immunoglobulin treatment of inclusion-body myositis stabilizes dysphagia. *Muscle Nerve* **2013**, *48*, 838–839. [CrossRef] [PubMed]
174. Joshi, D.; Mahmood, R.; Williams, P.; Kitchen, P. Dysphagia secondary to dermatomyositis treated successfully with intravenous immunoglobulin: A case report. *Int. Arch. Med.* **2008**, *1*, 12. [CrossRef]
175. Lee, K.-H.; Lim, S.-R.; Kim, Y.-J.; Lee, K.-J.; Myung, D.-S.; Jeong, H.-C.; Yoon, W.; Lee, S.-S.; Park, Y.-W. Acute dermatomyositis associated with generalized subcutaneous edema. *Rheumatol. Int.* **2008**, *28*, 797–800. [CrossRef] [PubMed]
176. Dalakas, M.C.; Sonies, B.; Dambrosia, J.; Sekul, E.; Cupler, E.; Sivakumar, K. Treatment of inclusion-body myositis with IVIg: A double-blind, placebo-controlled study. *Neurology* **1997**, *48*, 712–716. [CrossRef] [PubMed]

177. Cherin, P.; Delain, J.-C.; de Jaeger, C.; Crave, J.-C. Subcutaneous Immunoglobulin Use in Inclusion Body Myositis: A Review of 6 Cases. *Case Rep. Neurol.* **2015**, *7*, 227–232. [CrossRef]
178. Patrick, C.; Jean-Christophe, D.; Jean-Charles, C.; Odile, C. High-dose subcutaneous immunoglobulins for the treatment of severe treatment-resistant polymyositis. *Case Rep. Rheumatol.* **2014**, *2014*, 458231. [CrossRef]
179. Kwon, P.M.; Zhou, L.; Motiwala, R.; Kerr, L.D.; Shin, S.C. Immune Myopathy With Perimysial Pathology Associated With Interstitial Lung Disease and Anti-EJ Antibodies. *J. Clin. Neuromuscul. Dis.* **2017**, *18*, 223–227. [CrossRef]
180. Papakonstantinou, E.; Kapp, A.; Raap, U. A mild form of dermatomyositis as a prodromal sign of lung adenocarcinoma: A case report. *J. Med. Case Rep.* **2016**, *10*, 34. [CrossRef]
181. Dias, L.P.N.; Faria, A.L.A.; Scandiuzzi, M.M.; dos Santos Inhaia, C.L.; Shida, J.Y.; Gebrim, L.H. A rare case of severe myositis as paraneoplastic syndrome on breast cancer. *World J. Surg. Oncol.* **2015**, *13*, 134. [CrossRef]
182. Venhuizen, A.C.; Martens, J.E.; van der Linden, P.J. Dermatomyositis as first presentation of ovarian cancer. *Acta Obstet. Gynecol. Scand.* **2006**, *85*, 1271–1272. [CrossRef] [PubMed]
183. Yoshie, H.; Nakazawa, R.; Usuba, W.; Kudo, H.; Sato, Y.; Sasaki, H.; Chikaraishi, T. Paraneoplastic Dermatomyositis Associated with Metastatic Seminoma. *Case Rep. Urol.* **2016**, *2016*, 7050981. [CrossRef] [PubMed]
184. Nagano, Y.; Inoue, Y.; Shimura, T.; Fujikawa, H.; Okugawa, Y.; Hiro, J.; Toiyama, Y.; Tanaka, K.; Mohri, Y.; Kusunoki, M. Exacerbation of Dermatomyositis with Recurrence of Rectal Cancer: A Case Report. *Case Rep. Oncol.* **2015**, *8*, 482–486. [CrossRef]
185. Alenzi, F.M. Myositis Specific Autoantibodies: A Clinical Perspective. *Open Access Rheumatol.* **2020**, *12*, 9–14. [CrossRef] [PubMed]
186. Wang, L.; Huang, L.; Yang, Y.; Chen, H.; Liu, Y.; Liu, K.; Liu, M.; Xiao, Y.; Luo, H.; Zuo, X.; et al. Calcinosis and malignancy are rare in Chinese adult patients with myositis and nuclear matrix protein 2 antibodies identified by an unlabeled immunoprecipitation assay. *Clin. Rheumatol.* **2018**, *37*, 2731–2739. [CrossRef]
187. Costa, R.M.S.; Dumitrascu, O.M.; Gordon, L.K. Orbital myositis: Diagnosis and management. *Curr. Allergy Asthma Rep.* **2009**, *9*, 316–323. [CrossRef]
188. Kalf, J.G.; de Swart, B.J.M.; Bloem, B.R.; Munneke, M. Prevalence of oropharyngeal dysphagia in Parkinson's disease: A meta-analysis. *Parkinsonism Relat. Disord.* **2012**, *18*, 311–315. [CrossRef]
189. Leder, S.B.; Espinosa, J.F. Aspiration risk after acute stroke: Comparison of clinical examination and fiberoptic endoscopic evaluation of swallowing. *Dysphagia* **2002**, *17*, 214–218. [CrossRef]

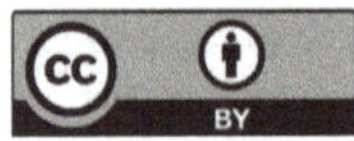

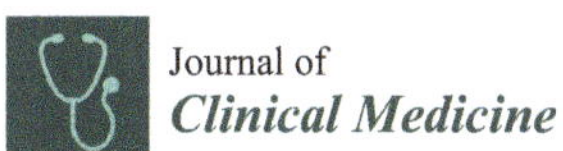

Journal of
Clinical Medicine

MDPI

Registered Report

Comparing the Clinical and Laboratory Features of Remitting Seronegative Symmetrical Synovitis with Pitting Edema and Seronegative Rheumatoid Arthritis: Stage 1

Misako Higashida-Konishi [1,*], Keisuke Izumi [1,2], Satoshi Hama [1], Hiroshi Takei [1], Hisaji Oshima [1] and Yutaka Okano [1]

1 Department of Connective Tissue Diseases, National Hospital Organization Tokyo Medical Center, Tokyo 1528902, Japan; izz@keio.jp (K.I.); shama@ntmc-hosp.jp (S.H.); htakei@ntmc-hosp.jp (H.T.); hoshimamac@mac.com (H.O.); yutakaokano@mac.com (Y.O.)

2 Division of Rheumatology, Department of Internal Medicine, Keio University School of Medicine, Tokyo 1608582, Japan

* Correspondence: higashidamisako@gmail.com; Tel.: +813-3411-0111

Abstract: In seronegative arthritis with extremity edema, the differential diagnosis between remitting seronegative symmetrical synovitis with pitting edema syndrome (RS3PE) and seronegative rheumatoid arthritis (SNRA) is difficult. We compared the clinical characteristics of RS3PE and SNRA and those of such patients with and without malignancies. We retrospectively examined patients diagnosed with RS3PE (McCarty criteria) and SNRA at our hospital in 2007–2020. Malignancy was diagnosed within 2 years before or after RS3PE or SNRA diagnosis. Overall, 24 RS3PE and 124 SNRA patients were enrolled. The mean ages were 79.0 and 66.5 years, and men comprised 54.2% and 37.1% of RS3PE and SNRA patients, respectively. RS3PE patients had higher inflammation levels ($p < 0.01$) and more incidences of malignancy ($p < 0.01$). Matching for age and sex, RS3PE patients had higher inflammation levels ($p < 0.01$) and more incidences of malignancy ($p = 0.02$). Overall, odds ratios (ORs) for malignancy were higher for older age (OR 1.06, $p = 0.04$), male sex (OR 4.34, $p = 0.02$), RS3PE patients (OR 4.83, $p = 0.01$), and patients with extremity edema (OR 4.83, $p = 0.01$). RS3PE patients had higher inflammation levels and associated factors of malignancy than SNRA patients. Patients who are older, male, with extremity edema, or with RS3PE should be screened for malignancies.

Keywords: rheumatoid arthritis; synovitis; neoplasms; edema; inflammation

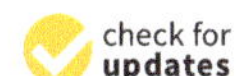

Citation: Higashida-Konishi, M.; Izumi, K.; Hama, S.; Takei, H.; Oshima, H.; Okano, Y. Comparing the Clinical and Laboratory Features of Remitting Seronegative Symmetrical Synovitis with Pitting Edema and Seronegative Rheumatoid Arthritis: Stage 1. *J. Clin. Med.* **2021**, *10*, 340. https://doi.org/10.3390/jcm10020340

Received: 3 December 2020
Accepted: 14 January 2021
Published: 18 January 2021

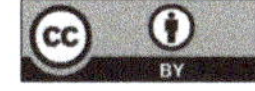

1. Introduction

Remitting seronegative symmetrical synovitis with pitting edema (RS3PE) was first reported by McCarty et al. in 1985 [1]. It is characterized by pitting edema of the extremities, sudden onset of polyarthritis, seronegativity for rheumatoid factor (RF), excellent response to glucocorticoids, and the absence of radiologically evident erosions [1]. RS3PE mainly affects the joints of the extremities, especially the metacarpophalangeal (MCP) and proximal interphalangeal (PIP) phalanges, wrists, shoulders, elbows, knees, and ankles [2]. Although the pathophysiology of RS3PE remains unclear, vascular endothelial growth factor (VEGF) serum levels have been found to be elevated in patients with RS3PE [3]. The increase in vascular permeability by VEGF is thought to be responsible for the development of pitting edema of the dorsum of both hands and both feet in patients with RS3PE [3].

Initially, RS3PE was thought to be a type of older-onset rheumatoid arthritis (RA) [4] and was considered the same disease as seronegative RA and polymyalgia rheumatica (PMR) [5]. Subsequently, comparisons between PMR and RS3PE have been reported [6]. Kawashiri et al. reported the differences in musculoskeletal ultrasound findings of both hands between RS3PE and "seropositive" elderly onset RA; however, to our knowledge, no reports have compared the characteristics of RS3PE and "seronegative" RA [7].

RS3PE is often described as a paraneoplastic disease [8] and has been reported to have a high rate of malignancy development [9]. Paraneoplastic arthritis often presents as symmetrical polyarthritis, mainly affecting the wrist and fingers, and is often negative for RF and anti-cyclic citrullinated peptide antibody (ACPA) [10]. Early diagnosis of malignancy is clinically important because it improves survival. Therefore, examination for malignancy is necessary in such cases.

The primary aim of this study was to compare the clinical characteristics of RS3PE and seronegative RA and evaluate the frequency of concurrent malignancy. The secondary aim was to compare the clinical features with and without malignancies in patients with RS3PE and to compare the clinical features with and without malignancies in patients with seronegative RA.

2. Materials and Methods

2.1. Compliance with Ethical Standards

All procedures were performed in accordance with the ethical standards of the institutional and national research committees and the 1975/1983 Helsinki Declaration and its later amendments.

2.2. Study Design

This was a retrospective medical record study.

2.3. Patients

Medical records of consecutive patients diagnosed with RS3PE and seronegative RA at our hospital between 2007 and 2020 were retrospectively examined. Patients who were both ACPA- and RF-negative were included. Patients who met the criteria for both PMR and RS3PE were included in the RS3PE group and those who met the criteria for both PMR and seronegative RA were included in the seronegative RA group. PMR was diagnosed according to the 2012 European League Against Rheumatism/American College of Rheumatology (EULAR/ACR) Provisional Classification Criteria for PMR [11]. For patients diagnosed with PMR before 2012, we retrospectively reviewed whether they met the 2012 PMR classification criteria. Patients who met the criteria for both RA and RS3PE were diagnosed with RS3PE. However, those who had erosion were diagnosed with seronegative RA. We defined RS3PE and seronegative RA patients by excluding those who met the criteria for PMR as "pure RS3PE" and "pure seronegative RA." Patients who met the criteria for both RA and PMR were diagnosed with seronegative RA. Patients with paraneoplastic polyarthritis were excluded from the group of patients with RS3PE or seronegative RA. Those with distal joint swelling that rapidly disappeared after tumor resection were diagnosed with paraneoplastic polyarthritis.

2.4. RS3PE Diagnosis

Patients were diagnosed with RS3PE when they met the McCarty et al. criteria [1]: (1) pitting edema of the dorsum of both hands and both feet, (2) sudden onset of polyarthritis, (3) seronegative for RF, and (4) no development of radiologically evident erosions.

2.5. Seronegative RA Diagnosis

Seronegative RA was diagnosed according to the 2010 EULAR/ACR criteria [12]. Patients who were first diagnosed with RS3PE or PMR and later diagnosed with seronegative RA were included in the seronegative RA group.

2.6. Clinical and Laboratory Features

We examined the affected joints and evaluated them for systemic signs and symptoms (temperature $\geq$ 38.0 °C, malaise or fatigue, weight loss, morning stiffness lasting at least 1 h, and edema). The affected joints were the shoulders, elbows, wrists, fingers (MCP and interphalangeal (IP)/PIP joints), hips, knees, ankles, and toes (MCP and IP/PIP joints).

Edema was evaluated separately as edema of only hands, only feet, and of both limbs. We also measured the erythrocyte sedimentation rate (ESR) and the levels of C-reactive protein (CRP), hemoglobin (Hb), albumin (Alb), lactate dehydrogenase (LDH), and matrix metalloproteinase 3 (MMP-3). Smokers were defined as those who had a smoking history within 2 years before and after RS3PE or seronegative RA diagnosis. If there were evaluable examinations, ultrasound imaging, breast imaging, joint X-ray imaging, chest computed tomography (CT), abdominal CT, pelvic CT, positron emission tomography/CT, joint magnetic resonance imaging, upper and lower gastrointestinal endoscopy, gynecological examination, and pathological tests were performed.

2.7. Statistical Analysis

The first analysis was performed on clinical and laboratory features of patients with RS3PE and seronegative RA. The secondary analysis was performed on the above evaluations with matching for age and sex. All data were analyzed using JMP version 14.0 (SAS Institute, Cary, NC, USA). The third analysis was performed to compare the clinical features of patients with or without malignancy among patients with RS3PE or seronegative RA. Univariate analysis, Fisher's exact test, and logistic regression analysis were applied to evaluate the associated factor of malignancy. A probability level less than 0.05 was used as the criterion of significance. Results that did not follow the Gaussian distribution were expressed as the median of the 25–75th percentile (interquartile range), and results that followed the Gaussian distribution were expressed as mean $\pm$ standard deviation.

Author Contributions: Conceptualization, M.H.-K. and K.I.; methodology, M.H.-K.; software, M.H.-K.; validation, M.H.-K., K.I., S.H., H.T. and H.O.; formal analysis, M.H.-K.; investigation, M.H.-K.; data curation, M.H.-K.; writing—original draft preparation, M.H.-K.; writing—review and editing, M.H.-K.; visualization, M.H.-K.; supervision, Y.O.; project administration, M.H.-K. All authors have read and agreed to the published version of the manuscript.

Funding: This research received no external funding.

Institutional Review Board Statement: The study was conducted according to the guidelines of the Declaration of Helsinki, and approved by the Ethics Committee of National Hospital Organization Tokyo Medical Center (approval number R19-011 and date of approval: 2 March 2015).

Informed Consent Statement: Informed consent was waived due to the retrospective study design.

Data Availability Statement: Not available.

Conflicts of Interest: The authors declare no conflict of interest.

References

1. McCarty, D.J.; O'Duffy, J.D.; Pearson, L.; Hunter, J.B. Remitting seronegative symmetrical synovitis with pitting edema. RS3PE syndrome. *JAMA* **1985**, *254*, 2763–2767. [CrossRef] [PubMed]
2. Olivé, A.; del Blanco, J.; Pons, M.; Vaquero, M.; Tena, X. The clinical spectrum of remitting seronegative symmetrical synovitis with pitting edema. The Catalán Group for the Study of RS3PE. *J. Rheumatol.* **1997**, *24*, 333–336.
3. Arima, K.; Origuchi, T.; Tamai, M.; Iwanaga, N.; Izumi, Y.; Huang, M.; Tanaka, F.; Kamachi, M.; Aratake, K.; Nakamura, H.; et al. RS3PE syndrome presenting as vascular endothelial growth factor associated disorder. *Ann. Rheum. Dis.* **2005**, *64*, 1653–1655. [CrossRef] [PubMed]
4. Mavragani, C.P.; Moutsopoulos, H.M. Rheumatoid arthritis in the elderly. *Exp. Gerontol.* **1999**, *34*, 463–471. [CrossRef]
5. Healy, L.A. RS3PE syndrome. *J. Rheumatol.* **1990**, *17*, 414.
6. Kimura, M.; Tokuda, Y.; Oshiawa, H.; Yoshida, K.; Utsunomiya, M.; Kobayashi, T.; Deshpande, G.A.; Matsui, K.; Kishimoto, M. Clinical characteristics of patients with remitting seronegative symmetrical synovitis with pitting edema compared to patients with pure polymyalgia rheumatica. *J. Rheumatol.* **2012**, *39*, 148–153. [CrossRef] [PubMed]
7. Kawashiri, S.; Suzuki, T.; Okada, A.; Tsuji, A.; Takatani, A.; Shimizu, T.; Koga, T.; Iwamoto, N.; Ichinose, K.; Nakamura, H.; et al. Differences in musculoskeletal ultrasound findings between RS3PE syndrome and elderly-onset rheumatoid arthritis. *Clin. Rheumatol.* **2020**, *39*, 1981–1988. [CrossRef] [PubMed]
8. Sibilia, J.; Friess, S.; Schaeverbeke, T.; Maloisel, F.; Bertin, P.; Goichot, B.; Kuntz, J.L. Remitting seronegative symmetrical synovitis with pitting edema (RS3PE): A form of paraneoplastic polyarthritis? *J. Rheumatol.* **1991**, *26*, 115–120.

9. Elizabeth, B.R. Remitting seronegative symmetrical synovitis with pitting edema syndrome: Followup for neoplasia. *J. Rheumatol.* **2005**, *32*, 1760–1761.
10. Morel, J.; Deschamps, V.; Toussirot, E.; Pertuiset, E.; Sordet, C.; Kieffer, P.; Berthelot, J.M.; Champagne, H.; Mariette, X.; Combe, B. Characteristics and survival of 26 patients with paraneoplastic arthritis. *Ann. Rheum. Dis.* **2008**, *67*, 244–247. [CrossRef] [PubMed]
11. Dasgupta, B.; Cimmino, M.A.; Maradit-Kremers, H.; Schmidt, W.A.; Schirmer, M.; Salvarani, C.; Bachta, A.; Dejaco, C.; Duftner, C.; Jensen, H.S.; et al. 2012 provisional classification criteria for polymyalgia rheumatica: A European League against Rheumatism/American College of Rheumatology collaborative initiative. *Ann. Rheum. Dis.* **2012**, *71*, 484–492. [CrossRef] [PubMed]
12. Aletaha, D.; Neogi, T.; Silman, A.J.; Funovits, J.; Felson, D.T.; Bingham, C.O., 3rd; Birnbaum, N.S.; Burmester, G.R.; Bykerk, V.P.; Cohen, M.D.; et al. 2010 Rheumatoid arthritis classification criteria: An American College of Rheumatology/European League against Rheumatism collaborative initiative. *Arthritis Rheumatol.* **2010**, *62*, 2569–2581. [CrossRef] [PubMed]

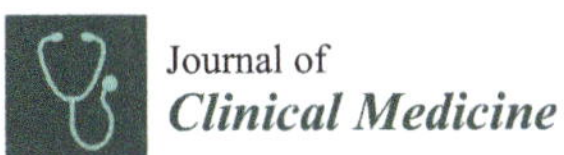
Journal of
Clinical Medicine

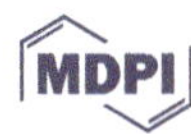

Registered Report

Comparing the Clinical and Laboratory Features of Remitting Seronegative Symmetrical Synovitis with Pitting Edema and Seronegative Rheumatoid Arthritis

Misako Higashida-Konishi [1,*], Keisuke Izumi [1,2], Satoshi Hama [1], Hiroshi Takei [1], Hisaji Oshima [1] and Yutaka Okano [1]

[1] Department of Connective Tissue Diseases, National Hospital Organization Tokyo Medical Center, Tokyo 1528902, Japan; izz@keio.jp (K.I.); shama@ntmc-hosp.jp (S.H.); htakei@ntmc-hosp.jp (H.T.); hoshimamac@mac.com (H.O.); yutakaokano@mac.com (Y.O.)

[2] Division of Rheumatology, Department of Internal Medicine, Keio University School of Medicine, Tokyo 1608582, Japan

* Correspondence: higashidamisako@gmail.com; Tel.: +81-3-3411-0111

Abstract: In seronegative arthritis with extremity edema, it is difficult to differentiate between remitting seronegative symmetrical synovitis with pitting edema syndrome (RS3PE) and seronegative rheumatoid arthritis (SNRA). We compared the clinical characteristics of RS3PE and SNRA in patients with and without malignancies. We retrospectively examined patients diagnosed with RS3PE (McCarty criteria) and SNRA at our hospital in 2007–2020. Malignancy was diagnosed within 2 years before or after RS3PE or SNRA diagnosis. Overall, 24 RS3PE and 124 SNRA patients were enrolled. The median ages were 79.5 and 68.5 years, and men comprised 54.2% and 37.1% of RS3PE and SNRA patients, respectively. RS3PE patients had higher inflammation levels ($p = 0.004$) and more incidences of malignancy ($p = 0.034$). Matching for age and sex, RS3PE patients had higher inflammation levels ($p = 0.021$) and more incidences of malignancy ($p = 0.005$). Overall, odds ratios (ORs) for malignancy were higher for older age (OR 1.06, $p = 0.037$), male sex (OR 4.34, $p = 0.007$), RS3PE patients (OR 4.83, $p = 0.034$), and patients with extremity edema (OR 4.83, $p = 0.034$). Inflammation levels and associated factors of malignancy were higher in RS3PE patients than in SNRA patients. Patients who are older, male, with extremity edema, or had RS3PE should be screened for malignancies.

Keywords: rheumatoid arthritis; synovitis; neoplasms; edema; inflammation

Citation: Higashida-Konishi, M.; Izumi, K.; Hama, S.; Takei, H.; Oshima, H.; Okano, Y. Comparing the Clinical and Laboratory Features of Remitting Seronegative Symmetrical Synovitis with Pitting Edema and Seronegative Rheumatoid Arthritis. *J. Clin. Med.* **2021**, *10*, 1116. https://doi.org/10.3390/jcm10051116

Academic Editor: Eugen Feist

Received: 25 January 2021
Accepted: 4 March 2021
Published: 7 March 2021

1. Introduction

Remitting seronegative symmetrical synovitis with pitting edema (RS3PE) was first reported by McCarty et al. in 1985 [1]. It is characterized by pitting edema of the extremities, sudden onset of polyarthritis, seronegativity for rheumatoid factor (RF), excellent response to glucocorticoids, and the absence of radiologically evident erosions [1]. RS3PE mainly affects the joints of the extremities, especially the metacarpophalangeal (MCP) and proximal interphalangeal (PIP) phalanges, wrists, shoulders, elbows, knees, and ankles [2]. Although the pathophysiology of RS3PE remains unclear, vascular endothelial growth factor (VEGF) serum levels have been found to be elevated in patients with RS3PE [3]. The increase in vascular permeability by VEGF is thought to be responsible for the development of pitting edema of the dorsum of both hands and both feet in patients with RS3PE [3].

Initially, RS3PE was thought to be a type of older-onset rheumatoid arthritis (RA) [4] and was considered the same disease as seronegative RA and polymyalgia rheumatica (PMR) [5]. Subsequently, comparisons between PMR and RS3PE have been reported [6]. Kawashiri et al. reported the differences in musculoskeletal ultrasound findings of both hands between RS3PE and "seropositive" elderly onset RA; however, to our knowledge, no reports have compared the characteristics of RS3PE and "seronegative" RA [7].

RS3PE is often described as a paraneoplastic disease [8] and has been reported to have a high rate of malignancy development [9]. Paraneoplastic arthritis often presents as symmetrical polyarthritis, mainly affecting the wrist and fingers, and is often negative for RF and anti-cyclic citrullinated peptide antibody (ACPA) [10]. Early diagnosis of malignancy is clinically important because it improves survival. Therefore, examination for malignancy is necessary in such cases.

The primary aim of this study was to compare the clinical characteristics of RS3PE and seronegative RA and evaluate the frequency of concurrent malignancy. The secondary aim was to compare the clinical features with and without malignancies in patients with RS3PE and to compare the clinical features with and without malignancies in patients with seronegative RA.

2. Materials and Methods

2.1. Compliance with Ethical Standards

All procedures were performed in accordance with the ethical standards of the institutional and national research committees and the 1975/1983 Helsinki Declaration and its later amendments.

2.2. Study Design

This was a retrospective medical record study.

2.3. Patients

Medical records of consecutive patients diagnosed with RS3PE and seronegative RA at our hospital between 2007 and 2020 were retrospectively examined. Patients who were both ACPA- and RF-negative were included. Patients who met the criteria for both PMR and RS3PE were included in the RS3PE group and those who met the criteria for both PMR and seronegative RA were included in the seronegative RA group. PMR was diagnosed according to the 2012 European League Against Rheumatism/American College of Rheumatology (EULAR/ACR) Provisional Classification Criteria for PMR [11]. For patients diagnosed with PMR before 2012, we retrospectively reviewed whether they met the 2012 PMR classification criteria. Patients who met the criteria for both RA and RS3PE were diagnosed with RS3PE. However, those who had erosion were diagnosed with seronegative RA. We defined RS3PE and seronegative RA patients by excluding those who met the criteria for PMR as "pure RS3PE" and "pure seronegative RA." Patients who met the criteria for both RA and PMR were diagnosed with seronegative RA. Patients with paraneoplastic polyarthritis were excluded from the group of patients with RS3PE or seronegative RA. Those with distal joint swelling that rapidly disappeared after tumor resection were diagnosed with paraneoplastic polyarthritis.

2.4. RS3PE Diagnosis

Patients were diagnosed with RS3PE when they met the McCarty et al. criteria [1]: (1) pitting edema of the dorsum of both hands and both feet, (2) sudden onset of polyarthritis, (3) seronegative for RF, and (4) no development of radiologically evident erosions.

2.5. Seronegative RA Diagnosis

Seronegative RA was diagnosed according to the 2010 EULAR/ACR criteria [12]. Patients who were first diagnosed with RS3PE or PMR and later diagnosed with seronegative RA were included in the seronegative RA group.

2.6. Clinical and Laboratory Features

We examined the affected joints and evaluated them for systemic signs and symptoms (temperature $\geq$38.0 °C, malaise or fatigue, weight loss, morning stiffness lasting at least 1 h, and edema). The affected joints were the shoulders, elbows, wrists, fingers (MCP and interphalangeal (IP)/PIP joints), hips, knees, ankles, and toes (MCP and IP/PIP joints).

Edema was evaluated separately as edema of only hands, only feet, and of both limbs. We also measured the erythrocyte sedimentation rate (ESR) and the levels of C-reactive protein (CRP), hemoglobin (Hb), albumin (Alb), lactate dehydrogenase (LDH), and matrix metalloproteinase 3 (MMP-3). Smokers were defined as those who had a smoking history within 2 years before and after RS3PE or seronegative RA diagnosis. If there were evaluable examinations, ultrasound imaging, breast imaging, joint X-ray imaging, chest computed tomography (CT), abdominal CT, pelvic CT, positron emission tomography/CT, joint magnetic resonance imaging, upper and lower gastrointestinal endoscopy, gynecological examination, and pathological tests were performed.

2.7. Statistical Analysis

The first analysis was performed on clinical and laboratory features of patients with RS3PE and seronegative RA. The secondary analysis was performed on the above evaluations with a 1:2 matching for age and sex. All data were analyzed using JMP version 14.0 (SAS Institute, Cary, NC, USA). The third analysis was performed to compare the clinical features of patients with or without malignancy among patients with RS3PE or seronegative RA. Univariate analysis, Fisher's exact test, and logistic regression analysis were applied to evaluate the associated factor of malignancy. A probability level less than 0.05 was used as the criterion of significance. Results that did not follow the Gaussian distribution were expressed as the median of the 25–75th percentile (interquartile range), and results that followed the Gaussian distribution were expressed as mean $\pm$ standard deviation. The odds ratio (OR) and its 95% confidence interval (95% CI) indicated the increased or decreased risk of malignancy associated with a one-unit change in the predictor variable for continuous variables. For dichotomous variables, the OR indicated the risk of malignancy associated with the presence of the feature compared to the absence of the characteristic. In the case of missing data, the number of patients with available data was specified.

3. Results

We enrolled 24 consecutive patients with RS3PE examined at our hospital between 2007 and 2020 (Supplementary Table S1). Initially, 25 patients were diagnosed with RS3PE according to the criteria of McCarty et al. [1]. However, one patient was later diagnosed with paraneoplastic polyarthritis with rapid remission of distal swelling with pitting edema after tumor resection and was excluded from the RS3PE group. Only one patient was diagnosed with paraneoplastic polyarthritis: an 81-year-old woman who presented with polyarthritis and edema of both hands and feet. Her blood test showed high levels of CRP (2.2 mg/dL). During examination, she was diagnosed with cancer of the pancreatic body and underwent surgery to remove the body and tail of the pancreas. The postoperative course is uneventful. One month after the operation, the polyarthritis resolved and the levels of CRP decreased (0.1 mg/dL) without the use of medication.

In the control group, 124 consecutive patients with seronegative RA during the same period were enrolled. Supplementary Figure S1 shows the patient diagnosis flow.

Figure 1 shows the breakdown of patients according to the criteria for RS3PE, RA, and PMR. The RS3PE group consisted of Group A, B, and C patients. The seronegative RA group consisted of Group D and E patients. In the RS3PE and seronegative RA groups, two and 17 patients, respectively, met the 2012 EULAR/ACR provisional criteria for PMR [11] (Figure 1). After excluding those patients, 22 patients (Groups A and B, Figure 1) with RS3PE and 107 patients (Group D, Figure 1) with seronegative RA were analyzed with similar results to those obtained at baseline, including the incidence of comorbid malignancies (Supplementary Table S2).

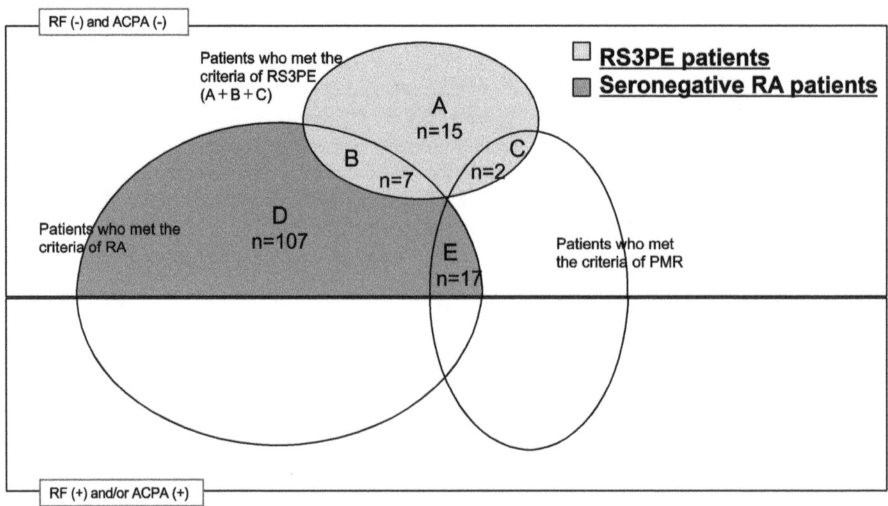

Group A: RS3PE patients who met only the criteria of RS3PE
Group B: RS3PE patients who met both the criteria of RS3PE and the criteria of RA
Group C: RS3PE patients who met both the criteria of RS3PE and the criteria of PMR
Group D: Seronegative RA patients who met only the criteria of RA
Group E: Seronegative RA patients who met both the criteria of RA and the criteria of PMR

Figure 1. Diagnostic criteria for RS3PE and seronegative RA, as used in this study. Patients in Group A met only the criteria for RS3PE. Patients in Group B met the criteria for both RS3PE and RA. Patients in Group C met the criteria for both RS3PE and PMR. Patients in Group D met only the criteria for RA. Patients in Group E met the criteria for both RA and PMR. The RS3PE group consisted of Group A + B + C patients. The seronegative RA group consisted of Group D + E patients. No patients met the criteria for RS3PE, RA, and PMR. ACPA, anti-cyclic citrullinated peptide antibody; PMR, polymyalgia rheumatica; RA, rheumatoid arthritis; RF, rheumatoid factor; RS3PE, remitting seronegative symmetrical synovitis.

3.1. Comparison of Clinical and Laboratory Features of RS3PE and Seronegative RA

In the first analysis, baseline characteristics at diagnosis of the 24 RS3PE patients were compared with those of the 124 seronegative RA patients (Table 1). The onset age of RS3PE was significantly higher than that of seronegative RA. The RS3PE patients had less swollen small joints and significantly higher levels of CRP, LDH, and MMP-3 than the seronegative RA patients. The numbers of swollen and/or tender joints were similar in both groups, except for the elbows and fingers, which were more affected in the seronegative RA patients. The ankles were more affected in the RS3PE patients than in the seronegative RA patients.

Malignancies were detected in six of 24 (25%) patients in the RS3PE group and in eight of 124 (6.5%) patients in the seronegative RA group within 2 years before and after RS3PE/seronegative RA diagnosis. The malignancy incidence rate in the RS3PE group was significantly higher than that in the seronegative RA group ($p = 0.034$). Table 2 presents the patients with malignancies and the types of malignancies. Advanced malignancies were not found in the RS3PE patients. There was one case of advanced malignancy (pancreatic cancer) in a seronegative RA patient.

Table 1. Patient baseline characteristics at diagnosis.

Characteristics	RS3PE Patients (n = 24)		Seronegative RA Patients (n = 124)		p Value
Age, median (IQR), years	79.5 (73.8–86.5)		68.5 (58.5–78.0)		<0.001
Length of follow-up, median (IQR), months	31.5 (12.0–109.0)		62.9 (30.7–98.4)		0.09
Male sex, n (%)	13 (54.2)		46 (37.1)		0.17
Smoking, n (%)	5 (20.8)		23 (18.6)		0.78
Diabetes, n (%)	6 (25.0)		14 (11.3)		0.10
Hypertension, n (%)	12 (50.0)		41 (33.1)		0.16
Hyperlipidemia, n (%)	5 (20.8)		33 (26.1)		0.62
Swollen or/and tender joints, n (%)					
Shoulders	8 (33.3)		67 (54.3)		0.08
Elbows	2 (8.3)		53 (42.7)		0.001
Wrists	17 (70.8)		100 (80.7)		0.28
Fingers	19 (79.2)		120 (96.8)		0.022
Hips	4 (16.7)		13 (10.5)		0.48
Knees	9 (37.5)		59 (47.6)		0.38
Ankles	18 (75.0)		65 (52.4)		0.046
Toes	8 (33.3)		35 (28.2)		0.63
Patients with swollen large joints, n (%)	17 (70.8)		64 (51.6)		0.12
Patients with swollen small joints, n (%)	21 (87.5)		124 (100.0)		0.024
Number of swollen large joints, median (IQR), n	2.0 (0.0–2.8)		1.0 (0.0–2.0)		0.17
Number of swollen small joints, median (IQR), n	3.0 (1.3–13.3)		9.0 (5.0–15.0)		0.33
28 swollen joints, median (IQR), n	4.0 (1.3–10.8)		8.0 (5.0–14.0)		0.29
28 tender joints, median (IQR), n	6.5 (4.3–12.0)		11.0 (7.3–15.0)		0.15
Patients with erosion, n (%)	0 (0.0)		39 (31.5)		<0.001
Systemic signs and symptoms, n (%)					
Temperature ≥38 °C	2 (8.3)		7 (5.7)		0.64
Malaise or fatigue	3 (12.5)		8 (6.5)		0.39
Weight loss	5 (20.8)		12 (9.7)		0.16
Morning stiffness (lasting at least 1 h)	2 (8.3)		31 (25.0)		0.11
Edema (both hands and feet)	24 (100.0)		0(0)		<0.001
Edema (only hands)	0 (0.0)		1 (0.8)		1.0
Edema (only feet)	0 (0.0)		19 (15.3)		<0.001
CRP, median (IQR), mg/dL	8.2 (4.0–14)		2.8 (0.7–6.6)		0.004
ESR, median (IQR), mm/h					
Men+Women	91.0 (59–112.5)		55.0 (32.0–90.0)		0.07
Men	85.0 (28.5–114.5)		57.0 (31.0–90.0)		0.36
Women	91.0 (82–113)		54.0 (32.0–88.0)		0.010
Alb, median (IQR), g/dL	3.5 (3.0–3.7)	(n = 23) *	3.9 (3.4–4.1)	(n = 100) *	0.012
LDH, median (IQR), U/L	197.0 (161–234)		176.0 (155.5–195)		0.07
MMP-3, median (IQR), ng/mL					

Table 1. *Cont.*

Characteristics	RS3PE Patients (*n* = 24)		Seronegative RA Patients (*n* = 124)		*p* Value
Men+Women	378.5(243.3–662.2)	(*n* = 16) *	162.0 (82.2–401.1)	(*n* = 115) *	0.022
Men	359.4(269.1–435.4)	(*n* = 7) *	211.0 (115.3–420.9)	(*n* = 45) *	0.08
Women	414.1(92.8–997.2)	(*n* = 9) *	151.0 (47.2–348.5)	(*n* = 70) *	0.07
Hb, mean ± SD, g/dL					
Men + Women	10.7 ± 1.8		11.9 ± 1.8		0.024
Men	10.8 ± 2.0		12.2 ± 1.7		0.10
Women	10.6 ± 1.5		11.7 ± 1.8		0.12
Malignancy (within 2 years before and after the diagnosis of RS3PE or seronegative RA), *n* (%)	6 (25.0)		8 (6.5)		0.034
Patients fulfilling the classification criteria for RA [11,12], *n* (%)	7 (29.2)		124 (100.0)		<0.001
Patients fulfilling the classification criteria for PMR [10], *n* (%)	2 (8.3)		17 (13.7)		0.74
Patients fulfilling the classification criteria for RA [11,12] + PMR [10], *n* (%)	0 (0.0)		17 (13.7)		0.08

Alb, albumin; CRP, C-reactive protein; ESR, erythrocyte sedimentation rate; Hb, hemoglobin; IQR, inter quartile range; LDH, lactate dehydrogenase; MMP-3, matrix metalloproteinase 3; PMR, polymyalgia rheumatica; RA, rheumatoid arthritis; RS3PE, remitting seronegative symmetrical synovitis with pitting edema; SD, standard deviation. * In the case of missing data, the number of patients with available data was specified.

Table 2. Patients with malignancies 2 years before and after RS3PE or seronegative RA diagnosis.

Sex, Age (years)	Interval between Diagnosis of RS3PE/Seronegative RA and Malignancies (Months)	Malignancy Type
RS3PE		
M, 81	−24	Prostate cancer
M, 78	−24	Prostate cancer
M, 78	−11	Rectal cancer
F, 87	0 (+5 days)	Pancreatic cancer
M, 79	0 (+6 days)	Stomach cancer
M, 80	3	Rectal cancer
Seronegative RA		
M, 84	−20	Rectal cancer
F, 64	−17	Uterine cancer
M, 82	−6	Ascending colon cancer
M, 69	−5	Small cell lung cancer
F, 58	−4	Breast cancer
F, 80	1	Breast cancer
M, 67	9	Diffuse large B cell lymphoma
M, 83	18	Pancreatic cancer

RA, rheumatoid arthritis; RS3PE, remitting seronegative symmetrical synovitis with pitting edema; M, male; F, female.

3.2. Comparison of Clinical and Laboratory Features of RS3PE and Seronegative RA with a 1:2 Matching for Age and Sex

Since the incidence of malignancies depends on age and sex, we performed a 1:2 matching in the second analysis. After matching for age and sex, 24 patients with RS3PE and 48 with seronegative RA were selected for comparison. Malignancies were significantly more common in the RS3PE than in the seronegative RA patients (Table 3). The RS3PE patients had less swollen and tender joints and significantly higher CRP levels than the seronegative RA patients.

Table 3. Baseline characteristics at diagnosis of RS3PE and seronegative RA patients with a 1:2 matching for age and sex.

Characteristic	RS3PE Patients (n = 24)	Seronegative RA Patients (n = 48)	p Value
Age, median (IQR), years	79.5 (73.8–86.5)	79.5 (73.3–85.3)	0.58
Male sex, n (%)	13 (54.2)	23 (47.9)	0.80
Swollen or/and tender joint, n (%)			
Shoulders	8 (33.3)	33 (68.8)	0.006
Elbows	2 (8.3)	19 (39.6)	0.006
Wrists	17 (70.8)	42 (87.5)	0.11
Fingers	19 (79.2)	46 (95.8)	0.037
Hips	4 (16.7)	6 (12.5)	0.72
Knees	9 (37.5)	19 (39.6)	1.00
Ankles	18 (75.0)	25 (52.1)	0.08
Toes	8 (33.3)	11 (22.9)	0.40
Patients with swollen large joints, n (%)	17 (70.8)	26 (54.2)	0.21
Patients with swollen small joints, n (%)	21 (87.5)	48 (100.0)	0.034
Number of swollen small joints, median (IQR), n	3.0 (1.3–13.3)	9.0 (6.0–15.0)	0.021
28 swollen joints, median (IQR), n	4.0 (1.3–10.8)	9.5 (6.0–15.0)	0.008
28 tender joints, median (IQR), n	6.5 (4.3–12.0)	11.0 (8.3–15.0)	0.019
Patients with erosion, n (%)	0 (0.0)	15 (31.3)	0.001
CRP, median (IQR), mg/dL	8.2 (4.0–14)	4.4 (1.3–8.4)	0.021
ESR, median (IQR), mm/h	91.0 (59–112.5)	75.0 (37.0–103.0)	0.25
LDH, median (IQR), U/L	197.0 (161–234)	184.5 (164.0–210.5)	0.26
MMP-3, median (IQR), ng/mL	378.5(243.3–662.2)	251.0 (124.0–555.0)	0.27
Hb, mean±SD, mg/dL	10.7 ± 1.8	11.5 ± 2.0	0.08
Malignancy (within 2 years before and after the diagnosis of RS3PE or seronegative RA), n (%)	6 (25.0)	1 (2.1)	0.005
Patients fulfilling the classification criteria for RA [11,12], n (%)	7 (29.2)	48 (100.0)	0.09
Patients fulfilling the classification criteria for PMR [10], n (%)	2 (8.3)	7 (14.6)	0.71
Patients fulfilling the classification criteria for RA [11,12] + PMR [10], n (%)	0 (0.0)	7 (14.6)	0.09

CRP, C-reactive protein; ESR, erythrocyte sedimentation rate; Hb, hemoglobin; IQR, interquartile range; LDH, lactate dehydrogenase; MMP-3, matrix metalloproteinase 3; PMR, polymyalgia rheumatica; RA, rheumatoid arthritis; RS3PE, remitting seronegative symmetrical synovitis with pitting edema; SD, standard deviation.

3.3. Comparison of Clinical Features of Patients with and without Malignancies among the RS3PE and Seronegative RA Patients

Table 4 shows a comparison of the clinical features of the patients with and without malignancies. There were 14 patients with malignancies and 134 patients without malignancies, with median ages of 79.5 and 69.5 years, respectively ($p = 0.032$). Furthermore, 71.4% and 36.6% of the patients, respectively, were men ($p = 0.011$). The RS3PE patients constituted 42.9% and 13.4% ($p = 0.034$) of the patients with and without malignancies, respectively. Patients with malignancies had more edema of both hands and both feet ($p = 0.034$) than those without malignancies. There was no difference between the groups in terms of percentage of patients who fulfilled the criteria for PMR ($p = 1.00$). In terms of overall ORs for malignant comorbidities among the patients with RS3PE or seronegative RA, older age (OR 1.06, 95% CI 1.002–1.11, $p = 0.037$), male sex (OR 4.34, 95% CI 1.29–14.57, $p = 0.007$), RS3PE (OR 4.83, 95% CI 1.50–15.56, $p = 0.034$), and edema of both hands and both feet (OR 4.83, 95% CI 1.50–15.56, $p = 0.034$) were associated with the presence of comorbid malignancies. Seronegative RA (OR 0.21, 95% CI 0.06–0.07, $p = 0.034$) and increased Hb levels in men (OR 0.51, 95% CI 0.33–0.81, $p = 0.005$) were associated with the absence of comorbid malignancies (Table 5).

Table 4. Patient baseline characteristics at diagnosis of RS3PE and seronegative RA patients with or without malignancies.

Characteristics	With Malignancy ($n = 14$)	Without Malignancy ($n = 134$)	p Value
Age, median (IQR), years	79.5 (68.5–82.3)	69.5 (60.0–79.0)	0.032
Length of follow-up, median (IQR), months	40.6 (7.9–87.7)	57.4 (27.4–97.7)	0.36
Male sex, n (%)	10 (71.4)	49 (36.6)	0.011
Smoking, n (%)	5 (35.7)	23 (17.2)	0.14
Diabetes, n (%)	4 (28.6)	16 (11.9)	0.10
Hypertension, n (%)	5 (35.7)	48 (35.8)	1.00
Hyperlipidemia, n (%)	4 (28.6)	34 (25.4)	0.76
Swollen or/and tender joints, n (%)			
Shoulders	5 (35.7)	70 (52.2)	0.27
Elbows	5 (35.7)	50 (37.3)	1.00
Wrists	11 (78.6)	106 (79.1)	1.00
Fingers	13 (92.9)	126 (94.0)	1.00
Hips	2 (14.3)	15 (11.2)	0.67
Knees	5 (35.7)	63 (47.0)	0.56
Ankles	8 (57.1)	75 (56.0)	1.00
Toes	4 (28.6)	39 (29.1)	1.00
Patients with swollen large joints, n (%)	6 (42.9)	75 (56.0)	0.41
Patients with swollen small joints, n (%)	13 (92.9)	132 (98.0)	0.26
Number of swollen large joints, median (IQR), n	0.0 (0.0–2.3)	1.0 (0.0–2.0)	0.44
Number of swollen small joints, median (IQR), n	12.5 (4.3–18.5)	8.0 (4.0–13.0)	0.46
28 swollen joints, median (IQR), n	9.5 (3.5–16.8)	8.0 (4.0–12.0)	0.62
28 tender joints, median (IQR), n	7.5 (5.8–19.3)	10.0 (7.0–14.3)	0.74
Patients with erosion, n (%)	5 (35.7)	34 (25.4)	0.52

Table 4. *Cont.*

Characteristics	With Malignancy (*n* = 14)		Without Malignancy (*n* = 134)		*p* Value
Systemic signs and symptoms, *n* (%)					
Temperature ≥ 38 °C	0 (0.0)		9 (6.7)		1.00
Malaise or fatigue	2 (14.3)		9 (6.7)		0.28
Weight loss	1 (7.1)		16 (12.0)		1.00
Morning stiffness (lasting at least 1 h)	4 (28.6)		29 (21.7)		0.55
Edema (both hands and feet)	6 (42.9)		18 (13.4)		0.034
Edema (only hands)	0 (0.0)		1 (0.8)		1.00
Edema (only feet)	0 (0.0)		19 (14.2)		0.22
CRP, median (IQR), mg/dL	6.1 (3.1–11.9)		3.1 (0.8–7.2)		0.08
ESR, median (IQR), mm/h					
Men + Women	46.0 (21.5–112.0)		59.0 (33.0–91.5)		0.88
Men	90.0 (35.0–114.0)		59.0 (31.0–90.5)		0.53
Women	22.5 (13.8–91.3)		59.0 (33.5–93.5)		0.15
Alb, median (IQR), g/dL	3.5 (3.1–4.0)		3.8 (3.3–4.1)	(*n* = 109) *	0.24
LDH, median (IQR), U/L	174.5 (166.8–214.8)		178.0 (155.0–206.3)		0.79
MMP-3, median (IQR), ng/mL					
Men+Women	220.0 (43.8–364.8)	(*n* = 13) *	181.0 (84.8–428.5)	(*n* = 118) *	0.75
Men	234.7 (133.0–364.8)	(*n* = 9) *	213.0 (116.0–426.2)	(*n* = 43) *	0.85
Women	37.7 (28.1–463.8)	(*n* = 4) *	162.0 (66.8–465.0)	(*n* = 75) *	0.13
Hb, mean ± SD, g/dL					
Men + Women	10.9 ± 2.0		11.8 ± 1.8		0.10
Men	10.3 ± 1.4		12.3 ± 1.7		0.001
Women	12.7 ± 2.3		11.5 ± 1.8		0.24
Patients diagnosed with RS3PE, *n* (%)	6 (42.9)		18 (13.4)		0.034
Patients diagnosed with RA [11,12], *n* (%)	8 (57.1)		116 (86.6)		0.034
Patients fulfilling the classification criteria for RA [11,12], *n* (%)	10 (71.4)		121 (90.0)		0.058
Patients fulfilling the classification criteria for PMR [10], *n* (%)	1 (7.1)		18 (13.4)		1.00

Alb, albumin; CRP, C-reactive protein; ESR, erythrocyte sedimentation rate; Hb, hemoglobin; IQR, interquartile range; LDH, lactate dehydrogenase; MMP-3, matrix metalloproteinase 3; RA, rheumatoid arthritis; RS3PE, remitting seronegative symmetrical synovitis with pitting edema; SD, standard deviation. * In the case of missing data, the number of patients with available data was specified.

Table 5. Risk factors for malignancy in patients with RS3PE or seronegative RA analyzed by univariate logistic regression analysis.

Characteristics	Odds Ratio	95% Confidence Interval	*p* Value
Age	1.06	1.002–1.11	0.037
Length of follow-up	0.999801	0.9994–1.0002	0.36
Male sex	4.34	1.29–14.57	0.007
Smoking	2.68	0.82–8.74	0.10
Diabetes	2.95	0.83–10.52	0.10
Hypertension	0.995	0.32–3.14	0.99
Hyperlipidemia	1.18	0.35–3.997	0.79
Swollen or/and tender joints			
Shoulders	0.51	0.16–1.60	0.25
Elbows	0.93	0.30–2.94	0.91
Wrists	0.97	0.25–3.71	0.96
Fingers	0.83	0.10–7.13	0.86
Hips	1.32	0.27–6.49	0.73
Knees	0.63	0.20–1.97	0.42
Ankles	1.05	0.34–3.19	0.93
Toes	0.97	0.29–3.29	0.97
Patients with swollen large joints	0.59	0.19–1.79	0.35
Patients with swollen small joints	0.20	0.02-2.32	0.20
Number of swollen large joints	0.87	0.60–1.25	0.44
Number of swollen small joints	1.04	0.98–1.10	0.22
28 swollen joints	1.03	0.95–1.11	0.50
28 tender joints	1.004	0.92–1.10	0.92
Patients with erosion	1.63	0.51–5.21	0.41
Systemic signs and symptoms			
Temperature ≥ 38 °C	8.20×10^{-7}	0–>10^6	0.99
Malaise or fatigue	2.31	0.45–11.97	0.32
Weight loss	0.57	0.07–4.63	0.60
Morning stiffness (lasting at least 1 h)	1.45	0.42–4.96	0.56
Edema (both hands and feet)	4.83	1.50–15.56	0.034
Edema (only hands)	6.45×10^{-7}	0–>10^5	0.99
Edema (only feet)	2.78×10^{-7}	0–>10^6	0.99
CRP	1.08	1.18–0.92	0.08
ESR			
Men+Women	0.999905	0.98–1.02	0.08
Men	1.006	0.988–1.02	0.51
Women	0.98	0.95–1.01	0.25
Alb	0.63	0.24–1.65	0.35
LDH	1.0009	0.99–1.02	0.90

Table 5. *Cont.*

Characteristics	Odds Ratio	95% Confidence Interval	p Value
MMP-3			
Men +Women	1.00009	0.9992–1.001	0.84
Men	1.0006	0.9993–1.002	0.34
Women	0.9985	0.99–1.003	0.50
Hb			
Male + Women	0.77	0.57–1.06	0.11
Men	0.51	0.33–0.81	0.005
Women	1.47	0.80–2.71	0.21
Patients with RS3PE	4.83	1.50–15.56	0.034
Patients with seronegative RA	0.21	0.06–0.07	0.034
Patients fulfilling the classification criteria for RA [11,12]	0.27	0.07–0.98	0.046
Patients fulfilling the classification criteria for PMR [10]	0.50	0.06–4.02	0.51
Patients fulfilling the classification criteria for RA [11,12] + PMR [10]	2.82×10^{-7}	0–>10^6	0.99

Alb, albumin; CRP, C-reactive protein; ESR, erythrocyte sedimentation rate; Hb, hemoglobin; IQR, interquartile range; LDH, lactate dehydrogenase; MMP-3, matrix metalloproteinase 3; PMR, polymyalgia rheumatica; RA, rheumatoid arthritis; RS3PE, remitting seronegative symmetrical synovitis with pitting edema; SD, standard deviation.

3.4. Comparison of Baseline Characteristics between RS3PE Patients with and without Malignancies

No clinical differences were noted between the RS3PE patients with and without malignancies (Supplementary Table S3).

3.5. Comparison of Baseline Characteristics between Seronegative RA Patients with and without Malignancies

The seronegative RA patients with malignancies had less swollen large joints ($p = 0.027$), lower MMP-3 levels (83.8 vs. 173.0 ng/mL, $p = 0.07$), lower ESRs in women (19.0 vs. 55.0 mm/h, $p = 0.020$), and higher Hb levels in women (13.7 ± 1.3 vs. 11.6 ± 1.8, $p = 0.045$) than those without malignancies (Supplementary Table S4).

4. Discussion

4.1. Comparison of Clinical and Laboratory Features of RS3PE and Seronegative RA

We found that patients with RS3PE were characterized by an older age at onset, higher affectation of the ankles compared to the elbows and fingers, higher levels of CRP and ESR, and a higher malignancy rate compared to patients with seronegative RA. These results (Table 1) are similar to those of Olive et al. [2], who reported that, in RS3PE patients, the MCP (81.5%) and PIP joints (70.4%), wrists (55.5%), shoulders (48%), knees (33.3%), and ankles (25.9%) were more frequently affected, while the elbows (11.1%) were less frequently affected. Patients with RS3PE had swollen and/or tender finger joints less frequently than those with seronegative RA (79.2% vs. 96.8%, $p = 0.022$). The reason for this is that patients with seronegative RA must present with 11 or more swollen or tender joints, including at least one small joint, to meet the 2010 EULAR/ACR criteria for RA [12]. This suggests that patients with seronegative RA tend to have many small joints affected. In our study, RS3PE more frequently affected the joints of the ankles than did seronegative RA. The high incidence of affected joints of the ankles in RS3PE patients may be due to attending physicians determining swelling in the ankle because of lower extremity edema in RS3PE patients.

The number of affected joints in the RS3PE patients was lower than that in the seronegative RA patients; however, the levels of CRP, and MMP-3 were higher. When analyzed with a 1:2 matching for age and sex, CRP levels were higher in the RS3PE group than in the seronegative RA group, while MMP-3 levels were comparable between the groups (Table 3). This implies that RS3PE and seronegative RA are essentially different diseases. Patients with RS3PE have often been reported to be positive for human leukocyte antigen (HLA)-B7, -Cw7, and -DQw2 [13], but not for HLA-DRB1, which is positive in RA [13,14]. Furthermore, RS3PE patients have higher levels of VEGF than RA patients [3]. This suggests that the pathogenesis of RS3PE is different from that of seronegative RA. Malignancies such as advanced cancers [15] and kidney cancers [16], which cause high levels of CRP, were not found in the RS3PE patients in this study.

PMR and seronegative RA have both positive HLA-DRB1, which may suggest that their etiologies may be the same; however, there are differences regarding their clinical manifestations. In PMR patients, there is significantly more frequent bilateral shoulder and hip pain and significantly less frequent peripheral arthritis (peripheral synovitis) than in RA patients [11]. Based on the distribution of the affected joints, it is not difficult to distinguish PMR from seronegative RA. Therefore, when the primary symptom of a patient who meets the criteria for PMR is peripheral arthritis; a diagnosis of RA is often made when the patient also meets the criteria for RA.

Compared to RS3PE, PMR has also been found to be significantly more common in male patients with a higher frequency of hip morning stiffness and pain [6]. Salvarani et al. [17] reported 19 cases of PMR with distal extremity swelling with pitting edema. However, edema in both hands and both feet was present in only three of the 19 cases, and all three cases met the criteria for RS3PE [1], although there are some missing data on RF. PMR with distal extremity swelling with pitting edema appears to identify a more benign disease subset than PMR without edema [18]. Patients who met the criteria for both PMR and RS3PE have previously been categorized as RS3PE [6,19]. Therefore, PMR with edema in all extremities could have been defined as RS3PE.

In our study, the patients who met the criteria for both RS3PE and PMR were defined as having RS3PE, and those who met the criteria for both seronegative RA and PMR were defined as having seronegative RA. Two (8.3%) and 17 (13.7%) patients with RS3PE and seronegative RA met the criteria for PMR [11], respectively. Excluding these patients who met the criteria for PMR, we reanalyzed 22 "pure RS3PE" and 107 "pure seronegative RA" patients. There were no differences in clinical characteristics and results between the "pure RS3PE" and "pure seronegative RA" groups, including the incidence of comorbid malignancies. These results suggest that it is not possible to differentiate RS3PE from seronegative RA regardless of the patients meeting the criteria for PMR. In paraneoplastic syndromes in rheumatology, musculoskeletal symptoms are known to occur in the joints and muscles [20] and PMR-like symptoms are also known to develop [21]. In our study, however, there was no relationship between meeting the PMR criteria and the presence or absence of malignancies (Table 5).

4.2. Comparison between RS3PE/Seronegative RA with and without Malignancies

Comorbid malignancies were found in 25.0% and 6.5% of the RS3PE and seronegative RA patients, respectively (Table 1). Based on data from the National Cancer Institute of Japan [22], the 4-year incidences of malignancies (2 years before and after the diagnosis of RS3PE/seronegative RA) in the Japanese population of the same age were 9.1% and 6.3% in RS3PE and seronegative RA patients, respectively. Thus, compared with the Japanese population, the incidence of comorbid malignancies was higher in the RS3PE group and comparable in the seronegative RA group. This is consistent with the findings of a previous report that the incidence of malignancies is higher in patients with RS3PE than in the general population [9]. The types of malignancies associated with RS3PE [23] include stomach, rectal, and prostate cancers, as observed in our study.

4.3. Comparison between RS3PE Patients with and without Malignancies

In the current study, there was no significant difference in the clinical characteristics of RS3PE between patients with and without malignancies (Supplementary Table S3). Origuchi et al. reported that RS3PE with malignancies has higher MMP-3 serum levels than RS3PE without malignancies, due to the abundant production of MMP-3 owing to malignancies [24]. In our study, there was no difference in MMP-3 levels. This discrepancy may have been due to the small number of cases both in the study by Origuchi et al. [24] and ours. These authors included eight patients with malignancy out of a total of 33 patients with RS3PE, and our study included six patients with malignancy out of a total of 24 patients with RS3PE. Due to the small number of cases to be analyzed, sufficient detection power may not have been obtained. These authors also included not only patients with edema of the hands and feet, but also that of only hands or only feet, which is different from our inclusion criteria that included patients with edema in both hands and both feet, similar to the study of McCarty et al. [1]. There was no difference in MMP-3 levels when analyzed separately by sex.

4.4. Comparison between Seronegative RA Patients with and without Malignancies

In our study, the seronegative RA patients with malignancies had lower MMP-3 levels and fewer swollen large joints than those without malignancies. Although MMP-3 serum levels can be elevated with steroids [25], all patients in this study had not used steroids before seronegative RA diagnosis. Additionally, patients with malignancies had fewer swollen large joints than those without malignancies (Supplementary Table S4). Serum levels of MMP-3 have been reported to be higher in RA patients with synovitis in large joints [26]. The MMP-3 serum levels did not correlate with the number of tender and swollen joints used in the core set of ACR, but they correlated with the Lansbury's joint scores, which have a high coefficient for large joints [27]. Therefore, in our study, the low circulating levels of MMP-3 in seronegative RA patients with malignancy may be due to the small number of swollen large joints.

4.5. Comparison between Seronegative RA and RS3PE Patients with and without Malignancies

We also examined the differences in the clinical characteristics of the overall patients with and without malignant comorbidities. The ORs of the patients with malignancies were higher for older age, male sex, RS3PE, and edema of both hands and both feet (Table 5). Regarding older and male patients, these results are consistent with data from the National Cancer Institute of Japan and the general Japanese trend. The high ORs of RS3PE and edema in both hands and both feet for malignancy also suggest that a thorough examination for malignancies should be performed in patients with RS3PE.

4.6. Limitations

Our study has several limitations. First, this was a retrospective study. Therefore, we employed matching to minimize selection bias. Second, 23 seronegative RA patients (one with malignancy, 22 without malignancies) and eight RS3PE patients (three with malignancies, five without malignancies) could not be followed for $\geq$2 years after the diagnosis of seronegative RA and RS3PE, respectively. Nevertheless, the results were not different after the exclusion of these patients. In our study, the incidence of malignancies was defined within 2 years before and after RS3PE or seronegative RA diagnosis; however, it is not clear within what year malignancy should be included. Some reports included comorbid malignancies within a definite period after the onset of RS3PE [6,24], while other reports did not present a definite period [9,28]. The significant difference in the incidence of comorbid malignancies between the RS3PE and seronegative RA groups was noted even when including malignancies within 1 or 3 years before or after the diagnosis of RS3PE/RA. Third, our study population was small. Since RS3PE is a rare disease and this was a single center study, multicenter validation studies are warranted. Finally, there were some missing data on Alb and MMP-3, but there were no missing data on important indices such as CRP and ESR.

5. Conclusions

Patients with RS3PE had higher CRP levels and a higher risk for malignancy than those with seronegative RA. As RS3PE patients are likely to have malignancies, it is necessary to thoroughly examine for malignancies at RS3PE diagnosis.

The seronegative RA patients with malignancies had lower MMP-3 levels and fewer swollen large joints at RA diagnosis than those without malignancy. Furthermore, among seronegative RA patients, it is recommended that patients with lower MMP-3 levels and fewer swollen large joints should be screened for malignancy.

These findings may enable the performance of a differential diagnosis between RS3PE and seronegative RA. Moreover, this may encourage clinicians to examine for malignancies in patients with RS3PE, contributing to improved patient outcomes.

Supplementary Materials: The following are available online at https://www.mdpi.com/2077-0383/10/5/1116/s1, Figure S1: Flow of patient diagnosis, Table S1: Clinical features of the 24 patients with RS3PE at the time of diagnosis, Table S2: Baseline characteristics at diagnosis of RS3PE and seronegative RA patients, excluding patients fulfilling the classification criteria for PMR, Table S3. Baseline characteristics in patients with RS3PE at diagnosis, Table S4: Baseline characteristics in patients with seronegative RA at diagnosis.

Author Contributions: Conceptualization, M.H.-K. and K.I.; methodology, M.H.-K.; software, M.H.-K.; validation, M.H.-K., K.I., S.H., H.T., and H.O.; formal analysis, M.H.-K.; investigation, M.H.-K.; data curation, M.H.-K.; writing—original draft preparation, M.H.-K.; writing—review and editing, M.H.-K.; visualization, M.H.-K.; supervision, Y.O.; project administration, M.H.-K. All authors have read and agreed to the published version of the manuscript.

Funding: This research received no external funding.

Institutional Review Board Statement: The study was conducted according to the guidelines of the Declaration of Helsinki, and approved by the Ethics Committee of National Hospital Organization Tokyo Medical Center (approval number R19-011 and date of approval: 2 March 2015).

Informed Consent Statement: Informed consent was waived due to the retrospective study de-sign.

Data Availability Statement: Not available.

Acknowledgments: The authors thank Manami Koyama for her assistance in data collection.

Conflicts of Interest: The authors declare no conflict of interest.

References

1. McCarty, D.J.; O'Duffy, J.D.; Pearson, L.; Hunter, J.B. Remitting seronegative symmetrical synovitis with pitting edema. RS3PE syndrome. *JAMA* **1985**, *254*, 2763–2767. [CrossRef]
2. Olivé, A.; Del Blanco, J.; Pons, M.; Vaquero, M.; Tena, X. The clinical spectrum of remitting seronegative symmetrical synovitis with pitting edema. The Catalán Group for the Study of RS3PE. *J. Rheumatol.* **1997**, *24*, 333–336.
3. Arima, K.; Origuchi, T.; Tamai, M.; Iwanaga, N.; Izumi, Y.; Huang, M.; Tanaka, F.; Kamachi, M.; Aratake, K.; Nakamura, H.; et al. RS3PE syndrome presenting as vascular endothelial growth factor associated disorder. *Ann. Rheum. Dis.* **2005**, *64*, 1653–1655. [CrossRef]
4. Mavragani, C.P.; Moutsopoulos, H.M. Rheumatoid arthritis in the elderly. *Exp. Gerontol.* **1999**, *34*, 463–471. [CrossRef]
5. Healy, L.A. RS3PE syndrome. *J. Rheumatol.* **1990**, *17*, 414.
6. Kimura, M.; Tokuda, Y.; Oshiawa, H.; Yoshida, K.; Utsunomiya, M.; Kobayashi, T.; Deshpande, G.A.; Matsui, K.; Kishimoto, M. Clinical characteristics of patients with remitting seronegative symmetrical synovitis with pitting edema compared to patients with pure polymyalgia rheumatica. *J. Rheumatol.* **2012**, *39*, 148–153. [CrossRef] [PubMed]
7. Kawashiri, S.; Suzuki, T.; Okada, A.; Tsuji, A.; Takatani, A.; Shimizu, T.; Koga, T.; Iwamoto, N.; Ichinose, K.; Nakamura, H.; et al. Differences in musculoskeletal ultrasound findings between RS3PE syndrome and elderly-onset rheumatoid arthritis. *Clin. Rheumatol.* **2020**, *39*, 1981–1988. [CrossRef] [PubMed]
8. Sibilia, J.; Friess, S.; Schaeverbeke, T.; Maloisel, F.; Bertin, P.; Goichot, B.; Kuntz, J.L. Remitting seronegative symmetrical synovitis with pitting edema (RS3PE): A form of paraneoplastic polyarthritis? *J. Rheumatol.* **1991**, *26*, 115–120.

9. Elizabeth, B.R. Remitting seronegative symmetrical synovitis with pitting edema syndrome: Follow up for neoplasia. *J. Rheumatol.* **2005**, *32*, 1760–1761.
10. Morel, J.; Deschamps, V.; Toussirot, E.; Pertuiset, E.; Sordet, C.; Kieffer, P.; Berthelot, J.M.; Champagne, H.; Mariette, X.; Combe, B. Characteristics and survival of 26 patients with paraneoplastic arthritis. *Ann. Rheum. Dis.* **2008**, *67*, 244–247. [CrossRef]
11. Dasgupta, B.; Cimmino, M.A.; Maradit-Kremers, H.; Schmidt, W.A.; Schirmer, M.; Salvarani, C.; Bachta, A.; Dejaco, C.; Duftner, C.; Jensen, H.S.; et al. Provisional classification criteria for polymyalgia rheumatica: A European League Against Rheumatism/American College of Rheumatology collaborative initiative. *Ann. Rheum. Dis.* **2012**, *71*, 484–492. [CrossRef]
12. Aletaha, D.; Neogi, T.; Silman, A.J.; Funovits, J.; Felson, D.T.; Bingham, C.O., 3rd; Birnbaum, N.S.; Burmester, G.R.; Bykerk, V.P.; Cohen, M.D.; et al. Rheumatoid arthritis classification criteria: An American College of Rheumatology/European League Against Rheumatism collaborative initiative. *Arthritis Rheum.* **2010**, *62*, 2569–2581. [CrossRef]
13. Yao, Q.; Su, X.; Altman, R.D. Is remitting seronegative symmetrical synovitis with pitting edema (RS3PE) a subset of rheumatoid arthritis? *Semin. Arthritis Rheum.* **2010**, *40*, 89–94. [CrossRef] [PubMed]
14. Gregersen, P.K.; Silver, J.; Winchester, R.J. The shared epitope hypothesis. An approach to understanding the molecular genetics of susceptibility to rheumatoid arthritis. *Arthritis Rheum.* **1987**, *30*, 1205–1213. [CrossRef] [PubMed]
15. Fan, Z.; Fan, K.; Gong, Y.; Huang, Q.; Yang, C.; Cheng, H.; Jin, K.; Ni, Q.; Yu, X.; Luo, G.; et al. The CRP/Albumin Ratio Predicts Survival and Monitors Chemotherapeutic Effectiveness in Patients With Advanced Pancreatic Cancer. *Cancer Manag. Res.* **2019**, *11*, 8781–8788. [CrossRef]
16. Saito, K.; Kihara, K. Role of C-reactive protein as a biomarker for renal cell carcinoma. *Expert Rev. Anticancer Ther.* **2010**, *10*, 1979–1989. [CrossRef]
17. Salvarani, C.; Gabriel, S.; Hunder, G. Distal extremity swelling with pitting edema in polymyalgia rheumatica. Report of nineteen cases. *Arthritis Rheum.* **1996**, *39*, 73–80. [CrossRef]
18. Salvarani, C.; Cantini, F.; Macchioni, P.; Olivieri, I.; Niccoli, L.; Padula, A.; Boiardi, L. Distal musculoskeletal manifestations in polymyalgia rheumatica: A prospective followup study. *Arthritis Rheum.* **1998**, *41*, 1221–1226. [CrossRef]
19. Bucaloiu, I.D.; Olenginski, T.P.; Harrington, T.M. Remitting seronegative symmetrical synovitis with pitting edema syndrome in a rural tertiary care practice: A retrospective analysis. *Mayo Clin. Proc.* **2007**, *82*, 1510–1515. [CrossRef]
20. Manger, B.; Schett, G. Paraneoplastic syndromes in rheumatology. *Nat. Rev. Rheumatol.* **2014**, *10*, 662–670. [CrossRef]
21. Muller, S.; Hider, S.; Helliwell, T.; Partington, R.; Mallen, C. The real evidence for polymyalgia rheumatica as a paraneoplastic syndrome. *Reumatismo* **2018**, *70*, 23–34. [CrossRef]
22. Cancer Statistics. Available online: https://ganjoho.jp/reg_stat/statistics/stat/index.html (accessed on 9 September 2020). (In Japanese).
23. Emamifar, A.; Hess, S.; Gildberg-Mortensen, R.; Hansen, I.M.J. Association of remitting seronegative symmetrical synovitis with pitting edema, polymyalgia rheumatica, and adenocarcinoma of the prostate. *Am. J. Case Rep.* **2016**, *17*, 60–64. [CrossRef] [PubMed]
24. Origuchi, T.; Arima, K.; Kawashiri, S.Y.; Tamai, M.; Yamasaki, S.; Nakamura, H.; Tsukada, T.; Aramaki, T.; Furuyama, M.; Miyashita, T.; et al. High serum matrix metalloproteinase 3 is characteristic of patients with paraneoplastic remitting seronegative symmetrical synovitis with pitting edema syndrome. *Mod. Rheumatol.* **2012**, *22*, 584–588. [CrossRef] [PubMed]
25. Sharif, M.; Salisbury, C.; Taylor, D.J.; Kirwan, J.R. Changes in biochemical markers of joint tissue metabolism in a randomized controlled trial of glucocorticoid in early rheumatoid arthritis. *Arthritis Rheum.* **1998**, *41*, 1203–1209. [CrossRef]
26. Ohuchi, E.; Iwata, K.; Yamanaka, H. Serum MMP-3 in rheumatoid arthritis. *Inflamm. Regenerat.* **2004**, *24*, 154–160. (In Japanese) [CrossRef]
27. Nagasawa, H.; Kameda, H.; Amano, K.; Takeuchi, T. Clinical significance of serum matrix metalloproteinase-3 level in patients with rheumatoid arthritis. *Inflamm. Regenerat.* **2004**, *25*, 60–64. (In Japanese) [CrossRef]
28. Karmacharya, P.; Donato, A.A.; Aryal, M.R.; Ghimire, S.; Pathak, R.; Shah, K.; Shrestha, P.; Poudel, D.; Wasser, T.; Subedi, A.; et al. RS3PE revisited: A systematic review and meta-analysis of 331 cases. *Clin. Exp. Rheumatol.* **2016**, *34*, 404–415.

MDPI
St. Alban-Anlage 66
4052 Basel
Switzerland
Tel. +41 61 683 77 34
Fax +41 61 302 89 18
www.mdpi.com

Journal of Clinical Medicine Editorial Office
E-mail: jcm@mdpi.com
www.mdpi.com/journal/jcm

www.ingramcontent.com/pod-product-compliance
Lightning Source LLC
LaVergne TN
LVHW070139170726
843515LV00007B/1832

* 9 7 8 3 0 3 6 5 2 5 6 0 0 *